RN Pharmacology for Nursing
REVIEW MODULE EDITION 9.0

W9-BAZ-350

Contributors

Alissa Althoff, Ed.D, MSN, RN

Mendy Gearhart, DNP, MSN, CCCE

Lori Grace, MSN, RN

Norma Jean Henry, MSN/Ed., RN

Honey C. Holman, MSN, RN

Janean Johnson, DNP, RN, CNE

Terri Lemon DNP, MSN, RN

Beth Cusatis Phillips, PhD,
RN, CNE, CHSE

Pamela Roland, MSN, MBA, RN

LaKeisha Wheless, MSN, RN

Debborah Williams, MSN, RN

Consultants

Lisa Bass, MSN, RN, CNE Ret.

Tracey Bousquet, BSN, RN

Lois Churchill, MN, RN

Penny Fauber, RN, BSN, MS, PhD

Brittney Fritzinger, Ed.D, MSN, RN

Jenni L. Hoffman, DNP, RN,
FNP-C, CLNC, FAANP

Deb Johnson-Schuh, MSN, RN, CNE

Lisa Kongable, MA, ARNP,
PMHCNS-BC, CNE

Virginia Tufano, Ed.D, MSN, RN

Sarah Veal, MSN, RN, CNE

INTELLECTUAL PROPERTY NOTICE

Director of content review: Kristen Lawler

Director of development: Derek Prater

Project management: Meri Ann Mason

Coordination of content review: Alissa Althoff, Honey C. Holman

*Copy editing: Kelly Von Lunen, Tricia Lunt, Bethany Robertson,
Kya Rodgers, Rebecca Her, Sam Shiel, Alethea Surland, Graphic World*

Layout: Bethany Robertson, Maureen Bradshaw, Haylee Hedge, scottie. o

Illustrations: Randi Hardy, Graphic World

Online media: Brant Stacy, Ron Hanson, Britney Frerking, Trevor Lund

Interior book design: Spring Lenox

IMPORTANT NOTICE TO THE READER

User's Guide

Welcome to the Assessment Technologies Institute® RN Pharmacology for Nursing Review Module Edition 9.0. The mission of ATI's Content Mastery Series® Review Modules is to provide user-friendly compendiums of nursing knowledge that will:
- Help you locate important information quickly.
- Assist in your learning efforts.
- Provide exercises for applying your nursing knowledge.
- Facilitate your entry into the nursing profession as a newly licensed nurse.

This newest edition of the Review Modules has been redesigned to optimize your learning experience. We've fit more content into less space and have done so in a way that will make it even easier for you to find and understand the information you need.

ORGANIZATION

This Review Module is organized into units covering pharmacological principles (Unit 1) and medications affecting the body systems and physiological processes (Units 2 to 13). Chapters within these units conform to one of two organizing principles for presenting the content.
- Nursing concepts
- Medications

Nursing concepts chapters begin with an overview describing the central concept and its relevance to nursing. Subordinate themes are covered in outline form to demonstrate relationships and present the information in a clear, succinct manner.

Medications chapters include an overview describing a disorder or group of disorders. Medications used to treat these disorders are grouped according to classification. A specific medication can be selected as a prototype or example of the characteristics of medications in this classification. These sections include information about how the medication works and its therapeutic uses. Next, you will find information about complications, contraindications/precautions, and interactions, as well as nursing interventions and client education to help prevent and/or manage these issues. Finally, the chapter includes information on nursing administration of the medication and evaluation of the medication's effectiveness.

ACTIVE LEARNING SCENARIOS AND APPLICATION EXERCISES

Each chapter includes opportunities for you to test your knowledge and to practice applying that knowledge. Active Learning Scenario exercises pose a nursing scenario and then direct you to use an ATI Active Learning Template (included at the back of this book) to record the important knowledge a nurse should apply to the scenario. An example is then provided to which you can compare your completed Active Learning Template. The Application Exercises include NCLEX-style questions, such as multiple-choice and multiple-select items, providing you with opportunities to practice answering the kinds of questions you might expect to see on ATI assessments or the NCLEX. After the Application Exercises, an answer key is provided, along with rationales.

NCLEX® CONNECTIONS

To prepare for the NCLEX-RN, it is important to understand how the content in this Review Module is connected to the NCLEX-RN test plan. You can find information on the detailed test plan at the National Council of State Boards of Nursing's website, www.ncsbn.org. When reviewing content in this Review Module, regularly ask yourself, "How does this content fit into the test plan, and what types of questions related to this content should I expect?"

To help you in this process, we've included NCLEX Connections at the beginning of each unit and with each question in the Application Exercises Answer Keys. The NCLEX Connections at the beginning of each unit point out areas of the detailed test plan that relate to the content within that unit. The NCLEX Connections attached to the Application Exercises Answer Keys demonstrate how each exercise fits within the detailed content outline. These NCLEX Connections will help you understand how the detailed content outline is organized, starting with major client needs categories and subcategories and followed by related content areas and tasks. The major client needs categories are:
- Safe and Effective Care Environment
  - Management of Care
  - Safety and Infection Control
- Health Promotion and Maintenance
- Psychosocial Integrity
- Physiological Integrity
  - Basic Care and Comfort
  - Pharmacological and Parenteral Therapies
  - Reduction of Risk Potential
  - Physiological Adaptation

An NCLEX Connection might, for example, alert you that content within a unit is related to:
- Pharmacological and Parenteral Therapies
  - Adverse Effects/Contraindications/Side Effects/Interactions
    - Identify a contraindication to the administration of a medication to the client.

QSEN COMPETENCIES

As you use the Review Modules, you will note the integration of the Quality and Safety Education for Nurses (QSEN) competencies throughout the chapters. These competencies are integral components of the curriculum of many nursing programs in the United States and prepare you to provide safe, high-quality care as a newly licensed nurse. Icons appear to draw your attention to the six QSEN competencies.

Safety: The minimization of risk factors that could cause injury or harm while promoting quality care and maintaining a secure environment for clients, self, and others.

Patient-Centered Care: The provision of caring and compassionate, culturally sensitive care that addresses clients' physiological, psychological, sociological, spiritual, and cultural needs, preferences, and values.

Evidence-Based Practice: The use of current knowledge from research and other credible sources, on which to base clinical judgment and client care.

Informatics: The use of information technology as a communication and information-gathering tool that supports clinical decision-making and scientifically based nursing practice.

Quality Improvement: Care related and organizational processes that involve the development and implementation of a plan to improve health care services and better meet clients' needs.

Teamwork and Collaboration: The delivery of client care in partnership with multidisciplinary members of the health care team to achieve continuity of care and positive client outcomes.

ICONS

Icons are used throughout the Review Module to draw your attention to particular areas. Keep an eye out for these icons.

(N) This icon is used for NCLEX Connections.

(G) This icon indicates gerontological considerations, or knowledge specific to the care of older adult clients.

Qs This icon is used for content related to safety and is a QSEN competency. When you see this icon, take note of safety concerns or steps that nurses can take to ensure client safety and a safe environment.

QPCC This icon is a QSEN competency that indicates the importance of a holistic approach to providing care.

QEBP This icon, a QSEN competency, points out the integration of research into clinical practice.

QI This icon is a QSEN competency and highlights the use of information technology to support nursing practice.

QQI This icon is used to focus on the QSEN competency of integrating planning processes to meet clients' needs.

QTC This icon highlights the QSEN competency of care delivery using an interprofessional approach.

SDoH This icon highlights content related to social determinants of health.

M◈ This icon appears at the top-right of pages and indicates availability of an online media supplement, such as a graphic, animation, or video. If you have an electronic copy of the Review Module, this icon will appear alongside clickable links to media supplements. If you have a hard copy version of the Review Module, visit www.atitesting.com for details on how to access these features.

FEEDBACK

ATI welcomes feedback regarding this Review Module. Please provide comments to comments@atitesting.com.

As needed updates to the Review Modules are identified, changes to the text are made for subsequent printings of the book and for subsequent releases of the electronic version. For the printed books, print runs are based on when existing stock is depleted. For the electronic versions, a number of factors influence the update schedule. As such, ATI encourages faculty and students to refer to the Review Module addendums for information on what updates have been made. These addendums, which are available in the Help/FAQs on the student site and the Resources/eBooks & Active Learning on the faculty site, are updated regularly and always include the most current information on updates to the Review Modules.

Table of Contents

When reviewing the following chapters, keep in mind the relevant topics and tasks of the NCLEX outline, in particular:

Management of Care

CLIENT RIGHTS: Recognize the client's right to refuse treatment/procedures.

Pharmacological and Parenteral Therapies

ADVERSE EFFECTS/CONTRAINDICATIONS/SIDE EFFECTS/INTERACTIONS

Identify a contraindication to the administration of a medication to the client.

Notify the primary health care provider of side effects, adverse effects, and contraindications of medications and parenteral therapy.

DOSAGE CALCULATIONS

Perform calculations needed for medication administration.

Use clinical decision-making/critical thinking when calculating dosages.

MEDICATION ADMINISTRATION

Prepare and administer medications, using rights of medication administration.

Evaluate appropriateness and accuracy of medication order for client.

Administer and document medications given by common routes (e.g., oral, topical).

PARENTERAL/INTRAVENOUS THERAPIES:

Apply knowledge and concepts of mathematics/nursing procedures/psychomotor skills when caring for a client receiving intravenous and parenteral therapy.

UNIT 1 PHARMACOLOGICAL PRINCIPLES

CHAPTER 1 *Pharmacokinetics and Routes of Administration*

Pharmacokinetics refers to how medications travel through the body. They undergo a variety of biochemical processes that result in absorption, distribution, metabolism, and excretion.

PHASES OF PHARMACOKINETICS

ABSORPTION

Absorption is the transmission of medications from the location of administration (gastrointestinal [GI] tract, muscle, skin, mucous membranes, or subcutaneous tissue) to the bloodstream. The most common routes of administration are enteral (through the GI tract) and parenteral (by injection). Each of these routes has a unique pattern of absorption.
- The rate of medication absorption determines how soon the medication will take effect.
- The amount of medication the body absorbs determines the intensity of its effects.
- The route of administration affects the rate and amount of absorption.

Oral

BARRIERS TO ABSORPTION: Medications must pass through the layer of epithelial cells that line the GI tract.

ABSORPTION PATTERN: Varies greatly due to:
- Stability and solubility of the medication
- GI and intestinal pH and emptying time
- Gastric emptying time
- Presence of food in the stomach or intestines
- Other concurrent medications
- Forms of medications (enteric-coated pills or sustained-release liquids)

Sublingual, buccal

BARRIERS TO ABSORPTION: Swallowing before dissolution allows gastric pH to inactivate the medication.

ABSORPTION PATTERN: Quick absorption systemically through highly vascular mucous membranes

Other mucous membranes (rectal, vaginal)

BARRIERS TO ABSORPTION: Presence of stool in the rectum or infectious material in the vagina limits tissue contact.

ABSORPTION PATTERN: Easy absorption with both local and systemic effects

Inhalation via mouth, nose

BARRIERS TO ABSORPTION: Inspiratory effort.

ABSORPTION PATTERN: Rapid absorption through alveolar capillary networks

Intradermal, topical

BARRIERS TO ABSORPTION: Close proximity of epidermal cells.

ABSORPTION PATTERN
- Slow, gradual absorption
- Effects primarily local, but systemic as well, especially with lipid-soluble medications passing through subcutaneous fatty tissue

Subcutaneous, intramuscular

BARRIERS TO ABSORPTION: Capillary walls have large spaces between cells. Therefore, there is no significant barrier.

ABSORPTION PATTERN
- Solubility of the medication in water: Highly soluble medications have rapid absorption (10 to 30 min); poorly soluble medications have slow absorption.
- Blood perfusion at the site of injection: sites with high blood perfusion have rapid absorption; sites with low blood perfusion have slow absorption.

Intravenous

BARRIERS TO ABSORPTION: No barriers.

ABSORPTION PATTERN
- **Immediate:** enters directly into the blood
- **Complete:** reaches the blood in its entirety

DISTRIBUTION

Distribution is the transportation of medications to sites of action by bodily fluids. Factors influencing distribution include the following.

Circulation: Conditions that inhibit blood flow or perfusion, such as peripheral vascular or cardiac disease, can delay medication distribution.

Permeability of the cell membrane: The medication must be able to pass through tissues and membranes to reach its target area. Medications that are lipid-soluble or have a transport system can cross the blood-brain barrier and the placenta.

Plasma protein binding: Medications compete for protein binding sites within the bloodstream, primarily albumin. The ability of a medication to bind to a protein can affect how much of the medication will leave and travel to target tissues. Two medications can compete for the same binding sites, resulting in toxicity.

METABOLISM

Metabolism (biotransformation) changes medications into less active or inactive forms by the action of enzymes. This occurs primarily in the liver, but it also takes place in the kidneys, lungs, intestines, and blood.

FACTORS INFLUENCING THE RATE OF MEDICATION METABOLISM

- **Age**: Infants have a limited medication-metabolizing capacity. The aging process also can influence medication metabolism, but varies with the individual. In general, hepatic medication metabolism tends to decline with age. Older adults require smaller doses of medications due to the possibility of accumulation in the body. ⑥
- **Increase in some medication-metabolizing enzymes**: This can metabolize a particular medication sooner, requiring an increase in dosage of that medication to maintain a therapeutic level. It can also cause an increase in the metabolism of other concurrent-use medications.
- **First-pass effect**: The liver inactivates some medications on their first pass through the liver, and thus they require a nonenteral route (sublingual, IV) because of their high first-pass effect.
- **Similar metabolic pathways**: When the same pathway metabolizes two medications, it can alter the metabolism of one or both of them. In this way, the rate of metabolism can decrease for one or both of the medications, leading to medication accumulation.
- **Nutritional status**: Clients who are malnourished can be deficient in the factors that are necessary to produce specific medication-metabolizing enzymes, thus impairing medication metabolism.

OUTCOMES OF METABOLISM

- Increased renal excretion of medication
- Inactivation of medications
- Increased therapeutic effect
- Activation of pro-medications (also called pro-drugs) into active forms
- Decreased toxicity when active forms of medications become inactive forms
- Increased toxicity when inactive forms of medications become active forms

EXCRETION

Excretion is the elimination of medications from the body, primarily through the kidneys. Elimination also takes place through the liver, lungs, intestines, and exocrine glands (such as in breast milk). Kidney dysfunction can lead to an increase in the duration and intensity of a medication's response, so it is important to monitor BUN and creatinine levels.

MEDICATION RESPONSES

Medication dosing attempts to regulate medication responses to maintain plasma levels between the minimum effective concentration (MEC) and the toxic concentration. A plasma medication level is in the therapeutic range when it is effective and not toxic. Nurses use therapeutic levels of many medications to monitor clients' responses.

THERAPEUTIC INDEX

Medications with a high therapeutic index (TI) have a wide safety margin. Therefore, there is no need for routine blood medication-level monitoring. Medications with a low TI require close monitoring of medication levels. Nurses should consider the route of administration when monitoring for peak levels (highest plasma level). For example, an oral medication can peak from 1 to 3 hr after administration. If the route is IV, the peak time might occur within 10 min. (Refer to a drug reference or a pharmacist for specific medication peak times.) For trough levels (lowest plasma level), obtain a blood sample immediately before the next medication dose, regardless of the route of administration. A plateau is a medication's concentration in plasma during a series of doses.

HALF-LIFE

Half-life (t½) refers to the time for the medication in the body to drop by 50%. Liver and kidney function affect half-life. It usually takes four half-lives to achieve a steady blood concentration (medication intake = medication metabolism and excretion).

SHORT HALF-LIFE

- Medications leave the body quickly (4 to 8 hr).
- Short-dosing interval or MEC drops between doses.

LONG HALF-LIFE

- Medications leave the body more slowly: over more than 24 hr, with a greater risk for medication accumulation and toxicity.
- Medications can be given at longer intervals without loss of therapeutic effects.
- Medications take a longer time to reach a steady state.

PHARMACODYNAMICS

Pharmacodynamics describes the interactions between medications and target cells, body systems, and organs to produce effects. These interactions result in functional changes that are the mechanism of action of the medication. Medications interact with cells in one of two ways or in both ways.

Agonists are medications that bind to or mimic the receptor activity that endogenous compounds regulate. For example, morphine is an agonist because it activates the receptors that produce analgesia, sedation, constipation, and other effects. (Receptors are the medication's target sites on or within the cells.)

Antagonists are medications that can block the usual receptor activity that endogenous compounds regulate or the receptor activity of other medications. For example, losartan, an angiotensin II receptor blocker, is an antagonist. It works by blocking angiotensin II receptors on blood vessels, which prevents vasoconstriction.

Partial agonists act as agonists and antagonists, with limited affinity to receptor sites. For example, nalbuphine acts as an antagonist at mu receptors and an agonist at kappa receptors, causing analgesia with minimal respiratory depression at low doses.

Routes of administration

ORAL OR ENTERAL

Tablets, capsules, liquids, suspensions, elixirs, lozenges

NURSING ACTIONS
- Contraindications for oral medication administration include vomiting, decreased GI motility, absence of a gag reflex, difficulty swallowing, and a decreased level of consciousness.
- Unless contraindicated, have clients sit upright at a 90° angle to facilitate swallowing.
- Administer irritating medications, such as analgesics, with small amounts of food.
- Do not mix with large amounts of food or beverages in case clients cannot consume the entire quantity.
- Avoid administration with interacting foods or beverages, such as grapefruit juice.
- Administer oral medications as prescribed, and follow directions for whether medication is to be taken on an empty stomach (30 min to 1 hr before meals, 2 hr after meals) or with food.
- Follow the manufacturer's directions for crushing, cutting, and diluting medications. Break or cut scored tablets only. (See the Institute for Safe Medication Practices website.)
- Make sure clients swallow enteric-coated or time-release medications whole.
- Use a liquid form of the medication to facilitate swallowing whenever possible.
- For liquids, including suspension and elixirs, follow directions for dilution and shaking. To prepare the medication, place a medicine cup on a flat surface before pouring, and ensure the base of the meniscus (lowest fluid line) is at the level of the dose.

ADVANTAGES
- Safe
- Inexpensive
- Easy and convenient

DISADVANTAGES
- Oral medications have highly variable absorption.
- Inactivation can occur in the GI tract or by first-pass effect.
- Clients must be cooperative and conscious.

Sublingual and buccal

Sublingual: under the tongue

Buccal: between the cheek and the gum
Directly enters the bloodstream and bypasses the liver

CLIENT EDUCATION
- Keep the medication in place until complete absorption occurs.
- Do not eat or drink while the tablet is in place or until it has completely dissolved.

Nasogastric and gastrostomy tubes
- Use liquid forms of medications; if not available, consider crushing medications if guidelines allow.
- Do not administer sublingual medications through the NG tube (can give sublingual medications under the tongue).
- Do not crush specifically-prepared oral medications (extended/time-release, fluid-filled, enteric-coated).
- Administer each medication separately.
- Do not mix medications with enteral feedings.
- Completely dissolve crushed tablets and capsule contents in 15 to 30 mL of sterile water prior to administration.

NURSING ACTIONS
- Verify proper tube placement.
- Use a syringe and allow the medication to flow in by gravity or push it in with the plunger of the syringe.
- To prevent clogging, flush the tubing before and after each medication and ending with a flush after instilling all the medications. Flush with another 15 to 30 mL of warm sterile water after instilling all the medications.

TOPICAL

Medications directly applied to the mucous membranes or skin, which can include powders, sprays, creams, ointments, pastes, oil-and suspension-based lotions.
- Painless
- Limited adverse effects

NURSING ACTIONS
- Apply with a glove, tongue blade, or cotton-tipped applicator.
- Do not apply with a bare hand.
- For skin applications, wash the skin with soap and water. Pat dry before application.
- Use surgical asepsis to apply topical medications to open wounds.

Transdermal

Medication in a skin patch for absorption through the skin, producing systemic effects

CLIENT EDUCATION
- Apply patches to ensure proper dosing.
- Wash the skin with soap and water, and dry thoroughly before applying a new patch.
- Place the patch on a hairless area, and rotate sites daily to prevent skin irritation.

Eye
- Have clients sit upright or lie supine, tilt their head slightly, and look up at the ceiling.
- Rest your dominant hand on the clients' forehead, hold the dropper above the conjunctival sac about 1 to 2 cm, drop the medication into the sac, avoid placing it directly on the cornea, and have them close the eye gently. If they blink during instillation, repeat the procedure.
- Apply gentle pressure with your finger and a clean facial tissue on the nasolacrimal duct for 30 to 60 seconds to prevent systemic absorption of the medication.
- If instilling more than one medication in the same eye, wait at least 5 min between them.
- For eye ointment, apply a thin ribbon to the edge of the lower eyelid from the inner to the outer canthus.

Ear

- Have clients sit upright or lie on their side.
- Straighten the ear canal by pulling the auricle upward and outward for adults or down and back for children less than 3 years of age. Hold the dropper 1 cm above the ear canal, instill the medication, and then gently apply pressure with your finger to the tragus of the ear unless it is too painful.
- Do not press a cotton ball deep into the ear canal. If necessary, gently place it into the outermost part of the ear canal.
- Have clients remain in the side-lying position if possible for 2 to 3 min after instilling ear drops.
- Drops may be warmed with hands as cold drops may cause dizziness.

Nose

- Use medical aseptic technique when administering medications into the nose.
- Have clients lie supine with their head positioned to allow the medication to enter the appropriate nasal passage.
- Use your dominant hand to instill nasal drops, supporting the head with your nondominant hand.
- Instruct clients to breathe through the mouth, stay in a supine position, and not blow their nose for 5 min after drop instillation.
- For nasal spray, prime the spray if indicated, insert tip into nare, and point nozzle away from the center of the nose.
- Spray into nose while the client inhales. Instruct the client not to blow their nose for several minutes.

Rectal suppositories

- Position clients in the left lateral or lateral semi–prone recumbent position.
- Insert the suppository just beyond the internal sphincter.
- Instruct clients to remain flat or in the left lateral position for at least 5 min after insertion to retain the suppository. Absorption times vary with the medication.

Vaginal

- Position clients supine with their knees bent and their feet flat on the bed and close to their hips (modified lithotomy or dorsal recumbent position).
- Provide perineal care, if needed.
- Lubricate the suppository or fill the applicator, depending on the formulation.
- Insert the medication along the posterior wall of the vagina (7.5 to 10 cm [3 to 4 in] for suppositories; 5 to 7.6 cm [2 to 3 in] for creams, jellies or foams) or instill irrigation as indicated.
- Instruct clients to remain supine for at least 5 min after insertion to retain the suppository.
- If using a reusable applicator, wash it with soap and water. (If it is disposable, discard it.)

INHALATION

Administered through metered dose inhalers (MDI) or dry-powder inhalers (DPI)

MDI

CLIENT EDUCATION
- Remove the cap from the inhaler's mouthpiece.
- Shake the inhaler vigorously five or six times.
- Hold the inhaler with the mouthpiece at the bottom.
- Hold the inhaler with your thumb near the mouthpiece and your index and middle fingers at the top.
- Hold the inhaler about 2 to 4 cm (1 to 2 in) away from the front of your mouth or close your mouth around the mouthpiece of the inhaler with the opening pointing toward the back of your throat.
- Take a deep breath and then exhale.
- Tilt your head back slightly, press the inhaler, and, at the same time, begin a slow, deep inhalation breath. Continue to breathe in slowly and deeply for 3 to 5 seconds to facilitate delivery to the air passages.
- Hold your breath for 10 seconds to allow the medication to deposit in your airways.
- Take the inhaler out of your mouth and slowly exhale through pursed lips.
- Resume normal breathing.
- Wait at least one minute between inhalations when two inhalations of the same medication are needed.
- Rinse the mouth out with water or brush the teeth if using a corticosteroid inhaler to reduce the risk of fungal infections of the mouth.
- A spacer keeps the medication in the device longer, thereby increasing the amount of medication the device delivers to the lungs and decreasing the amount of medication in the oropharynx.
- If using a spacer:
  ○ Remove the covers from the mouthpieces of the inhaler and of the spacer.
  ○ Insert the MDI into the end of the spacer.
  ○ Shake the inhaler five or six times.
  ○ Exhale completely, and then close your mouth around the spacer's mouthpiece. Continue as with an MDI.

DPI

CLIENT EDUCATION
- Do not shake the device.
- Take the cover off the mouthpiece.
- Follow the manufacturer's directions for preparing the medication, such as turning the wheel of the inhaler or loading a medication pellet.
- Exhale completely.
- Place the mouthpiece between your lips and take a deep inhalation breath through your mouth.
- Hold your breath for 5 to 10 seconds.
- Take the inhaler out of your mouth and slowly exhale through pursed lips.
- Resume normal breathing.

- If more than one puff is needed, wait the length of time the provider specifies before self-administering the second puff.
- Rinse the mouth out with water or brush the teeth if using a corticosteroid inhaler to reduce the risk of fungal infections of the mouth.
- Remove the canister and rinse the inhaler, cap, and spacer once a day with warm running water and dry them completely before using the inhaler again.

PARENTERAL

NURSING ACTIONS
- The vastus lateralis is best for infants (1 year and younger) and toddlers (12 months to 2 years).
- The ventrogluteal site is preferable for IM injections and for injecting volumes exceeding 2 mL.
- The deltoid site has a smaller muscle mass and can only accommodate up to 1 mL of fluid.
- Use a needle size and length appropriate for the type of injection and the client's size. Syringe size should approximate the volume of medication.
- Use a tuberculin syringe for solution volumes smaller than 0.5 mL.
- Rotate injection sites to enhance medication absorption, and document each site.
- Do not use injection sites that are edematous, inflamed, or have moles, birthmarks, or scars.
- For IV administration, immediately monitor clients for therapeutic and adverse effects.
- Discard all sharps (broken ampule bottles, needles) in leak- and puncture-proof containers.

INTRADERMAL

NURSING ACTIONS
- Use for tuberculin testing or checking for medication or allergy sensitivities.
- Use small amounts of solution (0.01 to 0.1 mL) in a tuberculin syringe with a fine-gauge needle (25- to 27-gauge) in lightly pigmented, thin-skinned, hairless sites (the inner surface of the mid-forearm or scapular area of the back) at a 10° to 15° angle.
- Insert the needle with the bevel up. A small bleb should appear.
- Do not massage the site after injection.

SUBCUTANEOUS AND INTRAMUSCULAR

NURSING ACTIONS

Subcutaneous
- Use for small doses of nonirritating, water-soluble medications, such as insulin and heparin.
- Use a 3/8- to 5/8-inch, 25- to 31-gauge needle. Use an insulin syringe when administering insulin. Inject no more than 1.5 mL of solution.
- Select sites that have an adequate fat-pad size (abdomen, upper hips, lateral upper arms, thighs).
- For average-size clients, pinch up the skin and inject at a 45° to 90° angle. For clients who are obese, use a 90° angle.

Intramuscular
- Use for irritating medications, solutions in oils, and aqueous suspensions.
- The most common sites are ventrogluteal, deltoid, and vastus lateralis (pediatric). The dorsogluteal is no longer recommended as a common injection site due to its close proximity to the sciatic nerve.
- Use a needle size 18- to 25-gauge, 5/8- to 1.5-inch long and inject at a 90° angle. Solution volume is usually 1 to 3 mL. Divide larger volumes into two syringes and use two different sites.

ADVANTAGES
- Use for poorly soluble medications.
- Use for administering medications that have slow absorption for an extended period of time (depot preparations).

DISADVANTAGES
- Injections are more costly.
- Injections are inconvenient.
- There can be pain with the risk for local tissue damage and nerve damage.
- There is a risk for infection at the injection site.

INTRAVENOUS

NURSING ACTIONS
- Use for administering medications, fluid, and blood products.
- Vascular access devices can be for short-term use (peripheral catheters) or long-term use (peripherally inserted central catheter, tunneled and non-tunneled catheter and implantable port. For peripheral access. The use of 16-gauge devices for clients who have trauma, 18-gauge during surgery and for blood administration, and 22- to 24-gauge for children, older adults, and clients who have medical issues or are stable postoperatively are general guidelines.
- Peripheral veins in the arm or hand are preferable. Ask clients which site they prefer. For newborns, use veins in the head, lower legs, and feet. After administration, immediately monitor for therapeutic and adverse effects.
- Use the Z-track technique for IM injections of irritating fluids or fluids that can stain the skin (iron preparations). This method prevents medication from leaking back into subcutaneous tissue.

ADVANTAGES
- Onset is rapid, and absorption into the blood is immediate, which provides an immediate response.
- This route allows control over the precise amount of medication to administer.
- It allows for administration of large volumes of fluid.
- It dilutes irritating medications in free-flowing IV fluid.

DISADVANTAGES
- IV injections are even more costly.
- IV injections are inconvenient.
- Absorption of the medication into the blood is immediate. This is potentially dangerous if giving the wrong dosage or the wrong medication.
- There is an increased risk for infection or embolism with IV injections.
- Poor circulation can inhibit the medication's distribution.

EPIDURAL

NURSING ACTIONS

- Use for IV opioid analgesia (morphine or fentanyl).
- The clinician advances the catheter through the needle into the epidural space at the level of the fourth or fifth vertebra.
- Use an infusion pump to administer medication.

Active Learning Scenario

A nurse is demonstrating the use a metered-dose inhaler (MDI) with a spacer to a client. What should the nurse include in the instructions? Use the *ATI Active Learning Template: Therapeutic Procedure* to complete this item.

INDICATIONS: Identify the medication absorption pattern and a barrier to absorption.

CLIENT EDUCATION: Describe the steps to follow when using an MDI with a spacer.

Application Exercises

1. Sort each of the following factors affecting the rate of medication metabolism to indicate if the factor results in the need for an increased medication dosage or a decreased medication dosage.

    A. Increased renal excretion

    B. Elevated medication-metabolizing enzymes

    C. Liver failure

    D. Peripheral vascular disease

    E. Concurrent medications using the same metabolization pathway

    F. Malnourishment

2. A nurse receives a prescription to obtain a trough level of the client's medication. Which of the following actions should the nurse take?

    A. Obtain a blood specimen immediately prior to administering the next dose of medication.

    B. Verify that the client has been taking the medication for 24 hr before obtaining a blood specimen.

    C. Ask the client to provide a urine specimen after the next dose of medication.

    D. Administer the medication, and obtain a blood specimen 30 min later.

3. A provider prescribes phenobarbital for a client who has a seizure disorder. The medication has a long half-life of 4 days. How many times per day should the nurse expect to administer this medication?

    A. One

    B. Two

    C. Three

    D. Four

4. A nurse is teaching a client about a new prescription for a transdermal patch. Which of the following client statements indicates an understanding?

    A. "I will clean the site with an alcohol swab before I apply the patch."

    B. "I will rotate the application sites weekly."

    C. "I will apply the patch to an area of skin with no hair."

    D. "I will place the new patch on the site of the old patch."

5. A nurse is preparing to administer eye drops to a client. Which of the following actions should the nurse take? (Select all that apply.)

    A. Have the client lie on one side.

    B. Ask the client to look up at the ceiling.

    C. Tell the client to blink when the drops enter the eye.

    D. Drop the medication into the client's conjunctival sac.

    E. Instruct the client to close the eye gently after instillation.

Application Exercises Key

1. **INCREASED DOSAGE:** A, B, D;
   DECREASED DOSAGE: C, E, F

2. A. **CORRECT:**

   To evaluate the therapeutic effectiveness of a client's medication by obtaining a trough level of the medication, the nurse should obtain a blood specimen immediately before administering the next dose of medication.

   Ⓝ *NCLEX® Connection: Pharmacological and Parenteral Therapies, Parenteral/Intravenous Therapies*

3. A. **CORRECT:** When evaluating outcomes, the nurse should recognize medications with long half-lives remain at their therapeutic levels between doses for long periods of time. The nurse should expect to administer this medication once a day.

   Ⓝ *NCLEX® Connection: Pharmacological and Parenteral Therapies, Medication Administration*

4. C. **CORRECT:** When evaluating a client's understanding of teaching about applying a transdermal patch, the nurse should ensure the client understands the need to apply the patch to a hairless area of skin to promote absorption of the medication.

   Ⓝ *NCLEX® Connection: Pharmacological and Parenteral Therapies, Medication Administration*

5. B, D, E. **CORRECT:** When taking actions to administer eye drops to a client, the nurse should drop the medication into the conjunctival sac to promote distribution and recognize that the client should look upward to keep the drops from falling onto the cornea and should close their eyes gently to promote distribution of the medication.

   Ⓝ *NCLEX® Connection: Pharmacological and Parenteral Therapies, Medication Administration*

Active Learning Scenario Key

Using the ATI Active Learning Template: Therapeutic Procedure

INDICATIONS

- Medication Absorption Pattern: rapid absorption through the alveolar capillary network. A spacer keeps the medication in the device longer, thereby increasing the amount of medication the device delivers to the lungs and decreasing the amount of medication in the oropharynx.
- Barrier to Absorption: Inadequate respiratory effort

CLIENT EDUCATION

- Remove the covers from the mouthpieces of the inhaler and of the spacer.
- Insert the MDI into the end of the spacer.
- Shake the inhaler five or six times.
- Exhale completely, and then close your mouth around the spacer's mouthpiece.
- Take a deep breath and then exhale.
- Tilt your head back slightly, press the inhaler, and, at the same time, begin a slow, deep inhalation breath. Continue to breathe in slowly and deeply for 3 to 5 seconds to facilitate delivery to the air passages.
- Hold your breath for 10 seconds to allow the medication to deposit in your airways.
- Take the mouthpiece out of your mouth and slowly exhale through pursed lips.
- Resume normal breathing.

Ⓝ *NCLEX® Connection: Pharmacological and Parenteral Therapies, Medication Administration*

UNIT 1   PHARMACOLOGICAL PRINCIPLES

CHAPTER 2
Safe Medication Administration and Error Reduction

The providers who can legally write prescriptions in the United States include physicians, advanced practice nurses, dentists, and physician assistants. These providers are responsible for obtaining clients' medical history, performing a physical examination, diagnosing, prescribing medications, monitoring response to therapy, and modifying prescriptions as necessary.

Nurses are responsible for having knowledge of federal, state (nurse practice act), and local laws, and facilities' policies that govern prescribing and dispensing medications; preparing and administering medications; and evaluating clients' responses to medications. Nurses should develop and maintain an up-to-date knowledge base of medications they administer, including uses, mechanisms of action, routes of administration, safe dosage range, adverse effects, precautions, contraindications, and interactions. Nurses can help reduce adverse events related to medications by determining the accuracy of medication prescriptions, reporting all medication errors, safeguarding and storing medications, following legal mandates when administering controlled substances, calculating medication doses accurately, and understanding the responsibilities of other members of the health care team regarding medications. Qs

MEDICATION CATEGORY AND CLASSIFICATION

NOMENCLATURE

Chemical name is the name of the medication that reflects its chemical composition and molecular structure (isobutylphenylpropanoic acid).

Generic name is the official or nonproprietary name the United States Adopted Names Council gives a medication. Each medication has only one generic name (ibuprofen).

Trade name is the brand or proprietary name the company that manufactures the medication gives it. One medication can have multiple trade names (Advil, Motrin).

CONSIDERATIONS

Nurses administer prescription medications under the supervision of providers. Some medications can be habit-forming, or have potential harmful effects and require more stringent supervision. Qs

Uncontrolled substances require monitoring by a provider, but do not generally pose risks of misuse and addiction. Antibiotics are an example of uncontrolled prescription medications.

Controlled substances have a potential for misuse and dependence and have a "Schedule" classification. Heroin is in Schedule I and has no medical use in the United States. Medications in Schedules II through V have legitimate applications. Each subsequent level has a decreasing risk of misuse and dependence. For example, morphine is a Schedule II medication that has a greater risk for misuse and dependence than phenobarbital, which is a Schedule IV medication.

FDA REGULATIONS

- New drugs in development undergo the rigorous testing procedures of the U.S. Food and Drug Administration (FDA) to determine both effectiveness and safety before approval. However, new drugs can have unidentified or unreported adverse effects. Nurses observing these can report them to MedWatch on the FDA's website.
- Implementation of newer FDA pregnancy labeling guidelines began in 2015. The Pregnancy and Lactation Labeling Rule (PLLR) mandates three sections for labeling: pregnancy, lactation, and females and males of reproductive potential. You may access the full report at www.fda.gov.
- Before administering any medication to a client who is pregnant or could be pregnant, determine whether it is safe for use during pregnancy.

MEDICATION PRESCRIPTIONS

Each facility has written policies for medication prescriptions, including which providers can write, receive, and transcribe medication prescriptions. Qᴛᴄ

Use verbal prescriptions only for emergencies, and follow the facility's protocol for telephone prescriptions. Nursing students cannot accept verbal or telephone prescriptions.

Types of medication prescriptions

Routine or standing prescriptions

Single or one-time prescriptions

Stat prescriptions

PRN prescriptions

Components of a medication prescription

- Client's full name
- Date and time of the prescription
- Name of the medication (generic or brand)
- Strength and dosage of the medication
- Route of administration
- Time and frequency of administration: exact times or number of times per day (according to the facility's policy or the specific qualities of the medication)
- Quantity to dispense and the number of refills
- Signature of the prescribing provider

Medication reconciliation

The Joint Commission requires policies and procedures for medication reconciliation. Nurses compile a list of each client's current medications, including all medications with their dosages and frequency. They compare the list with new medication prescriptions and reconcile it with the provider to resolve any discrepancies. This process should take place at admission, when transferring clients between units or facilities, and at discharge.

2.1 Knowledge required prior to medication administration

Medication category/class

Medications have a pharmacological action, therapeutic use, body system target, chemical makeup, and classification for use during pregnancy.

For example, lisinopril is an ACE inhibitor (pharmacological action) and an antihypertensive (therapeutic use).

Mechanism of action

This is how medications produce their therapeutic effect.

For example, glipizide is an oral hypoglycemic agent that lowers blood glucose levels primarily by stimulating pancreatic islet cells to release insulin.

Therapeutic effect

This is the expected effect (physiological response) for which the nurse administers a medication to a specific client. One medication can have more than one therapeutic effect.

One client might take diphenhydramine to relieve allergies while another takes it to induce sleep.

Adverse effects

These are undesirable and potentially dangerous responses to a medication.

For example, the antibiotic gentamicin can cause hearing loss. Adverse effects can be inadvertent or predictable. Some adverse effects are immediate and others take weeks or months to develop.

Toxic effects

Medications can have specific risks and manifestations of toxicity. They develop after taking a medication for a lengthy period of time or when toxic amounts build up due to faulty metabolism or excretion.

For example, nurses monitor clients taking digoxin for dysrhythmias, a manifestation of cardiotoxicity. Hypokalemia places these clients at greater risk for digoxin toxicity.

Medication interactions

Medications can interact with each other, resulting in beneficial or harmful effects.

For example, giving the beta blocker atenolol concurrently with the calcium channel blocker nifedipine helps prevent reflex tachycardia.

An example of an undesirable interaction is giving omeprazole, a proton pump inhibitor, concurrently with phenytoin, an anticonvulsant. This can increase the blood level of phenytoin.

Obtain a complete medication history, and be knowledgeable of clinically significant interactions.

Be aware that medications can also interact beneficially or harmfully with food and with herbal and dietary supplements.

Precautions/Contraindications

These are conditions (diseases, age, pregnancy, lactation) that make it risky or completely unsafe for clients to take specific medications.

For example, tetracyclines can stain developing teeth. Therefore, children younger than 8 years should not take these medications. Another example is that myasthenia gravis is a contraindication for fentanyl, an opioid analgesic.

Some medications require caution with some conditions.

For example, the kidneys excrete vancomycin without changing it. Therefore, renal impairment requires caution when administering this medication.

Preparation, dosage, administration

It is important to know any specific considerations for preparation, safe dosages, dosage calculations, and how to administer the medication.

For example, morphine is available in many formulations. Oral doses of morphine are generally higher than parenteral doses due to extensive first-pass effect. Clients who have chronic, severe pain (cancer) generally take oral doses of morphine.

Nursing implications

Know how to monitor therapeutic effects and adverse effects, prevent and treat adverse effects, provide comfort, and instruct clients about the safe use of medications.

RIGHTS OF SAFE MEDICATION ADMINISTRATION

Right client

Verify clients' identification before each medication administration. The Joint Commission requires two client identifiers.

- Acceptable identifiers include the client's name, an assigned identification number, telephone number, birth date, or another person-specific identifier (a photo identification card).
- Check identification bands for name and identification number.
- Check for allergies by asking clients, looking for an allergy bracelet or medal, and reviewing the MAR.
- Use barcode scanners to identify clients. Qₗ

Right medication

Correctly interpret medication prescriptions, verifying completeness and clarity.

- Read medication labels and compare them with the MAR three times: before removing the container, when removing the amount of medication from the container, and in the presence of the client before administering the medication.
- Leave unit-dose medication in its package until administration.
- When using automated medication dispensing systems, perform the same checks and adapt them as necessary. Qₗ

Right dose

- Use a unit-dose system to decrease errors. If not available, calculate the correct medication dose.
- Check a drug reference to ensure the dose is within the usual range.
- When performing medication calculations or conversions, have another qualified nurse check the calculated dose.
- Prepare medication dosages using standard measurement devices (graduated cups or syringes). Some medication dosages require a second verifier or witness (some cytotoxic medications). Automated medication dispensing systems use a machine to control the dispensing of medications.

Right time

Administer medication on time to maintain a consistent therapeutic blood level.

- Administer time-critical medications 30 min before or after the prescribed time. Facilities define which medications are time-critical; usually this includes medications that require a consistent blood level (antibiotics).
- Administer non-time-critical medications prescribed once daily, weekly, or monthly within 2 hr of the prescribed time.
- Administer non-time-critical medications prescribed more than once daily (but not more than every 4 hr) within 1 hr of the prescribed time.

Right route

The most common routes of administration are oral, topical, subcutaneous, IM, and IV. Additional routes include sublingual, buccal, intradermal, transdermal, epidural, inhalation, nasal, ophthalmic, otic, rectal, vaginal, intraosseous, and via enteral tubes.

- Select the correct preparation for the route the provider prescribed (otic versus ophthalmic topical ointment or drops).
- Always use different syringes for enteral and parenteral medication administration.
- Know how to administer medication safely and correctly.

Right documentation

- Immediately record the medication, dose, route, time, and any pertinent information, including the client's response to the medication. Document the medication after administration, not before.
- For some medications, in particular those to alleviate pain, evaluate the client's response and document it later, perhaps after 30 min.

Right client education

- Inform clients about the medication: its purpose, what to expect, how to take it, and what to report.
- To individualize the teaching, determine what the clients already know about the medication, need to know about the medication, and want to know about the medication.

Right to refuse

- Respect clients' right to refuse any medication.
- Explain the consequences, inform the provider, and document the refusal.

Right assessment

Collect any essential data before and after administering any medication. For example, measure apical heart rate before giving digoxin.

Right evaluation

Follow up with clients to verify therapeutic effects as well as adverse effects.

MEDICATION ERROR PREVENTION

COMMON MEDICATION ERRORS

- Wrong medication or IV fluid
- Incorrect dose or IV rate
- Wrong client, route, or time
- Administration of an allergy-inducing medication
- Omission of a dose or administration of extra doses
- Incorrect discontinuation of a medication or IV fluid
- Inaccurate prescribing
- Inadvertently giving a medication that has a similar name

USING THE NURSING PROCESS TO PREVENT MEDICATION ERRORS Qs

Assessment

- Be knowledgeable about the medications administered. Use appropriate resources.
  - Providers, including nurses, physicians, and pharmacists
  - Poison control: 1-800-222-1222 (24/7)
  - Sales representatives from drug companies
  - Nursing pharmacology textbooks and drug handbooks
  - Physicians' Desk Reference
  - Professional journals
  - Professional websites
- Obtain information about medical diagnoses and conditions affecting medication administration (ability to swallow; allergies; heart, liver, and kidney disorders).
- Obtain necessary pre-administration data (heart rate, blood pressure, blood levels) to assess the appropriateness of the medication and to obtain baseline data for evaluating the effectiveness of medications.
- Omit or delay doses as necessary due to clients' status.
- Determine whether the medication prescription is complete.
- Interpret the medication prescription accurately. The Institute for Safe Medication Practices (ISMP) is a nonprofit organization working to educate health care providers and consumers about safe medication practices. The ISMP and the FDA identify the most common medical abbreviations that result in misinterpretation, mistakes, and injury. For a complete list, go to the ISMP website.
  - **Error-Prone Abbreviation List:** abbreviations that have caused a high number of medication errors
  - **Confused Medication Name List:** sound-alike and look-alike medication names
  - **High-Alert Medication List:** medications that, if a nurse administers them in error, have a high risk for resulting in significant harm to clients. Strategies to prevent errors include limiting access; using auxiliary labels and automated alerts; standardizing the prescription, preparation, and administration; and using automated or independent double checks.
- Question the provider if the prescription is unclear or seems inappropriate for the client. Refuse to administer a medication if it seems unsafe, and notify the charge nurse or supervisor.
- Providers usually make dosage changes gradually. Question them about abrupt and excessive changes.

Planning

- Identify client outcomes for medication administration.
- Set priorities (which medications to give first or before specific treatments or procedures).

2.2 Confused medication name list

ESTABLISHED NAME	RECOMMENDED NAME
acetohexamide	acetoHEXAMIDE
acetazolamide	acetaZOLAMIDE
bupropion	buPROPion
buspirone	busPIRone
chlorpromazine	chlorproMAZINE
chlorpropamide	chlorproPAMIDE
clomiphene	clomiPHENE
clomipramine	clomiPRAMINE
cyclosporine	cycloSPORINE
cycloserine	cycloSERINE
daunorubicin	DAUNOrubicin
doxorubicin	DOXOrubicin
dimenhydrinate	dimenhyDRINATE
diphenhydramine	diphenhydrAMINE
dobutamine	DOBUTamine
dopamine	DOPamine
glipizide	glipiZIDE
glyburide	glyBURIDE
hydralazine	hydrALAZINE
hydromorphone	hYDROmorphone
hydroxyzine	hydrOXYzine
medroxyprogesterone	medroxyPROGESTERone
methylprednisolone	methylPREDNISolone
methyltestosterone	methylTESTOSTERone
mitoxantrone	mitoXANTRONE
nicardipine	niCARdipine
nifedipine	NIFEdipine
prednisone	predniSONE
prednisolone	prednisoLONE
risperidone	risperiDONE
ropinirole	ROPINIRole
sulfadiazine	sulfADIAZINE
sulfisoxazole	sulfiSOXAZOLE
tolazamide	TOLAZamide
tolbutamide	TOLBUTamide
vinblastine	vinBLAStine
vincristine	vinCRIStine

Implementation

- Avoid distractions during medication preparation (poor lighting, ringing phones). Interruptions can increase the risk of error.
- Prepare medications for one client at a time.
- Check the labels for the medication's name and concentration.
- Measure doses accurately, and double-check dosages of high-alert medications (insulin and heparin) with a colleague. Check the medication's expiration date.
- Doses are usually one to two tablets or one single-dose vial. Question multiple tablets or vials for a single dose.
- Follow the rights of medication administration consistently and carefully. Take the MAR to the bedside.
- Do not administer medications that someone else prepared.

- Encourage clients to become part of the safety net, teaching them about medications and the importance of proper identification before medication administration. Omit or delay a dose when clients question the size of a dose or the appearance of a medication.
- Follow correct procedures for all routes of administration.
- Follow all laws and regulations for preparing and administering controlled substances. Keep them in a secure area. Have another nurse witness the discarding of controlled substances.
- Do not leave medications at the bedside. Some facilities' policies allow exceptions (for topical medications).
- Educate the client and anyone who will be assisting in the client's care regarding medications. Provide verbal and written instructions.

Evaluation

- Evaluate clients' responses to medications, and document and report them.
- Use knowledge of the therapeutic effect and common adverse effects of medications to compare expected outcomes with actual findings.
- Identify adverse effects, and document and report them.
- Notify the provider of all errors, and implement corrective measures immediately.
  - Complete an incident report within the time frame the facility specifies, usually 24 hr. This report should include. Qↄ
    - Client's identification
    - Name and dose of the medication
    - Time and place of the incident
    - Accurate and objective account of the event
    - Who you notified
    - What actions you took
    - Your signature (or that of the person who completed the report)
  - Do not reference or include the incident report in the client's medical record.
  - Medication errors relate to systems, procedures, product design, or practice patterns. Report all errors to help the facility's risk managers determine how errors occur and what changes to make to avoid similar errors in the future.

2.3 High-alert medication list

The following medications and medication categories from the ISMP's list require specific safeguards to reduce the risk of errors. Strategies include limiting access; using auxiliary labels and automated alerts; standardizing the prescription, preparation, and administration; and using automated or independent double checks.

Class or category of medications

- Adrenergic agonists, IV (epinephrine)
- Adrenergic antagonists, IV (propranolol)
- Anesthetic agents, general, inhaled and IV (propofol)
- Cardioplegic solutions
- Chemotherapeutic agents, parenteral and oral
- Dextrose, hypertonic, 20% or greater
- Dialysis solutions, peritoneal and hemodialysis
- Epidural or intrathecal medications
- Glycoprotein IIb/IIIa inhibitors (eptifibatide)
- Hypoglycemics, oral
- Inotropic medications, IV (digoxin, milrinone)
- Liposomal forms of drugs (liposomal amphotericin B)
- Moderate sedation agents, IV (midazolam)
- Moderate sedation agents, oral, for children (chloral hydrate)
- Narcotics/opiates, IV and oral (including liquid concentrates, immediate- and sustained-release)
- Neuromuscular blocking agents (succinylcholine)
- Radiocontrast agents, IV
- Sodium chloride injection, hypertonic, more than 0.9% concentration
- Thrombolytics/fibrinolytics, IV (tenecteplase)
- Total parenteral nutrition solutions

Specific medications

- Epinephrine, subcutaneous
- Epoprostenol, IV
- Heparin, low molecular weight, injection
- Heparin, unfractionated, IV
- Insulin, subcutaneous and IV
- Lidocaine, IV
- Magnesium sulfate injection
- Methotrexate, oral, nononcologic use
- Opium tincture
- Oxytocin, IV
- Nitroprusside for injection
- Potassium chloride for injection concentrate
- Potassium phosphates injection
- Promethazine, IV
- Vasopressin, IV or intraosseous
- Warfarin

SOCIAL DETERMINANTS OF HEALTH (SDOH)

To fully implement safe medication administration and error prevention, the nurse should determine the SDOH for each individual client. Clients are born into SDOH conditions in the environment in which they live. These conditions affect their daily life and, eventually, their health.

Social determinants of health account for 90% of health outcomes, whereas medical care accounts for only 10 to 15%. It is imperative that a member of the client's healthcare team (nurse, pharmacist) collect the necessary data relating to the 6 determinants of health.

- Economic Stability (poverty level, employment, housing instability)
  - Clients who live at a low socioeconomic level or are unemployed, may not be able to afford the medications needed for treatment and or maintenance of health care issues.
  - Clients without adequate housing may not be able to store medications that require refrigeration such as insulin.
- Education (level of education, language and literacy, early childhood education and development)
  - Clients who have a low level of education might be suited for educational materials with visuals for better understanding.
- Health and Health Care (access to health care, access to primary care, health literacy)
  - Clients who have a low health literacy may not be able to comprehend a pamphlet so the nurse would need to find an alternative method for medication education.
- Neighborhood and Built Environment (access to foods that support healthy eating patterns, quality of housing, crime and violence, environmental conditions)
  - Clients who have limited access to transportation may need information regarding prescription delivery options.
- Social and Community Context (social cohesion, civic participation, discrimination, incarceration)
- Food Security (versus food insecurity)
  - Clients who are experiencing food insecurity will need assistance with medications that should be taken with food.

Health care team members should not only gather the necessary data regarding SDOH but should act on the findings to ensure safe medication practices for all clients.

2.4 Case study

Scenario introduction

Maggie is a nurse on the surgical unit who inadvertently administered a client's pain medication by the incorrect route. Rachel is the nursing supervisor on the unit.

Scene 1

Maggie: "Rachel, I need to speak with you in private please."

Rachel: "Certainly, Maggie. Let's go to my office and we can talk there."

Scene 2

Rachel: "You seem concerned, Maggie. How can I help you?"

Maggie: "I inadvertently administered a client's prescribed pain medication using the wrong route. The client is stable and in no distress. Will I need to complete an incident report since there was no harm done to the client?"

Scene 3

Rachel: "Yes, you will need to complete an incident report and forward it to risk management."

Scenario conclusion

Rachel assists Maggie with the completion of an incident report, and it is sent to the facility risk manager.

Case study exercises

1. A nurse is preparing to complete an incident report for a medication error. Which of the following information should the nurse include in the report? (Select all that apply.)

   A. Time of the incident

   B. Location in the chart of where the report is filed

   C. Who was notified of the incident

   D. Actions taken following the incident

   E. Opinion regarding why the incident occurred

   F. Client identification

2. Incident reports can assist the facility's risk manager to determine how errors occur and what changes can be made to avoid similar errors in the future. The nurse should identify that medication errors relate to what four entities within the facility?

Application Exercises

1. A nurse is preparing a client's medications. The nurse is responsible for gaining and maintaining knowledge about which of the following medication information? (Select all that apply.)

   A. Adverse effects

   B. Determining dose

   C. Mechanism of action

   D. Contraindications

   E. Insurance coverage

2. A nurse is preparing to administer digoxin to a client who states, "I don't want to take that medication. I do not want one more pill." Which of the following responses should the nurse make?

   A. "Your physician prescribed it for you, so you really should take it."

   B. "Well, let's just get it over quickly then."

   C. "Okay, I'll just give you your other medications."

   D. "Tell me your concerns about taking this medication."

3. A nurse is assessing a client before administering medications. Which of the following data should the nurse obtain? (Select all that apply.)

   A. Use of herbal products

   B. Ability to swallow

   C. Daily fluid intake

   D. Previous surgical history

   E. Allergies

4. A nurse is working with a newly licensed nurse who is administering medications to clients. Which of the following actions should the nurse identify as an indication that the newly hired nurse understands medication error prevention?

   A. Taking all medications out of the unit-dose wrappers before entering the client's room

   B. Checking the prescription when a single dose requires administration of multiple tablets

   C. Administering a medication, then looking up the usual dosage range

   D. Relying on another nurse to clarify a medication prescription

Active Learning Scenario

A staff educator is reviewing the prevention of medication errors with a group of newly licensed nurses. What should the educator include about using the nursing process to prevent medication errors? Use the *ATI Active Learning Template: Basic Concept* to complete this item.

NURSING INTERVENTIONS: Using the nursing process to prevent medication errors, list the following.

- Three assessment actions
- One planning action
- Four implementation actions
- Three evaluation actions

Application Exercises Key

1. A, C, D. **CORRECT:** The nurse should plan to generate solutions to address medication administration by developing and maintaining up-to-date knowledge regarding medication adverse effects, mechanism of action and contraindications.

   (N) *NCLEX® Connection: Pharmacological Therapies, Medication Administration*

2. D. **CORRECT:** Although clients have the right to refuse a medication, the nurse should take action by determining the reason for refusal by asking about the client's concerns. The nurse can provide education to the client regarding their health condition and care management so they can make an informed decision. At that point, if the client still wishes to exercise their right to refuse the medication, notify the provider and document the refusal and the actions taken.

   (N) *NCLEX® Connection: Pharmacological Therapies, Medication Administration*

3. A, B, E. **CORRECT:** The nurse should recognize cues by assessing the client for use of herbal products, ability to swallow and allergies prior to medication administration. This nurse can use this information to note for potential interactions or reactions, the best delivery route for medications and information to share with the healthcare team.

   (N) *NCLEX® Connection: Pharmacological Therapies, Medication Administration*

4. B. **CORRECT:** The nurse should analyze cues from the client's medication administration record and determine if the dose to administer is correct. If a single dose requires multiple tablets, it is possible that an error has occurred in the prescription or transcription of the medication. This action could prevent a medication error.

   (N) *NCLEX® Connection: Pharmacological Therapies, Medication Administration*

Active Learning Scenario Key

Using the ATI Active Learning Template: Basic Concept

NURSING INTERVENTIONS

Assessment
- Be knowledgeable about the medication to administer. Use appropriate resources.
- Obtain information about medical diagnoses and conditions that affect medication administration.
- Determine whether the medication prescription is complete.
- Interpret the medication prescription accurately.
- Question the provider if the prescription is unclear or seems inappropriate for the client.
- Question the provider about abrupt and excessive changes in dosage.

Planning
- Identify clients' outcomes for medication administration.
- Set priorities (which medications to give first or before specific treatments or procedures).

Implementation
- Avoid distractions and interruptions during medication preparation.
- Prepare medications for one client at a time.
- Check the labels for the medication's name and concentration.
- Question multiple tablets or vials for a single dose.
- Follow the rights of medication administration consistently and carefully.
- Do not administer medications that someone else prepared.
- Encourage clients to become part of the safety net.
- Follow correct procedures for all routes of administration.
- Communicate clearly both verbally and in writing.
- Use verbal prescriptions only for emergencies, and follow the facility's protocol for telephone prescriptions.
- Follow all laws and regulations for preparing and administering controlled substances.
- Do not leave medications at the bedside.
- Follow the principles of client and family education for medications.

Evaluation
- Evaluate clients' responses to medications, and document and report them.
- Use knowledge of the therapeutic effect and common side and adverse effects of medications to compare expected outcomes with actual findings.
- Identify side and adverse effects, and document and report them.
- Report all errors, and implement corrective measures immediately.

   (N) *NCLEX® Connection: Safety and Infection Control, Reporting of Incident/Event/Irregular Occurrence Variance*

Case Study Exercises Key

1. A, C, D, F. **CORRECT:** The nurse should take action to address the medication error by completing an incident report and forwarding it to the facility risk manager.

   (N) *NCLEX® Connection: Safety and Infection Control, Reporting of Incident/Event/Irregular Occurrence Variance*

2. When evaluating the outcomes of incident reporting, the nurse should identify that medication errors relate to systems, procedures, product designs or practice patterns.

   (N) *NCLEX® Connection: Safety and Infection Control, Reporting of Incident/Event/Irregular Occurrence Variance*

UNIT 1   PHARMACOLOGICAL PRINCIPLES

CHAPTER 3 # Dosage Calculations

Basic medication dose conversion and calculation skills are essential for providing safe nursing care. Qs

Nurses are responsible for administering the correct amount of medication by calculating the precise amount of medication to give. Nurses can use three different methods for dosage calculation: ratio and proportion, formula (desired over have), and dimensional analysis.

TYPES OF CALCULATIONS

- Solid oral medication
- Liquid oral medication
- Injectable medication
- Correct doses by weight
- IV infusion rates

STANDARD CONVERSION FACTORS

- 1 mg = 1,000 mcg
- 1 g = 1,000 mg
- 1 kg = 1,000 g
- 1 oz = 30 mL
- 1 L = 1,000 mL
- 1 tsp = 5 mL
- 1 tbsp = 15 mL
- 1 tbsp = 3 tsp
- 1 kg = 2.2 lb
- 1 gr = 60 mg

GENERAL ROUNDING GUIDELINES

ROUNDING UP: If the number to the right is equal to or greater than 5, round up by adding 1 to the number on the left.

ROUNDING DOWN: If the number to the right is less than 5, round down by dropping the number, leaving the number to the left as is.

For dosages less than 1.0: Round to the nearest hundredth.
- **For example (rounding up):** 0.746 mL = 0.75 mL. The calculated dose is 0.746 mL. Look at the number in the thousandths place (6). Six is greater than 5. To round to hundredths, add 1 to the 4 in the hundredths place and drop the 6. The rounded dose is 0.75 mL.
- **Or (rounding down):** 0.743 mL = 0.74 mL. The calculated dose is 0.743 mL. Look at the number in the thousandths place (3). Three is less than 5. To round to the hundredth, drop the 3 and leave the 4 as is. The rounded dose is 0.74 mL.

For dosages greater than 1.0: Round to the nearest tenth.
- **For example (rounding up):** 1.38 = 1.4. The calculated dose is 1.38 mg. Look at the number in the hundredths place (8). Eight is greater than 5. To round to the tenth, add 1 to the 3 in the tenth place and drop the 8. The rounded dose is 1.4 mg.
- **Or (rounding down):** 1.34 mL = 1.3 mL. The calculated dose is 1.34 mL. Look at the number in the hundredths place (4). Four is less than 5. To round to the tenth, drop the 4 and leave the 3 as is. The rounded dose is 1.3 mL.

Solid dosage

Example: A nurse is preparing to administer phenytoin 0.2 g PO every 8 hr. The amount available is phenytoin 100 mg/capsule. How many capsules should the nurse administer per dose? (Round the answer to the nearest whole number. Use a leading zero if it applies. Do not use a trailing zero.)

USING RATIO AND PROPORTION

STEP 1: What is the unit of measurement the nurse should calculate?

capsules

STEP 2: What is the dose the nurse should administer?
Dose to administer = Desired

0.2 g

STEP 3: What is the dose available? Dose available = Have

100 mg

STEP 4: Should the nurse convert the units of measurement?
Yes (g ≠ mg)
Set up an equation.

$$\frac{1\ g}{1{,}000\ mg} = \frac{0.2\ g}{X\ mg}$$

Solve for X.

X mg = 200 mg

Or you can use your knowledge of equivalents.

1 g = 1,000 mg (1 × 1,000)

0.2 g = 200 mg (0.2 × 1,000)

STEP 5: What is the quantity of the dose available?
= Quantity

1 capsule

STEP 6: Set up the equation and solve for X.

$$\frac{Have}{Quantity} = \frac{Desired}{X}$$

$$\frac{100\ mg}{1\ capsule} = \frac{200\ mg}{X\ capsule(s)}$$

X capsule(s) = 2 capsules

STEP 7: Round, if necessary.

STEP 8: Determine whether the amount to administer makes sense. If there are 100 mg/capsule and the prescription reads 0.2 g (200 mg), it makes sense to administer 2 capsules. The nurse should administer phenytoin 2 capsules PO.

USING DESIRED OVER HAVE

STEP 1: What is the unit of measurement the nurse should calculate?

capsules

STEP 2: What is the dose the nurse should administer?
Dose to administer = Desired

0.2 g

STEP 3: What is the dose available? Dose available = Have

100 mg

STEP 4: Should the nurse convert the units of measurement? Yes (g ≠ mg)
Set up an equation.

$$X \, mg \;=\; \frac{0.2 \, g \times 1{,}000 \, mg}{1 \, g}$$

$X \, mg = 200 \, mg$

Or you can use your knowledge of equivalents.

1 g = 1,000 mg (1 × 1,000)

0.2 g = 200 mg (0.2 × 1,000)

STEP 5: What is the quantity of the dose available?
= Quantity

1 capsule

STEP 6: Set up the equation and solve for X.

$$X \;=\; \frac{Desired \times Quantity}{Have}$$

$$X \, capsule(s) \;=\; \frac{200 \, mg \times 1 \, cap}{100 \, mg}$$

$X \, capsule(s) = 2 \, capsules$

STEP 7: Round, if necessary.

STEP 8: Determine whether the amount to administer makes sense. If there are 100 mg/capsule and the prescription reads 0.2 g (200 mg), it makes sense to administer 2 capsules. The nurse should administer phenytoin 2 capsules PO.

USING DIMENSIONAL ANALYSIS

STEP 1: What is the unit of measurement the nurse should calculate? (Place the unit of measure being calculated on the left side of the equation.)

X capsule(s) =

STEP 2: Determine the ratio that contains the same unit as the unit being calculated. (Place the ratio on the right side of the equation ensuring that the unit in the numerator matches the unit being calculated.)

$$X \, capsule(s) \;=\; \frac{1 \, capsule}{100 \, mg}$$

STEP 3: Place any remaining ratios that are relevant to the item on the right side of the equation along with any needed conversion factors to cancel out unwanted units of measure.

$$X \, capsule(s) \;=\; \frac{1 \, capsule}{100 \, mg} \times \frac{1{,}000 \, mg}{1 \, g} \times \frac{0.2 \, g}{1}$$

STEP 4: Solve for X.

$X \, capsule(s) = 2 \, capsules$

STEP 5: Round, if necessary.

STEP 6: Determine whether the amount to administer makes sense. If there are 100 mg/capsule and the prescription reads 0.2 g, it makes sense to administer 2 capsules. The nurse should administer phenytoin 2 capsules PO.

Liquid dosage

Example: A nurse is preparing to administer amoxicillin 0.25 g PO every 8 hr. The amount available is amoxicillin oral suspension 250 mg/5 mL. How many mL should the nurse administer per dose? (Round the answer to the nearest tenth. Use a leading zero if it applies. Do not use a trailing zero.)

USING RATIO AND PROPORTION

STEP 1: What is the unit of measurement the nurse should calculate?

mL

STEP 2: What is the dose the nurse should administer?
Dose to administer = Desired

0.25 g

STEP 3: What is the dose available? Dose available = Have

250 mg

STEP 4: Should the nurse convert the units of measurement? Yes (g ≠ mg) (Place the unit of measure being calculated on the left side of the equation.)
Set up an equation.

$$\frac{1 \, mg}{1{,}000 \, mg} \;=\; \frac{0.25 \, g}{X \, mg}$$

$X \, mg = 200 \, mg$

Or you can use your knowledge of equivalents.

1 g = 1,000 mg (1 × 1,000)

0.25 g = 250 mg (0.25 × 1,000)

STEP 5: What is the quantity of the dose available?
= Quantity

5 mL

STEP 6: Set up the equation and solve for X.

$$\frac{Have}{Quantity} = \frac{Desired}{X}$$

$$\frac{250 \text{ mg}}{5 \text{ mL}} = \frac{250 \text{ mg}}{X \text{ mL}}$$

X mL = 5 mL

STEP 7: Round, if necessary.

STEP 8: Determine whether the amount to administer makes sense. If there are 250 mg/5 mL and the prescription reads 0.25 g (250 mg), it makes sense to administer 5 mL. The nurse should administer amoxicillin 5 mL PO every 8 hr.

USING DESIRED OVER HAVE

STEP 1: What is the unit of measurement the nurse should calculate?

mL

STEP 2: What is the dose the nurse should administer? Dose to administer = Desired

0.25 g

STEP 3: What is the dose available? Dose available = Have

250 mg

STEP 4: Should the nurse convert the units of measurement? Yes (g ≠ mg)
Set up an equation:

$$X \text{ mg} = \frac{0.25 \text{ g} \times 1,000 \text{ mg}}{1 \text{ g}}$$

X mg = 250 mg

Or you can use your knowledge of equivalents.

1 g = 1,000 mg (1 × 1,000)

0.25 g = 250 mg (0.25 × 1,000)

STEP 5: What is the quantity of the dose available?
= Quantity

5 mL

STEP 6: Set up the equation and solve for X.

$$X \text{ mL} = \frac{Desired \times Quantity}{Have}$$

$$X \text{ mL} = \frac{250 \text{ mg} \times 5 \text{ mL}}{250 \text{ mg}}$$

X mL = 5 mL

STEP 7: Round, if necessary.

STEP 8: Determine whether the amount to administer makes sense. If there are 250 mg/5 mL and the prescription reads 0.25 g (250 mg), it makes sense to administer 5 mL. The nurse should administer amoxicillin 5 mL PO every 8 hr.

USING DIMENSIONAL ANALYSIS

STEP 1: What is the unit of measurement the nurse should calculate? (Place the unit of measure being calculated on the left side of the equation.)

X mL =

STEP 2: Determine the ratio that contains the same unit as the unit being calculated. (Place the ratio on the right side of the equation ensuring that the unit in the numerator matches the unit being calculated.)

$$X \text{ mL} = \frac{5 \text{ mL}}{250 \text{ mg}}$$

STEP 3: Place any remaining ratios that are relevant to the item on the right side of the equation along with any needed conversion factors to cancel out unwanted units of measurement.

$$X \text{ mL} = \frac{5 \text{ mL}}{250 \text{ mg}} \times \frac{1,000 \text{ mg}}{1 \text{ g}} \times \frac{0.25 \text{ g}}{1}$$

STEP 4: Solve for X.

X mL = 5 mL

STEP 5: Round, if necessary.

STEP 6: Determine whether the amount to administer makes sense. If there are 250 mg/5 mL and the prescription reads 0.25 g, it makes sense to administer 5 mL. The nurse should administer amoxicillin 5 mL PO every 8 hr.

Injectable dosage

Example: A nurse is preparing to administer heparin 8,000 units subcutaneously every 12 hr. Available is heparin injection 10,000 units/mL. How many mL should the nurse administer per dose? (Round the answer to the nearest tenth. Use a leading zero if it applies. Do not use a trailing zero.)

USING RATIO AND PROPORTION

STEP 1: What is the unit of measurement the nurse should calculate?

mL

STEP 2: What is the dose the nurse should administer? Dose to administer = Desired

8,000 units

STEP 3: What is the dose available? Dose available = Have

10,000 units

STEP 4: Should the nurse convert the units of measurement? No

STEP 5: What is the quantity of the dose available? = Quantity

> 1 mL

STEP 6: Set up the equation and solve for X.

$$\frac{Have}{Quantity} = \frac{Desired}{X}$$

$$\frac{10,000 \text{ units}}{1 \text{ mL}} = \frac{8,000 \text{ units}}{X \text{ mL}}$$

$$X \text{ mL} = 0.8 \text{ mL}$$

STEP 7: Round, if necessary.

STEP 8: Determine whether the amount to administer makes sense. If there are 10,000 units/mL and the prescription reads 8,000 units, it makes sense to administer 0.8 mL. The nurse should administer heparin injection 0.8 mL subcutaneously every 12 hr.

USING DESIRED OVER HAVE

STEP 1: What is the unit of measurement the nurse should calculate?

> mL

STEP 2: What is the dose the nurse should administer? Dose to administer = Desired

> 8,000 units

STEP 3: What is the dose available? Dose available = Have

> 10,000 units

STEP 4: Should the nurse convert the units of measurement? No

STEP 5: What is the quantity of the dose available? = Quantity

> 1 mL

STEP 6: Set up an equation and solve for X.

$$X = \frac{Desired \times Quantity}{Have}$$

$$X \text{ mL} = \frac{8,000 \text{ units} \times 1 \text{ mL}}{10,000 \text{ units}}$$

$$X \text{ mL} = 0.8 \text{ mL}$$

STEP 7: Round, if necessary.

STEP 8: Determine whether the amount to administer makes sense. If there are 10,000 units/mL and the prescription reads 8,000 units, it makes sense to administer 0.8 mL. The nurse should administer heparin injection 0.8 mL subcutaneously every 12 hr.

USING DIMENSIONAL ANALYSIS

STEP 1: What is the unit of measurement the nurse should calculate? (Place the unit of measure being calculated on the left side of the equation.)

> X mL =

STEP 2: Determine the ratio that contains the same unit as the unit being calculated. (Place the ratio on the right side of the equation ensuring that the unit in the numerator matches the unit being calculated.)

$$X \text{ mL} = \frac{1 \text{ mL}}{10,000 \text{ units}}$$

STEP 3: Place any remaining ratios that are relevant to the item on the right side of the equation along with any needed conversion factors to cancel out unwanted units of measurements.

$$X \text{ mL} = \frac{8,000 \text{ units}}{10,000 \text{ units}} \times \frac{1 \text{ mL}}{1 \text{ dose}}$$

STEP 4: Solve for X.

$$X \text{ mL} = 0.8 \text{ mL}$$

STEP 5: Round, if necessary.

STEP 6: Determine whether the amount to administer makes sense. If there are 10,000 units/mL and the prescription reads 8,000 units, it makes sense to administer 0.8 mL. The nurse should administer heparin injection 0.8 mL subcutaneously every 12 hr.

Dosages by weight

Example: A nurse is preparing to administer cefixime 8 mg/kg/day PO to divide equally every 12 hr to a toddler who weighs 22 lb. Available is cefixime suspension 100 mg/5 mL. How many mL should the nurse administer per dose? (Round the answer to the nearest whole number. Use a leading zero if it applies. Do not use a trailing zero.)

USING RATIO AND PROPORTION

STEP 1: What is the unit of measurement the nurse should calculate?

> kg

STEP 2: Set up an equation and solve for X.

$$\frac{2.2 \text{ lb}}{1 \text{ kg}} = \frac{Client's \ desired \ weight \ in \ lb}{X \text{ kg}}$$

$$\frac{2.2 \text{ lb}}{1 \text{ kg}} = \frac{22 \text{ lb}}{X \text{ kg}}$$

$$X \text{ kg} = 10 \text{ kg}$$

STEP 3: What is the unit of measurement the nurse should calculate?

mg

STEP 4: Set up an equation and solve for X.

X mg × kg/day =

X mg/day = mg/kg/day × Client's weight in kg

X mg/day = 8 mg/kg/day × 10 kg

X mg/day = 80 kg/day

STEP 5: The dose is divided equally every 12 hours. Divide X by 2.

$$X \text{ mg} = \frac{80 \text{ mg}}{2 \text{ doses}}$$

X mg = 40 mg/dose

STEP 6: What is the unit of measurement the nurse should calculate?

mL

STEP 7: What is the dose the nurse should administer? Dose to administer = Desired

40 mg

STEP 8: What is the dose available? Dose available = Have

100 mg

STEP 9: Should the nurse convert the units of measurement? No

STEP 10: What is the quantity of the dose available? = Quantity

5 mL

STEP 11: Set up the equation and solve for X.

$$\frac{Have}{Quantity} = \frac{Desired}{X}$$

$$\frac{100 \text{ mg}}{5 \text{ mL}} = \frac{40 \text{ mg}}{X \text{ mL}}$$

X mL = 2 mL

STEP 12: Round, if necessary.

STEP 13: Determine whether the amount to give makes sense. If there are 100 mg/5 mL and the prescription reads 40 mg, it makes sense to give 2 mL. The nurse should administer cefixime suspension 2 mL PO every 12 hr.

USING DESIRED OVER HAVE

STEP 1: What is the unit of measurement the nurse should calculate?

kg

STEP 2: Set up an equation and solve for X.

$$X \, kg = \frac{Client's \ weight \ in \ lb \times 1 \ kg}{2.2 \ lb}$$

$$X \text{ kg} = \frac{22 \text{ lb} \times 1 \text{ kg}}{2.2 \text{ lb}}$$

X kg = 10 kg

STEP 3: What is the unit of measurement the nurse should calculate?

mg

STEP 4: Set up an equation and solve for X.

X = Dose per kg × Client's weight in kg

X mg = 8 mg × 10 kg

X mg = 80 mg

The dose is divided equally every 12 hours; therefore, divide X by 2.

$$\frac{80 \text{ mg}}{2} = 40 \text{ mg}$$

STEP 5: What is the unit of measurement the nurse should calculate?

mL

STEP 6: What is the dose the nurse should administer? Dose to administer = Desired

40 mg

STEP 7: What is the dose available? Dose available = Have

100 mg

STEP 8: Should the nurse convert the units of measurement? No

STEP 9: What is the quantity of the dose available? = Quantity

5 mL

STEP 10: Set up an equation and solve for X.

$$X = \frac{Desired \times Quantity}{Have}$$

$$X \text{ mL} = \frac{40 \text{ mg} \times 5 \text{ mL}}{100 \text{ mg}}$$

X mL = 2 mL

STEP 11: Round, if necessary.

STEP 12: Determine whether the amount to give makes sense. If there are 100 mg/5 mL and the prescription reads 40 mg, it makes sense to give 2 mL. The nurse should administer cefixime suspension 2 mL PO every 12 hr.

USING DIMENSIONAL ANALYSIS

STEP 1: What is the unit of measurement the nurse should calculate? (Place the unit of measure being calculated on the left side of the equation.)

X mL/dose =

STEP 2: Determine the ratio that contains the same unit as the unit being calculated. (Place the ratio on the right side of the equation ensuring that the unit in the numerator matches the unit being calculated.)

$$\frac{X\ mL}{dose} = \frac{5\ mL}{100\ mg}$$

STEP 3: Place any remaining ratios that are relevant to the item on the right side of the equation along with any needed conversion factors to cancel out unwanted units of measurements.

X mL/dose =

$$\frac{X\ mL}{dose} = \frac{5\ mL}{100\ mg} \times \frac{8\ mg}{1\ kg} \times \frac{1\ kg}{2.2\ lb} \times \frac{22\ lb}{1\ day} \times \frac{1\ day}{2\ dose}$$

STEP 4: Solve for X.

X mL = 2 mL

STEP 5: Round, if necessary.

STEP 6: Determine whether the amount to give makes sense. If there are 100 mg/5 mL and the prescription reads 40 mg, it makes sense to give 2 mL. The nurse should administer cefixime suspension 2 mL PO every 12 hr.

IV flow rates

Nurses calculate IV flow rates for large-volume continuous IV infusions and intermittent IV bolus infusions using electronic infusion pumps (mL/hr) and manual IV tubing (gtt/min).

IV INFUSIONS WITH ELECTRONIC INFUSION PUMPS

Infusion pumps control an accurate rate of fluid infusion. Infusion pumps deliver a specific amount of fluid during a specific amount of time. For example, an infusion pump can deliver 150 mL in 1 hr or 50 mL in 20 min.

Example: A nurse is preparing to administer dextrose 5% in water (D₅W) 500 mL IV to infuse over 4 hr. The nurse should set the IV infusion pump to deliver how many mL/hr? (Round the answer to the nearest whole number. Use a leading zero if it applies. Do not use a trailing zero.)

USING RATIO AND PROPORTION AND DESIRED OVER HAVE

STEP 1: What is the unit of measurement the nurse should calculate?

mL/hr

STEP 2: What is the volume the nurse should infuse?

500 mL

STEP 3: What is the total infusion time?

4 hr

STEP 4: Should the nurse convert the units of measurement? No

STEP 5: Set up the equation and solve for X.

$$X\ mL/hr = \frac{Volume\ (mL)}{Time\ (hr)}$$

$$X\ mL/hr = \frac{500\ mL}{4\ hr}$$

X mL/hr = 125 mL/hr

STEP 6: Round, if necessary.

STEP 7: Determine whether the IV flow rate makes sense.

If the prescription reads 500 mL to infuse over 4 hr, it makes sense to administer 125 mL/hr. The nurse should set the IV pump to deliver D₅W 500 mL IV at 125 mL/hr.

USING DIMENSIONAL ANALYSIS

STEP 1: What is the unit of measurement the nurse should calculate? (Place the unit of measure being calculated on the left side of the equation.)

X mL/hr =

STEP 2: Determine the ratio that contains the same unit as the unit being calculated. (Place the ratio on the right side of the equation ensuring that the unit in the numerator matches the unit being calculated.)

$$X\ mL/hr = \frac{500\ mL}{4\ hr}$$

STEP 3: Place any remaining ratios that are relevant to the item on the right side of the equation along with any needed conversion factors to cancel out unwanted units of measurements.

$$X\ mL/hr = \frac{500\ mL}{4\ hr}$$

STEP 4: Solve for X.

X mL/hr = 125 mL/hr

STEP 5: Round, if necessary.

STEP 6: Determine whether the IV flow rate makes sense. If the prescription reads 500 mL to infuse over 4 hr, it makes sense to administer 125 mL/hr. The nurse should set the IV pump to deliver D₅W 500 mL IV at 125 mL/hr.

> Example: A nurse is preparing to administer cefotaxime 1 g intermittent IV bolus over 45 min. Available is cefotaxime 1 g in 100 mL 0.9% sodium chloride (0.9% NaCl). The nurse should set the IV infusion pump to deliver how many mL/hr? (Round the answer to the nearest whole number.)

USING RATIO AND PROPORTION

STEP 1: What is the unit of measurement the nurse should calculate?

mL/hr

STEP 2: What is the volume the nurse should infuse?

100 mL

STEP 3: What is the total infusion time?

45 min

STEP 4: Should the nurse convert the units of measurement?

Yes (min does not equal hr)

$$\frac{60 \text{ min}}{1 \text{ hr}} = \frac{45 \text{ min}}{X \text{ hr}}$$

X hr = 0.75 hr

STEP 5: Set up an equation and solve for X.

$$\frac{X \text{ mL}}{\text{hr}} = \frac{Volume\ (mL)}{Time\ (hr)}$$

$$X \text{ mL/hr} = \frac{100 \text{ mL}}{0.75 \text{ hr}}$$

X mL/hr = 133.333333 mL/hr

STEP 6: Round, if necessary.

133.3333 rounds to 133

STEP 7: Determine whether the IV flow rate makes sense.

If the prescription reads 100 mL to infuse over 45 min (0.75 hr), it makes sense to administer 133 mL/hr. The nurse should set the IV pump to deliver cefotaxime 1 g in 100 mL of 0.9% NaCl IV at 133 mL/hr.

USING DESIRED OVER HAVE

STEP 1: What is the unit of measure the nurse should calculate?

mL/hr

STEP 2: What is the volume the nurse should infuse?

100 mL

STEP 3: What is the total infusion time?

45 min

STEP 4: Should the nurse convert the units of measurement?

$$X \text{ hr} = \frac{45 \text{ min} \times 1 \text{ hr}}{60 \text{ min}}$$

X hr = 0.75 hr

STEP 5: Set up the equation and solve for X.

$$X \text{ mL/hr} = \frac{Volume\ (mL)}{Time}$$

$$X \text{ mL/hr} = \frac{100 \text{ mL}}{0.75 \text{ hr}}$$

X mL/hr = 133.333333 mL/hr

STEP 6: Round, if necessary.

133.333333 rounds to 133

STEP 7: Determine whether the amount to administer makes sense. If the prescription reads 100 mL to infuse over 45 min (0.75 hr), it makes sense to administer 133 mL/hr. The nurse should set the IV pump to deliver cefotaxime 1 g in 100 mL of 0.9% NaCl IV at 133 mL/hr.

USING DIMENSIONAL ANALYSIS

STEP 1: What is the unit of measurement the nurse should calculate? (Place the unit of measure being calculated on the left side of the equation.)

X mL/hr =

STEP 2: Determine the ratio that contains the same unit as the unit being calculated. (Place the ratio on the right side of the equation ensuring that the unit in the numerator matches the unit being calculated.)

$$X \text{ mL/hr} = \frac{100 \text{ mL}}{45 \text{ min}}$$

STEP 3 : Place any remaining ratios that are relevant to the item on the right side of the equation along with any needed conversion factors to cancel out unwanted units of measurements.

$$X \text{ mL/hr} = \frac{100 \text{ mL}}{45 \text{ min}} \times \frac{60 \text{ min}}{1 \text{ hr}}$$

STEP 4: Solve for X.

X mL/hr = 133.333333 mL/hr

STEP 5: Round, if necessary.

133.333333 rounds to 133

STEP 6: Determine whether the IV flow rate makes sense. If the prescription reads 100 mL to infuse over 45 min (0.75 hr), it makes sense to administer 133 mL/hr. The nurse should set the IV pump to deliver cefotaxime 1 g in 100 mL of 0.9% NaCl IV at 133 mL/hr.

MANUAL IV INFUSIONS

If an electronic infusion pump is not available, regulate the IV flow rate using the roller clamp on the IV tubing. When setting the flow rate, count the number of drops that fall into the drip chamber over 1 min. Then calculate the flow rate using the drop factor on the manufacturer's package containing the administration set. The drop factor is the number of drops per milliliter of solution.

> Example: A nurse is preparing to administer lactated Ringer's (LR) 1,500 mL IV to infuse over 10 hr. The drop factor of the manual IV tubing is 15 gtt/mL. The nurse should adjust the manual IV infusion to deliver how many gtt/min? (Round the answer to the nearest whole number. Use a leading zero if it applies. Do not use a trailing zero.)

USING RATIO AND PROPORTION

STEP 1: What is the unit of measurement the nurse should calculate?

> gtt/min

STEP 2: What is the volume the nurse should infuse?

> 1,500 mL

STEP 3: What is the total infusion time?

> 10 hr

STEP 4: Should the nurse convert the units of measurement? No (mL = mL) Yes (hr ≠ min)

$$\frac{1 \text{ hr}}{60 \text{ min}} = \frac{10 \text{ hr}}{X \text{ min}}$$

X min = 600 min

STEP 5: Set up the equation and solve for X.

$$X = \frac{Volume \text{ (mL)} \times drop \text{ factor (gtt/mL)}}{Time \text{ (min)}}$$

$$X \text{ gtt/min} = \frac{1{,}500 \text{ mL}}{600 \text{ min}} \times \frac{15 \text{ gtt}}{1 \text{ mL}}$$

X gtt/min = 37.5 gtt/min

STEP 6: Round, if necessary.

> 37.5 rounds to 38

STEP 7: Determine whether the IV flow rate makes sense.

> If the prescription reads 1,500 mL to infuse over 10 hr (600 min), it makes sense to administer 38 gtt/min. The nurse should adjust the manual IV infusion to deliver LR 1,500 mL IV at 38 gtt/min.

USING DESIRED OVER HAVE

STEP 1: What is the unit of measurement the nurse should calculate?

> gtt/min

STEP 2: What is the volume the nurse should infuse?

> 1,500 mL

STEP 3: What is the total infusion time?

> 10 hr

STEP 4: Should the nurse convert the units of measurement?
Yes (hr does not equal min)

$$X \text{ hr} = \frac{60 \text{ min} \times 10 \text{ hr}}{1 \text{ hr}}$$

X min = 600 min

STEP 5: Set up the equation and solve for X.

$$X = \frac{Volume \text{ (mL)} \times drop \text{ factor (gtt/mL)}}{Time \text{ (min)}}$$

$$X \text{ gtt/min} = \frac{1{,}500 \text{ mL} \times 15 \text{ gtt}}{600 \text{ min}}$$

X gtt/min = 37.5 gtt/min

STEP 6: Round, if necessary.

> 37.5 rounds to 38

STEP 7: Determine whether the IV flow rate makes sense.

> If the prescription reads 1,500 mL to infuse over 10 hr (600 min), it makes sense to administer 38 gtt/min. The nurse should adjust the manual IV infusion to deliver LR 1,500 mL IV at 38 gtt/min.

USING DIMENSIONAL ANALYSIS

STEP 1: What is the unit of measurement the nurse should calculate? (Place the unit of measure being calculated on the left side of the equation.)

> X gtt/min =

STEP 2: Determine the ratio that contains the same unit as the unit being calculated. (Place the ratio on the right side of the equation ensuring that the unit in the numerator matches the unit being calculated.)

$$X \text{ gtt/min} = \frac{15 \text{ gtt}}{1 \text{ mL}}$$

STEP 3: Place any remaining ratios that are relevant to the item on the right side of the equation along with any needed conversion factors to cancel out unwanted units of measurements.

$$X \text{ gtt/min} = \frac{15 \text{ gtt}}{1 \text{ mL}} \times \frac{1500 \text{ mL}}{10 \text{ hr}} \times \frac{1 \text{ hr}}{60 \text{ min}}$$

STEP 4: Solve for X.

> X gtt/min = 37.5 gtt/min

STEP 5: Round, if necessary.

37.5 rounds to 38

STEP 6: Determine whether the IV flow rate makes sense.

If the prescription reads 1,500 mL to infuse over 10 hr (600 min), it makes sense to administer 38 gtt/min. The nurse should adjust the manual IV infusion to deliver LR 1,500 mL IV at 38 gtt/min.

Example: A nurse is preparing to administer famotidine 120 mg by intermittent IV bolus. Available is famotidine 120 mg in 100 mL of 0.9% sodium chloride (0.9% NaCl) to infuse over 30 min. The drop factor of the manual IV tubing is 10 gtt/mL. The nurse should adjust the manual IV infusion to deliver how many gtt/min? (Round the answer to the nearest whole number. Use a leading zero if it applies. Do not use a trailing zero.)

USING RATIO AND PROPORTION AND DESIRED OVER HAVE

STEP 1: What is the unit of measurement the nurse should calculate?

gtt/min

STEP 2: What is the volume the nurse should infuse?

100 mL

STEP 3: What is the total infusion time?

30 min

STEP 4: Should the nurse convert the units of measurement? No

STEP 5: Set up the equation and solve for X.

$$X = \frac{Volume\ (mL) \times drop\ factor\ (gtt/mL)}{Time\ (min)}$$

$$X\ gtt/min = \frac{100\ mL \times 10\ gtt}{30\ min}$$

$X\ gtt/min = 33.333333\ gtt/min$

STEP 6: Round if necessary.

33.333333 rounds to 33

STEP 7: Determine whether the IV flow rate makes sense. If the amount prescribed is 100 mL to infuse over 30 min, it makes sense to administer 33 gtt/min. The nurse should adjust the manual IV infusion to deliver famotidine 120 mg in 100 mL of 0.9% NaCl IV at 33 gtt/min.

USING DIMENSIONAL ANALYSIS

STEP 1: What is the unit of measure to calculate? (Place the unit of measure being calculated on the left side of the equation.)

$X\ gtt/min =$

STEP 2: Determine the ratio that contains the same unit as the unit being calculated. (Place the ratio on the right side of the equation ensuring that the unit in the numerator matches the unit being calculated.)

$$X\ gtt/min = \frac{10\ gtt}{1\ mL}$$

STEP 3: Place any remaining ratios that are relevant to the item on the right side of the equation along with any needed conversion factors to cancel out unwanted units of measurements.

$$X\ gtt/min = \frac{10\ gtt}{1\ mL} \times \frac{100\ mL}{30\ min}$$

STEP 4: Solve for X.

$X\ gtt/min = 33.333333\ gtt/min$

STEP 5: Round if necessary.

33.333333 rounds to 33

STEP 6: Determine whether the IV flow rate makes sense.

If the amount prescribed is 100 mL to infuse over 30 min, it makes sense to administer 33 gtt/min. The nurse should adjust the manual IV infusion to deliver famotidine 120 mg in 100 mL of 0.9% NaCl IV at 33 gtt/min.

Application Exercises

1. A nurse is preparing to administer haloperidol 2 mg PO every 12 hr. The amount available is haloperidol 1 mg/tablet. How many tablets should the nurse administer? (Round the answer to the nearest whole number. Do not use a trailing zero.)

2. A nurse is preparing to administer furosemide 80 mg PO daily. The amount available is furosemide oral solution 10 mg/1 mL. How many mL should the nurse administer? (Round the answer to the nearest whole number. Do not use a trailing zero.)

3. A nurse is preparing to administer heparin 15,000 units subcutaneously every 12 hr. The amount available is heparin injection 20,000 units/mL. How many mL should the nurse administer per dose? (Round the answer to the nearest tenth. Do not use a trailing zero.)

4. A nurse is preparing to administer amoxicillin 20 mg/kg/day PO to divide equally every 12 hr to a preschooler who weighs 44 lb. The amount available is amoxicillin suspension 250 mg/5 mL. How many mL should the nurse administer per dose? (Round the answer to the nearest whole number. Do not use a trailing zero.)

5. A nurse is preparing to administer clindamycin 200 mg by intermittent IV bolus. The amount available is clindamycin injection 200 mg in 100 mL 0.9% sodium chloride (0.9% NaCl) to infuse over 30 min. The nurse should set the IV pump to deliver how many mL/hr? (Round the answer to the nearest whole number. Do not use a trailing zero.)

6. A nurse is preparing to administer vancomycin 1 g by intermittent IV bolus. Available is vancomycin 1 g in 100 mL of dextrose 5% in water (D_5W) to infuse over 45 min. The drop factor of the manual IV tubing is 10 gtt/mL. The nurse should adjust the manual IV infusion to deliver how many gtt/min? (Round the answer to the nearest whole number. Do not use a trailing zero.)

1. **2** tablets

Using Ratio and Proportion

STEP 1: What is the unit of measurement the nurse should calculate?   tablet

STEP 2: What is the dose the nurse should administer? Dose to administer = Desired = 2 mg

STEP 3: What is the dose available? Dose available = Have = 1 mg

STEP 4: Should the nurse convert the units of measurement?   No

STEP 5: What is the quantity of the dose available? = Quantity = 1 tablet

STEP 6: Set up the equation and solve for X.

$$\frac{Have}{Quantity} = \frac{Desired}{X}$$

$$\frac{1 \text{ mg}}{1 \text{ tablet}} = \frac{2 \text{ mg}}{X \text{ tablets}}$$

X tablet(s) = 2 tablets

STEP 7: Round, if necessary.

STEP 8: Determine whether the amount to administer makes sense. If there is 1 mg/tablet and the prescription reads 2 mg, it makes sense to administer 2 tablets. Administer haloperidol 2 tablets every 12 hr.

Using Desired Over Have

STEP 1: What is the unit of measurement the nurse should calculate?   tablet

STEP 2: What is the dose the nurse should administer? Dose to administer = Desired = 2 mg

STEP 3: What is the dose available? Dose available = Have = 1 mg

STEP 4: Should the nurse convert the units of measurement?   No

STEP 5: What is the quantity of the dose available? = Quantity = 1 tablet

STEP 6: Set up the equation and solve for X.

$$X = \frac{Desired \times Quantity}{Have}$$

$$X \text{ tablet(s)} = \frac{2 \text{ mg} \times 1 \text{ tablet}}{1 \text{ mg}}$$

X tablet(s) = 2 tablets

STEP 7: Round, if necessary.

STEP 8: Determine whether the amount to administer makes sense. If there is 1 mg/tablet and the prescription reads 2 mg, it makes sense to administer 2 tablets. Administer haloperidol 2 tablets every 12 hr.

Using Dimensional Analysis

STEP 1: What is the unit of measurement the nurse should calculate? (Place the unit of measure being calculated on the left side of the equation.)

X tablet(s)/dose =

STEP 2: Determine the ratio that contains the same unit as the unit being calculated. (Place the ratio on the right side of the equation ensuring that the unit in the numerator matches the unit being calculated.)

$$X \text{ tablet(s)/dose} = \frac{1 \text{ tablet}}{1 \text{ mg}}$$

STEP 3: Place the remaining ratios that are relevant to the item on the right side of the equation along with any needed conversion factors to cancel out unwanted units of measurement.

$$X \text{ tablet(s)/dose} = \frac{1 \text{ tablet}}{1 \text{ mg}} \times \frac{2 \text{ mg}}{1 \text{ dose}}$$

STEP 4: Solve for X.

X tablet(s)/dose = 2 tablets/dose

STEP 5: Round, if necessary.

STEP 6: Determine whether the amount to administer makes sense. If there is 1 mg/tablet and the prescription reads 2 mg, it makes sense to administer 2 tablets. Administer haloperidol 2 tablets every 12 hr.

Ⓝ NCLEX® Connection: Pharmacological and Parenteral Therapies, Dosage Calculations

2. **8** mL

Using Ratio and Proportion

STEP 1: What is the unit of measurement the nurse should calculate?   mL

STEP 2: What is the dose the nurse should administer? Dose to administer = Desired = 80 mg

STEP 3: What is the dose available? Dose available = Have = 10 mg

STEP 4: Should the nurse convert the units of measurement?   No

STEP 5: What is the quantity of the dose available? = Quantity = 1 mL

STEP 6: Set up the equation and solve for X.

$$\frac{Have}{Quantity} = \frac{Desired}{X}$$

$$\frac{10 \text{ mg}}{1 \text{ mL}} = \frac{80 \text{ mg}}{X \text{ mL}}$$

X mL = 8mL

STEP 7: Round, if necessary.

STEP 8: Determine whether the amount to administer makes sense. If there are 10 mg/1 mL and the prescription reads 80 mg, it makes sense to administer 8 mL. Administer furosemide 8 mL PO daily.

Using Desired Over Have

STEP 1: What is the unit of measurement the nurse should calculate?   mL

STEP 2: What is the dose the nurse should administer? Dose to administer = Desired = 80 mg

STEP 3: What is the dose available? Dose available = Have = 10 mg

STEP 4: Should the nurse convert the units of measurement? No

STEP 5: What is the quantity of the dose available? = Quantity = 1 mL

STEP 6: Set up the equation and solve for X.

$$X = \frac{Desired \times Quantity}{Have}$$

$$X \text{ mL} = \frac{80 \text{ mg} \times 1 \text{ mL}}{10 \text{ mg}}$$

X mL = 8 mL

STEP 7: Round, if necessary.

STEP 8: Determine whether the amount to administer makes sense. If there are 10 mg/1 mL and the prescription reads 80 mg, it makes sense to administer 8 mL. Administer furosemide 8 mL PO daily.

Using Dimensional Analysis

STEP 1: What is the unit of measurement the nurse should calculate? (Place the unit of measure being calculated on the left side of the equation.)

X mL =

STEP 2: Determine the ratio that contains the same unit as the unit being calculated. (Place the ratio on the right side of the equation ensuring that the unit in the numerator matches the unit being calculated.)

$$X \text{ mL} = \frac{1 \text{ mL}}{10 \text{ mg}}$$

STEP 3: Place any remaining ratios that are relevant to the item on the right side of the equation along with any needed conversion factors to cancel out unwanted units of measurements.

$$X \text{ mL} = \frac{1 \text{ mL}}{10 \text{ mg}} \times \frac{80 \text{ mg}}{1}$$

STEP 4: Solve for X.

X mL = 8 mL

STEP 5: Round, if necessary.

STEP 6: Determine whether the amount to administer makes sense. If there are 10 mg/1 mL and the prescription reads 80 mg, it makes sense to administer 8 mL. Administer furosemide 8 mL PO daily.

Ⓝ NCLEX® Connection: Pharmacological and Parenteral Therapies, Dosage Calculations

3. **0.8** mL

Using Ratio and Proportion

STEP 1: What is the unit of measurement the nurse should calculate?   mL

STEP 2: What is the dose the nurse should administer? Dose to administer = Desired = 15,000 units

STEP 3: What is the dose available? Dose available = Have = 20,000 units

STEP 4: Should the nurse convert the units of measurement?   No

STEP 5: What is the quantity of the dose available? = Quantity = 1 mL

STEP 6: Set up the equation and solve for X.

$$\frac{Have}{Quantity} = \frac{Desired}{X}$$

$$\frac{20,000\ units}{1\ mL} = \frac{15,000\ units}{X\ mL}$$

X mL = 0.75 mL

STEP 7: Round, if necessary.   0.75 rounds to 0.8

STEP 8: Determine whether the amount to administer makes sense. If there are 20,000 units/mL and the prescription reads 15,000 units, it makes sense to administer 0.8 mL. Administer heparin injection 0.8 mL subcutaneously every 12 hr.

Using Desired Over Have

STEP 1: What is the unit of measurement the nurse should calculate?   mL

STEP 2: What is the dose the nurse should administer? Dose to administer = Desired = 15,000 units

STEP 3: What is the dose available? Dose available = Have = 20,000 units

STEP 4: Should the nurse convert the units of measurement?   No

STEP 5: What is the quantity of the dose available? = Quantity = 1 mL

STEP 6: Set up an equation and solve for X.

$$X = \frac{Desired \times Quantity}{Have}$$

$$X\ mL = \frac{15,000\ units \times 1\ mL}{20,000\ units}$$

X mL = 0.75 mL

STEP 7: Round, if necessary.   0.75 rounds to 0.8

STEP 8: Determine whether the amount to administer makes sense. If there are 10,000 units/mL and the prescription reads 8,000 units, it makes sense to administer 0.8 mL. Administer heparin injection 0.8 mL subcutaneously every 12 hr.

Using Dimensional Analysis

STEP 1: What is the units of measurement the nurse should calculate? (Place the unit of measure being calculated on the left side of the equation.)

X mL =

STEP 2: Determine the ratio that contains the same units as the unit being calculated. (Place the ratio on the right side of the equation ensuring that the unit in the numerator matches the unit being calculated.)

$$X\ mL = \frac{1\ mL}{20,000\ units}$$

STEP 3: Place any remaining ratios that are relevant to the item on the rights side of the equation along with any needed conversion factors to cancel out unwanted units of measurements.

$$X\ mL = \frac{1\ mL}{20,000\ units} \times \frac{15,000\ units}{1}$$

STEP 4: Solve for X.

X mL = 0.75 mL

STEP 5: Set up the equation and solve for X.

$$\frac{Have}{Quantity} = \frac{Desired}{X}$$

$$\frac{20,000\ units}{1\ mL} = \frac{15,000\ units}{X\ mL}$$

X mL = 0.75 mL

STEP 6: Round, if necessary.   0.75 rounds to 0.8

STEP 7: Determine whether the amount to administer makes sense. If there are 10,000 units/mL and the prescription reads 8,000 units, it makes sense to administer 0.8 mL. Administer heparin injection 0.8 mL subcutaneously every 12 hr.

Ⓝ *NCLEX® Connection: Pharmacological and Parenteral Therapies, Dosage Calculations*

4. 4 mL

Using Ratio and Proportion

STEP 1: What is the unit of measurement the nurse should calculate? kg

STEP 2: Set up an equation and solve for X.

$$\frac{2.2 \text{ lb}}{1 \text{ kg}} = \frac{\text{Client's weight in kg}}{X \text{ kg}}$$

$$\frac{2.2 \text{ lb}}{1 \text{ kg}} = \frac{44 \text{ lb}}{X \text{ kg}}$$

X kg = 20 kg

STEP 3: What is the unit of measurement the nurse should calculate? mg

STEP 4: Set up an equation and solve for X

X = Dose per kg x Client's weight in kg

X mg = 20 mg/kg/day x 20 kg

X mg = 400 mg/day

The dose is divided equally every 12 hr; therefore, divide X by 2.

$$\frac{400 \text{ mg}}{2} = 200 \text{ mg}$$

STEP 5: What is the unit of measurement the nurse should calculate? mL

STEP 6: What is the dose the nurse should administer? Dose to administer = Desired = 200 mg

STEP 7: What is the dose available? Dose available = Have = 250 mg

STEP 8: Should the nurse convert the units of measurement? No

STEP 9: What is the quantity of the dose available? = Quantity = 5 mL

STEP 10: Set up the equation and solve for X.

$$\frac{Have}{Quantity} = \frac{Desired}{X}$$

$$\frac{250 \text{ mg}}{5 \text{ mL}} = \frac{200 \text{ mg}}{X \text{ mL}}$$

X mL = 4 mL

STEP 11: Round, if necessary.

STEP 12: Determine whether the amount to give makes sense. If there are 250 mg/5 mL and the prescription reads 200 mg, it makes sense to give 4 mL. Administer amoxicillin suspension 4 mL PO every 12 hr.

Using Desired Over Have

STEP 1: What is the unit of measurement the nurse should calculate? kg

STEP 2: Set up an equation and solve for X.

$$X \text{ kg} = \frac{\text{Client's weight in lb} \times 1 \text{ kg}}{2.2 \text{ lb}}$$

$$X \text{ kg} = \frac{44 \text{ lb} \times 1 \text{ kg}}{2.2 \text{ lb}}$$

X kg = 20 kg

STEP 3: What is the unit of measurement the nurse should calculate? mg

STEP 4: Set up an equation and solve for X.

X = Dose per kg x Client's weight in kg

X mg = 20 mg/kg/day x 20 kg

X mg = 400 mg/day

The dose is divided equally every 12 hr; therefore, divide X by 2.

$$\frac{400 \text{ mg}}{2} = 200 \text{ mg}$$

STEP 5: What is the unit of measurement the nurse should calculate? mL

STEP 6: What is the dose the nurse should administer? Dose to administer = Desired 200 mg

STEP 7: What is the dose available? Dose available = Have = 250 mg

STEP 8: Should the nurse convert the units of measurement? No

STEP 9: What is the quantity of the dose available? = Quantity = 5 mL

STEP 10: Set up an equation and solve for X.

$$X = \frac{Desired \times Quantity}{Have}$$

$$X \text{ mL} = \frac{200 \text{ mg} \times 5 \text{ mL}}{250 \text{ mg}}$$

X mL = 4 mL

STEP 11: Round, if necessary.

STEP 12: Determine whether the amount to give makes sense. If there are 250 mg/5 mL and the prescription reads 200 mg, it makes sense to give 4 mL. Administer amoxicillin suspension 4 mL PO every 12 hr.

Using Dimensional Analysis

STEP 1: What is the unit of measurement the nurse should calculate? (Place the unit of measure being calculated on the left side of the equation.)

X mL/dose=

STEP 2: Determine the ratio that contains the same unit as the unit being calculated. (Place the ratio on the right side of the equation ensuring that the unit in the numerator matches the unit being calculated.)

$$X \text{ mL/dose} = \frac{5 \text{ mL}}{250 \text{ mg}}$$

STEP 3: Place any remaining ratios that are relevant to the item on the right side of the equation along with any needed conversion factors to cancel out unwanted units of measurements.

$$\frac{X \text{ mL}}{\text{dose}} = \frac{5 \text{ mL}}{250 \text{ mg}} \times \frac{20 \text{ mg}}{1 \text{ kg}} \times \frac{1 \text{ kg}}{2.2 \text{ lb}} \times \frac{44 \text{ lb}}{1 \text{ day}} \times \frac{1 \text{ day}}{24 \text{ hr}} \times \frac{12 \text{ hr}}{1 \text{ dose}}$$

STEP 4: Solve for X.

X mL/dose = 4 mL/dose

STEP 5: Round, if necessary.

STEP 6: Determine whether the amount to give makes sense. If there are 250 mg/5 mL and the prescription reads 200 mg, it makes sense to give 4 mL. Administer amoxicillin suspension 4 mL PO every 12 hr.

(N) *NCLEX® Connection: Pharmacological and Parenteral Therapies, Dosage Calculations*

5. **200** mL/hr

Using Ratio and Proportion

STEP 1: What is the unit of measurement the nurse should calculate?   mL/hr

STEP 2: What is the volume the nurse should infuse?   100 mL

STEP 3: What is the total infusion time?   30 min

STEP 4: Should the nurse convert the units of measurement? Yes (min does not equal hr)

$$\frac{60 \text{ min}}{1 \text{ hr}} = \frac{30 \text{ min}}{X \text{ hr}}$$

X hr = 0.5 hr

STEP 5: Set up an equation and solve for X.

$$X \text{ mL/hr} = \frac{Volume \text{ (mL)}}{Time \text{ (hr)}}$$

$$X \text{ mL/hr} = \frac{100 \text{ mL}}{0.5 \text{ hr}}$$

X mL = 200 mL

STEP 6: Round, if necessary.

STEP 7: Determine whether the IV flow rate makes sense. If the prescription reads 100 mL to infuse over 30 min (0.5 hr), it makes sense to administer 200 mL/hr. Set the IV pump to deliver clindamycin 200 mg in 100 mL of 0.9% NaCl IV at 200 mL/hr.

Using Desired Over Have

STEP 1: What is the unit of measurement the nurse should calculate?   mL/hr

STEP 2: What is the volume the nurse should infuse?   100 mL

STEP 3: What is the total infusion time?   30 min

STEP 4: Should the nurse convert the units of measure? Yes (min does not equal hr)

$$X \text{ mL/hr} = \frac{30 \text{ min} \times 1 \text{ hr}}{60 \text{ min}}$$

X hr = 0.5 hr

STEP 5: Set up an equation and solve for X.

$$X \text{ mL/hr} = \frac{Volume \text{ (mL)}}{Time \text{ (hr)}}$$

$$X \text{ mL/hr} = \frac{100 \text{ mL}}{0.5 \text{ hr}}$$

X mL = 200 mL

STEP 6: Round, if necessary.

STEP 7: Determine whether the IV flow rate makes sense. If the prescription reads 100 mL to infuse over 30 min (0.5 hr), it makes sense to administer 200 mL/hr. Set the IV pump to deliver clindamycin 200 mg in 100 mL of 0.9% NaCl IV at 200 mL/hr.

Using Dimensional Analysis

STEP 1: What is the unit of measurement the nurse should calculate? (Place the unit of measure on the left side of the equation.)

X mL/hr =

STEP 2: Determine the ratio that contains the same unit as the unit being calculated. (Place the ratio on the right side of the equation ensuring that the unit in the numerator matches the unit being calculated.)

$$X \text{ mL/hr} = \frac{100 \text{ mL}}{30 \text{ min}}$$

STEP 3: Place any remaining ratios that are relevant to the item on the right side of the equation along with any needed conversion factors to cancel out unwanted units of measurements.

$$X \text{ mL/hr} = \frac{100 \text{ mL}}{30 \text{ min}} \times \frac{60 \text{ min}}{1 \text{ hr}}$$

STEP 4: Solve for X.

X mL/hr = 200 mL/hr

STEP 5: Round, if necessary.

STEP 6: Determine whether the IV flow rate makes sense. If the prescription reads 100 mL to infuse over 30 min (0.5 hr), it makes sense to administer 200 mL/hr. Set the IV pump to deliver clindamycin 200 mg in 100 mL of 0.9% NaCl IV at 200 mL/hr.

Ⓝ *NCLEX® Connection: Pharmacological and Parenteral Therapies, Parenteral/Intravenous Therapies*

6. **22** gtt/min

Using Ratio and Proportion and Desired Over Have

STEP 1: What is the unit of measurement the nurse should calculate?   gtt/min

STEP 2: What is the total infusion time?   45 min

STEP 3: What is the volume the nurse should infuse?   100 mL

STEP 4: Should the nurse convert the units of measure?   No

STEP 5: Set up an equation and solve for X.

$$X \text{ gtt/mL} = \frac{Volume \text{ (mL)}}{Time \text{ (min)}} \times Drop factor \text{ (gtt/mL)}$$

$$X \text{ gtt/mL} = \frac{100 \text{ mL}}{45 \text{ min}} \times 10 \text{ gtt/mL}$$

X gtt/mL = 22.222222 gtt/mL

STEP 6: Round, if necessary.   22.2222 rounds to 22

STEP 7: Determine whether the IV flow rate makes sense. If the amount prescribed is 100 mL to infuse over 45 min, it makes sense to administer 22 gtt/min. Adjust the manual IV infusion to deliver vancomycin 1 g in 100 mL of D₅W IV at 22 gtt/min.

Using Dimensional Analysis

STEP 1: What is the unit of measurement the nurse should calculate? (Place the unit of measure being calculated on the left side of the equation.)

X gtt/min =

STEP 2: Determine the ratio that contains the same unit as the unit being calculated. (Place the ratio on the right side of the equation ensuring that the unit in the numerator matches the unit being calculated.)

$$X \text{ gtt/min} = \frac{10 \text{ gtt}}{1 \text{ mL}}$$

STEP 3: Place any remaining ratios that are relevant to the item on the right side of the equation along with any needed conversion factors to cancel out unwanted units of measurements.

$$X \text{ mL/min} = \frac{100 \text{ mL}}{45 \text{ min}} \times \frac{10 \text{ gtt}}{1 \text{ mL}}$$

STEP 4: Solve for X.

X gtt/min = 22.222222 gtt/min

STEP 5: Round if necessary.   22.2222 rounds to 22

STEP 6: Determine whether the IV flow rate makes sense. If the amount prescribed is 100 mL to infuse over 45 min, it makes sense to administer 22 gtt/min. Adjust the manual IV infusion to deliver vancomycin 1 g in 100 mL of D₅W IV at 22 gtt/min.

Ⓝ *NCLEX® Connection: Pharmacological and Parenteral Therapies, Parenteral/Intravenous Therapies*

UNIT 1   PHARMACOLOGICAL PRINCIPLES

CHAPTER 4 *Intravenous Therapy*

Intravenous therapy involves administering fluids via an IV catheter to administer medications, supplement fluid intake, or give fluid replacement, electrolytes, or nutrients.

Nurses administer large-volume IV infusions on a continuous basis.

Nurses or pharmacists mix IV medication in a large volume of fluid to give as a continuous IV infusion or intermittently in a small amount of fluid. Nurses also administer medications as an IV bolus, giving the medication in a small amount of solution, concentrated, or diluted, and injecting it over a short time (1 to 2 min or longer, depending on the medication).

Refer to Fundamentals for Nursing, Chapter 49: Intravenous Therapy for IV procedural guidelines.

DESCRIPTION OF PROCEDURE

The provider prescribes the type of IV fluid, the volume to infuse, and either the rate at which to infuse the IV fluid or the total amount of time it should take to infuse the fluid. The nurse regulates the IV infusion, either with an IV pump or manually, to be sure to deliver the right amount.

ADVANTAGES

- Rapid effects
- Precise amounts
- Less discomfort after initial insertion
- Constant therapeutic blood levels
- Less irritation to subcutaneous and muscle tissue
- Permits the use of large volumes of fluid for medications that are poorly soluble and need larger amounts of fluid to dissolve
- Permits the use of medications that contain irritant properties, such as chemotherapy

DISADVANTAGES

- Circulatory fluid overload is possible if the infusion is large or too rapid.
- Immediate absorption leaves little time to correct errors.
- IV fluid administration can irritate the lining of the vein.
- Failure to maintain surgical asepsis can lead to local and systemic infection.

WAYS TO ADMINISTER IV MEDICATIONS

- Give the medication the pharmacist mixed in a large volume of fluid (500 to 1,000 mL) as a continuous IV infusion, such as potassium chloride and vitamins.
- Deliver the medication in premixed solution bags from the medication's manufacturer.
- Administer volume-controlled infusions.
- Give an IV bolus dose.

TYPES OF IV ACCESS

Peripheral or central venous access

GUIDELINES FOR SAFE IV MEDICATION ADMINISTRATION

- Use an infusion pump to administer medications that can cause serious adverse reactions. Never administer them by IV bolus. Double-check the dose prescribed, the dilution or amount of fluid, and the rate at which to give the medication.
- Add medications to a new IV fluid container, not to an IV container that is already hanging.
- Never administer IV medications through tubing that is infusing blood, blood products, or parenteral nutrition solutions.
- Verify the compatibility of medications with IV solutions before infusing a medication through tubing that is infusing an IV solution.
- Perform any assessments required prior to administration, based on the medication, and determine if continuous monitoring is required during administration (ECG).
- Use the IV port closest to the client to administer the medication.
- Ensure the IV is patent prior to administration. If the client does not have IV fluids infusing or has fluids that are not compatible with the medication, flush the IV access before and following administration.

Specific considerations

- Older adult clients, clients who are taking anticoagulants, and clients who have fragile veins Ⓖ
  - Avoid tourniquets. Use a blood pressure cuff to help visualize, but not over distend, the veins to help prevent hematoma formation.
  - Do not slap the extremity to visualize veins.
  - Instruct the client to hold their hand below the level of the heart to help distend and thus visualize the veins.
  - Avoid using the back of the client's hand.
  - Avoid rigorous friction while cleaning the site.
- Edema in extremities
  - Apply digital pressure over the selected vein to displace edema.
  - Apply pressure with an alcohol pad.
  - Cannulate the vein quickly.
- Clients who have a BMI greater than 30: Use anatomical landmarks to find veins.

Tourniquet

Avoid the use of a tourniquet with older adult clients who often have fragile veins or veins that easily bruise to prevent damage and bruising.

Blood pressure cuff

Use a blood pressure cuff to help visualize, but not over distend, the veins to help prevent hematoma formation and skin trauma.

Hand slapping veins

Hard tapping or slapping on the vein of an older adult client can cause venous constriction and possibly bruising and hematoma formation.

Veins on back of client's hand

Avoid the fragile dorsal veins of the older adult client. These veins have a greater risk for tissue damage and developing an infiltration or thrombophlebitis.

Client with hand below the level of the heart

Ask the client to hold their hand below heart level as gravity promotes vascular distention making the vein more visible.

Vigorous friction with cleaning

Vigorous friction on the vein of an older adult client can cause venous constriction and possibly bruising and hematoma formation.

COMPLICATIONS

Complications require notification of the provider and complete documentation. Use new tubing and catheters for restarting IV infusions after detecting complications.

Infiltration (infiltration of a nonvesicant solution)

FINDINGS: Pallor, local swelling at the site, decreased skin temperature around the site, damp dressing, slowed infusion

TREATMENT
- Stop the infusion and remove the catheter.
- Elevate the extremity.
- Encourage active range of motion.
- Apply a cold or warm compress depending on the type of solution that infiltrated the tissue.
- Check with the provider to determine whether the client still needs IV therapy. If so, restart the infusion proximal to the site or in another extremity.

PREVENTION
- Carefully select the site and catheter.
- Secure the catheter.
- Inspect IV infusion site frequently for any findings of infiltration.

Extravasation (infiltration of a vesicant or tissue-damaging medication)

FINDINGS: Pain, burning, redness, swelling

TREATMENT
- Stop the infusion and notify the provider.
- Follow the facility's protocol, which can include withdrawing the vesicant solution from the IV access and infusing an antidote through the catheter before removal.
- Further treatment is the same as for IV infiltration.

PREVENTION
- Closely monitor the IV site and dressing.
- Always use an infusion pump.

Fluid overload

FINDINGS
- Distended neck veins
- Increased blood pressure
- Tachycardia
- Shortness of breath
- Crackles in the lungs
- Edema
- Additional findings varying with the IV solution

TREATMENT
- Slow the IV rate or stop the infusion.
- Raise the head of the bed.
- Monitor vital signs and oxygen saturation.
- Adjust the rate after correcting fluid.
- Anticipate administering diuretics.

PREVENTION
- Use an infusion pump.
- Monitor I&O.

Phlebitis/thrombophlebitis

FINDINGS
- Edema, erythema
- Throbbing, burning, or pain at the site
- Increased skin temperature
- Red line up the arm with a palpable band at the vein site
- Slowed infusion

TREATMENT
- Promptly discontinue the infusion and remove the catheter.
- Elevate the extremity.
- Apply a cold compress to minimize the flow of blood, then apply a warm compress to increase circulation.
- Check with the provider to determine whether the client still needs IV therapy. If so, restart the infusion proximal to the site or in another extremity.
- Obtain a specimen for culture at the site and prepare the catheter for culture if drainage is present.

PREVENTION
- Rotate sites at least every 72 hr according to facility policy.
- Monitor IV sites using a phlebitis scale.
- Avoid the lower extremities.
- Use hand hygiene.
- Use surgical aseptic technique.

Other complications

Catheter embolus, cellulitis

NURSING ACTIONS: Assist with providing treatment according to facility protocol.

Application Exercises

1. A nurse is preparing to initiate IV therapy for an older adult client. Which of the following actions should the nurse plan to take?

    A. Use a disposable razor to remove excess hair on the extremity.

    B. Select the back of the client's hand to insert the IV catheter.

    C. Distend the veins by using a blood pressure cuff.

    D. Direct the client to raise their arm above the heart.

2. A nurse assessing the IV catheter insertion site for a client receiving a nonvesicant solution and notes swelling at the site with decreased skin temperature. Which of the following actions should the nurse take? (Select all that apply.)

    A. Stop the infusion.

    B. Start a new IV access distal to this site.

    C. Apply warm compresses to the insertion site

    D. Obtain a specimen for culture at the insertion site.

    E. Elevate the client's extremity.

3. A nurse is caring for a client experiencing IV extravasation. The facility requires the administration of an antidote for the prescribed IV solution. After stopping the IV infusion, which of the following actions should the nurse take first?

    A. Remove the IV catheter.

    B. Withdraw the solution from the IV access.

    C. Administer the antidote to the vesicant.

    D. Insert a new IV access in a different extremity.

Active Learning Scenario

A nurse on a medical-surgical unit is providing care for a group of clients who are receiving IV therapy. The nurse is assessing the clients for complications. Use the *ATI Active Learning Template: Nursing Skill* to complete this item.

INDICATIONS: Identify three indications for IV therapy.

POTENTIAL COMPLICATIONS: Identify four potential complications of IV therapy.

Active Learning Scenario Key

Using the ATI Active Learning Template: Nursing Skill

INDICATIONS
- To administer medications
- To supplement fluid intake
- To replace electrolytes and nutrients

POTENTIAL COMPLICATIONS
- Infiltration
- Extravasation
- Cellulitis
- Fluid overload
- Catheter embolus
- Phlebitis, thrombophlebitis

Ⓝ *NCLEX® Connection: Pharmacological and Parenteral Therapies, Parenteral/Intravenous Therapies*

Application Exercises Key

1. C. **CORRECT:** The nurse should plan to generate solutions to address the IV therapy needs of the older adult client by distending the veins using a blood pressure cuff to reduce overfilling of the vein, which can result in a hematoma.

   Ⓝ *NCLEX® Connection: Pharmacological and Parenteral Therapies, Parenteral/Intravenous Therapies*

2. A, C, E. **CORRECT:** The nurse should recognize the cues from the client's assessment and take action by stopping the infusion, applying a compress to the insertion site (can be warm or cool according to facility policy depending on the type of solution that infiltrated), and elevating the client's arm.

   Ⓝ *NCLEX® Connection: Pharmacological and Parenteral Therapies, Parenteral/Intravenous Therapies*

3. B. **CORRECT:** When taking actions, the nurse should recognize that according to evidence-based practice, the first action is to withdraw the solution from the IV access. This reduces the amount of vesicant in the body and lowers the risk of tissue damage.

   Ⓝ *NCLEX® Connection: Pharmacological and Parenteral Therapies, Parenteral/Intravenous Therapies*

UNIT 1 PHARMACOLOGICAL PRINCIPLES

CHAPTER 5 *Adverse Effects, Interactions, and Contraindications*

To ensure safe medication administration and prevent errors, the nurse must know why a medication is prescribed and its intended therapeutic effect. In addition, the nurse must be aware of potential side/adverse effects, interactions, contraindications, and precautions.

Every medication has the potential to cause side and adverse effects. Side effects occur when the medication is given at a therapeutic dose. Discontinuation of the medication is usually not warranted. Adverse effects are undesired, inadvertent, and unexpected severe responses to the medication. Adverse effects can occur at both therapeutic and higher-than-therapeutic doses. Providers will discontinue the medication immediately. Adverse effects are reported to the FDA using the MedWatch program.

Medications are chemicals that affect the body. When more than one medication is given, there is a potential for an interaction. In addition, medications can interact with foods, herbal medicines, or other unconventional remedies.

Contraindications and precautions of specific medications refer to client conditions that make it unsafe or potentially harmful to administer these medications.

Response to medications differs for individuals based on multiple factors (age, sex, disease process, and ethnic/genetic variations). These factors can be responsible for many expected and unexpected adverse effects.

ADVERSE MEDICATION EFFECTS

These effects can be classified according to body systems.

Central nervous system

Can result from central nervous system (CNS) stimulation (excitement) or CNS depression

NURSING ACTIONS
• If CNS stimulation is expected, clients can be at risk for seizures, and precautions should be taken.
• If CNS depression is likely, advise clients not to drive, operate heavy machinery, or participate in other activities that can be dangerous.

Anticholinergic

• Effects that are a result of muscarinic receptor blockade.
• Most are seen in eyes, smooth muscle, exocrine glands, and the heart.

CLIENT EDUCATION
• Manage these effects to minimize danger and discomfort.

  For example, dry mouth can be relieved by sipping on liquids; photophobia can be managed by use of sunglasses; and urinary retention can be reduced by urinating before taking the medication.

• Avoid activities that could lead to overheating, because there is a decreased ability to produce sweat to cool the body.

Cardiovascular

• Can involve blood vessels and the heart.
• Antihypertensives can cause orthostatic hypotension.

CLIENT EDUCATION: Monitor for indications of postural hypotension (lightheadedness, dizziness). If these occur, sit or lie down. Postural hypotension can be minimized by getting up and changing position slowly.

Gastrointestinal (GI)

• Can result from local irritation of the GI tract.
• Stimulation of the vomiting center also results in adverse effects.

CLIENT EDUCATION
• NSAIDs can cause GI upset. Take these medications with food.
• Opioid analgesics slow peristalsis and can cause nausea and sedation. Perform methods to avoid constipation and GI irritation, and promote safety.

Hematologic

Relatively common and potentially life-threatening with some groups of medications.

NURSING ACTIONS: Bone marrow depression/suppression is generally associated with anticancer medications and hemorrhagic disorders with anticoagulants and thrombolytics.

CLIENT EDUCATION: Monitor for bleeding (bruising, discolored urine/stool, petechiae, bleeding gums). Notify the provider if these effects occur.

TOXICITY

- An adverse medication effect that is considered severe and can be life-threatening.
- It can be caused by an excessive dose, but it also can occur at therapeutic dose levels.

NURSING ACTIONS: Liver damage will occur with an acetaminophen overdose. There is a greater risk of liver damage with chronic alcohol use. The antidote, acetylcysteine, can be used to minimize liver damage.

Hepatotoxicity

- Can occur with many medications.
- Because most medications are metabolized in the liver, the liver is particularly vulnerable to drug-induced injury.
- Damage to liver cells can impair metabolism of many medications, causing medication accumulation in the body and producing adverse effects.
- Many medications can alter normal values of liver function tests with no obvious clinical indications of liver dysfunction.

NURSING ACTIONS
- When two or more medications that are hepatotoxic are combined, the risk for liver damage is increased.
- Liver function tests are indicated when clients start a medication known to be hepatotoxic and periodically thereafter.
- Monitor clients for manifestations of hepatotoxicity (nausea, vomiting, jaundice, dark urine, abdominal discomfort, and anorexia). Advise clients to monitor for these manifestations.

Nephrotoxicity

- Can occur with a number of medications, but it is primarily the result of certain antimicrobial agents and NSAIDs.
- Damage to the kidneys can interfere with medication excretion, leading to medication accumulation and adverse effects.

NURSING ACTIONS: Aminoglycosides can injure cells in the renal tubules of the kidneys. Monitor blood creatinine and BUN, as well as peak and trough medication levels for clients taking medication that is nephrotoxic (acyclovir, aminoglycosides, cyclosporine, NSAIDs, amphotericin B).

HYPERSENSITIVITY/ALLERGIES

- Hypersensitivity and allergy are terms used interchangeably.
- Occurs when an individual develops an immune response to a medication.
- The individual has been previously exposed to the medication and has developed antibodies.
- Hypersensitivity or allergies can result in a mild reaction (itching, rash, watery eyes, sneezing, rhinosinusitis) or a severe reaction resulting in anaphylaxis.

Rapid or immediate hypersensitivity

- Rapid or immediate hypersensitivity called atopic allergy causes an overproduction of immune-globulin E antibodies, resulting in acute inflammation, histamine release, and vasoactive amines release (basophils, eosinophils, and mast cells).
- Atopic allergies can result in hay fever, rhinosinusitis and can become severe. Severe reaction can result in angioedema, anaphylaxis, or allergic asthma. This can occur by inhaling, ingesting, injection, or direct contact with an allergen.
- Mild allergies (rash, hives, rhinosinusitis) is often treated with diphenhydramine.

Angioedema

- A severe allergic reaction that affects deep tissues (blood vessels, skin, subcutaneous tissue, mucous membranes).
- Generally, angioedema involves the lips, face, oropharyngeal cavity, and neck, but can also affect the intestinal system and other parts of the body.
- NSAIDs and angiotensin-converting enzyme inhibitors (ACE inhibitors) are the most common medications that can cause angioedema and can occur within 24 hr or anytime thereafter.

NURSING ACTIONS
- Obtain a complete medical history to determine the type of medication the client is taking.
- Intervention is to apply oxygen, alleviate anxiety with reassurance, and if needed, maintain an open airway with intubation or tracheostomy if laryngeal edema, stridor, and inability to swallow develops.
- Treatment is with corticosteroids, diphenhydramine, and epinephrine depending on the severity of the client's condition. Monitor for recurrence when medications wear off.

Anaphylaxis and Allergic asthma

- Anaphylaxis is a life-threatening, immediate systemic reaction caused from an allergic response to a medication, dye, food, or insect bite or sting. Allergic asthma also has a rapid onset with similar causes.
- Manifestations of anaphylaxis can start with anxiety, weakness, generalized itching and hives that progress to erythema and angioedema of the head and neck. Crackles, wheezing, decreased breath sounds, a feeling of a lump in the throat, hoarseness, and stridor can develop into a life-threatening condition that results in respiratory failure, hypoxemia, hypotension, tachycardia, and death. Allergic asthma has similar manifestations that involve the pulmonary system that can become life-threatening.
- Allergic asthma is the production of an asthma response following exposure to an allergen.

NURSING ACTIONS
- Prevention and rapid intervention are vital to avoid a fatal outcome. If the allergy is known, the client should wear a medical alert bracelet. The client should have available at all time injectable epinephrine.
- Stop the medication immediately if that is the antigen and notify the Rapid Response team.
- Establish an airway to maintain ventilation. Administer bronchodilators if needed.

- Treat with epinephrine IM or IV to constrict blood vessels, improve cardiac contraction, and promote bronchodilation of the pulmonary system, every 5 to 15 minutes as needed.
- Administer diphenhydramine, an antihistamine, to decrease manifestations of the angioedema and urticaria.
- Continue to administer oxygen, obtain arterial blood gases, plan for the client to receive inhaled beta-adrenergic agonist or bronchodilators (albuterol, metaproterenol) every 2 to 4 hr.
- Administer corticosteroids for late recurrence of manifestations.
- Monitor hemodynamics; watch for fluid overload from too rapid of IV fluid infusions, and pulmonary status.

EXTRAPYRAMIDAL SYMPTOMS (EPSs)

- Abnormal body movements that can include involuntary fine-motor tremors, rigidity, uncontrollable restlessness, and acute dystonia (spastic movements and/or muscle rigidity affecting the head, neck, eyes, face, tongue, back, and limbs).
- Can occur within a few hours or take months to develop.

NURSING ACTIONS
- EPSs are more often associated with medications affecting the CNS (those used to treat mental health disorders).
- Most EPSs can be treated with anticholinergic medications.

Immunosuppression

Decreased or absent immune response.

NURSING ACTIONS
- Immunosuppressant medications (glucocorticoids) can mask the usual manifestations of infection (fever).
- Monitor clients taking an immunosuppressant (a glucocorticoid) for delayed wound healing and subtle manifestations of infection (sore throat).

CLIENT EDUCATION: Avoid contact with anyone who has a communicable disease.

INTERACTIONS

DRUG-DRUG INTERACTIONS

Increased therapeutic effects

NURSING ACTIONS: Some medications can be given together to potentiate their action and increase therapeutic effects.

CLIENT EDUCATION: If with asthma, use albuterol, a beta2-adrenergic agonist inhaler, 5 min prior to using triamcinolone acetonide, a glucocorticoid inhaler, to increase the absorption of triamcinolone acetonide.

Increased adverse effects

NURSING ACTIONS: Clients can take two medications that have the same adverse effect. Taking these medications together increases the risk of potentiating these findings. Diazepam and hydrocodone bitartrate 5 mg/acetaminophen 500 mg both have CNS depressant effects. When these medications are used together, clients have an increased risk for CNS depression.

Decreased therapeutic effects

NURSING ACTIONS: One medication can increase the metabolism or block the effects of a second medication and therefore decrease the blood level and effectiveness of the second medication.

> For example: Phenytoin increases hepatic medication-metabolizing enzymes that affect warfarin and thereby decreases the blood level and the effect of warfarin.

Decreased side/adverse effects

NURSING ACTIONS: One medication can be given to counteract the side/adverse effects of another medication. Ondansetron hydrochloride, an antiemetic, can be administered to counteract the side effects of nausea and vomiting for clients receiving chemotherapy.

5.1 Over-the-counter (OTC) medication interactions

INTERACTIONS

Ingredients in OTC medications or herbal supplements can interact with other OTC or prescription medications.

Inactive ingredients (dyes, alcohol, or preservatives) can cause adverse reactions.

Potential for overdose exists because of the use of several preparations (including prescription medications and herbal supplements) with similar ingredients.

NURSING IMPLICATIONS

Obtain a complete medication history and include any prescription medications, OTC medications, illicit drug use, as well as herbal and other dietary supplements.

Instruct clients to follow the manufacturer's recommendation for dosage.

INTERACTION

Interactions of certain prescription and OTC medications can interfere with therapeutic effects.

NURSING IMPLICATIONS: Advise clients to use caution and to check with the provider before using any OTC preparations (antacids, laxatives, decongestants, herbal supplements, or cough syrups). For example, antacids can interfere with the absorption of cimetidine and other medications. Advise client to follow provider and pharmacist guidelines for separating administration of antacids and other medications.

Increased blood levels, leading to toxicity

NURSING ACTIONS: One medication can decrease the metabolism of a second medication and therefore increase the blood level of the second medication. This can lead to toxicity. Fluconazole inhibits hepatic medication-metabolizing enzymes that affect aripiprazole and thereby increases blood levels of this medication.

MEDICATION-FOOD INTERACTIONS

Food can alter medication absorption and/or can contain substances that react with certain medications.

EXAMPLES

- Consuming foods with tyramine while taking monoamine oxidase inhibitors (MAOIs) can lead to hypertensive crisis. Clients taking MAOIs should be aware of foods containing tyramine (cheese and processed meats) and avoid them.
- Vitamin K can decrease the therapeutic effects of warfarin and place clients at risk for developing blood clots. Clients taking warfarin should include a consistent amount of vitamin K in their diet.
- Tetracycline can interact with a chelating agent (milk), and form an insoluble, unabsorbable compound. Instruct clients not to take tetracycline within 2 hr of consuming dairy products.
- Grapefruit juice seems to act by inhibiting medication metabolism in the small bowel, thus increasing the amount of medication available for absorption of certain oral medications. This increases either the therapeutic effects or the adverse reactions. Instruct clients to not drink grapefruit juice if they are taking such a medication. QEBP

- Food often decreases the rate of medication absorption. However, some foods increase the rate of absorption of certain medications.

CONTRAINDICATIONS AND PRECAUTIONS

- A specific medication can be contraindicated for a client based on the client's condition. For example, penicillin and its derivatives are contraindicated for a client who has an allergy to penicillin.
- Precautions should be taken for a client who is more likely to have an adverse reaction than another client.

Morphine depresses respiratory function, so it should be used with caution for clients who have asthma or impaired respiratory function.

PREGNANCY LABELING

Implementation of newer FDA pregnancy labeling guidelines began in 2015. The Pregnancy and Lactation Labeling Rule (PLLR) mandates three sections for labeling: pregnancy, lactation, and females and males of reproductive potential. You may access the full report at the FDA website.

Before administering any medication to a client who is pregnant or could be pregnant, determine whether it is safe for use during pregnancy.

Active Learning Scenario

A nurse is planning care for a client who is receiving gentamicin IV bolus twice daily. The client has a history of musculoskeletal pain and takes naproxen daily for relief. What information should the nurse include in the client's plan of care? Use the *ATI Active Learning Template: Medication* to complete this item.

THERAPEUTIC USES: Describe the use of gentamicin.

COMPLICATIONS: Describe two adverse effects.

NURSING INTERVENTIONS

- Describe two laboratory findings to monitor.
- Describe two nursing actions.

Active Learning Scenario Key

Using the ATI Active Learning Template: Medication

THERAPEUTIC USES: Gentamicin is a narrow-spectrum aminoglycoside antibiotic prescribed to treat serious infections caused by aerobic bacilli.

COMPLICATIONS
- Gentamicin can injure cells of the proximal renal tubules.
- Naproxen and other NSAIDs can cause renal insufficiency.
- The glomerular filtration rate of the kidneys decreases with advanced age, making this client at increased risk for nephrotoxicity.

NURSING INTERVENTIONS
- Laboratory Findings to Monitor
  ○ BUN
  ○ Blood creatinine
  ○ Peak and trough levels of gentamicin
  ○ Specific gravity of urine
  ○ Urinalysis
- Nursing Actions
  ○ Monitor intake and output.
  ○ Notify the provider of low urinary output.
  ○ Ensure that the client is adequately hydrated, and monitor for fluid overload.
  ○ Assess for manifestations of ototoxicity.

Ⓝ *NCLEX® Connection: Pharmacological and Parenteral Therapies, Adverse Effects/Contraindications/Side Effects Interactions*

Application Exercises

1. A nurse is providing discharge instructions for a client who has a new prescription for an antihypertensive medication. Which of the following statements should the nurse give?

   A. "You will need to limit your potassium intake while taking this medication."

   B. "You should check your blood pressure every 8 hours while taking this medication."

   C. "Your medication dosage will be increased if you develop tachycardia."

   D. "Change positions slowly when you move from sitting to standing."

2. A nurse is reviewing a client's medical record and notes that the client experienced permanent extrapyramidal effects caused by a previous medication. The nurse should recognize that the medication affected which of the following systems in the client?

   A. Cardiovascular

   B. Immune

   C. Central nervous

   D. Gastrointestinal

3. A nurse is caring for a client who is taking oral oxycodone. The client is also taking ibuprofen in three recommended doses daily. The nurse should identify that an interaction between these two medications will cause which of the following findings?

   A. A decrease in blood levels of ibuprofen, possibly leading to a need for increased doses of this medication

   B. A decrease in blood levels of oxycodone, possibly leading to a need for increased doses of this medication

   C. An increase in the expected therapeutic effect of both medications

   D. An increase in expected adverse effects for both medications

4. A nurse is preparing to administer an IM dose of penicillin to a client who has a new prescription. The client states when they took penicillin 3 years ago, they developed a rash. Which of the following actions should the nurse take?

   A. Administer the prescribed dose.

   B. Withhold the medication.

   C. Ask the provider to change the prescription to an oral form.

   D. Administer an oral antihistamine at the same time.

5. A nurse in a clinic is caring for a group of clients. The nurse should contact the provider about a potential contraindication to a medication for which of the following clients? (Select all that apply.)

   A. A client at 8 weeks of gestation who asks for an influenza immunization

   B. A client who takes prednisone and has a possible fungal infection

   C. A client who has chronic liver disease and is taking hydrocodone/acetaminophen

   D. A client who has peptic ulcer disease, takes sucralfate, and has started taking OTC aluminum hydroxide

   E. A client who has a prosthetic heart valve, takes warfarin, and reports a suspected pregnancy

1. D. **CORRECT:** When taking actions, the nurse should instruct the client that orthostatic hypotension is a common adverse effect of antihypertensive medications. The client should move slowly to a sitting or standing position and should be taught to sit or lie down if lightheadedness or dizziness occurs.

   Ⓝ *NCLEX® Connection: Pharmacological and Parenteral Therapies, Adverse Effects/Contraindications/Side Effects/Interactions*

2. C. **CORRECT:** The nurse should analyze the cues from the client's medical record and determine that extrapyramidal effects are movement disorders that can be caused by a number of central nervous system medications (typical antipsychotic medications).

   Ⓝ *NCLEX® Connection: Pharmacological and Parenteral Therapies, Adverse Effects/Contraindications/Side Effects/Interactions*

3. C. **CORRECT:** The nurse should analyze the cues from the client's history and determine these medications can work together to increase the pain-relieving effects of both medications and can result in a lower dosage requirement. Oxycodone is a narcotic analgesic, and ibuprofen is an NSAID. They work by different mechanisms, but pain can have improved relief when they are taken together.

   Ⓝ *NCLEX® Connection: Pharmacological and Parenteral Therapies, Adverse Effects/Contraindications/Side Effects/Interactions*

4. B. **CORRECT:** The nurse should take actions to address the potential contraindication to taking the penicillin. The nurse should withhold the medication and notify the provider of the client's previous reaction to penicillin so that an alternative antibiotic can be prescribed. Allergic reactions to penicillin can range from mild to severe anaphylaxis, and prior sensitization should be reported to the provider.

   Ⓝ *NCLEX® Connection: Pharmacological Therapies, Adverse Effects/Contraindications/Side Effects/Interactions*

5. B. **CORRECT:** When taking actions, the nurse should identify that glucocorticoids should not be taken by a client who has a possible fungal infection.
   C. **CORRECT:** The nurse should also identify that acetaminophen is contraindicated due to toxicity for a client who has a liver disorder and notify the provider, who can prescribe a medication that does not contain acetaminophen.
   E. **CORRECT:** Lastly, the nurse should report to the provider of a client's suspected pregnancy because warfarin can cross the placenta and result in fetal hemorrhage as well as causing congenital malformation.

   Ⓝ *NCLEX® Connection: Pharmacological and Parenteral Therapies, Adverse Effects/Contraindications/Side Effects/Interactions*

NCLEX® Connections

When reviewing the following chapters, keep in mind the relevant topics and tasks of the NCLEX outline, in particular:

Psychosocial Integrity

CHEMICAL AND OTHER DEPENDENCIES/SUBSTANCE USE DISORDER
Plan and provide care to clients experiencing substance-related withdrawal or toxicity.

Provide symptom management for clients experiencing withdrawal or toxicity.

Pharmacological and Parenteral Therapies

ADVERSE EFFECTS/CONTRAINDICATIONS/SIDE EFFECTS/ INTERACTIONS
Provide information to the client on common side effects/adverse effects/ potential interaction of medications and inform the client when to notify the primary health provider.

Monitor for anticipated interactions among the client's prescribed medications and fluids.

Identify a contraindication to the administration of a medication to the client.

EXPECTED ACTIONS/OUTCOMES: Use clinical decision-making/ critical thinking when addressing expected effects/outcomes of medications.

MEDICATION ADMINISTRATION: Educate client about medications.

Reduction of Risk Potential

LABORATORY VALUES: Notify primary health care provider about laboratory test results.

Physiological Adaptation

MEDICAL EMERGENCIES: Notify primary health care provider about unexpected client response/emergency situation.

UNIT 2   MEDICATIONS AFFECTING THE NERVOUS SYSTEM

CHAPTER 6 # Anxiety and Trauma- and Stressor-Related Disorders

Anxiety disorders include generalized anxiety disorder, panic disorder, obsessive-complusive disorder, agoraphobia, social anxiety disorder, separation anxiety disorder, and specific phobia. Trauma- and stressor-related disorders include acute stress disorder and posttraumatic stress disorder. Persistent anxiety can become disabling and can require intervention with therapy, biofeedback, relaxation techniques, and the use of medications. Psychological manifestations of anxiety disorders can include fear and apprehension. Physical manifestations can include palpitations, tachycardia, and shortness of breath.

Sedative hypnotic anxiolytics: Benzodiazepines

SELECT PROTOTYPE MEDICATION: Alprazolam

OTHER MEDICATIONS
- Diazepam
- Lorazepam
- Clonazepam
- Chlordiazepoxide
- Clorazepate
- Oxazepam

PURPOSE

EXPECTED PHARMACOLOGICAL ACTION
Benzodiazepines enhance the inhibitory effects of gamma–aminobutyric acid (GABA) in the CNS. Relief from anxiety occurs rapidly following administration. Short-term use recommended due to potential for dependence.

THERAPEUTIC USES
Generalized anxiety disorder (GAD) and panic disorder

OTHER USES FOR BENZODIAZEPINES
- Trauma- and stressor-related disorders: Acute stress disorder (ASD) and posttraumatic stress disorder (PTSD)
- Hyperarousal manifestations of dissociative disorders
- Seizure disorders
- Insomnia

- Muscle spasm
- Alcohol withdrawal (for prevention and treatment of acute manifestations)
- Induction of anesthesia
- Amnesic prior to surgery or procedures

COMPLICATIONS

CNS depression

Sedation, lightheadedness, ataxia, decreased cognitive function

CLIENT EDUCATION
- Observe for CNS depression. Notify the provider if effects occur.
- Avoid activities that require alertness (driving, operating heavy equipment/machinery).
- Avoid alcohol and other antianxiety medications due to potentiated depressant effects such as severe respiratory depression.

Anterograde amnesia

Difficulty recalling events that occur after dosing

CLIENT EDUCATION: Observe for manifestations. Notify the provider if effects occur.

6.1 Medications at a glance

Major medications used to treat anxiety disorders

Benzodiazepine sedative hypnotic anxiolytics, such as lorazepam, alprazolam, diazepam, and clonazepam

Atypical anxiolytic/nonbarbiturate anxiolytics, such as buspirone

SELECTED ANTIDEPRESSANTS
- **Selective serotonin reuptake inhibitors (SSRIs):** paroxetine, sertraline, fluoxetine, citalopram, escitalopram, and fluvoxamine
- **Serotonin-norepinephrine reuptake inhibitors (SNRIs):** venlafaxine, duloxetine, and desvenlafaxine

OTHER ANTIDEPRESSANTS: **Tricyclic antidepressants (TCAs):** amitriptyline, imipramine, clomipramine

Other medications used less frequently
- Monoamine oxidase inhibitor (MAOI): phenelzine
- Mirtazapine
- Trazodone
- Antihistamines, such as hydroxyzine pamoate and hydroxyzine hydrochloride
- Beta blockers, such as propranolol
- Alpha blockers, such as prazosin
- Centrally-acting alpha$_2$ agonist, such as clonidine
- Anticonvulsants, such as gabapentin and pregabalin
- Antipsychotics, such as quetiapine

  In addition to anxiety disorders, some of these medications are used to treat adjustment disorders, dissociative disorders, and depressive disorders.

Toxicity

Acute toxicity

Oral toxicity: drowsiness, lethargy, confusion

IV toxicity: can lead to respiratory depression, severe hypotension, or cardiac/respiratory arrest
Benzodiazepines for IV use include:
- Diazepam
- Lorazepam

NURSING ACTIONS
- For oral toxicity, gastric lavage is used, followed by the administration of activated charcoal or saline cathartics.
- Administer flumazenil for benzodiazepine toxicity to counteract sedation and reverse adverse effects.
- Monitor vital signs, maintain patent airway, and provide fluids to maintain blood pressure.
- Have resuscitation equipment available.

CLIENT EDUCATION: Watch for manifestations. Notify the provider if these occur.

Paradoxical response

Insomnia, excitation, euphoria, anxiety, rage

CLIENT EDUCATION: Watch for manifestations. Notify the provider if these occur.

Withdrawal effects

Include anxiety, insomnia, diaphoresis, tremors, lightheadedness, delirium, hypertension, muscle twitching, and seizures

CLIENT EDUCATION
- Withdrawal effects are not common with short-term use.
- If taking benzodiazepines regularly and in high doses, taper the dose over several weeks. Qᴇʙᴘ

CONTRAINDICATIONS/PRECAUTIONS

- Warnings
  - Pregnancy: Benzodiazepines contraindicated.
  - Lactation: Benzodiazepines contraindicated.
- Benzodiazepines are classified under Schedule IV of the Controlled Substances Act.
- Benzodiazepines are contraindicated in clients who have sleep apnea, respiratory depression, or glaucoma.
- Use benzodiazepines cautiously in older adult clients and those who have liver disease, kidney impairment, or a history of substance use disorder.
- Benzodiazepines are generally used short-term due to the risk for dependence. Qs

INTERACTIONS

CNS depressants (alcohol, barbiturates, opioids) can result in respiratory depression. Anticonvulsants and antihistamines can cause increased CNS depression.

CLIENT EDUCATION
- Avoid alcohol and other substances that cause CNS depression.
- Avoid activities that require alertness (driving, operating heavy equipment/machinery).

Grapefruit juice can reduce metabolism.
CLIENT EDUCATION: Avoid the use of grapefruit juice.

High-fat meals can reduce absorption.
CLIENT EDUCATION: Do not take with fatty foods.

NURSING ADMINISTRATION

- Administer the medication with meals or snacks if gastrointestinal upset occurs.
- Administer the medication at bedtime if possible due to sedation.
- Advise clients to swallow sustained-release tablets and to avoid chewing or crushing the tablets.

CLIENT EDUCATION

- Do not take benzodiazepines in larger amounts or more often than prescribed without consulting the provider.
- Dependency can develop during or after treatment. Notify the provider if indications of withdrawal occur.
- Store benzodiazepines in a secure place to prevent misuse by others.
- Swallow sustained-release tablets and do not crush or chew them.

Atypical anxiolytic/ nonbarbiturate anxiolytic

SELECT PROTOTYPE MEDICATION: Buspirone

PURPOSE

EXPECTED PHARMACOLOGICAL ACTION
- The exact antianxiety mechanism of this medication is unknown. This medication binds to serotonin and dopamine receptors. Dependency is much less likely than with other anxiolytics, and use of buspirone does not result in sedation or potentiate the effects of other CNS depressants. It carries no risk of misuse.
- The major disadvantage is that antianxiety effects develop slowly. Initial responses take a week, and at least 2 to 4 weeks for it to reach its full effects. As a result of this pharmacological action, buspirone is taken on a scheduled basis, and is not suitable for PRN usage.

THERAPEUTIC USES
- Panic disorder
- Social anxiety disorder
- Obsessive-compulsive and related disorders
- Trauma- and stressor-related disorders, PTSD
- Generalized anxiety disorder (GAD)
- Bruxism

COMPLICATIONS

Dizziness, nausea, headache, lightheadedness, agitation
CLIENT EDUCATION
- Take with food to decrease nausea.
- Avoid activities that require alertness until effects are known.
- Most adverse effects are self-limiting.

Constipation
CLIENT EDUCATION: Increase fiber and fluid.

Suicidal ideation
NURSING ACTIONS: Monitor and report manifestations of depression and thoughts of suicide.

CONTRAINDICATIONS/PRECAUTIONS

- Warnings
  - Pregnancy: Buspirone safety not established.
  - Lactation: Buspirone safety not established.
- Use buspirone cautiously in older adult clients and clients who have liver and/or renal dysfunction.
- Buspirone is contraindicated for concurrent use with MAOI antidepressants or for 14 days after MAOIs are discontinued. Hypertensive crisis can result. Qs

INTERACTIONS

Erythromycin, ketoconazole, St. John's wort, and grapefruit juice can increase the effects of buspirone.

CLIENT EDUCATION
- Avoid the use of these antimicrobial agents.
- Avoid herbal preparations containing St. John's wort, and SAMe which can increase the risk of serotonin syndrome.
- Avoid drinking grapefruit juice

NURSING ADMINISTRATION

Labeled for short-term treatment of anxiety, but has shown therapeutic benefit for as long as a year

CLIENT EDUCATION
- Take the medication with meals to prevent gastric irritation.
- Effects do not occur immediately. It can take a week to notice the first therapeutic effects and 2 to 4 weeks for the full benefit. Take on a regular basis and not PRN. QEBP
- Tolerance, dependence, or withdrawal effects are not an issue with this medication.

Selective serotonin reuptake inhibitors (SSRI antidepressants)

SELECT PROTOTYPE MEDICATION: Paroxetine

OTHER MEDICATIONS
- Sertraline
- Citalopram
- Escitalopram
- Fluoxetine
- Fluvoxamine

PURPOSE

EXPECTED PHARMACOLOGICAL ACTION
- These medications are the first line treatment for anxiety disorders.
- Paroxetine selectively inhibits serotonin reuptake, allowing more serotonin to stay at the junction of the neurons.
- It does not block uptake of dopamine or norepinephrine.
- The medication has a long effective half-life. A time frame of up to 4 weeks is necessary to produce therapeutic medication levels.

THERAPEUTIC USES

Paroxetine
- Generalized anxiety disorder (GAD)
- Panic disorder: Decreases both the frequency and intensity of panic attacks and also prevents anticipatory anxiety about attacks
- Obsessive-compulsive disorder (OCD): Reduces manifestations by increasing serotonin
- Social anxiety disorder
- Trauma- and stressor-related disorders
- Dissociative disorders
- Depressive disorders
- Adjustment disorders

Sertraline: indicated for panic disorder, OCD, social anxiety disorder, and PTSD.

Escitalopram: indicated for GAD and OCD.

Fluoxetine: used for panic disorder, OCD, and PTSD.

Fluvoxamine: used for OCD and social anxiety disorder.

COMPLICATIONS

Early adverse effects

First few days/weeks: Nausea, diaphoresis, tremor, fatigue, drowsiness

CLIENT EDUCATION
- Report adverse effects to the provider.
- Take the medication as prescribed.
- These effects should soon subside.

Later adverse effects

After 5 to 6 weeks of therapy: Insomnia, headache, and sexual dysfunction (impotence, delayed or absent orgasm, delayed or absent ejaculation, decreased sexual interest)

CLIENT EDUCATION: Report problems with sexual function (managed with dose reduction, medication holiday, changing medications).

Weight changes

Occurrence of weight loss early in therapy that can be followed by weight gain with long-term treatment

NURSING ACTIONS: Monitor the client's weight.

CLIENT EDUCATION: Follow a well-balanced diet and exercise regularly.

GI bleeding

NURSING ACTIONS: Use caution in clients who have a history of GI bleed or ulcers and in clients taking other medications that affect blood coagulation.

CLIENT EDUCATION: Report indications of bleeding (dark stool, coffee-ground emesis).

Hyponatremia

More likely in older adult clients taking diuretics

NURSING ACTIONS: Obtain baseline blood sodium level and monitor level periodically throughout treatment.

Serotonin syndrome

Agitation, confusion, disorientation, difficulty concentrating, anxiety, hallucinations, myoclonus (spastic, jerky muscle contractions), hyperreflexia, incoordination, tremors, fever, diaphoresis, hostility, delirium, seizures, tachycardia, labile blood pressure, nausea, vomiting, diarrhea, abdominal pain, coma leading to apnea, and death in severe cases

NURSING ACTIONS

- Serotonin syndrome usually begins 2 to 72 hr after initiation of treatment.
- This resolves when the medication is discontinued.
- Watch for and advise clients to withhold the medication and report any of these manifestations, which could indicate a lethal problem.

Bruxism

Grinding and clenching of teeth, usually during sleep

NURSING ACTIONS

- Report bruxism to the provider, who might switch the client to another class of medication.
- Treat bruxism with low-dose buspirone.

CLIENT EDUCATION: Use a mouth guard during sleep.

Withdrawal syndrome

Nausea, sensory disturbances, anxiety, tremor, malaise, unease

NURSING ACTIONS: Minimized by tapering the medication slowly.

CLIENT EDUCATION: Do not discontinue use abruptly but slowly taper the dose of medication before stopping, especially with long-term use.

Postural hypotension

NURSING ACTIONS: Monitor for hypotension and advise client to change positions slowly.

Suicidal ideation

NURSING ACTIONS: Monitor and report manifestations of depression and thoughts of suicide.

CONTRAINDICATIONS/PRECAUTIONS

- Warnings
  - Client should notify provider if pregnancy occurs or is planned or if breastfeeding.
  - Pregnancy: Administer paroxetine only if benefit to client outweighs risk to fetus. First-trimester use can result in cardiac malformations and use in third trimester can result in neonatal serotonin syndrome.
  - Lactation: Use paroxetine with caution—present in breast milk, can cause agitation and anorexia
- Paroxetine is contraindicated in clients taking MAOIs or a TCA.
- Clients taking paroxetine should avoid alcohol.
- Use paroxetine cautiously in clients who have liver and renal dysfunction, seizure disorders, or a history of GI bleeding. Qs

INTERACTIONS

Use of St. John's wort, SAMe, MAOI antidepressants, or TCAs can cause serotonin syndrome.
NURSING ACTIONS: Educate the client about this combination. Avoid concurrent use.

Antiplatelet medications and anticoagulants can increase risk for bleeding
NURSING ACTIONS: Monitor for bleeding. Avoid concurrent use.

NURSING ADMINISTRATION

Administer with food.

CLIENT EDUCATION

- It can take up to 4 weeks to achieve therapeutic effects.
- Taking the medication at the same time daily promotes therapeutic levels.
- Taking the medication in the morning can prevent sleep disturbances.

Herbal and Dietary Supplements

6.2 Herbal/dietary supplements and potential uses with psychiatric manifestations/disorders

SUPPLEMENT	POTENTIAL USES
St. John's wort	Depression
Kava	Insomnia, Anxiety
Lavender	Anxiety, Insomnia, Depression
SAMe	Depression
Melatonin	Insomnia
Chamomile	Anxiety

NURSING EVALUATION OF MEDICATION EFFECTIVENESS

Depending on therapeutic intent, effectiveness is evidenced by the following.

- Verbalizing feeling less anxious and more relaxed
- Description of improved mood
- Improved memory retrieval
- Maintaining regular sleep pattern
- Greater ability to participate in social and occupational interactions
- Improved ability to cope with manifestations and identified stressors

Application Exercises

1. A nurse in the emergency department is caring for a client who has benzodiazepine toxicity. Which of the following medications should the nurse expect to administer?

   A. Chlordiazepoxide

   B. Citalopram

   C. Flumazenil

   D. Fluoxetine

2. A nurse is caring for a client who has been newly prescribed alprazolam for the treatment of panic disorder. Which of the following statements by the client would prompt the nurse to notify the physician?

   A. "I will take this medication only if I need it."

   B. "I need to stop this medication if I become pregnant.'

   C. "I will take this medication in the morning with a cup of grape juice."

   D. "I have had less panic attacks during my Alcoholics Anonymous meetings since starting this medication."

3. A nurse is providing teaching to a client who has been newly prescribed buspirone for treatment of anxiety. Sort the following information by what the nurse should include vs what not to include.

   A. "This mediation has a high risk for dependency."

   B. "Expect optimal therapeutic effects within 24 hours."

   C. "Take this medication on a scheduled basis."

   D. "Take this medication on an empty stomach."

   E. "Avoid drinking grapefruit juice."

   F. "Avoid activities that require alertness when initially taking."

   G. "Herbal preparations can be combined with this medication."

   H. "Increase fiber and fluid in your diet."

4. A nurse is caring for a client who has recently initiated sertraline for treatment of posttraumatic stress disorder. Which of the following signs or symptoms reported by the client will the nurse note as concern for serotonin syndrome? (Select all that apply.)

   A. Bradycardia

   B. Fever

   C. Somnolence

   D. Hyperreflexia

   E. Anxiety

   F. Tremors

5. A nurse is teaching a client who was newly prescribed escitalopram for treatment of generalized anxiety disorder. Which of the following statements by the client indicates understanding of the teaching?

   A. "I should take the medication on an empty stomach."

   B. "I will follow a low-sodium diet while taking this medication."

   C. "I need to discontinue this medication slowly."

   D. "I should not crush this medication before swallowing."

6. Sort each Herbal/Dietary Supplement to the manifestation/disorder for which it is taken. Some may be taken for more than one manifestation/disorder: Depression; Insomnia, Anxiety, Depression; Insomnia, Anxiety; Insomnia

   A. Melatonin

   B. Kava

   C. Valerian Root

   D. SAMe

   E. St. John's Wort

Application Exercises Key

1. C. **CORRECT:** Flumazenil is administered for benzodiazepine toxicity to counteract sedation and reverse adverse effects.

2. D. **CORRECT:** Benzodiazepines, including alprazolam, are contraindicated for persons who have a history of substance abuse disorder.

3. **INCLUDE:** C, E, F, H,
   DO NOT INCLUDE: A, B, D, G

   Buspirone has a low risk for dependency and needs to be taken on a regular, scheduled, rather than PRN basis. It may take at least 2 to 4 weeks to reach its therapeutic effect. It is advised to take with food to decrease GI irritation, and to increase fiber and fluid to decrease constipation. Drinking grapefruit juice and herbal preparations, such as St. John's wort and SAMe should be avoided due to them increasing the effects of buspirone. It is also advised to avoid activities that require alertness until effects are known.

   Ⓝ *NCLEX® Connection: Pharmacological and Parenteral Therapies, Medication Administration*

4. B, D, E, F. **CORRECT:**

   Serotonin syndrome is a rare, but potentially life-threatening adverse reaction to SSRIs and usually begins 2 to 72 hr after initiation of treatment. Signs and symptoms can include: Agitation, confusion, disorientation, difficulty concentrating, anxiety, hallucinations, myoclonus (spastic, jerky muscle contractions), hyperreflexia, incoordination, tremors, fever, diaphoresis, hostility, delirium, seizures, tachycardia, labile blood pressure, nausea, vomiting, diarrhea, abdominal pain, coma leading to apnea, and death in severe cases.

5. A. The client can take this medication with food for GI distress or without food.
   B. The client is at risk for hyponatremia while taking escitalopram.
   C. **CORRECT:** When discontinuing escitalopram, the client should taper the medication slowly according to a prescribed tapered dosing schedule to reduce the risk of withdrawal syndrome.
   D. The client can crush escitalopram before swallowing.

   Ⓝ *NCLEX® Connection: Pharmacological and Parenteral Therapies, Medication Administration*

6. **DEPRESSION:** D, E
   INSOMNIA, ANXIETY, DEPRESSION: C
   INSOMNIA, ANXIETY: B
   INSOMNIA: A

Active Learning Scenario

A nurse is assessing a client 4 hr after receiving an initial dose of fluoxetine. The nurse is concerned that the client is developing serotonin syndrome. Use the *ATI Active Learning Template: System Disorder* and the *Mental Health Nursing Review Module* to complete this item.

ALTERATIONS IN HEALTH (DIAGNOSIS)

EXPECTED FINDINGS: Identify at least six.

RISK FACTORS: Describe at least one risk factor.

Active Learning Scenario Key

Using the ATI Active Learning Template: System Disorder and Mental Health Nursing Review Module

ALTERATION IN HEALTH (DIAGNOSIS): Serotonin syndrome is a potentially lethal complication that usually begins 2 to 72 hr after initiation of treatment with an SSRI. The syndrome resolves when the medication is discontinued.

EXPECTED FINDINGS
- Agitation
- Confusion
- Disorientation
- Difficulty concentrating
- Anxiety
- Hallucinations
- Hyperreflexia
- Incoordination
- Tremors
- Fever
- Diaphoresis
- Hostility
- Delirium
- Seizures
- Tachycardia
- Labile blood pressure
- Nausea
- Vomiting
- Diarrhea
- Abdominal pain
- Coma leading to apnea
- Death

RISK FACTORS
- Onset of treatment with an SSRI within the last 2 to 72 hr
- Concurrent use of an SSRI with an MAOI
- Concurrent use of an SSRI with a TCA

Ⓝ *NCLEX® Connection: Pharmacological and Parenteral Therapies, Adverse Effects/Contraindications/Side Effects/Interactions*

UNIT 2   MEDICATIONS AFFECTING THE NERVOUS SYSTEM

CHAPTER 7 *Depressive Disorders*

Depressive disorders are a widespread problem, ranking high among causes of disability. Clients who have major depression can require hospitalization with close observation and suicide precautions until antidepressant medications reach their peak effect.

Antidepressant medications are classified into five main groups: selective serotonin reuptake inhibitors (SSRIs), serotonin-norepinephrine reuptake inhibitors (SNRIs), atypical antidepressants, tricyclic antidepressants (TCAs), and monoamine oxidase inhibitors (MAOIs).

Atypical antipsychotic medications to treat depression are used as monotherapy, and adjunct therapy for depression, and bipolar depressive disorders.

Selective Serotonin Reuptake Inhibitors

SELECT PROTOTYPE MEDICATION: Fluoxetine

OTHER MEDICATIONS
- Citalopram
- Escitalopram
- Paroxetine
- Sertraline
- Fluvoxamine

SEROTONIN/NOREPINEPHRINE REUPTAKE INHIBITORS
- Venlafaxine
- Desvenlafaxine
- Duloxetine
- Levomilnacipran

PURPOSE

EXPECTED PHARMACOLOGICAL ACTION
- SSRIs selectively block reuptake of the monoamine neurotransmitter serotonin in the synaptic space, thereby intensifying the effects of serotonin.
- SSRIs are considered first-line treatment for depression. They can take 1 to 3 weeks or longer before pharmacological benefits take effect. Q EBP

THERAPEUTIC USES
- Major depression
- Obsessive-compulsive disorders
- Bulimia nervosa
- Premenstrual dysphoric disorders
- Panic disorders
- Posttraumatic stress disorder
- Social anxiety disorder
- Generalized anxiety disorder
- Bipolar disorder

COMPLICATIONS

Sexual dysfunction

Anorgasmia, impotence, decreased libido

CLIENT EDUCATION
- Remain aware of possible adverse effects and to notify the provider if intolerable.
- Utilize ways to manage sexual dysfunction, which can include lowering dosage, discontinuing medication temporarily (medication holiday), and using adjunct medications to improve sexual function (sildenafil, buspirone).
- An atypical antidepressant (bupropion) has fewer sexual dysfunction adverse effects.

CNS stimulation

Inability to sleep, agitation, anxiety

CLIENT EDUCATION
- Notify the provider. Dose might need to be lowered.
- Take dose in the morning.
- Avoid caffeinated beverages.
- Perform relaxation techniques to promote sleep.

Neuroleptic malignant syndrome

NURSING ACTIONS
- Monitor client for manifestations (fever, respiratory distress, and tachycardia).
- Monitor client for seizure activity.

Suicidal thoughts

NURSING ACTIONS
- Observe client for suicidal tendencies, (especially during early therapy).
- Children, adolescents, and adults 24 or under in age may be at higher risk.
- Monitor client for torsades de pointes.

Weight loss early in therapy

Can be followed by weight gain with long-term treatment

NURSING ACTIONS
- Monitor the client's weight.
- Encourage clients to participate in regular exercise and to follow a healthy, well-balanced diet.

Serotonin syndrome

Can begin 2 to 72 hr after starting treatment and can be lethal. Qs

MANIFESTATIONS

- Confusion, agitation, poor concentration, hostility
- Disorientation, hallucinations, delirium
- Seizures leading to status epilepticus
- Tachycardia leading to cardiovascular shock
- Labile blood pressure
- Diaphoresis
- Fever leading to hyperpyrexia
- Incoordination, hyperreflexia, tremors
- Nausea, vomiting, diarrhea, abdominal pain
- Coma leading to apnea (and death in severe cases)
- Anxiety

NURSING ACTIONS: Start symptomatic treatment (medications to create serotonin-receptor blockade and muscle rigidity, cooling blankets, anticonvulsants, artificial ventilation)

CLIENT EDUCATION: Observe for manifestations. If any occur, notify the provider, and withhold the medication.

Withdrawal syndrome

Resulting in headache, nausea, visual disturbances, anxiety, dizziness, and tremors

Manifestation begin days to weeks following the last dose and can last for 1 to 3 weeks

CLIENT EDUCATION: Taper dose gradually.

Hyponatremia

More likely in older adult clients taking diuretics

NURSING ACTIONS: Obtain baseline blood sodium and monitor level periodically throughout treatment.

Rash

CLIENT EDUCATION: A rash is treatable with an antihistamine or withdrawal of medication.

Sleepiness, faintness, lightheadedness

CLIENT EDUCATION

- These adverse effects are not common but can occur.
- Avoid driving if these adverse effects occur.

Gastrointestinal bleeding

NURSING ACTIONS: Use caution in clients who have a history of GI bleed and ulcers, and those taking other medications that affect blood coagulation.

Bruxism

NURSING ACTIONS: Changing to a different classification of antidepressants or adding a low dose of buspirone can decrease this adverse effect.

CLIENT EDUCATION

- Report to the provider.
- Use a mouth guard.

CONTRAINDICATIONS/PRECAUTIONS

- The use of SSRIs during late pregnancy can cause pulmonary hypertension of the newborn.
- Most are considered safe during lactation.

> Paroxetine increases the risk of birth defects. Therefore, other SSRIs are recommended. Safety is not established during lactation.

- SSRIs are contraindicated in clients taking MAOIs or TCAs. SSRIs need to be discontinued at least 2 weeks before initiating a MAOI.
- Use cautiously in clients who have liver and kidney dysfunction, cardiac disease, seizure disorders, diabetes, ulcers, and a history of GI bleeding.

INTERACTIONS

TCAs, MAOIs, or St. John's wort: MAOIs, TCAs, and St. John's wort increase the risk of serotonin syndrome.
NURSING ACTIONS

- MAOIs should be discontinued for 14 days prior to starting an SSRI. If already taking fluoxetine, an SSRI, the client should wait 5 weeks before starting an MAOI.
- Avoid concurrent use of TCAs and St. John's wort due to suppression of platelet aggregations that can increase the risk of gastrointestinal bleeding.

Warfarin: Fluoxetine can displace warfarin from bound protein and result in increased risk of bleeding.
NURSING ACTIONS

- Monitor PT and INR levels.
- Assess for indications of bleeding and the need for dosage adjustment.

Tricyclic antidepressants and lithium: Fluoxetine can increase the levels of tricyclic antidepressants and lithium.
NURSING ACTIONS: Avoid concurrent use.

NSAIDs and anticoagulants: Fluoxetine suppresses platelet aggregation and thus increases the risk of bleeding when used concurrently with NSAIDs and anticoagulants.
CLIENT EDUCATION: Monitor for indications of bleeding (bruising, hematuria) and notify the provider if they occur.

Serotonin-norepinephrine reuptake inhibitors

SELECT PROTOTYPE MEDICATION: Venlafaxine

OTHER MEDICATIONS

- Desvenlafaxine
- Duloxetine
- Venlafaxine
- Levomilnacipran

PURPOSE

EXPECTED PHARMACOLOGICAL ACTION
SNRIs block reuptake of norepinephrine as well as serotonin with effects similar to the SSRIs.

THERAPEUTIC USES
- Major depression
- Generalized anxiety disorder (duloxetine, venlafaxine, desvenlafaxine, levomilnacipran unlabeled use)
- Social anxiety disorder (venlafaxine, desvenlafaxine unlabeled use)
- Panic disorder (venlafaxine, desvenlafaxine unlabeled use)
- Pain due to fibromyalgia, osteoarthritis, low-back pain, diabetic neuropathy (duloxetine, unlabeled use for venlafaxine, desvenlafaxine, levomilnacipran)

COMPLICATIONS

Nausea, anorexia, weight loss

NURSING ACTIONS: Monitor weight and food intake.

Headache, insomnia, anxiety

NURSING ACTIONS: Monitor for these findings.

Hypertension, tachycardia

NURSING ACTIONS: Monitor vital signs and report changes.

Neuroleptic malignant syndrome

NURSING ACTIONS
- Monitor client for manifestations (fever, respiratory distress, and tachycardia),
- Monitor client for seizure activity

Suicidal thoughts

NURSING ACTIONS
- Observe client for suicidal tendencies, (especially during early therapy).
- Children, adolescents, and adults 24 or under in age may be at higher risk.
- Monitor client for torsades de pointes.

Dizziness, blurred vision

CLIENT EDUCATION
- Avoid driving, use of machinery until effects are known.
- Venlafaxine can cause mydriasis and can increase ocular damage if taken when the client has glaucoma.

Withdrawal syndrome

Resulting in headache, nausea, visual disturbances, anxiety, agitation,tachycardia, tinnitus, dizziness, tremors, and worsening of pretreatment manifestations

CLIENT EDUCATION: Withdraw from medication gradually.

Risk for suicide in children and adolescents

NURSING ACTIONS: Assess children/adolescents carefully for suicidal ideation, thought disorders. Qs

Sexual dysfunction

Anorgasmia, decreased libido, impotence, menstrual changes

CLIENT EDUCATION
- Report sexual dysfunction to provider.
- Utilize ways to manage sexual dysfunction, which can include lowering dosage, discontinuing medication temporarily (medication holiday), and using adjunct medications to improve sexual function (sildenafil, buspirone).
- An atypical antidepressant (bupropion) has fewer sexual dysfunction adverse effects.

Serotonin syndrome

See information under SSRIs (above)

CONTRAINDICATIONS/PRECAUTIONS

- Avoid during the third trimester due to the risk of withdrawal syndrome for the newborn.
- Avoid if client is lactating.
- Precautions are needed for older adults, and clients who have bipolar disorder, mania, seizure disorder, recent MI, hypertension, liver/kidney impairment, or interstitial lung disease.
- Taper slowly when discontinuing antidepressant medication, especially venlafaxine, which can cause severe withdrawal syndrome if stopped abruptly.

INTERACTIONS

Serotonin syndrome if given concurrently with MAOIs
NURSING ACTIONS: Stop MAOI at least 14 days before beginning a SNRI.

NSAIDs, anticoagulants increase risk for bleeding with venlafaxine
NURSING ACTIONS: Review client's medications with provider, including over-the-counter medications.

Alcohol and other medications affecting the CNS increase risk for CNS effects
CLIENT EDUCATION
- Avoid alcohol and other CNS depressants.
- Use caution when driving or using machinery. Qs

Kava, valerian increase risk for CNS depression; St. John's wort can cause serotonin syndrome.
CLIENT EDUCATION: Avoid these supplements.

Atypical antidepressants

SELECT PROTOTYPE MEDICATION: Bupropion

OTHER MEDICATIONS
- Vilazodone
- Mirtazapine
- Nefazodone
- Trazodone ER

PURPOSE

EXPECTED PHARMACOLOGICAL ACTION
Bupropion acts by inhibiting norepinephrine and dopamine uptake and is referred to as a norepinephrine-dopamine reuptake inhibitor.

THERAPEUTIC USES
- Treatment of depression, major depressive disorder, and seasonal affective disorder
- Alternative to SSRIs and SNRIs for clients unable to tolerate sexual dysfunction adverse effects of these antidepressants
- Aid for smoking cessation
- Prevention of seasonal pattern depression
- Alternative treatment choice for attention-deficit disorder

COMPLICATIONS

Headache, dry mouth, GI distress, constipation, increased heart rate, hypertension, restlessness, and insomnia

NURSING ACTIONS: Treat headache with mild analgesic.

CLIENT EDUCATION
- Observe for effects and notify the provider if intolerable.
- Sip on fluids to treat dry mouth and increase dietary fiber to prevent constipation.

Nausea, vomiting, anorexia, weight loss

NURSING ACTIONS: Monitor weight and food intake.

Seizures

NURSING ACTIONS
- Avoid administering to clients at risk for seizures (a clients who have head injuries).
- Monitor for seizures, and treat accordingly.

CONTRAINDICATIONS/PRECAUTIONS

- If client is pregnant, use only if the benefit to the client outweighs the risks to the fetus.
- Contraindicated if client is lactating, serious adverse reactions to nursing infants.
- Contraindicated in clients taking MAOIs.
- Contraindicated for clients who have seizure disorders or eating disorders.
- Use cautiously in clients who have renal/hepatic impairment.

INTERACTIONS

MAOIs (phenelzine) increase the risk of toxicity.
NURSING ACTIONS: MAOIs should be discontinued 2 weeks prior to beginning treatment with bupropion.

Other atypical antidepressants

Vilazodone

PHARMACOLOGICAL ACTION: Both blocks serotonin and works as a serotonin agonist at receptor sites (first medication to work in this way)

NURSING ACTIONS
- Contraindicated with SSRIs and SNRIs (serotonin syndrome), and other serotonin receptor agonists (buspirone and phenothiazines). Stop MAOI at least 14 days before starting vilazodone.
- Teach manifestations of serotonin syndrome to client and instruct when to notify provider.
- Monitor for suicidal ideation.
- Many adverse effects are similar to those of SSRIs and SNRIs.
- Take with food to help increase absorption.

CLIENT EDUCATION: Avoid grapefruit juice while taking vilazodone because grapefruit juice inhibits CYP3A4 metabolism resulting in an increase in the medication blood level.

Mirtazapine

PHARMACOLOGICAL ACTION: Referred to as a serotonin-norepinephrine disinhibitor. It increases the release of serotonin and norepinephrine by blocking presynaptic receptors, and thereby increases the number of neurotransmitters available for impulse transmission.

NURSING ACTIONS
- Therapeutic effects can occur sooner with less sexual dysfunction than with SSRIs.
- Mirtazapine is generally well tolerated. Clients can experience sleepiness that can be exacerbated by other CNS depressants (alcohol, benzodiazepines), weight gain, and elevated cholesterol.

CLIENT EDUCATION
- Take at bedtime; can be used as a sleep aid.
- Report sudden onset of anxiety, agitation, and panic.

Nefazodone

PHARMACOLOGICAL ACTION: Selectively inhibits the reuptake of serotonin and norepinephrine.

NURSING ACTIONS
- Rapidly absorbed within 1 hr when taken without food.
- Adverse effects are sleepiness, headache, dizziness, blurred vision, dry mouth, nausea, constipation, weight gain, and sexual dysfunction.
- Stop MAOI at least 14 days before starting nefazodone.

Trazodone ER

PHARMACOLOGICAL ACTION: Moderate selective blockade of serotonin receptors, which allows more serotonin to be available for impulse transmission.

NURSING ACTIONS
- Usually used with another antidepressant agent.
- Sedation is a potential problem; can be indicated for a client who has insomnia.
- Priapism is a potential adverse effect. Instruct clients to seek medical attention immediately if this occurs.
- Grapefruit juice inhibits CYP3A4 metabolism resulting in an increase in the medication blood level resulting in toxicity.
- Monitor client for serotonin syndrome (agitation, tachycardia, hyperthermia, or gastrointestinal symptoms).
- Monitor client for suicidal tendencies.

Tricyclic antidepressants

SELECT PROTOTYPE MEDICATION: Amitriptyline

OTHER MEDICATIONS
- Imipramine
- Doxepin
- Nortriptyline
- Amoxapine
- Trimipramine
- Desipramine
- Clomipramine

PURPOSE

EXPECTED PHARMACOLOGICAL ACTION
- These medications block reuptake of norepinephrine and serotonin in the synaptic space, thereby intensifying the effects of these neurotransmitters.
- It can take 10 to 14 days or longer before TCAs begin to work, and maximum effects might be not seen until 4 to 8 weeks.

THERAPEUTIC USES
- Depression
- Depressive episodes of bipolar disorders

OTHER USES

- Neuropathic pain
- Fibromyalgia
- Anxiety disorders
- Obsessive-compulsive disorder
- Insomnia
- Attention-deficit/hyperactivity disorder (ADHD)
- Bipolar disorder

7.1 Medications used to treat depression, but not classified as antidepressants

Atypical antipsychotics

ARIPIPRAZOLE: used as an augmenting antidepressant agent in conjunction with SSRIs.

QUETIAPINE: approved for treatment of depression and bipolar depression.

BREXPIPRAZOLE: used as adjunct agent for treatment of resistant depression such as major depressive disorder.

CARIPRAZINE: used for acute bipolar mania, mixed episodes of bipolar disorder.

LURASIDONE: used for acute depressive bipolar disorder by blocking receptors for dopamine and serotonin. Take with food for best absorption.

VORTIOXETINE: used for major depressive disorder. Is a serotonin antagonist and reuptake inhibitor. Weight gain, sedation, headache, and dizziness are adverse effects of the medication.

COMPLICATIONS

Orthostatic hypotension

Nursing Actions: Monitor blood pressure and heart rate for clients in the hospital for orthostatic changes before administration and 1 hr after. If a significant decrease in blood pressure or increase in heart rate is noted, do not administer the medication, and notify the provider.

NURSING ACTIONS
- Be aware of the effects of postural hypotension (lightheadedness, dizziness). If these occur, advise the client to sit or lie down. Orthostatic hypotension is minimized by changing positions slowly.
- Avoid dehydration, which increases the risk of hypotension.
- Monitor the client for suicidal tendencies.

Anticholinergic effects

- Dry mouth
- Blurred vision
- Photophobia
- Urinary hesitancy or retention
- Constipation
- Tachycardia

CLIENT EDUCATION
- Minimize anticholinergic effects.
  - Chewing sugarless gum
  - Sipping on water
  - Wearing sunglasses when outdoors
  - Eating foods high in fiber
  - Participating in regular exercise
  - Increasing fluid intake to at least 2 to 3 L a day from beverages and food sources
  - Voiding just before taking medication
- Notify the provider if effects persist.

Sedation

This effect usually diminishes over time.

CLIENT EDUCATION
- Avoid hazardous activities (driving) if sedation is excessive.
- Take medication at bedtime to minimize daytime sleepiness and to promote sleep.

Toxicity

Resulting in cholinergic blockade and cardiac toxicity evidenced by dysrhythmias, mental confusion, and agitation, followed by seizures, coma, and possible death

NURSING ACTIONS
- Obtain baseline ECG.
- Monitor vital signs frequently.
- Monitor manifestations of toxicity.
- Notify the provider if manifestations of toxicity occur.

Decreased seizure threshold

NURSING ACTIONS: Monitor clients who have seizure disorders.

Excessive sweating

CLIENT EDUCATION: Be aware of adverse effects. Perform frequent linen changes.

CONTRAINDICATIONS/PRECAUTIONS

- If the client is pregnant, use only if the benefit to the client outweighs the risks to the fetus.
- Caution with lactating clients; can cause sedation in infants.
- Contraindicated in clients who have seizure disorders or who have recently experienced a myocardial infarction.
- Use cautiously in clients who are elderly or who have coronary artery disease; diabetes, liver, kidney, or respiratory disorders; urinary retention or obstruction; angle-closure glaucoma; benign prostatic hyperplasia; and hyperthyroidism. Ⓖ
- Clients at an increased risk for suicide should receive a 1-week supply of medication at a time due to the lethality of a toxic dose. Ⓠs

INTERACTIONS

Concurrent use with MAOIs or St. John's wort can lead to serotonin syndrome.
NURSING ACTIONS: Avoid concurrent use.

Concurrent use with MAOIs can cause severe hypertension.
NURSING ACTIONS: Avoid concurrent use.

Antihistamines and other anticholinergic agents have additive anticholinergic effects.
NURSING ACTIONS: Avoid concurrent use.

Increased effects of epinephrine, dopamine (direct-acting sympathomimetics) occur because uptake into the nerve terminals is blocked by TCAs, and they remain for a longer amount of time in the synaptic space.
NURSING ACTIONS: Avoid concurrent use.

TCAs decrease the effects of ephedrine, amphetamine (indirect-acting sympathomimetics) because uptake into the nerve terminals is blocked, and they are unable to reach their site of action.
NURSING ACTIONS: Avoid concurrent use.

Alcohol, benzodiazepines, opioids, and antihistamines cause additive CNS depression when used concurrently.
CLIENT EDUCATION: Avoid other CNS depressants.

Monoamine oxidase inhibitors

SELECT PROTOTYPE MEDICATION: Phenelzine

OTHER MEDICATIONS
- Isocarboxazid
- Tranylcypromine
- Selegiline (transdermal MAOI)

PURPOSE

EXPECTED PHARMACOLOGICAL ACTION: These medications block MAOI enzymes in the brain, thereby increasing the amount of norepinephrine, dopamine, serotonin, and tyramine available for transmission of impulses. An increased amount of these neurotransmitters at nerve endings intensifies responses and relieves depression. However, the increase in tyramine can cause heightened blood pressure or hypertensive crisis if dietary and medication restrictions are not implemented.
- Onset of therapeutic action is not immediate, and usually takes 2 to 4 weeks.
- Less frequently used in comparison to other antidepressants due to food/drug interactions and adverse effects.

THERAPEUTIC USES
- Depression
- Bulimia nervosa
- Panic disorder
- Social anxiety disorder
- Generalized anxiety disorder
- Obsessive-compulsive disorder
- Posttraumatic stress disorder

COMPLICATIONS

CNS stimulation

Anxiety, agitation, mania, or hypomania

CLIENT EDUCATION: Observe for effects and notify the provider if they occur.

Orthostatic hypotension

NURSING ACTIONS: Monitor blood pressure and heart rate for orthostatic changes. Hold medication and notify the provider of significant changes. Instruct the client to change positions slowly.

Hypertensive crisis, severe hypertension, headache, nausea, increased heart rate, and increased blood pressure

- Hypertensive crisis resulting from intake of dietary tyramine, which could lead to a cerebral vascular accident
- Severe hypertension as a result of intensive vasoconstriction and stimulation of the heart
- Headache, nausea, and increased heart rate and blood pressure

NURSING ACTIONS
- Administer phentolamine IV (a rapid-acting alpha-adrenergic blocker) or nifedipine SL.
- Provide continuous cardiac monitoring and respiratory support as indicated.

Local rash with transdermal preparation

NURSING ACTIONS
- Choose a clean, dry area for each application.
- Apply a topical glucocorticoid on the affected area.
- Avoid hairy, irritated, calloused areas.
- Wash hands after applying new and disposing old patch.

CONTRAINDICATIONS/PRECAUTIONS

- If the client is pregnant, use only if the benefit to the client outweighs the risks to the fetus.
- Safety not established for clients who are lactating. Qs
- Contraindicated in clients taking SSRIs and in those who have pheochromocytoma, heart failure, cardiovascular and cerebral vascular disease, and severe renal insufficiency.
- Use cautiously in clients who have diabetes and seizure disorders or those taking TCAs.
- Transdermal selegiline is contraindicated for clients taking carbamazepine or oxcarbazepine, which can increase blood levels of the MAOI.

INTERACTIONS

Indirect-acting sympathomimetic medications (ephedrine, amphetamine) promote the release of norepinephrine and can lead to hypertensive crisis.
CLIENT EDUCATION: Avoid over-the-counter decongestants and cold remedies, which frequently contain medications with sympathomimetic action.

Use of tricyclic antidepressants can lead to hypertensive crisis.
NURSING ACTIONS: Use MAOIs and TCAs cautiously.

Use of SSRIs can lead to serotonin syndrome.
NURSING ACTIONS: Avoid concurrent use.

Antihypertensives have an additive hypotensive effect.
NURSING ACTIONS
- Monitor blood pressure.
- Notify the provider if there is a significant drop in blood pressure. A reduced dosage of antihypertensive can be indicated.

Use of meperidine can lead to hyperpyrexia.
NURSING ACTIONS: Use an alternative analgesic.

Tyramine-rich foods can lead to hypertensive crisis.
- Clients will most likely experience headache, nausea, increased heart rate, and increased blood pressure
- Tyramine-rich foods include aged cheese, pepperoni, salami, avocados, figs, bananas, smoked fish, protein dietary supplements, soups, soy sauce, some beers, and red wine.
- The MAOI transdermal patch does not seem to affect tyramine sensitivity at its low dose, but tyramine restriction is recommended at higher doses.

NURSING ACTIONS
- Assess for ability to follow strict adherence to dietary restrictions.
- Provide clients with written instructions regarding foods and beverages to avoid.

CLIENT EDUCATION
- Monitor for manifestations and notify the provider if they occur.
- Avoid taking any medications without approval of the provider.
- Dietary and medication restrictions should be continued for 2 weeks after the MAOI has been discontinued.

Concurrent use of vasopressors (phenylethylamine, caffeine) can result in hypertension.
CLIENT EDUCATION: Avoid foods that contain these agents (caffeinated beverages, chocolate, fava beans, ginseng).

General anesthetics
CLIENT EDUCATION: MAOIs should not be used within 10 to 14 days before or after surgery.

For all medications in this chapter

NURSING ADMINISTRATION

- Assist with medication regimen adherence by informing clients that it can take 1 to 3 weeks to begin experiencing therapeutic effects. Full therapeutic effects can take 2 to 3 months. Qpcc
- Assess for suicide risk. Antidepressant medications can increase a client's risk for suicide, particularly during initial treatment. Antidepressant-induced suicide is mainly associated with clients younger than age 25. Qs

CLIENT EDUCATION
- Take these medications as prescribed on a daily basis to establish therapeutic plasma levels.
- Continue therapy after achieving therapeutic effects. Sudden discontinuation of medication can result in relapse.
- Therapy usually continues for 6 months after resolution of manifestations and can continue for a year or longer.

SSRIs and SNRIs

Avoid use of MAOIs.

- Obtain baseline sodium levels for older adult clients taking diuretics, and monitor periodically. Ⓖ

CLIENT EDUCATION
- Take medication in the morning to minimize sleep disturbances.
- Take medications with food to minimize GI disturbances.
- These medications can cause sexual adverse effects.

Atypical antidepressants

For all atypical antidepressant medications, avoid use with MAOIs.

CLIENT EDUCATION: If taking bupropion for prevention of seasonal pattern depression, take medication beginning in the autumn each year and gradually taper dose and discontinue by spring.

TCAs

- Monitor for toxicity manifested by cardiac dysrhythmias.
- Administer at bedtime due to sedation and risk for orthostatic hypotension.
- Monitor for clients "cheeking" or hoarding TCAs due to potential lethality in toxicity.

MAOIs

Give clients a list of tyramine-rich foods so hypertensive crises can be avoided.

CLIENT EDUCATION: Avoid taking any other prescription or nonprescription medications unless approved by the provider.

NURSING EVALUATION OF MEDICATION EFFECTIVENESS

Depending on therapeutic intent, effectiveness is evidenced by the following.
- Verbalizing improvement in mood
- Increased hopefulness and will to live
- Ability to perform ADLs
- Improved sleeping and eating habits
- Increased interaction with peers

1. A nurse is providing discharge teaching to a client who has a new prescription for fluoxetine for posttraumatic stress disorder. Which of the following statements should the nurse include in the teaching?

   A. "You can have a decreased desire for intimacy while taking this medication."

   B. "You should take this medication at bedtime to help promote sleep."

   C. "You will have fewer urinary adverse effects if you urinate just before taking this medication."

   D. "You'll need to wear sunglasses when outdoors due to the light sensitivity caused by this medication."

2. A nurse is caring for a client who has been taking sertraline for the past 2 days. Which of the following assessment findings should alert the nurse to the possibility that the client is developing serotonin syndrome?

   A. Bruising

   B. Fever

   C. Tinnitus

   D. Rash

3. A nurse is caring for a client who has depression and a new prescription for venlafaxine. The nurse should monitor the client for which of the following manifestations as an adverse effect of this medication? (Select all that apply.)

   A. Mydriasis

   B. Dizziness

   C. Decreased libido

   D. Alopecia

   E. Hypotension

4. A nurse is providing teaching to a client who has a new prescription for amitriptyline for treatment of depression. Which of the following should the nurse include in the teaching? (Select all that apply.)

   A. Expect therapeutic effects in 24 to 48 hr.

   B. Discontinue the medication after a week of improved mood.

   C. Change positions slowly to minimize dizziness.

   D. Decrease dietary fiber intake to control diarrhea.

   E. Chew sugarless gum to prevent dry mouth.

5. A nurse is caring for a client who has a new prescription for phenelzine for the treatment of depression. Which of the following indicates that the client has developed an adverse effect of this medication?

   A. Orthostatic hypotension

   B. Hearing loss

   C. Gastrointestinal bleeding

   D. Weight loss

Active Learning Scenario

A nurse in an emergency department is caring for a client who is experiencing hypertensive crisis. The client reports taking tranylcypromine for the treatment of depression and that they ate pepperoni pizza shortly before the manifestations began. Use the *ATI Active Learning Template: System Disorder* and the ATI Mental Health Review Module to complete this item.

ALTERATIONS IN HEALTH (DIAGNOSIS)

EXPECTED FINDINGS: Identify at least three.

MEDICATIONS: Identify at least one medication appropriate for treatment.

CLIENT EDUCATION: Identify four dietary sources of tyramine the client should avoid.

Active Learning Scenario Key

Using the ATI Active Learning Template: System Disorder

ALTERATIONS IN HEALTH (DIAGNOSIS): Hypertensive crisis results from intensive vasoconstriction due to the intake of dietary tyramine while taking an MAOI.

EXPECTED FINDINGS
- Severe hypertension
- Headache
- Nausea
- Increased heart rate

MEDICATIONS
- Phentolamine IV, a rapid-acting alpha-adrenergic blocker
- Nitroprusside (a vasodilator)

CLIENT EDUCATION
- Aged cheeses
- Smoked or preserved fish or meats (pepperoni and salami)
- Avocados
- Figs
- Bananas
- Protein dietary supplements
- Soups containing meat extracts
- Soy sauce
- Some beers
- Red wine

ⓝ *NCLEX® Connection: Pharmacological and Parenteral Therapies, Medication Administration*

Application Exercises Key

1. A. **CORRECT:** The nurse should take actions when teaching a client who has a new prescription for fluoxetine and instruct the client that a decreased libido is a potential adverse effect of fluoxetine and other SSRIs.

   ⓝ *NCLEX® Connection: Pharmacological and Parenteral Therapies, Medication Administration*

2. B. **CORRECT:** The nurse should analyze the cues from the client's assessment and identify that fever is a manifestation of serotonin syndrome which can result from taking an SSRI such as sertraline.

   ⓝ *NCLEX® Connection: Pharmacological and Parenteral Therapies, Adverse Effects/Contraindications/Side Effects/Interactions*

3. A, B, C. **CORRECT:** The nurse should plan to generate solutions to address the client's safety from potential adverse effects of this medication. The nurse should monitor the client for potential adverse effect manifestations, which can include: mydriasis, a dilation of the pupil; dizziness, which is a common adverse effect; and sexual dysfunction, which includes decreased libido, decreased orgasm, and menstrual changes.

   ⓝ *NCLEX® Connection: Pharmacological and Parenteral Therapies, Adverse Effects/Contraindications/Side Effects/Interactions*

4. C, E. **CORRECT:** The nurse should take actions when teaching a client who has a new prescription for amitriptyline and instruct the client to change positions slowly to decrease the risk of orthostatic hypotension or a sudden drop in blood pressure.

   ⓝ *NCLEX® Connection: Pharmacological and Parenteral Therapies, Medication Administration*

5. A. **CORRECT:** The nurse should analyze cues from the client's assessment findings and determine that orthostatic hypotension can be an adverse effect. The nurse should report this finding to the provider.

   ⓝ *NCLEX® Connection: Pharmacological and Parenteral Therapies, Adverse Effects/Contraindications/Side Effects/Interactions*

UNIT 2   MEDICATIONS AFFECTING THE NERVOUS SYSTEM

CHAPTER 8 *Bipolar Disorders*

Bipolar disorders are primarily managed with mood-stabilizing medications (lithium carbonate). Other medications used to treat bipolar disorders include antiepileptic drugs (AEDs) (valproic acid, carbamazepine, lamotrigine, oxcarbazepine, and topiramate).

Atypical antipsychotics (olanzapine) can be useful in early treatment to promote sleep and to decrease anxiety and agitation. These medications also demonstrate mood-stabilizing properties. Antipsychotics approved for treatment of bipolar depression include lurasidone and quetiapine, and a combination medication that includes olanzapine and fluoxetine.

Anxiolytics (clonazepam, lorazepam) can be useful in treating acute mania and managing the psychomotor agitation often seen in mania.

Antidepressant medications (bupropion, sertraline) can be useful during the depressive phase. These are typically prescribed in combination with a mood stabilizer to prevent rebound mania.

Bipolar disorder is primarily managed with mood-stabilizing medications (lithium carbonate). Bipolar disorder also can be treated with certain antiepileptic medications.

Antiepileptic medications for bipolar disorder

- Valproic acid
- Carbamazepine
- Lamotrigine
- Oxcarbazepine
- Topiramate

OTHER MEDICATIONS USED FOR BIPOLAR DISORDER

Antipsychotics: These can be useful in early treatment to promote sleep and to decrease anxiety and agitation. These medications also demonstrate mood-stabilizing properties.

Anxiolytics: Clonazepam and lorazepam can be useful in treating acute mania and managing the psychomotor agitation often seen in mania.

Antidepressants: Medications (bupropion, venlafaxine, and selective serotonin reuptake inhibitors [SSRIs]) are useful during the depressive phase. These are typically prescribed in combination with a mood stabilizer to prevent rebound mania.

Mood stabilizer

SELECT PROTOTYPE MEDICATION: Lithium carbonate

PURPOSE

EXPECTED PHARMACOLOGICAL ACTION
- Lithium produces neurochemical changes in the brain, including serotonin receptor blockade.
- There is evidence that the use of lithium can show a decrease in neuronal atrophy and/or an increase in neuronal growth.

THERAPEUTIC USES: Lithium is used in the treatment of bipolar disorders. Lithium controls episodes of acute mania and helps prevent the return of mania or depression.

COMPLICATIONS

Effects with therapeutic lithium levels (some resolve within a few weeks)

Gastrointestinal (GI) distress

Nausea, diarrhea, abdominal pain

NURSING ACTIONS: Administer medication with meals or milk.

CLIENT EDUCATION: Effects are usually transient.

Fine hand tremors

Can interfere with purposeful motor skills and can be exacerbated by factors (stress and caffeine)

NURSING ACTIONS
- Administer beta-adrenergic blocking agents (propranolol).
- Adjust to the lowest possible dosage, give in divided doses, or use long-acting formulations.

CLIENT EDUCATION: Report an increase in tremors, which could be a manifestation of lithium toxicity.

Polyuria, mild thirst

NURSING ACTIONS: Use a potassium-sparing diuretic (spironolactone).

CLIENT EDUCATION: Maintain adequate fluid intake by consuming 1,500 to 3,000 mL fluid from beverages and food sources.

Weight gain

NURSING ACTIONS: Assist clients to follow a healthy diet and regular exercise regimen.

Renal toxicity

NURSING ACTIONS
- Monitor I&O.
- Adjust dosage and keep dose low.
- Assess baseline kidney function and monitor kidney function periodically.

Goiter and hypothyroidism

With long–term treatment

NURSING ACTIONS
- Obtain baseline T_3, T_4, and TSH levels prior to starting treatment, and then annually.
- Administer levothyroxine to manage hypothyroid effects.

CLIENT EDUCATION: Monitor for manifestations of hypothyroidism (cold, dry skin; decreased heart rate; weight gain).

Bradydysrhythmia, hypotension, and electrolyte imbalances

CLIENT EDUCATION: Maintain adequate fluid and sodium intake.

Lithium toxicity

Common adverse effects
LITHIUM LEVEL: Below 1.5 mEq/L
- **MANIFESTATIONS:** Diarrhea, nausea, vomiting, thirst, polyuria, muscle weakness, fine hand tremor, slurred speech, lethargy
- **CLIENT EDUCATION:** Manifestations at low levels often improve over time.

Early indications
LITHIUM LEVEL: 1.5 to 2.0 mEq/L
- **MANIFESTATIONS:** Ongoing gastrointestinal distress, including nausea, vomiting, and diarrhea; mental confusion; poor coordination; coarse tremors; sedation
- **NURSING ACTIONS**
  ○ Administer new dosage based on blood lithium levels and sodium levels.
  ○ If manifestations are severe, it can be necessary to promote excretion.
- **CLIENT EDUCATION:** Withhold medication and notify the provider.

Advanced indications
LITHIUM LEVEL: 2.0 to 2.5 mEq/L
- **MANIFESTATIONS:** Extreme polyuria of dilute urine, tinnitus, involuntary extremity movements, blurred vision, ataxia, seizures, severe hypotension leading to coma and possibly death from respiratory complications
- **NURSING ACTIONS:** Whole bowl irrigation may be prescribed.

8.1 Case study

Scenario introduction

Tammy is a nurse caring for Brian who has bipolar disease and is taking lithium. Brian has come to the clinic for an appointment today.

Scene 1

Tammy: Hello Brian, I am glad to see you. How have you been feeling.

Brian: I have not been feeling very good at all. I noticed my hands are really shaky. I go to the bathroom to pee a lot more often, but I have also been constipated. My vision is blurry at times

Tammy: Let me talk with Dr. Smith about these new symptoms, I expect he will want to have some tests and bloodwork done if that is okay with you.

Brian: Okay, sure. I just want to feel better.

Scene 2

Tammy: Dr. Smith has prescribed and ECG and some bloodwork.

Brian: Good. Can I lie down? I feel a bit dizzy.

Tammy: Certainly, let me help you get comfortable.

Scene 3

Tammy: Dr. Smith will be in shortly to share your results with you and determine a treatment plan for you. Let me check your blood pressure.

Brian: Okay.

Scenario conclusion

ECG indicates significant changes, blood pressure 80/45, lithium level 2.2 mEq/L. Dr. Smith discusses results with Brian and a diagnosis and treatment plan are made.

Case study questions

1. Tammy is assessing Brian who takes lithium carbonate for the treatment of bipolar disorder. The nurse should identify which of the following findings is a possible indication of toxicity to this medication? (Select all that apply.)

   A. Severe hypertension

   B. Coarse tremors

   C. Constipation

   D. Blurred vision

   E. Increased urine output

2. Tammy is reviewing laboratory findings and notes that the client's lithium level is 2.1 mEq/L. Which of the following actions should the nurse take?

   A. Perform immediate gastric lavage.

   B. Prepare the client for hemodialysis.

   C. Administer an additional dose of lithium.

   D. Request a stat repeat of the laboratory test.

Severe toxicity

LITHIUM LEVEL: Greater than 2.5 mEq/L
- MANIFESTATIONS: Oliguria, seizures, rapid progression of manifestations leading to coma and death
- NURSING ACTIONS: Hemodialysis

CONTRAINDICATIONS/PRECAUTIONS

- Warnings
  - Pregnancy: Not recommended for use during pregnancy; however, avoid during the first trimester unless the benefits to the client outweigh the risks to the fetus.
  - Lactation: Contraindicated
  - Reproductive: Recommend avoiding the use of lithium for clients who are considering pregnancy
- Use cautiously in clients who have renal dysfunction, heart disease, sodium depletion, hypovolemia, schizophrenia, or dehydration.
- Use cautiously in older adult clients and clients who have thyroid disease, seizure disorder, or diabetes.

INTERACTIONS

Diuretics

Sodium is excreted with the use of diuretics. Reduced blood sodium decreases lithium excretion, which can lead to toxicity.

NURSING ACTIONS: Monitor for indications of toxicity.

CLIENT EDUCATION
- Observe for indications of toxicity and notify the provider.
- Maintain a diet adequate in sodium, and drink replace with 1.5 to 3 L of water each day from food and beverage sources.

NSAIDs (ibuprofen and celecoxib)

Concurrent use will increase renal reabsorption of lithium, leading to toxicity.

NURSING ACTIONS
- Avoid use of NSAIDs to prevent toxic accumulation of lithium.
- Use aspirin as a mild analgesic.

Anticholinergics

Antihistamines and tricyclic antidepressants can induce urinary retention and polyuria, leading to abdominal discomfort.

CLIENT EDUCATION: Avoid medications with anticholinergic effects.

NURSING ADMINISTRATION

Monitor plasma lithium levels during treatment.
- Obtain a lithium level with each dosage change and after beginning lithium therapy every 2 to 3 days. Once a therapeutic level is obtained, monthly monitoring can occur, then every 3 to 6 months after a period of stability.
- Older adult clients often require more frequent monitoring because of increased risk for toxicity. Ⓖ
- Lithium blood levels should be obtained in the morning, 10 to 12 hr after the last dose.
- During initial treatment of a manic episode, higher levels can be required (1 to 1.5 mEq/L).
- Maintenance level range is between 0.6 to 1.2 mEq/L.
- Plasma levels at or greater than 1.5 mEq/L can result in toxicity.

Severe toxicity
- Care for clients who have advanced or severe lithium toxicity in an acute care setting, and provide supportive measures. Hemodialysis can be indicated.
- Monitor CBC, blood electrolytes, renal function tests, and thyroid function tests during lithium therapy.
- Advise clients that effects begin within 5 to 7 days.
- Advise clients to take lithium as prescribed. Lithium must be administered in 2 to 3 doses daily due to a short half-life. Taking lithium with food will help decrease GI distress.
- Encourage clients to adhere to laboratory appointments needed to monitor lithium effectiveness and adverse effects. Emphasize the high risk of toxicity due to the narrow therapeutic range.
- Provide nutritional counseling. Stress the importance of adequate fluid and sodium intake. Ｑᴘᴄᴄ
- Instruct clients to monitor for manifestations of toxicity and when to contact the provider. Clients should withhold medication and seek medical attention if experiencing diarrhea, vomiting, or excessive sweating.
- Conditions that cause dehydration (exercising in hot weather or diarrhea) put client at risk for lithium toxicity.

Mood-stabilizing antiepileptics

SELECT PROTOTYPE MEDICATIONS
- Carbamazepine
- Valproic acid
- Lamotrigine

Oxcarbazepine and topiramate are less frequently used and recommended for maintenance treatment of bipolar disorder.

PURPOSE

EXPECTED PHARMACOLOGICAL ACTION: Help treat and manage bipolar disorders by various mechanisms.

- Slowing the entrance of sodium and calcium back into the neuron and, thus, extending the time it takes for the nerve to return to its active state.
- Potentiating the inhibitory effects of gamma butyric acid (GABA).
- Inhibiting glutamic acid (glutamate), which in turn suppresses CNS excitation.

THERAPEUTIC USES: Treatment and prevention of relapse of mania and depressive episodes. Especially useful for clients who have mixed mania and rapid cycling bipolar disorders.

COMPLICATIONS

CARBAMAZEPINE

CNS effects

Cognitive function is minimally affected, but CNS effects can include nystagmus, double vision, vertigo, staggering gait, and headache.

NURSING ACTIONS
- Administer low doses initially, then gradually increase dosage.
- Administer dose at bedtime.

CLIENT EDUCATION
- Avoid driving and other activities that require alertness at the beginning of treatment. Qs
- CNS effects should subside within a few weeks.

Blood dyscrasias

Leukopenia, anemia, thrombocytopenia

NURSING ACTIONS
- Obtain baseline CBC and platelets, and perform ongoing monitoring.
- Observe for indications of thrombocytopenia, including bruising and bleeding of gums.

CLIENT EDUCATION: Monitor for and report sore throat, fatigue, or other indications of infection or bleeding.

Teratogenesis

CLIENT EDUCATION: Avoid use in pregnancy.

Hypo-osmolality

Promotes secretion of ADH, which inhibits water excretion by the kidneys and places clients who have heart failure at risk for fluid overload Ⓖ

NURSING ACTIONS
- Monitor blood levels of sodium levels.
- Monitor for edema, decrease in urine output, and hypertension.

Skin disorders

Dermatitis, rash, and Stevens–Johnson syndrome, which is potentially life-threatening

NURSING ACTIONS: Treat mild reactions with anti-inflammatory or antihistamine medications.

CLIENT EDUCATION
- Wear sunscreen.
- Notify the provider if Stevens–Johnson syndrome rash occurs and withhold medication.

Hepatotoxicity

Evidenced by anorexia, nausea, vomiting, fatigue abdominal pain, and jaundice

NURSING ACTIONS
- Assess baseline liver function, and monitor liver function regularly.
- Avoid using in children younger than 2 years old.
- Administer lowest effective dose.

CLIENT EDUCATION: Observe for indications and notify the provider if they occur.

LAMOTRIGINE

Double or blurred vision, dizziness, headache, nausea, and vomiting

NURSING ACTIONS: Caution clients about performing activities requiring concentration or visual acuity.

Serious skin rashes

Include Stevens–Johnson syndrome

NURSING ACTIONS: Instruct clients to withhold medication and notify provider if rash occurs. To minimize the risk of serious rash, the initial dosage should be low and advanced slowly.

VALPROIC ACID

GI effects

Nausea, vomiting, indigestion

CLIENT EDUCATION
- Manifestations are usually self-limiting.
- Take medication with food or switch to enteric-coated pills to reduce GI effects.

Hepatotoxicity

Anorexia, nausea, vomiting, fatigue abdominal pain, jaundice

NURSING ACTIONS
- Assess baseline liver function, and monitor liver function regularly.
- Avoid using in children younger than 2 years old.
- Administer lowest effective dose.

CLIENT EDUCATION: Observe for indications and notify the provider if they occur.

Pancreatitis

Nausea, vomiting, and abdominal pain

NURSING ACTIONS
- Monitor amylase levels.
- Discontinue medication if pancreatitis develops.

CLIENT EDUCATION: Observe for indications and notify the provider immediately if they occur.

Thrombocytopenia

NURSING ACTIONS: Monitor platelet counts.

CLIENT EDUCATION: Observe for manifestations (bruising) and notify the provider if these occur.

Teratogenesis

CLIENT EDUCATION: Avoid use in pregnancy.

Weight gain

CLIENT EDUCATION: Follow a healthy low-calorie diet, engage in regular exercise, and monitor weight.

CONTRAINDICATIONS/PRECAUTIONS

- Warnings
  - Pregnancy
    - Carbamazepine should be used only if the benefits to the client outweigh the risks to the fetus. Recommend vitamin K during the last week of pregnancy.
    - Lamotrigine may increase the risk of cleft lip/palate if used during the first trimester.
    - Valproic acid should be avoided during pregnancy; however, can use for migraines.
  - Lactation
    - Carbamazepine and valproic acid: Contraindicated.
    - Lamotrigine: Use with caution.
- Carbamazepine is contraindicated in clients who have bone marrow suppression or bleeding disorders. Clients should avoid breastfeeding. Qs
- Valproic acid is contraindicated in clients who have liver disorders. Clients of child-bearing potential should use contraception while taking valproic acid.
- Monitor plasma valproic acid and carbamazepine levels while undergoing treatment.
  - The therapeutic blood level range for carbamazepine is 4 to 12 mcg/mL.
  - The therapeutic blood level range for valproic acid is 50 to 125 mcg/mL.

INTERACTIONS

CARBAMAZEPINE

Oral contraceptives, warfarin

Concurrent use causes a decrease in the effects of these medications due to stimulation of hepatic drug-metabolizing enzymes.

NURSING ACTIONS
- Monitor for therapeutic effects of warfarin.
- Dosages can need to be adjusted.

CLIENT EDUCATION: Use a non-hormonal form of birth control.

Grapefruit juice

Inhibits metabolism, thus increasing carbamazepine levels.

CLIENT EDUCATION: Avoid intake of grapefruit juice.

Phenytoin and phenobarbital

Decrease the effects of carbamazepine by stimulating metabolism.

NURSING ACTIONS
- Monitor phenytoin and phenobarbital levels.
- Adjust dosage of medications as prescribed.

LAMOTRIGINE

Carbamazepine, phenytoin, and phenobarbital

These promote liver drug-metabolizing enzymes, thereby decreasing the effect of lamotrigine.

NURSING ACTIONS
- Monitor for therapeutic effects.
- Adjust dosage of medications as prescribed.

Valproic acid

Inhibits medication-metabolizing enzymes and thus increases the half-life of lamotrigine.

NURSING ACTIONS
- Monitor for adverse effects.
- Adjust dosage of medications as prescribed.

Oral contraceptives

Lamotrigine can reduce progestin levels; estrogen-containing contraceptives can reduce levels of lamotrigine.

CLIENT EDUCATION: Lamotrigine dosage change can be required when beginning or stopping oral contraceptive therapy.

VALPROIC ACID

Phenytoin and phenobarbital

Blood levels of these medications are increased when used concurrently with valproic acid.

NURSING ACTIONS
- Monitor phenytoin and phenobarbital levels.
- Adjust dosage of medications as prescribed.

NURSING EVALUATION OF MEDICATION EFFECTIVENESS

Depending on therapeutic intent, effectiveness is evidenced by the following.
- Relief of manifestations of acute mania (flight of ideas, excessive talking, agitation) or depression (fatigue, poor appetite, psychomotor retardation)
- Mood stability
- Ability to perform ADLs
- Improved sleeping and eating habits
- Appropriate interaction with peers

Antipsychotics

- Lurasidone, olanzapine, quetiapine, aripiprazole, risperidone, asenapine, cariprazine, and ziprasidone are useful during acute mania with or without valproate or lithium.
- Ziprasidone, olanzapine, and aripiprazole can be used long-term as prophylaxis against mood episodes.
- Lurasidone is approved for bipolar depression.

Active Learning Scenario

A nurse is reviewing discharge instructions with a client who has a new diagnosis of bipolar disorder. The client has a new prescription for lithium carbonate 600 mg PO three times a day. Use the *ATI Active Learning Template: Medication* to complete this item.

CLIENT EDUCATION: Include three adverse effects the nurse should include in the teaching.

Application Exercises

1. A nurse is caring for a client who has a new prescription for lithium carbonate. When teaching the client about ways to prevent lithium toxicity, the nurse should advise the client to do which of the following?

   A. Avoid the use of acetaminophen for headaches.

   B. Restrict intake of foods rich in sodium.

   C. Decrease fluid intake to less than 1,500 mL daily.

   D. Limit aerobic activity in hot weather.

2. A nurse is caring for a client who has a new prescription for valproic acid. The nurse should instruct the client to have which of the following blood laboratory tests completed periodically? (Select all that apply.)

   A. Thrombocyte count

   B. Glucose

   C. Sodium

   D. Liver function tests

   E. Potassium

3. A nurse is preparing a teaching plan for a client who has bipolar disorder and a new prescription for carbamazepine. Which of the following instructions should the nurse include in the teaching?

   A. "This medication can safely be taken during pregnancy."

   B. "Eliminate grapefruit juice from your diet."

   C. "You will need to have a complete blood count and carbamazepine levels drawn periodically."

   D. "Notify your provider if you develop a rash."

   E. "Avoid driving for the first few days after starting this medication."

Application Exercises Key

1. A. Instruct the client to use acetaminophen, rather than NSAIDs such as ibuprofen, for headaches because NSAIDs interact with lithium and can cause increased blood levels of lithium.
   B. Restrict intake of foods rich in sodium. Also, the client should increase, rather than decrease, sodium intake to reduce the risk for toxicity.
   C. The client should increase, rather than decrease, fluid intake to reduce the risk for toxicity.
   D. **CORRECT:** The nurse should instruct the client to avoid activities that have the potential to cause sodium/water/deletion, which can increase the risk for toxicity.

   Ⓝ NCLEX® Connection: Pharmacological and Parenteral Therapies, Adverse Effects/Contraindications/Side Effects/Interactions

2. A, D. **CORRECT:** The nurse should instruct the client to have thrombocyte counts periodically. Treatment with valproic acid can result in thrombocytopenia. Also, liver function studies should be monitored periodically because it can cause hepatoxicity.
   B, C, E. Blood glucose, potassium, and glucose levels are not known to have an effect on the client.

   Ⓝ NCLEX® Connection: Pharmacological and Parenteral Therapies, Expected Actions/Outcomes

3. A. Carbamazepine is a Pregnancy Category Risk D medication. The client should be instructed to avoid pregnancy while taking carbamazepine.
   B. **CORRECT:** When taking actions and teaching a client about a new prescription for carbamazepine, the nurse should instruct the client about how grapefruit juice affects carbamazepine metabolism and that it should be avoided.
   C. **CORRECT:** The nurse should instruct the client that carbamazepine blood levels and CBCs will be monitored during therapy. The client is at risk for bone marrow depression while taking carbamazepine and the nurse should instruct the client to notify the provider for a sore throat or other manifestations of an infection.
   D. **CORRECT:** Carbamazepine can cause Stevens-Johnson syndrome, which can be fatal. The nurse should teach the client to notify the provider promptly if a rash occurs.
   E. **CORRECT:** CNS effects (drowsiness or dizziness) can occur early in treatment with carbamazepine, and the client should be instructed to avoid activities requiring alertness until these effects subside.

   Ⓝ NCLEX® Connection: Pharmacological and Parenteral Therapies, Medication Administration

Case Study Exercises Key

1. B, D, E. **CORRECT:** When analyzing cues, the nurse should identify coarse tremors, blurred vision, increased urinary output can be indications of lithium toxicity.

   Ⓝ NCLEX® Connection: Pharmacological and Parenteral Therapies, Adverse Effects/Contraindications/Side Effects/Interactions

2. A. **CORRECT:** When taking actions to address the client's lithium level, the nurse should prepare the client for gastric lavage due to severe toxicity , as evidenced by a plasma lithium level of 2.1 mEq/L. This action will lower the client's lithium level.

   Ⓝ NCLEX® Connection: Pharmacological and Parenteral Therapies, Adverse Effects/Contraindications/Side Effects/Interactions

Active Learning Scenario Key

Using the ATI Active Learning Template: Medication

CLIENT EDUCATION
- Gastrointestinal distress: nausea, diarrhea, abdominal pain
- Fine hand tremors
- Polyuria
- Mild thirst
- Weight gain
- Renal toxicity
- Goiter and hypothyroidism
- Dysrhythmias
- Hypotension
- Electrolyte imbalances

Ⓝ NCLEX® Connection: Pharmacological and Parenteral Therapies, Medication Administration

CHAPTER 9 *Psychotic Disorders*

Schizophrenia spectrum disorders are the primary reason for the administration of antipsychotic medications. The clinical course of schizophrenia usually involves acute exacerbations with intervals of semi-remission.

Medications are used to treat positive manifestations related to behavior, thought, perception, and speech (agitation, bizarre behavior, delusions, hallucinations, flight of ideas, illogical thinking patterns, tangential speech patterns) and negative manifestations (social withdrawal, lack of emotion, lack of energy [anergia], flattened affect, decreased motivation, decreased pleasure in activities).

The goals of psychopharmacological treatment for schizophrenia spectrum and other psychotic disorders include suppressing acute episodes, preventing acute recurrence, and promoting the highest possible level of functioning. Qᴇʙᴘ

Antipsychotics: First-generation (conventional)

These medications control mainly positive manifestations of psychotic disorders (hallucinations, delusions, bizarre behavior).

SELECT PROTOTYPE MEDICATION:
Chlorpromazine: low potency

OTHER MEDICATIONS
- Haloperidol: high potency
- Fluphenazine: high potency
- Thiothixene: medium potency
- Perphenazine: medium potency
- Loxapine: medium potency
- Trifluoperazine: high potency

PURPOSE

EXPECTED PHARMACOLOGICAL ACTION
- Block dopamine (D_2), acetylcholine, histamine, and norepinephrine receptors in the brain and periphery.
- Inhibition of psychotic manifestations, believed to be a result of D_2 blockade in the brain.

THERAPEUTIC USES
- Acute and chronic psychotic disorders
- Schizophrenia spectrum disorders
- Bipolar disorders (primarily the manic phase)
- Tourette syndrome
- Agitation
- Prevention of nausea/vomiting through blocking of dopamine in the chemoreceptor trigger zone of the medulla

COMPLICATIONS

EXTRAPYRAMIDAL SIDE EFFECTS (EPSs)

Acute dystonia

The client experiences severe spasms of tongue, neck, face, or back. If the laryngeal muscles are affected, respiration can decrease. This is a crisis situation, which requires rapid treatment. Qs

NURSING ACTIONS
- Monitor for acute dystonia between a few hours to 5 days after administration of the first dose.
- Treat with anticholinergic agents, such as benztropine IM or IV. Expect improvement within 5 min (IV dosing) to 20 min (IM dosing).

Parkinsonism

Findings include bradykinesia, rigidity, shuffling gait, drooling, and tremors.

NURSING ACTIONS
- Observe for parkinsonism within 1 month of initiation of therapy.
- Treat with benztropine, diphenhydramine, or amantadine. Discontinue these medications to determine if they are still needed. If manifestations return, administer atypical antipsychotic as prescribed.

Akathisia

The client is unable to stand still or sit, and is continually pacing and agitated.

NURSING ACTIONS
- Observe for akathisia within 2 months of the initiation of treatment.
- Manage effects with beta blocker, benzodiazepine, or anticholinergic medication.

Tardive dyskinesia (TD)

- Manifestations include involuntary movements of the tongue and face, such as lip-smacking, which cause speech and/or eating disturbances.
- Can also include involuntary movements of arms, legs, or trunk.

NURSING ACTIONS
- TD is a late EPS that can occur months to years after the start of therapy and can improve following medication change or can be permanent.
- Administer the lowest dosage possible to control manifestations.
- Evaluate the client after 12 months of therapy and then every 3 months. If indications of TD appear, dosage should be lowered, or the client should be switched to an atypical agent.
- Valbenazine can be prescribed to treat TD for adult clients.

OTHER ADVERSE EFFECTS

Neuroleptic malignant syndrome

! Life-threatening medical emergency.

Manifestations include sudden high-grade fever, blood pressure fluctuations, dysrhythmias, muscle rigidity, diaphoresis, tachycardia, and change in level of consciousness developing into coma. Qs

NURSING ACTIONS
- Stop antipsychotic medication.
- Monitor vital signs.
- Apply cooling blankets.
- Administer antipyretics (aspirin, acetaminophen).
- Increase fluid intake.
- Administer diazepam to control anxiety.
- Administer dantrolene and bromocriptine to induce muscle relaxation.
- Administer medication as prescribed to treat dysrhythmias.
- Assist with immediate transfer to intensive care.
- Wait 2 weeks before resuming therapy. Consider switching to an atypical agent.

Anticholinergic effects

- Dry mouth
- Blurred vision
- Photophobia
- Urinary hesitancy/retention
- Constipation
- Tachycardia

NURSING ACTIONS: Suggest strategies to decrease anticholinergic effects.
- Chew sugarless gum
- Sip water
- Avoid hazardous activities
- Wear sunglasses when outdoors

- Eat foods high in fiber
- Participate in regular exercise
- Maintain fluid intake of 2 to 3 L water daily from food and beverage sources
- Void prior to taking medication

Neuroendocrine effects

Effects include gynecomastia (breast enlargement), galactorrhea, and menstrual irregularities.

CLIENT EDUCATION: Observe for manifestations and notify the provider if these occur.

Seizures

The greatest risk for developing seizures is existing seizure disorders.

NURSING ACTIONS: An increase in antiseizure medication can be necessary.

CLIENT EDUCATION: Report seizure activity to the provider.

Skin effects

Effects include photosensitivity resulting in severe sunburn, and contact dermatitis from handling medications.

CLIENT EDUCATION
- Avoid excessive exposure to sunlight, use sunscreen, and wear protective clothing.
- Avoid direct contact with medication.

Orthostatic hypotension

NURSING ACTIONS: In the hospital setting, monitor blood pressure and heart rate for orthostatic changes. If a significant decrease in blood pressure or increase in heart rate is noted, do not administer the medication, and notify the provider.

CLIENT EDUCATION
- Tolerance to orthostatic hypotension should develop in 2 to 3 months.
- If findings of postural hypotension (lightheadedness, dizziness) occur, sit or lie down. Orthostatic hypotension can be minimized by getting up or changing positions slowly.

Sedation

CLIENT EDUCATION
- Effects should diminish within a few weeks.
- Take this medication at bedtime to avoid daytime sleepiness.
- Do not drive until sedation has subsided. Qs

Sexual dysfunction

Altered libido, difficulty achieving orgasm, erectile and ejaculatory dysfunction.

CLIENT EDUCATION
- Report these effects to the provider.
- A lower dosage or changing to a high-potency agent can minimize these effects.

Agranulocytosis

NURSING ACTIONS: If indications of infection appear, obtain a baseline WBC. Medication should be discontinued if laboratory tests indicate the presence of infection.

CLIENT EDUCATION: Observe for indications of infection (fever, sore throat), and notify the provider if these occur.

Severe dysrhythmias

NURSING ACTIONS
- Obtain baseline ECG and potassium level prior to treatment and periodically throughout the treatment period.
- Avoid concurrent use with other medications that prolong QT interval.

Liver impairment

NURSING ACTIONS: Assess baseline liver function, and monitor liver function regularly.

CLIENT EDUCATION: Observe for indications (anorexia, nausea, vomiting, fatigue, abdominal pain, jaundice) and notify the provider.

CONTRAINDICATIONS/PRECAUTIONS

- Contraindicated in clients in a coma, and clients who have Parkinson's disease, liver damage, prolactin-dependent cancer of the breast, and severe hypotension.
- Contraindicated in older clients who have dementia. Ⓖ
- Use cautiously in clients who have glaucoma, paralytic ileus, prostate enlargement, heart disorders, liver or kidney disease, and seizure disorders.

INTERACTIONS

Anticholinergic agents

Concurrent use with other anticholinergic medications will increase anticholinergic effects.

CLIENT EDUCATION: Avoid over-the-counter medications that contain anticholinergic agents, such as sleep aids and antihistamines.

CNS depressants

Alcohol, opioids, and antihistamines have additive CNS depressant effects.

CLIENT EDUCATION
- Avoid alcohol and other medications that cause CNS depression.
- Avoid hazardous activities, such as driving.

Levodopa

By activating dopamine receptors, levodopa counteracts the effects of antipsychotic agents.

NURSING ACTIONS: Avoid concurrent use of levodopa and other direct dopamine receptor agonists.

NURSING ADMINISTRATION

- These medications are reserved for clients who are:
  - Using them successfully and can tolerate the adverse effects.
  - Violent or particularly aggressive.
- Use the Abnormal Involuntary Movement Scale (AIMS) to screen for the presence of EPS. Ⓠᴇʙᴾ
- Assess clients to differentiate between EPSs and worsening of psychotic disorder.
- Administer anticholinergics, beta blockers, and benzodiazepines to control early EPSs. If adverse effects are intolerable, the client can be switched to a low-potency or an atypical antipsychotic agent.
- Consider depot preparations administered IM once every 2 to 4 weeks for clients who have difficulty maintaining medication regimen. Inform the client that lower doses can be used with depot preparations, which will decrease the risk of adverse effects and the development of tardive dyskinesia. Ⓠᴾᶜᶜ
- Start oral administration with twice-a-day dosing, then switch to daily dosing at bedtime to decrease daytime drowsiness and promote sleep.

CLIENT EDUCATION
- Antipsychotic medications do not cause addiction.
- Some therapeutic effects can be noticeable within a few days, but significant improvement can take 2 to 4 weeks, and possibly several months for full effects.

Antipsychotics: Second- and third-generation (atypical)

These agents are often chosen as first-line treatment for schizophrenia. They are medications of choice for clients receiving initial treatment and for treating breakthrough episodes in clients on conventional medication therapy, because they are more effective with fewer adverse effects.

SELECT PROTOTYPE MEDICATION:
Risperidone (second-generation antipsychotic)

OTHER MEDICATIONS (9.1)
- Olanzapine
- Quetiapine
- Ziprasidone
- Clozapine
- Asenapine
- Lurasidone
- Paliperidone
- Iloperidone
- Aripiprazole, brexpiprazole, cariprazine (third-generation)

PURPOSE

EXPECTED PHARMACOLOGICAL ACTION:
Second–generation antipsychotic agents work mainly by blocking serotonin, and to a lesser degree, dopamine receptors. These medications also block receptors for norepinephrine, histamine, and acetylcholine. The third–generation medications work by stabilizing the dopamine system as both an agonist and antagonist.

THERAPEUTIC USES

- Schizophrenia spectrum disorders (negative and positive manifestations)
- Psychotic episodes induced by levodopa therapy
- Bipolar disorders
- Impulse control disorders

ADVANTAGES

- Relief of both the positive and negative manifestations of the disease
- Decrease in affective manifestations (depression, anxiety) and suicidal behaviors
- Improvement of neurocognitive deficits, such as poor memory
- Fewer or no EPSs, including TD, because of less dopamine blockade
- Fewer anticholinergic adverse effects because most atypical antipsychotics, with the exception of clozapine, cause little or no blockade of cholinergic receptors
- Less relapse

FORMULATIONS

- Tablets
- Quick–dissolving tablets
- Oral solution
- IM depot preparations

9.1 Other atypical antipsychotic agents

Olanzapine

FORMULATIONS: Tablets, orally disintegrating tablets, short-acting injectable, extended-release injection

COMPLICATIONS

- Low risk of EPS
- High risk for diabetes mellitus, weight gain, and dyslipidemia
- Other adverse effects: sedation, orthostatic hypotension, anticholinergic effects

Quetiapine

FORMULATIONS: Tablets, extended-release tablets

COMPLICATIONS

- Low risk of EPS
- Moderate risk for diabetes mellitus, weight gain, and dyslipidemia
- Other effects: cataracts, sedation, orthostatic hypotension, anticholinergic effects
- Clients should have screening eye exam and then every 6 months.

Ziprasidone

Affects both dopamine and serotonin; can be used for clients who have concurrent depression

FORMULATIONS: Capsules, short-acting injectable

COMPLICATIONS

- Low risk of EPS, diabetes mellitus, weight gain, dyslipidemia
- Other effects: sedation, orthostatic hypotension, anticholinergic effects, rash
- ECG changes and QT prolongation can lead to torsades de pointes.

Clozapine

The first atypical antipsychotic developed. Despite its effectiveness for schizophrenia spectrum disorders, it is no longer considered a first-line medication because of its serious adverse effects.

FORMULATIONS: Tablets, orally disintegrating tablets

COMPLICATIONS

- Low risk of EPS
- High risk of weight gain, diabetes mellitus, dyslipidemia
- Agranulocytosis can occur. Obtain baseline WBC and monitor weekly, bi-weekly, to monthly per protocol.
- Monitor for indications of infection (fever, sore throat, lesions in mouth), and notify the provider if manifestations occur.
- Other adverse effects: sedation, hypersalivation, orthostatic hypotension, and anticholinergic effects
- Pregnancy Risk Category B

Asenapine

FORMULATION: Sublingual tablets

COMPLICATIONS

- Drowsiness, prolonged QT interval, EPS (higher doses)
- Causes temporary numbing of the mouth
- Low risk of diabetes mellitus, weight gain, dyslipidemia, anticholinergic effects

Lurasidone

FORMULATION: Tablets

COMPLICATIONS

- Common adverse effects: sedation, akathisia, parkinsonism, agitation, anxiety
- Low risk for diabetes mellitus, weight gain, dyslipidemia
- Does not cause anticholinergic effects
- Pregnancy Risk Category B

Paliperidone

FORMULATIONS: Extended-release tablets, extended-release injections

COMPLICATIONS

- High risk for diabetes mellitus, weight gain, dyslipidemia
- Other adverse effects: sedation, prolonged QT interval, orthostatic hypotension, anticholinergic effects, mild EPS

Iloperidone

FORMULATION: Tablets

COMPLICATIONS

- Common adverse effects: dry mouth, sedation, fatigue, nasal congestion
- Significant risk for weight gain, prolonged QT interval, orthostatic hypotension
- Advise clients to follow titration schedule during initial therapy to minimize hypotension.
- Low risk for diabetes mellitus, dyslipidemia, EPS

Aripiprazole (third-generation antipsychotic)

FORMULATIONS: Tablets, orally disintegrating tablets, oral solution, sustained-release injectable

COMPLICATIONS

Common adverse effects: sedation, headache, anxiety, insomnia, gastrointestinal distress

COMPLICATIONS

Diabetes mellitus

New onset of diabetes mellitus or loss of glucose control in clients who have diabetes (referred to as metabolic syndrome and also includes weight gain and dyslipidemia)

NURSING ACTIONS: Obtain baseline fasting blood glucose and monitor throughout treatment.

CLIENT EDUCATION: Report indications (increased thirst, urination, and appetite).

Weight gain

CLIENT EDUCATION: Follow a healthy low-calorie diet, engage in regular exercise, and monitor weight gain.

Hypercholesterolemia

With increased risk for hypertension and other cardiovascular disease

NURSING ACTIONS: Monitor cholesterol and triglycerides.

Orthostatic hypotension

NURSING ACTIONS: Monitor blood pressure and heart rate for orthostatic changes.

CLIENT EDUCATION: Change positions slowly.

Anticholinergic effects

Include urinary hesitancy or retention, and dry mouth

NURSING ACTIONS: Monitor for effects and report occurrence to the provider.

CLIENT EDUCATION: Practice measures to relieve dry mouth, such as sipping fluids.

Agitation, dizziness, sedation, sleep disruption

NURSING ACTIONS
- Monitor for effects and report to the provider if they occur.
- Administer alternative medication if prescribed.

Mild EPSs, such as tremor or akathisia

NURSING ACTIONS
- Monitor for and teach clients to recognize EPSs.
- Use AIMS assessment to screen for EPSs.

Elevated prolactin levels

NURSING ACTIONS: Obtain prolactin level if indicated.

CLIENT EDUCATION: Observe for galactorrhea, gynecomastia, and amenorrhea. Notify the provider if these occur.

Sexual dysfunction (anorgasmia, impotence, low libido)

CLIENT EDUCATION
- Observe for possible sexual adverse effects and notify the provider if they are intolerable.
- Talk to the provider about ways to manage sexual dysfunction, which can include using adjunct medications to improve sexual function (such as sildenafil).

CONTRAINDICATIONS/PRECAUTIONS

- Warnings
  - Pregnancy
    - Clozapine, lurasidone: Use only if the benefit to the client outweighs the risks to the fetus.
    - Risperidone: Safety not established.
  - Lactation
    - Clozapine, risperidone: Contraindicated.
    - Lurasidone: Considered only if the benefit justifies the risk to the newborn.
- Contraindicated for clients who have dementia. All atypical antipsychotic medications can cause death related to cerebrovascular accident or infection. Ⓖ
- Clients should avoid use of alcohol.
- Use cautiously in clients who have cardiovascular or cerebrovascular disease, seizures, or diabetes mellitus. Obtain a fasting blood glucose for clients who have diabetes mellitus and monitor blood glucose carefully.

INTERACTIONS

Immunosuppressive medications

Immunosuppressants, such as anticancer medications, can further suppress immune function in clients taking clozapine.

NURSING ACTIONS: Avoid use in clients taking clozapine.

Alcohol, opioids, and antihistamines

Have additive CNS depressant effects.

CLIENT EDUCATION
- Avoid alcohol and medications that cause CNS depression.
- Avoid hazardous activities, such as driving.

Antipsychotic agents

By activating dopamine receptors, levodopa counteracts the effects of antipsychotic agents.

NURSING ACTIONS: Avoid concurrent use of levodopa and other direct dopamine receptor agonists.

Tricyclic antidepressants, amiodarone, and clarithromycin

Prolong QT interval and thus increase the risk of cardiac dysrhythmias in clients taking ziprasidone.

NURSING ACTIONS: Atypical antipsychotics that prolong the QT interval should not be used concurrently with other medications that have the same effect.

Barbiturates and phenytoin

Stimulate hepatic medication–metabolizing enzymes and thereby decrease drug levels of aripiprazole, quetiapine, and ziprasidone.

NURSING ACTIONS: Monitor medication effectiveness.

Fluconazole

Inhibits hepatic medication–metabolizing enzymes and thereby increases levels of aripiprazole, quetiapine, and ziprasidone

NURSING ACTIONS: Monitor for adverse effects or toxicity.

NURSING ADMINISTRATION

- Administer by PO or IM route. Therapeutic effect occurs up to several weeks following the first depot injection. Clients often require oral preparations until effectiveness is achieved. Advise clients that low doses of medication are given initially and are then gradually increased.
  - Risperidone is also available as a depot injection administered IM once every 2 weeks, and the long-acting injectable of paliperidone is administered every 28 days.
  - Aripiprazole also has a long-acting injectable, which is administered monthly. Use for clients who have difficulty adhering to medication regimen. Qpcc
- Use oral disintegrating tablets for clients who might attempt to "cheek" (or pocket) tablets or have difficulty swallowing them.
- Administer lurasidone and ziprasidone with food (at least 350 calories) to increase absorption.
- The cost of antipsychotic medications can be a factor for some clients. Assess the need for case management intervention. Qtc
- After administering olanzapine extended-release injection, monitor the client for at least 3 hr for adverse effects.

CLIENT EDUCATION: While taking asenapine, avoid eating or drinking for 10 min after each dose.

NURSING EVALUATION OF MEDICATION EFFECTIVENESS

- Depending on therapeutic intent, effectiveness can be evidenced by improvement in the following.
- Positive and negative manifestations (prevention of acute psychotic manifestations, absence of hallucinations, delusions, anxiety, and hostility)
- Ability to perform ADLs
- Ability to interact socially with peers
- Sleeping and eating habits

Application Exercises Key

1. B. **CORRECT:** The greatest risk to the client is from respiratory insufficiency if the laryngeal muscles are affected. Neck spasms are an indication of acute dystonia which is an emergent crisis. Therefore, this is the priority finding for the nurse to report to the provider.
   A, C, D. Shuffling gait, hand tremors and smacking of the lips could indicate parkinsonism or tardive dyskinesia which are adverse effects of haloperidol. However, these are not priority findings.

   Ⓝ *NCLEX® Connection: Pharmacological and Parenteral Therapies, Adverse Effects/Contraindications/Side Effects/Interactions*

2. B. **CORRECT:** When taking action, the nurse should instruct the client who is taking fluphenazine and is experiencing anticholinergic effects to chew sugarless gum. This instruction would provide moisture to the client's mouth and decrease the severity of dry mouth which is an anticholinergic adverse effect.
   A, C, D. Using cooling measures, taking an antacid, and taking the medication in the morning are actions that would not decrease the other anticholinergic adverse effects such as blurry vision, photophobia, tachycardia, constipation, and urinary hesitancy/retention.

   Ⓝ *NCLEX® Connection: Pharmacological Therapies, Medication Administration*

3. A. Risperidone can cause weight gain and the nurse should instruct the client to maintain a lower-calorie diet.
   B. **CORRECT:** When taking action, the nurse should instruct the client who has a new prescription for risperidone that they may experience difficulty sleeping, agitation, or irritability.
   C. Seizures are not an adverse effect of risperidone.
   D. It can cause sexual dysfunction such as decreased libido and impotence.

   Ⓝ *NCLEX® Connection: Pharmacological and Parenteral Therapies, Medication Administration*

4. A. Clozapine increases the client's risk of developing diabetes mellitus and weight. Therefore, it is not appropriate to increase carbohydrate intake.
   B. Clozapine has a low risk of EPS such as hand tremors.
   C. Asenapine, rather than clozapine, causes temporary numbing of the mouth.
   D. **CORRECT:** When taking action, the nurse should instruct the client who has a new prescription for clozapine to obtain weekly monitoring of their WBC count due to the risk for fatal agranulocytosis.

   Ⓝ *NCLEX® Connection: Pharmacological and Parenteral Therapies, Adverse Effects/Contraindications/Side Effects/Interactions*

5. **HIGH:** A, B, C; **LOW:** D
   When evaluating outcomes, the nurse should identify that a client who is taking prescribed quetiapine will have an increased risk for drowsiness, dyslipidemia, and weight. Quetiapine has a decreased risk of developing EPS.

   Ⓝ *NCLEX® Connection: Pharmacological and Parenteral Therapies, Expected Actions/Outcomes*

Active Learning Scenario

A nurse caring for a client who has neuroleptic malignant syndrome. Use the ATI Active Learning Template: System Disorder to complete this item to include the following sections.

DESCRIPTION OF DISORDER/DISEASE PROCESS

ASSESSMENT: Identify at least four expected objective findings.

MEDICATIONS: Identify two medications appropriate for treatment and their purpose.

NURSING CARE: Identify at least three appropriate interventions.

Active Learning Scenario Key

Using the ATI Active Learning Template: System Disorders
DESCRIPTION OF DISORDER/DISEASE PROCESS:
Neuroleptic malignant syndrome is a potential adverse effect of antipsychotic medications, although incidence with second-generation medications is rare.

ASSESSMENT
- Sudden high fever
- Blood pressure fluctuations
- Diaphoresis
- Dysrhythmias
- Muscle rigidity
- Changes in level of consciousness
- Coma

MEDICATIONS
- Aspirin: antipyretic
- Acetaminophen: antipyretic
- Dantrolene: induces muscle relaxation
- Bromocriptine: induces muscle relaxation

NURSING CARE
- Notify the provider immediately.
- Withhold the conventional antipsychotic medication.
- Monitor vital signs.
- Apply cooling blankets.
- Increase fluid intake.
- Discuss with the provider the need to wait 2 weeks before resuming therapy.
- Discuss with the provider the possible need to switch to an atypical agent.

Ⓝ *NCLEX® Connection: Pharmacological and Parenteral Therapies, Expected Actions/Outcomes*

CHAPTER 10

Medications for Children and Adolescents Who Have Mental Health Issues

Medications are available to manage various behavioral disorders in children and adolescents, including attention deficit-hyperactivity disorder, conduct disorder, intermittent explosive disorder, and autism spectrum disorders. Parents/guardians should understand that pharmacological management is most effective when accompanied by techniques to modify behavior.

Central nervous system stimulants

10.1 Select prototypes and other medications

	SHORT-ACTING	INTERMEDIATE-ACTING	LONG-ACTING
Methylphenidate	3 to 5 hr	6 to 8 hr	8 to 16 hr
Dexmethylphenidate	4 to 5 hr	n/a	8 to 12 hr
Dextroamphetamine	4 to 6 hr	n/a	6 to 10 hr
Amphetamine mixture	4 to 6 hr	n/a	10 to 12 hr
Lisdexamfetamine dimesylate	n/a	n/a	10 to 12 hr

PURPOSE

EXPECTED PHARMACOLOGICAL ACTION: Raise the levels of norepinephrine and dopamine in the central nervous system (CNS)

THERAPEUTIC USES
- ADHD
- Narcolepsy
- Obesity

COMPLICATIONS

CNS stimulation

Insomnia, restlessness

NURSING ACTIONS: Administer the last dose before 4 p.m. Q EBP

CLIENT EDUCATION: Observe for effects and notify the provider if they occur.

Decreased appetite, weight loss, growth suppression

NURSING ACTIONS
- Monitor the client's height and weight and compare to baseline height and weight.
- Administer medication immediately during or after meals.
- Promote good nutrition in children.
- Encourage children to eat at regular meal times and avoid unhealthy foods for snacks.
- Consult with prescriber about possible "drug holidays."

Cardiovascular effects

Dysrhythmias, chest pain, high blood pressure

NURSING ACTIONS
- These medications can increase the risk of sudden death in clients who have heart abnormalities.
- Monitor vital signs and ECG.

CLIENT EDUCATION: Observe for effects (shortness of breath, chest pain, dizziness) and notify the provider if they occur.

Development of psychotic manifestations

Hallucinations and paranoia

CLIENT EDUCATION: Report manifestations immediately and discontinue the medication if they occur.

Physical tolerance and withdrawal reaction

Headache, nausea, vomiting, and muscle weakness, depression

CLIENT EDUCATION: Do not stop taking medication suddenly. Doing so can lead to depression and severe fatigue. Taper medication gradually.

Hypersensitivity skin reaction to transdermal methylphenidate

Hives, papules

NURSING ACTIONS: Remove the patch and notify the provider.

Toxicity

Dizziness, palpitations, hypertension, hallucinations, seizures

NURSING ACTIONS
- Treat hallucinations with chlorpromazine.
- Treat seizures with diazepam.
- Administer fluids.

CONTRAINDICATIONS/PRECAUTIONS

- Warnings
  - Pregnancy: Methylphenidate safety not established.
  - Lactation: Use methylphenidate with caution (present in breast milk, can cause agitation and anorexia).
- Use with caution in clients who have hypertension or depression.
- These medications are contraindicated in clients who have a history of substance use disorder, hypertension, hyperthyroidism, cardiovascular disorders, glaucoma, severe anxiety, and psychosis.

INTERACTIONS

Concurrent use of MAOIs can cause hypertensive crisis.
NURSING ACTIONS: Avoid concurrent use. Do not use within 14 days of MAOIs.

Concurrent use of caffeine can increase CNS stimulant effects.
CLIENT EDUCATION: Avoid foods and beverages that contain caffeine.

Methylphenidate inhibits metabolism of phenytoin warfarin and phenobarbital, leading to increased blood levels.
NURSING ACTIONS
- Monitor clients for adverse effects (CNS depression, toxicity, indications of bleeding).
- Concurrent use of these medications is done with caution.

OTC cold and decongestant medications with sympathomimetic action can increase CNS stimulant effects.
CLIENT EDUCATION: Avoid use of OTC medications.

NURSING ADMINISTRATION

- Instruct parents and clients in safety and storage of medications.
- Therapeutic effects begin rapidly and their duration varies according to release form of medication.
- These are Schedule II medications.

CLIENT EDUCATION
- Swallow sustained-release tablets whole. Do not chew or crush the tablets.
- Administer the medication on a regular schedule.
- For transdermal medication, place the patch on alternating hips daily in the morning and leave it in place no longer than 9 hr.
- ADHD is not cured by medication. Management with an overall treatment plan that includes family therapy and cognitive-behavioral therapy will improve outcomes. Q_EBP
- These medications have specific handling procedures controlled by federal law. Handwritten prescriptions are required for medication refills.
- These medications have a high potential for development of a substance use disorder, especially in adolescents. Use strictly as prescribed.
- Avoid alcohol use while taking this medication.
- Avoid activities that require alertness until medication effects are known.

NURSING EVALUATION OF MEDICATION EFFECTIVENESS

Depending on therapeutic intent, effectiveness is evidenced by the following.
- Improvement of manifestations of ADHD (increased ability to focus and complete tasks, interact with peers, and manage impulsivity)
- Improved ability to stay awake

Norepinephrine selective reuptake inhibitors

SELECT PROTOTYPE MEDICATION: Atomoxetine

OTHER MEDICATION: Bupropion

PURPOSE

EXPECTED PHARMACOLOGICAL ACTION
- Block reuptake of norepinephrine at synapses in the CNS. Atomoxetine is not a stimulant medication.
- Bupropion blocks the synaptic reuptake of norepinephrine and dopamine. It is considered a second-line medication for ADHD.

THERAPEUTIC USES
- ADHD
- Depression

COMPLICATIONS

Atomoxetine is usually tolerated well with minimal adverse effects.

Appetite suppression, weight loss, growth suppression

NURSING ACTIONS
- Monitor the client's height and weight and compare to baseline height and weight.
- Administer medication with or without meals.

CLIENT EDUCATION: Eat at regular meal times and avoid unhealthy foods for snacks.

GI effects

Nausea and vomiting

CLIENT EDUCATION: Take with food if these occur.

Suicidal ideation

In children and adolescents

NURSING ACTIONS: Monitor for indications of depression.

CLIENT EDUCATION: Report change in mood, excessive sleeping, agitation, and irritability. Q_s

Hepatotoxicity

CLIENT EDUCATION: Report indications of liver damage (flu-like manifestations, yellowing skin, abdominal pain).

Seizure activity

NURSING ACTIONS: Use low doses, and monitor for seizure activity. Do not use in clients who have a seizure disorder.

CONTRAINDICATIONS/PRECAUTIONS

- Use cautiously in clients who have cardiovascular or hepatic disorders, and hypo/hypertension.
- Atomoxetine is contraindicated in clients who have angle-closure glaucoma, heart failure, and jaundice.
- Bupropion increases seizure risk at high dosages. It is contraindicated in clients who have seizure risk factors and eating disorders.

INTERACTIONS

Concurrent use of MAOIs can cause hypertensive crisis.
NURSING ACTIONS: Avoid concurrent use. Do not use within 14 days of MAOIs.

Paroxetine, fluoxetine, and quinidine gluconate inhibit hepatic metabolizing enzymes, thereby increasing levels of atomoxetine.
NURSING ACTIONS: Reduce dosage of atomoxetine if used concurrently with these medications.

CLIENT EDUCATION: Watch for and report increased adverse reactions of atomoxetine.

NURSING ADMINISTRATION

- Note any changes in the child's behavior related to dosing and timing of medications.
- Administer the medication in a daily dose in the morning, or in two divided doses (morning and afternoon), with or without food.
- Initial response takes a few days to develop, but maximal therapeutic effects can take 6 weeks to fully develop.

NURSING EVALUATION OF MEDICATION EFFECTIVENESS

Depending on therapeutic intent, effectiveness is evidenced by improvement of manifestations of ADHD (increase in ability to focus and complete tasks, interact with peers, and manage impulsivity).

Tricyclic antidepressants

SELECT PROTOTYPE MEDICATION: Desipramine

OTHER MEDICATIONS
- Imipramine
- Clomipramine

PURPOSE

EXPECTED PHARMACOLOGICAL ACTION: These medications block reuptake of the monoamine neurotransmitters norepinephrine and serotonin in the synaptic space, thereby intensifying the effects that these neurotransmitters produce.

THERAPEUTIC USES IN CHILDREN
- Depression
- Autism spectrum disorder
- ADHD (considered less effective than CNS stimulants and used as second-line treatment for ADHD)
- Panic, social phobia, separation anxiety disorder
- Obsessive compulsive disorder (OCD)

COMPLICATIONS

Increased suicide risk

- Risk is higher in clients who have depression (high risk early in treatment).
- Greatest risk during childhood, adolescence, and young adulthood.

NURSING ACTIONS: Ensure clients are screened for depression prior to therapy, and monitor for suicidal ideations.

Orthostatic hypotension

NURSING ACTIONS: Monitor blood pressure with first dose. Instruct client to change positions slowly. Qs

Anticholinergic effects

Dry mouth, blurred vision, photophobia, urinary hesitancy or retention, constipation, tachycardia

CLIENT EDUCATION
- Utilize ways to minimize anticholinergic effects.
  - Chewing sugarless gum
  - Sipping on water
  - Wearing sunglasses when outdoors
  - Eating foods high in fiber
  - Increasing fluid intake to at least 2 to 3 L/day from beverages or food sources
  - Voiding just before taking medication
- Notify the provider if anticholinergic effects are intolerable.

Weight gain

NURSING ACTIONS: Monitor client weight.

CLIENT EDUCATION: Participate in regular exercise and follow a healthy, low-calorie diet.

Sedation

CLIENT EDUCATION
- This adverse effect usually diminishes over time.
- Avoid activities that require alertness (driving if sedation is excessive).
- Take medication at bedtime to minimize daytime sleepiness and to promote sleep.

Toxicity

Resulting in cholinergic blockade and cardiac toxicity evidenced by dysrhythmias, mental confusion, and agitation, followed by seizures and coma or sudden death

NURSING ACTIONS
- Give clients who are acutely ill a 1-week supply of medication.
- Obtain baseline ECG.
- Monitor vital signs frequently.
- Monitor for toxicity and notify the provider if indications of toxicity occur.

Decreased seizure threshold

NURSING ACTIONS: Monitor clients who have seizure disorders.

Excessive sweating

NURSING ACTIONS: Inform clients of this adverse effect and assist with frequent linen changes.

CONTRAINDICATIONS/PRECAUTIONS

- Warnings
  - Pregnancy: Use desipramine only if benefits to the client outweigh the risk to the fetus.
  - Lactation: Use desipramine with caution (present in breast milk, can cause neonatal sedation).
- Use cautiously in clients who have seizure disorders; diabetes mellitus; liver, kidney and respiratory disorders; and hyperthyroidism
- Contraindicated in clients who have closed-angle glaucoma, and acute MI

INTERACTIONS

Concurrent use of monoamine oxidase inhibitors (MAOIs) causes hypertension.
NURSING ACTIONS
- Avoid concurrent use.
- Do not use within 14 days of MAOIs.

Antihistamines and other anticholinergic agents have additive anticholinergic effects.
NURSING ACTIONS: Avoid concurrent use.

Tricyclic antidepressants (TCAs) block uptake of epinephrine and NE (direct-acting sympathomimetics) in the synaptic space, leading to decreased intensity of their effects.
NURSING ACTIONS: Avoid concurrent use.

TCAs inhibit uptake of ephedrine and amphetamine (indirect-acting sympathomimetics) and reduce their ability to get to the site of action in the nerve terminal, leading to decreased responses to these medications.
NURSING ACTIONS: Avoid concurrent use.

Alcohol, benzodiazepines, opioids, and antihistamines cause additive CNS depression when used concurrently.
CLIENT EDUCATION: Avoid concurrent use with CNS depressants.

NURSING ADMINISTRATION

- Assist with medication regimen compliance by informing clients and parents that it can take 2 to 3 weeks to experience therapeutic effects. Full therapeutic effects can initially take around 6 weeks.
- Give only 1 week worth of medication at a time for an acutely ill client. Tricyclics have high lethality in overdosage. **Qs**
- Desipramine passes into breast milk and can cause neonatal sedation. Discontinue imipramine or offer alternate infant nutrition during lactation.

CLIENT EDUCATION
- Administer this medication as prescribed on a daily basis to establish therapeutic plasma levels.
- Understand the importance of continuing therapy after improvement in manifestations. Sudden discontinuation of the medication can result in relapse.
- Take medication at bedtime to prevent daytime drowsiness.

NURSING EVALUATION OF MEDICATION EFFECTIVENESS

Depending on therapeutic intent, effectiveness is evidenced by the following.

For depression
- Verbalizing improvement in mood
- Improved sleeping and eating habits
- Increased interaction with peers

For autism spectrum disorder: Decreased anger, agitation, and compulsive behavior

For ADHD: Less hyperactivity, greater ability to pay attention

For anxiety: Increased ability to recognize triggers, manage episodes, and increased ability for self care and social interactions.

Alpha₂ adrenergic agonists

SELECT PROTOTYPE MEDICATION: Guanfacine

OTHER MEDICATION: Clonidine

PURPOSE

EXPECTED PHARMACOLOGICAL ACTION: The action of alpha₂ adrenergic agonists is not completely understood. However, they are known to activate presynaptic alpha₂ adrenergic receptors within the brain.

THERAPEUTIC USES
- ADHD
- Tic disorders
- Conduct and oppositional defiant disorders

COMPLICATIONS

CNS effects

Sedation, drowsiness, fatigue

NURSING ACTIONS: Monitor for these adverse effects and report their occurrence to the provider.

CLIENT EDUCATION: Avoid activities that require alertness.

Cardiovascular effects

Hypotension, bradycardia

NURSING ACTIONS: Monitor blood pressure and pulse especially during initial treatment.

CLIENT EDUCATION: Do not abruptly discontinue medication which can cause rebound hypertension.

Weight gain

NURSING ACTIONS: Monitor client weight.

CLIENT EDUCATION: Participate in regular exercise and follow a healthy, well-balanced diet.

CONTRAINDICATIONS/PRECAUTIONS

- Extended-release clonidine is contraindicated for children younger than 6 years old.
- Use cautiously in clients who have cardiac disease, cerebrovascular disease, kidney or liver impairment.

INTERACTIONS

CNS depressants, including alcohol, can increase CNS effects.
NURSING ACTIONS: Avoid concurrent use.

Antihypertensives can worsen hypotension.
NURSING ACTIONS: Avoid concurrent use.

Foods with high-fat content will increase guanfacine absorption.
CLIENT EDUCATION: Avoid taking medication with a high-fat meal. QEBP

NURSING ADMINISTRATION

- Assess use of alcohol and CNS depressants, especially with adolescent clients.
- Monitor blood pressure and pulse at baseline, with initial treatment, and with each dosage change.

CLIENT EDUCATION
- Do not chew, crush, or split extended-release preparations.
- Avoid abrupt discontinuation of medication, which can result in rebound hypertension. Medication should be tapered according to a prescribed dosage schedule when discontinuing treatment. QPCC

NURSING EVALUATION OF MEDICATION EFFECTIVENESS

Depending on therapeutic intent, effectiveness is evidenced by improvement of manifestations of ADHD (increase in ability to focus and complete tasks, interact with peers, and manage impulsivity).

Antipsychotics: Atypical

SELECT PROTOTYPE MEDICATION: Risperidone

OTHER MEDICATIONS
- Olanzapine
- Quetiapine
- Aripiprazole

PURPOSE

EXPECTED PHARMACOLOGICAL ACTION
- Second-generation antipsychotic agents (risperidone, olanzapine, quetiapine) work mainly by blocking serotonin, and to a lesser degree, dopamine receptors. These medications also block receptors for norepinephrine, histamine, and acetylcholine.
- Aripiprazole is a third-generation antipsychotic and acts as a dopamine system stabilizer. It not only blocks dopamine and serotonin receptors, but it also is a partial agonist at these receptors. Thus, net effects on receptor activity will depend on how much dopamine and serotonin is present.

THERAPEUTIC USES
- Autism spectrum disorder
- Conduct disorder
- Posttraumatic stress disorder (PTSD)
- Relief of psychotic manifestations
- Intermittent explosive disorder
- OCD
- Tic disorders (including Tourette syndrome)

COMPLICATIONS

Diabetes mellitus

New onset of diabetes mellitus or loss of glucose control in clients who have diabetes

NURSING ACTIONS: Obtain baseline fasting blood glucose and monitor periodically throughout treatment.

CLIENT EDUCATION: Report indications (increased thirst, urination, and appetite).

Weight gain

CLIENT EDUCATION: Follow a healthy, low-caloric diet, engage in regular exercise, and monitor weight gain.

Hypercholesterolemia

With increased risk for hypertension and other cardiovascular disease

NURSING ACTIONS: Monitor cholesterol, triglycerides, and blood glucose if weight gain is more than 14 kg (30 lb).

Orthostatic hypotension

NURSING ACTIONS: Monitor blood pressure with first dose. Instruct client to change positions slowly.

Anticholinergic effects

Urinary hesitancy or retention, dry mouth

NURSING ACTIONS: Monitor for these adverse effects and report their occurrence to the provider.

CLIENT EDUCATION: Use measures to relieve dry mouth (sipping fluids) throughout the day.

Agitation, dizziness, sedation, sleep disruption

NURSING ACTIONS
- Monitor for these adverse effects and report their occurrence to the provider. Avoid activities that require alertness until effects are known.
- Administer an alternative medication if prescribed.

Mild extrapyramidal adverse effects (tremor)

NURSING ACTIONS: Monitor for and teach clients to recognize extrapyramidal adverse effects. These are usually dose-related.

Agranulocytosis, neutropenia

NURSING ACTIONS: Monitor WBC periodically and advise clients to monitor and report manifestations of an infection (a sore throat). Qs

Hyperprolactinemia

NURSING ACTIONS: Monitor and report gynecomastia and amenorrhea.

CONTRAINDICATIONS/PRECAUTIONS

- Be aware of possible alcohol use in the adolescent client. Instruct clients to avoid the use of alcohol.
- Use cautiously in clients who have cardiovascular disease, seizures, dehydration, kidney/hepatic disease, or diabetes mellitus. Obtain a baseline fasting glucose for clients who have diabetes mellitus and monitor carefully.

INTERACTIONS

Alcohol, opioids, and antihistamines cause additive CNS depressant effects.
CLIENT EDUCATION
- Avoid alcohol and other medications that cause CNS depression.
- Avoid hazardous activities (driving).

By activating dopamine receptors, levodopa counteracts effects of antipsychotic agents.
NURSING ACTIONS: Avoid concurrent use of levodopa and other direct dopamine receptor agonists.

Tricyclic antidepressants, amiodarone and clarithromycin prolong QT interval and thus increase the risk of cardiac dysrhythmias.
NURSING ACTIONS: Avoid concurrent use.

Barbiturates promote hepatic medication-metabolizing enzymes, thereby decreasing medication levels of quetiapine.
NURSING ACTIONS: Monitor medication effectiveness.

Medications that inhibit CYP3A4 (fluconazole) inhibit hepatic medication-metabolizing enzymes, thereby increasing medication levels of aripiprazole, quetiapine, and ziprasidone.
NURSING ACTIONS: Monitor for adverse effects.

NURSING ADMINISTRATION

- Administer by oral or IM route.
  - Risperidone and aripiprazole are available in an oral solution and quick-dissolving tablets for ease in administration.
  - Olanzapine is available in an orally disintegrating tablet for ease in administration.

CLIENT EDUCATION: Low doses of medication are given initially and are then gradually increased.

NURSING EVALUATION OF MEDICATION EFFECTIVENESS

Depending on therapeutic intent, effectiveness is evidenced by the following.

For autism spectrum disorder: reduction of hyperactivity, agitation, and improvement in mood

For conduct disorder: decrease in aggressiveness

For ADHD: reduction in hyperactivity and impulsivity

For OCD: reduced anxiety; increased ability for self-care, social interactions, and management of compulsions

Selective serotonin reuptake inhibitors

SELECT PROTOTYPE MEDICATION: Fluoxetine

OTHER MEDICATION: Sertraline, fluvoxamine

PURPOSE

EXPECTED PHARMACOLOGICAL ACTION: Selectively blocks the reuptake of serotonin, intensifying monoamine effects in the CNS.

THERAPEUTIC USES
- Autism spectrum disorder
- Obsessive compulsive disorder
- Major depressive disorder
- Intermittent explosive disorder
- Bulimia nervosa
- ADHD

COMPLICATIONS

Serotonin syndrome

Agitation, confusion, hallucinations

NURSING ACTIONS: Do not use within 14 days of MAOIs. Monitor for effects and discontinue.

Weight changes

CLIENT EDUCATION: Weight loss can occur initially, but there is a risk of weight gain with long-term use. Follow a healthy diet, engage in regular exercise, and monitor weight gain.

Withdrawal syndrome

Dizziness, nausea, tremors

NURSING ACTIONS: Do not discontinue abruptly.

Suicidal ideation

NURSING ACTIONS: Monitor and report any thoughts of suicide. Children, adolescents, and young adults should have follow-up visits weekly during first 4 weeks, then every 3 weeks, with long-term frequency to be determined by the provider.

Extrapyramidal effects

Ataxia, tremors

NURSING ACTIONS: Monitor and report manifestations.

Dizziness, fatigue, insomnia, agitation

CLIENT EDUCATION: Avoid activities that require alertness until effects are known. Reduce dosage if needed.

Dysrhythmias

NURSING ACTIONS: Monitor for dysrhythmias. Reduce dosage as needed.

CONTRAINDICATIONS/PRECAUTIONS

- Warnings
  - Pregnancy: Use fluoxetine with caution during first trimester due to increased risk of cardiovascular malformations and in third trimester due to increased risk for neonatal serotonin syndrome.
  - Lactation
    - Fluoxetine: Avoid breastfeeding; can cause sedation in infant.
  - Reproductive
    - Fluoxetine: Clients should advise their provider if pregnant, planning to become pregnant, or lactating.
- Use cautiously in clients who have narrow-angle glaucoma

INTERACTIONS

Concurrent use of MAOIs, St. John's wort, and other medications that can cause serotonin syndrome (SNRIs, buspirone, phenothiazines) increases the risk for serotonin syndrome.
NURSING ACTIONS
- Avoid concurrent use.
- Do not use within 14 days of MAOIs.

CLIENT EDUCATION: Do not take St. John's wort while taking this medication.

Elevation of plasma levels of TCAs and lithium can occur.
NURSING ACTIONS
- Avoid concurrent use.
- Monitor for toxicity.

Antiplatelet medications and anticoagulants increase risk for bleeding.
NURSING ACTIONS
- Avoid concurrent use.
- Monitor for bleeding.

NURSING ADMINISTRATION

- Administer orally with or without meals.
- Therapeutic effects can take 1 to 3 weeks with maximum effectiveness developing by around 12 weeks.
- Notify provider if pregnancy is suspected.

NURSING EVALUATION OF MEDICATION EFFECTIVENESS

Depending on therapeutic intent, effectiveness is evidenced by the following.

Improvement in mood, decreased manifestations of obsessive compulsive disorder, decrease in aggressiveness

For depression
- Verbalizing improvement in mood
- Improved sleeping and eating habits
- Increased interaction with peers

For autism spectrum disorder, intermittent explosive disorder: Decreased anger, agitation, and compulsive behavior

For bulimia nervosa: Decrease in bing-eating and vomiting episodes.

For anxiety disorders: Decrease in the frequency of panic attacks and increased sense of well-being.

Active Learning Scenario

A nurse working in a pediatric mental health clinic is caring for a client who has a new prescription for risperidone for the treatment of conduct disorder. Use the ATI Active Learning Template: Medication to complete this item.

COMPLICATIONS: Identify at least four adverse effects of this medication.

NURSING INTERVENTIONS: Identify at least four nursing interventions to prevent or minimize the adverse effects of this medication.

Application Exercises

1. A nurse is teaching the guardians and their school-age child about a new prescription for lisdexamfetamine. Which of the following information should the nurse include in the teaching? (Select all that apply.)

   A. An adverse effect of this medication is CNS stimulation.

   B. Administer the medication before bedtime.

   C. Monitor blood pressure while taking this medication.

   D. Therapeutic effects of this medication will take 1 to 3 weeks to fully develop.

   E. This medication raises the levels of dopamine in the brain.

2. A nurse is teaching the caregiver of a school-age child about transdermal methylphenidate. Which of the following instructions should the nurse include?

   A. Apply one patch twice per day.

   B. Leave the patch on for 9 hr.

   C. Apply the patch to the child's waist.

   D. Use opened tray within 6 months.

3. A nurse is caring for a school-age child who has a new prescription for atomoxetine. The nurse should monitor the client for which of the following manifestations as an adverse effect of this medication?

   A. Kidney toxicity

   B. Liver damage

   C. Seizure activity

   D. Adrenal insufficiency

4. A nurse is teaching the guardians of a child who has a new prescription for desipramine. The nurse should include that which of the following adverse effects is the priority to report to the provider?

   A. Constipation

   B. Suicidal thoughts

   C. Photophobia

   D. Dry mouth

Application Exercises Key

1. A. **CORRECT:** When taking action, the nurse should instruct the guardians and their school-age child about lisdexamfetamine. An adverse effect of lisdexamfetamine is CNS stimulation such as insomnia and restlessness.
   B. It should be given in the morning to reduce insomnia.
   C. **CORRECT:** It is important to monitor their blood pressure due to potential cardiovascular effects.
   D. The therapeutic effects of lisdexamfetamine begins immediately and last 10 to 12 hours.
   E. **CORRECT:** It is a CNS stimulant which works by raising the levels of norepinephrine and dopamine in the CNS.

   Ⓝ *NCLEX® Connection: Pharmacological and Parenteral Therapies, Medication Administration*

2. A. Transdermal methylphenidate is administered once per day.
   B. **CORRECT:** When taking action the nurse should instruct the caregiver of a school-age child to administered transdermal methylphenidate for 9 hr/day.
   C, D. It should be applied to the child's hip and use the opened tray of the transdermal patch within 2 months.

   Ⓝ *NCLEX® Connection: Pharmacological and Parenteral Therapies, Medication Administration*

3. A. Atomoxetine can cause urinary retention, but not kidney toxicity. Bupropion increases seizure risk at high dosages.
   B. **CORRECT:** When evaluating for adverse effects of atomoxetine, the nurse should identify that liver damage is a complication. The nurse should monitor for manifestations (jaundice, upper abdominal tenderness, darkening of urine, and elevated liver enzymes).
   C. Seizure activity is not an adverse effect of atomoxetine. Atomoxetine can cause suicidal ideation and mood swings.
   D. Adrenal insufficiency is not an adverse effect of atomoxetine.

   Ⓝ *NCLEX® Connection: Pharmacological and Parenteral Therapies, Adverse Effects/Contraindications/Side Effects/Interactions*

4. B. **CORRECT:** When taking action, the nurse should teach the guardians of a child who has a new prescription for desipramine, the greatest risk to this client is injury from a suicide attempt, therefore, this is the priority adverse effect to report to the provider. Desipramine can cause suicidal thoughts and behaviors which puts the client at risk. The guardians should monitor and report any indication of increase depression or thoughts of suicidal behavior.
   A, C, D. The client is at risk for constipation, photophobia, and dry mouth because of the anticholinergic effects desipramine. The client should increase fluid intake to reduce the risk of constipation and consume hard candy to reduce dry mouth. They should wear sunglasses when exposed to sunlight. However, another adverse effect is the priority.

   Ⓝ *NCLEX® Connection: Pharmacological and Parenteral Therapies, Adverse Effects/Contraindications/Side Effects/Interactions*

Active Learning Scenario Key

Using the ATI Active Learning Template: Medication

COMPLICATIONS
- New onset of diabetes mellitus or loss of glucose control in clients who have diabetes
- Weight gain
- Hypercholesterolemia
- Orthostatic hypotension
- Anticholinergic effects (urinary hesitancy or retention, dry mouth)
- Agitation
- Dizziness
- Sedation
- Sleep disruption
- Tremors
- Agranulocytosis, neutropenia
- Hyperprolactinemia

NURSING INTERVENTIONS
- Obtain the client's fasting blood glucose prior to and periodically throughout treatment.
- Instruct the client to report indications of diabetes mellitus including increased thirst, urination, and appetite.
- Advise clients to follow a healthy, low-caloric diet.
- Recommend regular exercise.
- Monitor weight throughout treatment.
- Monitor cholesterol and triglycerides, especially if weight gain is more than 30 lb.
- Monitor blood pressure with first dose and instruct client to change positions slowly.
- Encourage the client to sip fluids throughout the day.
- Monitor and report manifestations of an infection (a sore throat).
- Monitor and report gynecomastia and amenorrhea.

Ⓝ *NCLEX® Connection: Pharmacological and Parenteral Therapies, Adverse Effects/Contraindications/Side Effects/Interactions*

UNIT 2   MEDICATIONS AFFECTING THE NERVOUS SYSTEM

CHAPTER 11 *Substance Use Disorders*

Abstinence syndrome occurs when clients abruptly withdraw from a substance to which they are physically dependent.

Clients who have a substance use disorder can experience tolerance and withdrawal. Tolerance requires increased amounts of the substance to achieve the desired effect. Physiological manifestations of withdrawal occur when the concentration of the substance in the client's bloodstream declines.

Withdrawing from a substance that has the potential to cause physical dependence can cause abstinence syndrome. The client can experience distressing manifestations that can lead to coma and death.

Major substances associated with substance use disorder include alcohol, caffeine, cannabis, hallucinogens, inhalants, opioids, sedatives/ hypnotics/anxiolytics, stimulants, tobacco, and other (or unknown) substances (anabolic steroids, betel nut, and unidentified black market substances).

The severity of substance withdrawal varies depending on the substance and can produce a variety of manifestations, including gastrointestinal distress, neurologic and behavioral changes, cardiovascular changes, and seizures.

Medications to support withdrawal/abstinence from alcohol

- Effects of withdrawal usually start within 4 to 12 hr of the last intake of alcohol and can continue 5 to 7 days.
- Manifestations include nausea; vomiting; tremors; restlessness and inability to sleep; depressed mood or irritability; increased heart rate, blood pressure, respiratory rate, and temperature; diaphoresis; tonic-clonic seizures; and illusions.
- Alcohol withdrawal delirium can occur 2 to 3 days after cessation of alcohol and is considered a medical emergency. Findings include severe disorientation, psychotic manifestations (severe auditory or visual hallucinations), severe hypertension, and cardiac dysrhythmias that can progress to death. Qs

WITHDRAWAL

Benzodiazepines

First-line treatment for treatment of alcohol withdrawal

EXAMPLES: Chlordiazepoxide, diazepam, lorazepam

INTENDED EFFECTS
- Maintenance of vital signs within expected limits
- Decrease in the risk of seizures
- Decrease in the intensity of withdrawal manifestations
- Substitution therapy during alcohol withdrawal

NURSING ACTIONS
- Administer around the clock or PRN.
- Obtain baseline vital signs.
- Monitor vital signs and neurologic status on an ongoing basis.
- Provide seizure precautions.

ANTIDOTE: Flumazenil, a competitive benzodiazepine receptor antagonist, can reverse sedative effects and is approved for benzodiazepine toxicity. It is administered IV.

Adjunct medications to treatment with benzodiazepines

EXAMPLES: Carbamazepine, clonidine, propranolol, and atenolol

INTENDED EFFECTS
- Decrease in seizures: carbamazepine
- Depression of autonomic response (decrease in blood pressure, heart rate): clonidine, propranolol, and atenolol
- Decrease in craving: propranolol and atenolol

NURSING ACTIONS
- Provide seizure precautions.
- Obtain baseline vital signs, and continue to monitor on an ongoing basis.
- Check heart rate prior to administration of propranolol and withhold if less than 60/min.

ABSTINENCE MAINTENANCE (FOLLOWING WITHDRAWAL)

Disulfiram

INTENDED EFFECTS

- Disulfiram is a daily oral medication that is a type of aversion (behavioral) therapy.
- Disulfiram used concurrently with alcohol will cause acetaldehyde syndrome to occur.
- Effects include nausea, vomiting, weakness, sweating, palpitations, and hypotension.
- Acetaldehyde syndrome can progress to respiratory depression, cardiovascular suppression, seizures, and death.

NURSING ACTIONS: Monitor liver function tests to detect hepatotoxicity.

CLIENT EDUCATION

- Be aware of the dangers and potentially fatal reaction of drinking any alcohol.
- Avoid ingesting or applying any products that contain alcohol (cough syrups, sauces, mouthwash, aftershave lotion, colognes, and hand sanitizer).
- Wear a medical alert bracelet.
- Participate in a 12-step self-help program.
- Medication effects (potential for acetaldehyde syndrome with alcohol ingestion) persist for 2 weeks following discontinuation of disulfiram.

Naltrexone

INTENDED EFFECTS: Naltrexone is a pure opioid antagonist that suppresses the craving and pleasurable effects of alcohol (also used for opioid withdrawal).

NURSING ACTIONS

- Take an accurate history to determine whether clients are also dependent on opioids. Concurrent use of naltrexone and opiates results in withdrawal reactions. Qs
- Clients must abstain from alcohol before starting naltrexone.

CLIENT EDUCATION

- Take the medication with meals to decrease gastrointestinal distress.
- Utilize monthly IM injections of depot naltrexone if having difficulty adhering to an oral treatment regimen.

Acamprosate

INTENDED EFFECTS: Acamprosate decreases unpleasant effects resulting from abstinence (dysphoria, anxiety, restlessness).

CLIENT EDUCATION

- Inform clients that diarrhea can result.
- Advise clients to maintain adequate fluid intake and receive adequate rest.
- Advise clients to take medication three times a day with meals.
- Advise clients to avoid use in pregnancy.

Medications to support withdrawal/abstinence from opioids

- Characteristic withdrawal syndrome occurs within 1 hr to several days after cessation of substance use.
- Findings include agitation, insomnia, flu-like manifestations, rhinorrhea, yawning, sweating, piloerection, abdominal cramping, and diarrhea.
- Manifestations are non-life-threatening, although suicidal ideation can occur.

Methadone substitution

INTENDED EFFECTS

- Methadone substitution is an oral opioid agonist that replaces the opioid to which the client has a physical dependence.
- This will prevent abstinence syndrome from occurring and remove the need for the client to obtain illegal substances.
- It is used for withdrawal and long-term maintenance.
- Dependence will be transferred from the illegal opioid to methadone.

NURSING ACTIONS: Observe the client to make sure the dosage is adequate to suppress withdrawal. (Client's report of prior opiate usage can be unreliable.)

CLIENT EDUCATION

- The methadone dose must be slowly tapered to produce withdrawal.
- Participate in a 12-step self-help program. Qpcc
- Medication must be administered from an approved treatment center.

Clonidine

INTENDED EFFECTS

- Clonidine assists with withdrawal effects related to autonomic hyperactivity (diarrhea, nausea, vomiting).
- Clonidine therapy does not reduce the craving for opioids.

NURSING ACTIONS: Obtain baseline vital signs.

CLIENT EDUCATION

- Avoid activities that require mental alertness until drowsiness subsides.
- Chew sugarless gum or suck on hard candy, and sip small amounts of water or suck on ice chips to treat dry mouth.

Buprenorphine

INTENDED EFFECTS

- Buprenorphine is an agonist-antagonist opioid used for withdrawal and maintenance.
- It is substituted for the opioid to which the client has a physical dependence and prevents withdrawal manifestations.
- Decreases feelings of craving and can be effective in maintaining adherence

- Considered safer than methadone due to a decreased risk for respiratory depression and potential for dependence
- FDA has approved a variety of schedule III buprenorphine products, some containing naloxone, and are available as sublingual tablets, buccal film, or a surgical skin implant.

NURSING ACTIONS: Unlike methadone, a primary care provider can prescribe and dispense buprenorphine. Administer sublingually (tablets or films).

ANTIDOTE

Naloxone, a specific opioid antagonist, can be given IM, SQ, IV, or inhaled to reverse respiratory depression, coma, and other signs of opioid toxicity.

Medications to support withdrawal/abstinence from nicotine

Abstinence syndrome is evidenced by irritability, nervousness, restlessness, insomnia, and difficulty concentrating.

Bupropion

INTENDED EFFECTS: Bupropion decreases nicotine craving and manifestations of withdrawal.

NURSING ACTIONS: Avoid use in clients who have an increased risk for seizures.

CLIENT EDUCATION
- To treat dry mouth, chew sugarless gum or suck on hard candy, and sip small amounts of water or suck on ice chips.
- Avoid caffeine and other CNS stimulants to control insomnia.

Varenicline

INTENDED EFFECTS
- Varenicline is a nicotinic receptor agonist that promotes the release of dopamine to simulate the pleasurable effects of nicotine.
- Reduces cravings for nicotine as well as the severity of withdrawal manifestations
- Reduces the incidence of relapse by blocking the desired effects of nicotine

NURSING ACTIONS
- Monitor blood pressure during treatment.
- Monitor clients who have diabetes mellitus for loss of glycemic control.
- Follow instructions for titration to minimize adverse effects.

CLIENT EDUCATION
- Take medication after a meal.
- Notify the provider if nausea, vomiting, insomnia, new-onset depression, or suicidal thoughts occur. Can cause neuropsychiatric effects (unpredictable behavior, mood changes, and thoughts of suicide). Due to potential adverse effects, varenicline is banned for use in clients who are commercial truck or bus drivers, air traffic controllers, or airplane pilots. Qs

NICOTINE REPLACEMENT THERAPY

INTENDED EFFECTS
- These nicotine replacements are pharmaceutical product substitutes for the nicotine in cigarettes or chewing tobacco.
- The use of nicotine replacement therapy approximately doubles the success rate of smoking cessation.

NURSING ACTIONS: Clients should avoid using any nicotine products while pregnant or breastfeeding.

Nicotine lozenge

CLIENT EDUCATION
- Allow the lozenge to slowly dissolve in the mouth (20 to 30 min).
- Avoid oral intake 15 min prior to or during lozenge use.
- Follow product directions for dosage strength and recommended titration.
- Limit lozenge use to five in a 6 hr period or a maximum of 20/day.

Nicotine gum

NURSING ACTION: Use of nicotine gum is not recommended for longer than 6 months.

CLIENT EDUCATION
- Chew gum slowly and intermittently over 30 min.
- Avoid eating or drinking 15 min prior to and while chewing the gum.

Nicotine patch

NURSING ACTIONS: Remove the patch prior to MRI scan, and replace when the scan is completed.

CLIENT EDUCATION
- Apply a nicotine patch to an area of clean, dry skin each day.
- Avoid using any nicotine products while the patch is on.
- Follow product directions for dosage times.
- Stop using patches and notify the provider if local skin reactions occur.

Nicotine nasal spray

NURSING ACTIONS
- Provides pleasurable effects of smoking due to rapid rise of nicotine in the client's blood level
- One spray in each nostril delivers the amount of nicotine in one cigarette.
- Not recommended for clients who have disorders affecting the upper respiratory system (chronic sinus problems, allergies, or asthma)

CLIENT EDUCATION: Follow product instructions for dosage frequency.

Nicotine inhaler

NURSING ACTIONS
- Simulates smoking by puffing on the inhaler, which delivers nicotine
- Contains menthol, which creates sensation in the back of the throat similar to smoking
- Avoid in clients who have asthma.

CLIENT EDUCATION: Gradually taper use over 2 to 3 months and then discontinue. Ⓠ**EBP**

Electronic cigarettes (e-cigarettes)

NURSING ACTIONS
- Battery-powered device that releases a puff of vaporized nicotine (can also include flavorings and other chemicals)
- Dose of nicotine is unpredictable; safety and efficacy data is lacking.
- Not approved by FDA for any use including as an aid for smoking cessation

CLIENT EDUCATION: Avoid the use of these products.

NURSING EVALUATION OF MEDICATION EFFECTIVENESS

Depending on therapeutic intent, effectiveness is evidenced by the following.
- Absence of injury
- Decreased cravings for substance
- Abstinence from substance

Application Exercises

1. A nurse is providing teaching for a client who is withdrawing from alcohol and has a new prescription for propranolol. Which of the following information should the nurse include in the teaching?
   - A. Increases the risk for seizure activity
   - B. Provides a form of aversion therapy
   - C. Decreases cravings
   - D. Can increase blood pressure

2. A charge nurse is planning a staff education session to discuss medications used during the care of a client experiencing alcohol withdrawal. Which of the following medications should the charge nurse include in the discussion? (Select all that apply.)
   - A. Lorazepam
   - B. Diazepam
   - C. Disulfiram
   - D. Naltrexone
   - E. Acamprosate

3. A nurse is teaching a client who has a new prescription for clonidine to assist with maintenance of abstinence from opioids. The nurse should instruct the client to monitor for which of the following adverse effects?
   - A. Diarrhea
   - B. Dry mouth
   - C. Insomnia
   - D. Hypertension

4. A nurse in an acute mental health facility is caring for a client who is experiencing withdrawal from opioid use and has a new prescription for clonidine. Which of the following actions should the nurse identify as the priority?
   - A. Administer the clonidine on the prescribed schedule.
   - B. Provide ice chips at the client's bedside.
   - C. Educate the client on the effects of clonidine.
   - D. Obtain baseline vital signs.

5. A nurse is teaching a client who has tobacco use disorder about nicotine replacement therapy. Which of the following statements by the client indicates understanding of the teaching?
   - A. "I should avoid eating right before I chew a piece of nicotine gum."
   - B. "I will need to stop using the nicotine gum after 1 year."
   - C. "I know that nicotine gum is a safe alternative to smoking if I become pregnant."
   - D. "I must chew the nicotine gum quickly for about 15 minutes."

Application Exercises Key

1. A. Seizure activity is a potential effect of alcohol withdrawal. However, propranolol does not increase this risk.
    B. Disulfiram, rather than propranolol, provides a form of aversion therapy.
    C. **CORRECT:** When taking action, the nurse should instruct a client who is withdrawing from alcohol and has a prescription for propranolol that propranolol is an adjunct medication used during withdrawal to decrease the client's craving for alcohol.
    D. Propranolol is an antihypertensive medication that can result in hypotension rather than hypertension.

    Ⓝ *NCLEX® Connection: Pharmacological and Parenteral Therapies, Medication Administration*

2. A, B. **CORRECT:** When taking action, the nurse should plan to discuss medications used during the care of a client experiencing alcohol withdrawal. Lorazepam and Diazepam are benzodiazepines used during alcohol withdrawal to decrease anxiety and reduce the risk for seizures.
    C. Disulfiram is administered to assist the client in maintaining abstinence from alcohol following withdrawal.
    D. Naltrexone is administered to assist the client in maintaining abstinence from alcohol following withdrawal.
    E. Acamprosate decreases unpleasant effects (anxiety or restlessness) resulting from abstinence following withdrawal.

    Ⓝ *NCLEX® Connection: Pharmacological and Parenteral Therapies, Expected Actions/Outcomes*

3. A. Constipation, rather than diarrhea, is a common adverse effect associated with clonidine use.
    B. **CORRECT:** When taking action, the nurse should instruct the client who has a prescription for clonidine that dry mouth can be an adverse effect associated with clonidine use.
    C. Sedation, rather than insomnia, can be an adverse effect associated with clonidine use.
    D. Clonidine is more likely to cause hypotension than hypertension.

    Ⓝ *NCLEX® Connection: Pharmacological and Parenteral Therapies, Adverse Effects/Contraindications/Side Effects/Interactions*

4. A. Administering clonidine as prescribed is an important nursing action. However, it is not the priority action.
    B, C. Providing ice chips and educating the client about the medication are important nursing actions. However, they are not priority.
    D. **CORRECT:** When using the nursing process, the nurse should identify assessment is the initial step. Obtaining the client's baseline vital signs is the priority nursing action.

    Ⓝ *NCLEX® Connection: Pharmacological and Parenteral Therapies, Medication Administration*

5. A. **CORRECT:** When taking action, the nurse should instruct the client who is prescribed nicotine replacement therapy to avoid eating or drinking 15 min prior to and while chewing the nicotine gum.
    B, C. The client should not use nicotine gum for longer than 6 months, and should avoid all nicotine products, including nicotine gum, while pregnant or during lactation.
    D. The client should chew the nicotine gum slowly and intermittently over 30 min.

    Ⓝ *NCLEX® Connection: Pharmacological and Parenteral Therapies, Medication Administration*

Active Learning Scenario

A nurse is teaching a client who has tobacco use disorder about a new prescription for varenicline to promote smoking cessation. Use the ATI Active Learning Template: Medication to complete this item.

EXPECTED PHARMACOLOGICAL ACTION

THERAPEUTIC USES

COMPLICATIONS: Identify at least three adverse effects.

CLIENT EDUCATION: Identify at least two teaching points.

EVALUATION OF MEDICATION EFFECTIVENESS: Identify a client outcome to indicate medication effectiveness.

Active Learning Scenario Key

Using the ATI Active Learning Template: Medication

EXPECTED PHARMACOLOGICAL ACTION: Varenicline is a nicotinic receptor agonist that promotes the release of dopamine to simulate the pleasurable effects of nicotine.

THERAPEUTIC USES: Varenicline is indicated to reduce nicotine cravings and block the desired effects of nicotine in clients who have tobacco use disorder.

COMPLICATIONS
- New-onset hypertension
- Loss of glycemic control in clients who have diabetes mellitus
- Nausea
- Vomiting
- Insomnia
- New-onset depression
- Suicidal thoughts

CLIENT EDUCATION
- Clients who are commercial truck or bus drivers, airplane pilots, or air traffic controllers should not take varenicline.
- Take medication after a meal.
- Titrate as prescribed to minimize adverse effects.
- Notify the provider if adverse effects occur.

EVALUATION OF MEDICATION EFFECTIVENESS
- The client will maintain smoking cessation.
- The client will report reduced cravings for nicotine.

Ⓝ *NCLEX® Connection: Pharmacological and Parenteral Therapies, Medication Administration*

CHAPTER 12

Chronic Neurologic Disorders

Chronic neurologic disorders include Parkinson's disease and seizure disorders. Medications administered for chronic neurologic disorders are used to manage manifestations and improve quality of life.

Cholinesterase inhibitors

Cholinesterase inhibitors are known as anticholinesterase agents and have two categories.

Irreversible inhibitors (such as echothiophate): Therapeutic effect is long-acting and they are highly toxic. The only clinical indication is to treat glaucoma. Pralidoxime is used to reverse the effect of echothiophate.

Reversible inhibitors: Therapeutic effect lasts for a moderate duration (2 to 4 hr) and is used to treat Alzheimer's disease and Parkinson's disease and reverse the effects of nondepolarizing neuromuscular blocking agents following surgery.

SELECT PROTOTYPE MEDICATION: Neostigmine (reversible inhibitor)

OTHER MEDICATIONS
- Physostigmine
- Edrophonium
- Donepezil
- Pyridostigmine
- Galantamine
- Rivastigmine

PURPOSE

EXPECTED PHARMACOLOGICAL ACTION

Cholinesterase inhibitors prevent the enzyme cholinesterase from inactivating acetylcholine (ACh), thereby increasing the amount of ACh available at receptor sites. Transmission of nerve impulses is increased at all sites responding to ACh as a transmitter.

THERAPEUTIC USES

12.1 Therapeutic uses for cholinesterase inhibitors	NEOSTIGMINE	ECHOTHIOPHATE	PHYSOSTIGMINE	EDROPHONIUM	DONEPEZIL
Treatment of myasthenia gravis	✓				
Reversal of muscarinic antagonists			✓		
Treatment of glaucoma		✓			
Reversal of nondepolarizing neuromuscular blocking agents	✓			✓	
Treatment of Alzheimer's disease					✓

COMPLICATIONS

Excessive muscarinic stimulation

As evidenced by increased gastrointestinal (GI) motility, increased GI secretions, diaphoresis, increased salivation, bradycardia, and urinary urgency

NURSING ACTIONS
- Advise the client of potential adverse effects. If effects become intolerable, instruct the client to notify the provider.
- Treat severe adverse effects with atropine.

Cholinergic crisis

- Excessive muscarinic stimulation and respiratory depression from neuromuscular blockade
- Paralysis of the respiratory muscles is a possibility and can be fatal.
- Mnemonic to assist with the identification of cholinergic crisis manifestation: SLUDGE and the Killer Bs:
  - Salivation
  - Lacrimation
  - Urination
  - Diaphoresis/Diarrhea
  - Gastrointestinal cramping
  - Emesis
  - Bradycardia
  - Bronchospasm
  - Bronchorrhea

NURSING ACTIONS
- Provide respiratory support through mechanical ventilation and oxygen, and administer atropine to reverse muscarinic stimulation. Qs
- Have resuscitation equipment available.

CONTRAINDICATIONS/PRECAUTIONS

- **Warnings**
  - Pregnancy: Safety not established
  - Lactation: Safety not established
- Cholinesterase inhibitors contraindicated for clients receiving succinylcholine
- Obstruction of GI and renal system
- Used cautiously in clients who have seizure disorders, hyperthyroidism, peptic ulcer disease, asthma, bradycardia, and hypotension

INTERACTIONS

Atropine counteracts the effects of cholinesterase inhibitors.

- Atropine is used to treat toxicity from cholinesterase inhibitors (increased muscarinic stimulation and respiratory depression).

NURSING ACTIONS: Monitor the client closely and provide mechanical ventilation until the client has regained full muscle function.

Neostigmine and edrophonium reverse neuromuscular blockade caused by nondepolarizing neuromuscular blocking agents after surgical procedures and toxicity.
NURSING ACTIONS: Monitor for return of respiratory function. Support respiratory function as necessary. If used to treat toxicity, provide mechanical ventilation until the client has regained full muscle function.

Succinylcholine is a depolarizing short-acting neuromuscular blocker used for surgical procedures.

- Cholinesterase inhibitors increase the neuromuscular blockage of depolarizing neuromuscular blockers.

NURSING ACTIONS: Avoid concurrent use.

NURSING ADMINISTRATION

- Monitor the client for manifestations of toxicity (salivation, diaphoresis, diarrhea) and notify the provider if these occur.
- Neostigmine can be given PO, IM, IV, or subcutaneously.
- Advise clients that dosage is very individualized, starts at very low doses, and is titrated until desired muscle function is achieved.
- Advise clients to wear a medical alert bracelet.

NURSING EVALUATION OF MEDICATION EFFECTIVENESS

Depending on therapeutic intent, effectiveness is evidenced by the following.
- Recovery of muscle strength
- Improved cognition and slow disease progression

Anti-Parkinson's medications

SELECT PROTOTYPE MEDICATIONS

Dopaminergic medications promote dopamine synthesis, activate dopamine receptors, prevent dopamine breakdown, promote dopamine release, or block the degradation of levodopa.

- **Dopamine synthesis medications** (levodopa) are prepared in combination with a dopamine agonist (carbidopa), or listed as levodopa/carbidopa.
  - Levodopa crosses the blood-brain barrier, whereas dopamine alone cannot cross this barrier and has a very short half-life. Levodopa is taken up by dopaminergic nerve terminals and converted to dopamine (DA). This newly-synthesized DA is released into the synaptic space and causes stimulation of DA receptors thus restoring a proper balance between dopamine and acetylcholine.
  - Carbidopa is used to augment levodopa by decreasing the amount of levodopa that is converted to DA in the intestine and periphery. This results in larger amounts of levodopa reaching the CNS.
- **Dopamine agonists** activate dopamine receptors: pramipexole; bromocriptine; ropinirole, a first-line supplement to levodopa. Apomorphine is a rescue medication for "off" times.
- **Catecholamine-O-methyltransferase (COMT) inhibitors** enhance the effect of levodopa by blocking its breakdown: entacapone, tolcapone
- **Monoamine oxidase-B (MAO-B)** inhibitors prevent dopamine breakdown: selegiline, rasagiline
- **Dopamine releaser** prevents dopamine reuptake: amantadine

Anticholinergic medications block the muscarinic receptors, which assist in maintaining balance between dopamine and acetylcholine receptors in the brain.

Dopamine agonists, COMT inhibitors, MAO-B inhibitors, dopamine releasers, and centrally acting anticholinergic antagonists are used concurrently to increase the beneficial effects of levodopa/carbidopa.

PURPOSE

EXPECTED PHARMACOLOGICAL ACTION

These medications do not halt the progression of Parkinson's disease (PD). However, they do offer relief from dyskinesias (bradykinesia, resting tremors, and muscle rigidity) and an increase in the ability to perform ADLs by maintaining the balance between dopamine and acetylcholine in the extrapyramidal nervous system.

THERAPEUTIC USES

Levodopa/carbidopa

- Most effective for PD treatment, but the beneficial effects diminish by the end of year five.
- "Wearing off" effect may occur at the end of the dosing interval, indicating medication levels are subtherapeutic.
- "On-off" phenomena can occur any time during the dosing interval, lasting minutes to hours at a time and becoming more frequent and intense over time.

Dopamine agonist

Pramipexole, ropinirole, apomorphine, Rotigotine
- Administered as monotherapy in early-stage PD and used in conjunction with levodopa/carbidopa in late-stage PD to allow for lower dosage of levodopa/carbidopa and to reduce fluctuations in motor control
- Administered more often in younger clients who are better able to tolerate daytime drowsiness and postural hypotension

Bromocriptine, an ergot derivative, is poorly tolerated and has a high incidence of valvular heart injury. This medication is administered less frequently.

Dopamine releaser

Amantadine releases dopamine where it is stored in the neurons, prevents dopamine reuptake, and can block cholinergic and glutamate receptors.

COMT inhibitors

Beneficial in combination with levodopa/carbidopa to inhibit the metabolism of levodopa in the intestines and peripheral tissues: entacapone, tolcapone

MAO-B inhibitors

MAO-B is a first-line medication in combination with levodopa/carbidopa to decrease the "wear-off" effect.

Selegiline can preserve dopamine produced from levodopa and prolong the effects of levodopa but only up to one or two years.

Rasagiline preserves dopamine in the brain and is not converted into amphetamine or methamphetamine like selegiline does.

Centrally acting anticholinergics

Centrally acting anticholinergic antagonists diminish cholinergic effect (neuron excitability) due to decreased dopamine: benztropine, trihexyphenidyl.

ADVERSE EFFECTS

Levodopa/carbidopa

Usually dose-dependent

Nausea and vomiting, drowsiness
INTERACTIONS: Administration with foods containing large amounts of pyridoxine (Vitamin B_6) can reduce the effects of levodopa.

CLIENT EDUCATION
- Eat protein in several small portions during the day.
- Avoid vitamin preparations and foods containing pyridoxine (wheat germ, green vegetables, bananas, whole-grain cereals, liver, legumes), which reduce the therapeutic effects of levodopa/carbidopa.

Dyskinesias
- Head bobbing, tics, grimacing, tremors

NURSING ACTIONS
- Decrease the dosage. The decrease can result in resumption of PD manifestations.
- Administer amantadine (releases and uptakes DA) to decrease dyskinesias.
- Surgical or electrical stimulation

Orthostatic hypotension
NURSING ACTIONS
- Monitor blood pressure.
- Hypotension can be reduced by increasing intake of salt and water.

CLIENT EDUCATION: Monitor for indications of postural hypotension (lightheadedness, dizziness), and avoid sudden changes of position.

Cardiovascular effects from beta$_1$ stimulation
- Tachycardia, palpitations, irregular heartbeat

NURSING ACTIONS
- Monitor vital signs.
- Monitor ECG.
- Notify the provider if manifestations occur.
- Use cautiously in clients who have cardiovascular disorders.

Psychosis
- Visual hallucinations, nightmares, paranoid ideation

NURSING ACTIONS
- Administer second-generation antipsychotic medications (clozapine) as prescribed to decrease psychotic effects without increasing the manifestations of Parkinson's disease.
- Second-generation antipsychotic medications do not block dopamine receptors in the striatum.
- Avoid concurrent use of conventional antipsychotic agents (haloperidol), which block dopamine receptors and intensify manifestations of PD.
- Assess for the concurrent use of antidepressant MAOI medications, which can result in hypertensive crisis. Do not use levodopa/carbidopa within 2 weeks of MAOI use.

Discoloration of sweat and urine
CLIENT EDUCATION: This finding is harmless.

Activation of malignant melanoma
NURSING ACTIONS
- Avoid use of medication in clients who have skin lesions that have not been diagnosed.
- Perform a careful skin assessment of clients who are prescribed levodopa.

Dopamine agonist

Sudden inability to stay awake
CLIENT EDUCATION: Notify the provider immediately if this occurs.

Daytime sleepiness
CLIENT EDUCATION
- Remain aware of the potential for drowsiness, and avoid activities that require alertness.
- Avoid other CNS depressants (alcohol).

Orthostatic hypotension
CLIENT EDUCATION: Monitor for manifestations of postural hypotension (lightheadedness, dizziness), and avoid sudden changes of position.

Psychosis
- Visual hallucinations, nightmares, especially in older adults ©

NURSING ACTIONS: Administer second-generation antipsychotic medications (clozapine) if manifestations occur.

Impulse control disorder
- Gambling, shopping, binge eating, and hypersexuality

NURSING ACTIONS
- Manifestations appear 9 months after initial dose. Manifestations subside when medication is discontinued.
- Screen for compulsive behavior before initiating therapy.

Dyskinesias
- Head bobbing, tics, grimacing, tremors

NURSING ACTIONS: Decrease dosage of medication.

Nausea
CLIENT EDUCATION: Take medication with food (slows absorption of medication).

Dopamine releaser

CNS effects
- Confusion, dizziness, restlessness

CLIENT EDUCATION: Avoid activities that require alertness while taking the medication.

Atropine-like effects
- Dry mouth, blurred vision, mydriasis (dilated pupils), urinary hesitancy or retention, constipation

NURSING ACTIONS: Monitor I&O, and assess the client for hesitancy or urinary retention.

CLIENT EDUCATION
- Observe for manifestations and notify the provider.
- Chew sugarless gum, eat high-fiber foods, and increase fluid intake to 2 to 3 L/day from beverage and food.

Discoloration of skin, also called livedo reticularis
CLIENT EDUCATION: Discoloration of the skin will subside when the medication is discontinued.

COMT inhibitors

NURSING ACTIONS: Interventions are the same as for pramipexole when administered with levodopa/carbidopa.

GI: vomiting, diarrhea, constipation
NURSING ACTIONS: Treat adverse effects according to manifestations.

Discoloration of urine to a yellow-orange
NURSING CONSIDERATIONS: Assure the client that the urine color is harmless.

Rhabdomyolysis: muscle pain, tendon weakness
CLIENT EDUCATION: Monitor and report manifestations to provider.

Liver failure
NURSING ACTIONS
- Monitor liver function periodically.
- Monitor for manifestations of liver failure (nausea, fatigue, jaundice, abdominal pain).
- Use with caution if hepatic function is impaired.

MAO-B inhibitors

Insomnia (selegiline)
NURSING ACTIONS: Administer selegiline no later than noon.

Hypertensive crisis triggered from foods containing tyramine
CLIENT EDUCATION: Avoid eating foods that contain tyramine (avocados, soybeans, figs, smoked meats, dried or cured fish, cheese, yeast products, beer, chianti wine, chocolate, caffeinated beverages). Continue to avoid these foods for 2 weeks after stopping medication.

Hypertensive crisis and death from some medications
NURSING ACTIONS: Provide a list of medications to avoid (meperidine, fluoxetine, MAO inhibitors, antidepressants, sympathomimetics).

Nausea, diarrhea
NURSING ACTIONS: Take with meals and limit protein intake to increase absorption

Centrally acting anticholinergics

Nausea, vomiting

CLIENT EDUCATION: Take medication with food, but avoid high-protein snacks.

Atropine-like effects

- Dry mouth, blurred vision, mydriasis (dilated pupils), urinary retention, constipation

NURSING ACTIONS: Monitor I&O and assess clients for urinary retention.

CLIENT EDUCATION

- Observe for manifestations and notify the provider if they occur.
- Chew sugarless gum, eat foods high in fiber, and increase fluid intake to 2 to 3 L/day from beverage and food sources.
- Schedule periodic eye exam to measure for increased intraocular pressure that can result in glaucoma.

Antihistamine effects (sedation, drowsiness)

NURSING ACTIONS: Avoid administering to older adult clients due to CNS adverse effects (sedation, confusion, delusions and hallucinations).

CLIENT EDUCATION: Avoid activities that require alertness while taking the medication.

CLIENT EDUCATION

- Nausea and vomiting can be reduced by taking medications with food.
- Family members can assist clients with the medication at home.
- Monitor for the possible sudden loss of the effects of medication, and notify the provider if manifestations occur.
- Effects might not be noticeable for several weeks to several months.
- Medication "holidays" must be monitored in a hospital setting.
- If applicable, avoid pregnancy when taking levodopa or pramipexole.
- The use of pramipexole with cimetidine can increase the amount of pramipexole in blood levels.
- Do not discontinue medications abruptly.

NURSING EVALUATION OF MEDICATION EFFECTIVENESS

Depending on therapeutic intent, effectiveness is evidenced by the following.

- Improvement of manifestations as demonstrated by absence of tremors and reduction of irritability and stiffness.
- Increase in ability to perform ADLs

Antiepileptics (AEDs)

TRADITIONAL ANTIEPILEPTIC MEDICATIONS

- Phenobarbital
- Primidone
- Phenytoin
- Carbamazepine: administered also for bipolar disorder, trigeminal and glossopharyngeal neuralgias
- Valproic acid: can be used for bipolar disorder and migraine headaches
- Ethosuximide

NEWER ANTIEPILEPTIC MEDICATIONS

- Lamotrigine
- Levetiracetam
- Topiramate
- Oxcarbazepine
- Gabapentin
- Pregabalin
- Tiagabine
- Zonisamide
- Lacosamide
- Vigabatrin
- Ezogabine

OTHER MEDICATIONS: Benzodiazepines used for status epilepticus (acute prolonged seizure)

- Diazepam
- Lorazepam

12.2 Antiepileptic medications

	Traditional antiepileptic medications	PHENOBARBITAL	PRIMIDONE	PHENYTOIN	CARBAMAZEPINE	VALPROIC ACID	ETHOSUXIMIDE	Newer antiepileptic medications	LAMOTRIGINE	LEVETIRACETAM	TOPIRAMATE	OXCARBAZEPINE	GABAPENTIN	PREGABALIN	TIAGABINE	ZONISAMIDE	LACOSAMIDE	VIGABATRIN	EZOGABINE
Simple partial, complex partial, secondarily generalized seizures		✓	✓	✓	✓	✓			✓	✓	✓	✓	✓	✓	✓	✓	✓	✓	✓
Primary generalized seizures	Tonic-clonic	✓	✓	✓	✓	✓			✓	✓	✓								
	Absence					✓	✓		✓										
	Myoclonic					✓			✓	✓	✓								

PURPOSE

EXPECTED PHARMACOLOGICAL ACTION

AEDs control seizure disorders by various mechanisms. **(12.2)**

- Slowing the entrance of sodium and calcium back into the neuron, thus extending the time it takes for the nerve to return to its active state and slows the frequency of neuron firing
- Suppressing neuronal firing, which decreases seizure activity and prevents propagation of seizure activity into other areas of the brain
- Decreasing seizure activity by enhancing the inhibitory effects of gamma butyric acid (GABA)

COMPLICATIONS

TRADITIONAL ANTIEPILEPTIC MEDICATIONS

Barbiturates: phenobarbital, primidone

CNS effects
- In adults, CNS effects manifest as drowsiness, sedation, and depression, and in the older adult can cause confusion and anxiety.
- In children, CNS effects manifest as irritability and hyperactivity.

NURSING ACTIONS
- Never administer primidone with phenobarbital because phenobarbital is an active metabolic (stimulates medication metabolism cell porphyria).
- Primidone is generally administered with phenytoin or carbamazepine.
- Avoid administering other CNS depressants (alcohol, benzodiazepines, opioids).

CLIENT EDUCATION
- Observe for manifestations, and notify the provider if they occur.
- Avoid activities that require alertness (driving).

Physical dependence
- May cause physical dependence

NURSING ACTIONS
- Discontinue slowly

Toxicity
Nystagmus, ataxia, respiratory depression, coma, pinpoint pupils, hypotension, death

NURSING ACTIONS
- Stop medication. Administer oxygen and maintain respiratory function with ventilatory support. Qs
- Monitor vital signs.
- Have resuscitation equipment available.

Decreased synthesis of vitamins K and D, and decreased effectiveness of warfarin
NURSING ACTIONS: Monitor laboratory values (INR, calcium, vitamin D).

Hydantoins: phenytoin

CNS effects
- Nystagmus, sedation, ataxia, double vision, cognitive impairment

NURSING ACTIONS: Monitor for manifestations of CNS effects, and notify the provider if they occur.

Gingival hyperplasia
- Softening and overgrowth of gum tissue, tenderness, and bleeding gums

NURSING ACTIONS: Advise clients to maintain good oral hygiene (dental flossing, massaging gums). Folic acid supplements can decrease the occurrence.

Skin rash
NURSING ACTIONS: Stop medication if rash develops.

Cardiovascular effects: dysrhythmias, hypotension
NURSING ACTIONS
- Administer at slow IV rate (no faster than 50 mg/min) and in dilute solution to prevent adverse cardiovascular effects.
- Avoid administering to a client who has sinus bradycardia, sinoatrial block, or Stokes–Adams syndrome.
- Use a large peripheral or central vein with direct IV administration to decrease infiltration and extravasation.

Endocrine and other effects
- Coarsening of facial features, hirsutism, and interference with vitamin D metabolism

CLIENT EDUCATION
- Report changes.
- Consume adequate amounts of calcium and vitamin D.

Interference with vitamin K–dependent clotting factors causing bleeding in newborns
NURSING ACTIONS: Administer prophylactic vitamin K to the client for 1 month before the infant is delivered.

Carbamazepine

CNS effects
- Nystagmus, double vision, vertigo, staggering gait, and headache can occur, but cognitive function is minimally affected.

NURSING ACTIONS
- Administer in low doses initially and then gradually increase dosage.
- Administer the largest portion of the daily dose at bedtime.

Blood dyscrasias
- Leukopenia, anemia, thrombocytopenia

NURSING ACTIONS
- Obtain baseline CBC and platelets. Perform ongoing monitoring of CBC and platelets.
- Observe for manifestations of bruising and bleeding of gums, sore throat, fever, pallor, weakness, and infection.
- Avoid administering to a client who has bone marrow suppression or bleeding disorders.

Hypo-osmolarity

- Carbamazepine promotes secretion of ADH, which inhibits water excretion by the kidneys and places clients who have heart failure at risk for fluid overload.

NURSING ACTIONS

- Monitor blood sodium periodically.
- Monitor for edema, decrease in urine output, and hypertension.

Skin disorders

- Dermatitis, rash, Stevens-Johnson syndrome, morbilliform rash, and photosensitivity reactions

NURSING ACTIONS

- Treat mild reactions with anti-inflammatory or antihistamine medications.
- Medication should be discontinued if there is a severe reaction.

Valproic acid

GI effect

Nausea, vomiting, indigestion

CLIENT EDUCATION: Take medication with food. Enteric-coated formulation can decrease manifestations.

Hepatotoxicity

Anorexia, abdominal pain, jaundice

NURSING ACTIONS

- Assess baseline liver function and monitor liver function periodically.
- This medication should not be used for children younger than 2 years old.
- Medication should be prescribed in lowest effective dose.
- Avoid administering to a client who has liver disease.

CLIENT EDUCATION: Observe for manifestations of hepatotoxicity (anorexia, nausea, vomiting, abdominal pain, and jaundice), and notify the provider if they occur.

Pancreatitis

NURSING ACTIONS

- As evidenced by nausea, vomiting, and abdominal pain
- Monitor amylase levels.
- Medication should be discontinued if pancreatitis develops.

CLIENT EDUCATION: Observe for manifestations, and notify the provider immediately if these occur.

Thrombocytopenia

NURSING ACTIONS: Monitor platelet counts and bleeding time.

CLIENT EDUCATION: Observe for manifestations (bruising), and notify the provider if these occur.

CNS effects from hyperammonemia

Vomiting, lethargy, impaired cognitive function, and altered level of consciousness

NURSING ACTIONS

- Monitor blood ammonia levels periodically.
- Discontinue the medication.

Ethosuximide

GI effects: Nausea, vomiting
NURSING ACTIONS: Administer with food.

CNS effects: Sleepiness, lightheadedness, fatigue
NURSING ACTIONS: Administer low initial dosage.

CLIENT EDUCATION: Avoid hazardous activities (driving).

Note: Ethosuximide is indicated only for absence seizures.

NEWER ANTIEPILEPTIC MEDICATIONS

Lamotrigine

CNS effects

- CNS effects include dizziness, somnolence, aphasia, double or blurred vision, headache, nausea or vomiting, and depression.
- Risk for suicide can be greater than with other AEDs.

NURSING ACTIONS

- Avoid activities that require alertness until effects are stabilized.
- Discontinue medication if manifestations are severe.
- Monitor for suicidality before starting treatment and during the course of treatment.

Aseptic meningitis: Aseptic meningitis effects include headache, fever, stiff neck, nausea, vomiting, rash, and sensitivity to light.

NURSING ACTIONS

- Monitor for and report manifestations to the provider.
- Discontinue medication.

Skin disorders: Can include life-threatening rashes (Stevens-Johnson syndrome and toxic epidermal necrolysis).

NURSING ACTIONS

- Treat mild reactions with anti-inflammatory or antihistamine medications.
- Discontinue medication if there is a severe reaction.
- Concurrent use with valproic acid increases risk of skin disorder development.

Levetiracetam

CNS effects: Dizziness, asthenia (loss of strength, weakness) agitation, anxiety, depression, suicidal ideation

NURSING ACTIONS

- Discontinue medication if there is a severe reaction.
- Monitor for suicidal ideation.

Topiramate

Suicidal ideation: Risk for suicide greater than with most other antiseizure medications
NURSING ACTIONS: Screen for suicidality prior to administration and during course of treatment.

CNS effects: Somnolence, dizziness, ataxia, nervousness, diplopia, confusion, impaired cognitive function, nausea, anorexia, and weight loss

NURSING ACTIONS: Discontinue medication if there is a severe reaction.

Reduced sweating and increased body temperature
CLIENT EDUCATION: Monitor amount of strenuous activity while taking medication.

Metabolic acidosis
NURSING ACTIONS
- Monitor blood bicarbonate levels.
- Discontinue medication or reduce the dosage as prescribed by the provider.

CLIENT EDUCATION: Report hyperventilation, fatigue, anorexia.

Angle-closure glaucoma
CLIENT EDUCATION
- Monitor for manifestations of glaucoma (ocular pain, redness, blurring of vision).
- Have periodic eye exams to measure intraocular pressure.

Oxcarbazepine

CNS effects: Dizziness, drowsiness, double vision, nystagmus, headache, nausea, vomiting, and ataxia

NURSING ACTIONS
- Administer low initial dosage.
- Monitor blood sodium levels if having nausea and vomiting.

CLIENT EDUCATION: Avoid activities that require alertness, such as driving.

Skin disorders: Can include life-threatening rashes (Stevens-Johnson syndrome and toxic epidermal necrolysis

NURSING ACTIONS
- Treat mild reactions with anti-inflammatory or antihistamine medications.
- Discontinue medication if there is a severe reaction.

Hyponatremia: Nausea, drowsiness, headache, and confusion

NURSING ACTIONS
- Monitor blood sodium laboratory values.
- Use caution when the client is administered diuretic medication.

Hypothyroidism: Lethargy, cold intolerance, dry skin, brittle hair, constipation

NURSING ACTIONS
- Monitor laboratory testing.
- Discontinue medication if diagnosis confirmed.

Multiorgan hypersensitivity reactions: Fever and rash with some of the following: lymphadenopathy, hepatorenal syndrome, hematologic abnormalities

NURSING ACTIONS: Discontinue medication if manifestations develop or are suspected.

Gabapentin

CNS effects: Somnolence, dizziness, ataxia, fatigue, nystagmus, and peripheral edema diminish in time.

NURSING ACTIONS: Advise the client to avoid driving if experiencing a high degree of drowsiness.

Pregabalin

CNS effects
- Somnolence, dizziness, adverse cognitive effect, headache
- Blurred vision can develop early in therapy, but resolves with continued drug use.

NURSING ACTIONS: Discontinue medication if there is a severe reaction.

CLIENT EDUCATION: Avoid driving if experiencing a high degree of drowsiness.

Weight gain, peripheral edema, dry mouth
NURSING ACTIONS: Monitor daily weight, and report significant increase to the provider.

CLIENT EDUCATION: Chew gum or suck on hard candy to increase salivation.

Hypersensitivity reactions (angioedema)
CLIENT EDUCATION: Immediately discontinue use and contact provider if manifestations develop.

CONTRAINDICATIONS/PRECAUTIONS

TRADITIONAL ANTIEPILEPTIC MEDICATIONS

Barbiturates: phenobarbital, primidone

Warnings
- Pregnancy: Phenobarbital not recommended during pregnancy due to increased risk of fetus developing malformations. Abrupt withdrawal of phenobarbital can trigger seizures

CLIENT EDUCATION: Be aware of the potential risk of pregnancy, and consult with the provider.

Hydantoins: phenytoin

- Warnings
  - Pregnancy
    - Teratogenic: Cleft palate, heart defects, developmental deficiencies
    - Administer only if the benefits outweigh the risks.
- IV phenytoin is contraindicated for clients who have sinus bradycardia, sinoatrial block, 2nd or 3rd degree AV block, or Stokes-Adams Syndrome.

Carbamazepine

Warnings
- Pregnancy
  - Birth defects: Associated with spina bifida, neural tube defect, and delays in growth
  - Administer only if the benefits outweigh the risks.

Valproic acid

Warnings
- Pregnancy
  - Highly teratogenic: cleft palate, heart defects, neural tube defects
  - Increased risk for autism
  - Administer only if other alternatives are not effective and if the benefits outweigh the risks to the fetus.

NEWER ANTIEPILEPTIC MEDICATIONS

Lamotrigine

Warnings
- Pregnancy
  - Teratogenic: Cleft palate, cleft lip are low risk.
  - Administer only if the benefits outweigh the risks.

Topiramate

Warnings
- Pregnancy
  - Teratogenic: Cleft lip, cleft palate, heart defects
  - Administer only if the benefits outweigh the risks.

Oxcarbazepine

Warnings
- Pregnancy
  - Teratogenic: Cleft palate, heart defects.
  - Administer only if the benefits outweigh the risks.

Pregabalin

Warnings
- Pregnancy
- Birth defects: Can cause skeletal and visceral malformations
- Administer only if the benefits outweigh the risks.

INTERACTIONS

TRADITIONAL ANTIEPILEPTIC MEDICATIONS

Barbiturates: phenobarbital, primidone

Decreased effectiveness of oral contraceptives and warfarin
NURSING ACTIONS: Warfarin dosage might need to be increased.

CLIENT EDUCATION: Consider other forms of contraceptives.

Hydantoins: phenytoin

Warnings
- Pregnancy: Phenytoin causes a decrease in the effects of oral contraceptives, warfarin, and glucocorticoids due to stimulation of hepatic medication-metabolizing enzymes.

NURSING ACTIONS
- Dose of oral contraceptives might need to be adjusted, or an alternative form of birth control used.
- Monitor for therapeutic effects of warfarin and glucocorticoids (INR, blood glucose levels). Adjust dosage as needed.

Alcohol (when used acutely), diazepam, cimetidine, and valproic acid increase phenytoin levels.
NURSING ACTIONS: Monitor blood levels.

CLIENT EDUCATION: Avoid alcohol use.

Carbamazepine, phenobarbital, and chronic alcohol use decrease phenytoin levels.
CLIENT EDUCATION: Avoid use of alcohol.

Additive CNS depressant effects can occur with concurrent use of CNS depressants (barbiturates, alcohol).
CLIENT EDUCATION: Avoid concurrent use of alcohol and other CNS depressants.

Carbamazepine causes a decrease in the effects of oral contraceptives and warfarin due to stimulation of hepatic medication-metabolizing enzymes.
NURSING ACTIONS
- Adjust dose of oral contraceptives or use an alternative form of birth control.
- Monitor for therapeutic effects of warfarin with PT and INR.
- Adjust dose as needed.

Grapefruit juice inhibits metabolism, and thus increases carbamazepine levels.
CLIENT EDUCATION: Avoid intake of grapefruit juice.

Phenytoin and phenobarbital decrease effects of carbamazepine.
NURSING ACTIONS: Concurrent use is not recommended.

Concurrent use of valproic acid increases levels of phenytoin and phenobarbital.
NURSING ACTIONS
- Monitor phenytoin and phenobarbital levels.
- Adjust dosage of medications as prescribed.

NEWER ANTIEPILEPTIC MEDICATIONS

Topiramate

Phenytoin and carbamazepine can decrease topiramate level. Topiramate can increase phenytoin levels.
NURSING ACTIONS: Consult provider before administering phenytoin or carbamazepine with topiramate.

Oxcarbazepine

Decreases oral contraceptive levels.
CLIENT EDUCATION: Use alternate forms of contraception.

Phenytoin levels increase when administered with oxcarbazepine
NURSING ACTIONS: Consult provider before administering with phenytoin.

Alcohol can intensify CNS depression caused by oxcarbazepine
CLIENT EDUCATION: Avoid alcohol.

Pregabalin

Benzodiazepines, alcohol, and opioids intensify the depressive effects of pregabalin
CLIENT EDUCATION: Avoid medications that affect the CNS.

CLIENT EDUCATION

- Monitoring therapeutic plasma levels is recommended as prescribed by the provider.
- Monitor therapeutic plasma levels for medications prescribed and be aware of therapeutic levels for each medication. Notify the provider of results.
- If taking antiepileptic medications, treatment provides for control of seizures, not cure of disorder.
- Encourage the client to keep a seizure frequency diary to monitor effectiveness of therapy.
- Take medications as prescribed and do not stop medications without consulting the provider. Sudden cessation of medication can trigger seizures.
- Avoid activities that require alertness (driving, operating heavy machinery) until seizures are fully controlled and medication effects are known.
- If traveling, carry extra medication to avoid interruption of treatment.
- If of childbearing age, avoid pregnancy, because medications can cause birth defects and congenital abnormalities.
- Phenytoin doses must be individualized. Dosing usually starts three times a day and can be switched to once-a-day dosing with an extended-release form when maintenance dose has been established.
- Phenytoin has a narrow therapeutic range, and strict adherence to the medication regimen is imperative to prevent toxicity or therapeutic failure.
- Do not use phenobarbital, carbamazepine, topiramate, oxcarbazepine, or pregabalin while breastfeeding. If taking phenytoin, valproic acid, or lamotrigine, talk to the provider to weigh the risks and benefits of breastfeeding while taking the medication.

NURSING EVALUATION OF MEDICATION EFFECTIVENESS

Depending on therapeutic intent, effectiveness is evidenced by:
- Absence or decreased occurrence of seizures
- Ability to perform ADLs
- Absence of injury

Application Exercises

1. A nurse in the post-anesthesia recovery unit is caring for a client who received a nondepolarizing neuromuscular blocking agent and has muscle weakness. The nurse should expect a prescription for which of the following medications?

   A. Neostigmine

   B. Naloxone

   C. Dantrolene

   D. Vecuronium

2. A nurse is providing information to a client who has early Parkinson's disease and a new prescription for pramipexole. The nurse should instruct the client to monitor for which of the following adverse effects of this medication?

   A. Hallucinations

   B. Increased salivation

   C. Diarrhea

   D. Discoloration of urine

3. Match each medication to the type of seizure it can be prescribed as treatment for.

   A. Tonic-Clonic
   B. Absence Circle
   C. Tonic-clonic and Myoclonic
   D. Absence, Tonic-clonic and Myoclonic

   1. Ethosuximide
   2. Valproate
   3. Topiramate
   4. Phenobarbital

4. A nurse is reviewing a new prescription for oxcarbazepine with a client who has partial seizures. Which of the following instructions should the nurse include? (Select all that apply.)

   A. "Talk with your provider before taking a prescription for a diuretic medication."

   B. "Consider using an alternate form of contraception if you are using oral contraceptives."

   C. "Chew gum to increase saliva production."

   D. "Avoid driving until you see how the medication affects you."

   E. "Notify your provider if you develop a skin rash."

Active Learning Scenario

A nurse is planning care for a client who has tonic-clonic seizures and a new prescription for phenytoin. Considering the adverse effects and nursing interventions, what should the nurse include in the plan of care? Use the ATI Active Learning Template: Medication to complete this item to include the following:

THERAPEUTIC USES: Describe.

COMPLICATIONS: Describe two adverse effects and two medication interactions.

NURSING INTERVENTIONS: Include two interventions that relate to the two adverse effects, and two interventions that relate to the two medication interactions.

Active Learning Scenario Key

Using the ATI Active Learning Template: Medication

THERAPEUTIC USES: Phenytoin is a hydantoin medication that suppresses partial seizure and primary generalized seizure activity in the affected neurons.

COMPLICATIONS
- CNS effects
- Gingival hyperplasia
- Teratogenic birth defects
- Decreases effectiveness of oral contraceptives, warfarin, and glucocorticoids
- Causes stimulation of hepatic medication-metabolizing enzymes
- Alcohol (acute use), diazepam, cimetidine, and valproic acid increase phenytoin levels.
- Carbamazepine, phenobarbital, and chronic alcohol use decrease phenytoin levels.
- Additive CNS depressant effects can occur with concurrent use of CNS depressants.

NURSING INTERVENTIONS
- Instruct the client to refrain from alcohol and other medications that cause CNS depression, such as barbiturates.
- Encourage the client to use dental floss and massage gums daily.
- Instruct the client to avoid pregnancy and use an alternate form of contraception.
- Monitor INR if on warfarin and blood glucose levels if taking a glucocorticoid.
- Monitor therapeutic effects of warfarin and glucocorticoids.
- Never abruptly discontinue antiepileptic medications.
- Advise clients to avoid use of alcohol and other CNS depressants
- Monitor blood phenytoin levels

Ⓝ *NCLEX® Connection: Pharmacological and Parenteral Therapies, Adverse Effects/Contraindications/Side Effects/Interactions*

Application Exercises Key

1. A. **CORRECT:** The nurse should analyze cues from the client's recent surgical procedure and expect a prescription for neostigmine, a cholinesterase inhibitor used to reverse the effects of nondepolarizing neuromuscular blockers.

   Ⓝ *NCLEX® Connection: Pharmacological and Parenteral Therapies, Medication Administration*

2. A. **CORRECT:** When taking actions and providing information to a client who has a new prescription for pramipexole, the nurse should instruct the client that this medication can cause hallucinations within 9 months of the initial dose and might require discontinuation.

   Ⓝ *NCLEX® Connection: Pharmacological and Parenteral Therapies, Adverse Effects/Contraindications/Side Effects/Interactions*

3. A, 4; B, 1; C, 3; D, 2

   Ⓝ *NCLEX® Connection: Pharmacological and Parenteral Therapies, Adverse Effects/Contraindications/Side Effects/Interactions*

4. A. **CORRECT:** When taking actions and reviewing a new prescription for oxcarbazepine with a client, the nurse should remind the client to talk with their provider before taking a diuretic medication due to the high risk for hyponatremia when taking oxcarbazepine.
   B. **CORRECT:** The nurse should talk with the client about alternate forms of contraception for clients taking oral contraceptives because oxcarbazepine decreases oral contraceptive levels.
   D, E. **CORRECT:** Instruct the client to avoid driving due to potential CNS effects of dizziness, drowsiness, and double vision and to notify the provider if a skin rash occurs because life-threatening skin disorders can develop.

   Ⓝ *NCLEX® Connection: Pharmacological and Parenteral Therapies, Medication Administration*

CHAPTER 14

UNIT 2   MEDICATIONS AFFECTING THE NERVOUS SYSTEM

CHAPTER 13 # Eye and Ear Disorders

Eye disorders

Glaucoma is a frequent cause of blindness. Damage to the optic nerve occurs when aqueous humor does not exit from the anterior chamber of the eye. This results in the buildup of aqueous humor, increased intraocular pressure (IOP), and loss of vision.

TYPES OF GLAUCOMA

Primary open-angle glaucoma (POAG)

- POAG is the most common form of glaucoma.
- Peripheral vision is lost gradually, with central visual field loss occurring if damage to the optic nerve continues.
- Clients typically do not experience manifestations until there is widespread damage. Manifestations can include halos seen around lights, loss of peripheral vision, and headaches.
- The expected reference range for IOP is 10 to 21 mm Hg. IOP greater than 21 mm Hg is a major risk factor for POAG. However, it can occur at therapeutic IOP levels.
- Treatment includes medication therapy to reduce IOP. Surgical intervention is indicated if IOP cannot be reduced by medications.
- POAG is treated with the following medications.
  - Beta adrenergic blockers
  - Alpha$_2$ adrenergic agonists
  - Prostaglandin analogs
  - Cholinergic agonists
  - Carbonic anhydrase inhibitors

Angle-closure (narrow-angle) glaucoma

- This is an acute disorder with a sudden onset, resulting in irreversible blindness within 1 to 2 days without emergency treatment.
- Findings include acute onset of ocular pain, seeing halos around lights, brow pain, nausea, blurred vision, and photophobia. The optic nerve is damaged when the aqueous humor builds up as a result of displacement of the iris.
- Treatment includes medication therapy to reduce IOP, with subsequent corrective surgery for restoration of the iris.
- Although several other classes of glaucoma medications are used to treat angle-closure glaucoma, osmotic agents are first-line medications used to control the condition until corrective surgery can be implemented.

Beta-adrenergic blockers

NONSELECTIVE BETA BLOCKERS (which have both beta$_1$ and beta$_2$ properties)
- Timolol
- Carteolol
- Metipranolol
- Levobunolol

CARDIOSELECTIVE BETA$_1$ BLOCKERS: Betaxolol

PURPOSE

EXPECTED PHARMACOLOGICAL ACTION
Beta blockers decrease IOP by decreasing the amount of aqueous humor produced.

THERAPEUTIC USES
- Topical beta blockers are used primarily to treat POAG. They can be prescribed in combination with other topical medications to lower IOP.
- These medications are occasionally used to treat acute closed-angle glaucoma on an emergency basis.

COMPLICATIONS

Stinging discomfort

Reports of temporary stinging discomfort in the eye immediately after drop is instilled

CLIENT EDUCATION: This effect is transient.

Occasional conjunctivitis, blurred vision, photophobia, dry eyes

CLIENT EDUCATION: Report these effects to the provider.

Systemic effects of beta blockade on heart and lungs

Heart block, bradycardia, bronchospasms, and hypotension

CLIENT EDUCATION
- Avoid excessive dosing to prevent systemic effects.
- When taking beta$_1$ blockers, monitor for bradycardia. Notify the provider for heart rate less than 50/min.

CONTRAINDICATIONS/PRECAUTIONS

- **Warnings**
  - Pregnancy: Safety not established
  - Lactation: Use lowest effective dose if the benefits to the client outweigh the risk to the newborn.
- Do not use beta$_2$ blockers for clients who have chronic respiratory disease because they can constrict airway and cause bronchospasms. Use beta$_1$ blockers with caution in clients who have chronic respiratory disease.
- Do not use beta blockers for clients who have sinus bradycardia, or AV heart block, and use with caution in clients who have heart failure.

INTERACTIONS

Oral beta blockers and calcium channel blockers can increase cardiovascular and respiratory effects.
CLIENT EDUCATION: Inform the provider if taking any of these medications.

Beta blockers can interfere with some effects of insulin.
CLIENT EDUCATION: If diabetic, monitor blood glucose.

NURSING ADMINISTRATION

- Instill one drop in the affected eye once or twice daily.
- Review the proper method of instilling eye drops, and provide instruction to a family member if indicated. Qpcc
- Avoid touching any part of the applicator, and keep the lid in place when not in use.
- Hold gentle pressure on the nasolacrimal duct for 30 to 60 seconds immediately after instilling the drop(s) to prevent or minimize any expected systemic effect.
- Monitor pulse rate/rhythm as indicated for beta blocker. Qs

Alpha₂ adrenergic agonists

SELECT PROTOTYPE MEDICATION: Brimonidine

OTHER MEDICATION: Apraclonidine

ALPHA₂ AGONIST/BETA BLOCKER COMBINATION: Brimonidine and timolol

PURPOSE

EXPECTED PHARMACOLOGICAL ACTION
Brimonidine decreases production while increasing outflow of aqueous humor to lower IOP.

THERAPEUTIC USES
- Brimonidine is used as a first-line medication for long-term topical treatment of POAG.
- Apraclonidine is a short-term therapy for POAG only and is also used preoperatively for laser eye surgeries.

COMPLICATIONS

Stinging discomfort, pruritus

- Localized stinging discomfort and pruritus of conjunctiva
- Sensation that a foreign body is in the eye

CLIENT EDUCATION: Do not rub the eyes.

Dilated pupils, blurred vision, headache, dry mouth

CLIENT EDUCATION: Report these effects.

Reddened sclera

Caused by blood-vessel engorgement

CLIENT EDUCATION: Be aware of the possibility of this effect.

Hypotension, drowsiness

Brimonidine crosses the blood-brain barrier

CLIENT EDUCATION: Use caution with driving and other tasks, and inform the provider if dizziness and/or weakness occur.

CONTRAINDICATIONS/PRECAUTIONS

- **Warnings**
  - Pregnancy: Safety not established
  - Lactation: Use lowest effective dose if the benefits to the client outweigh the risk to the newborn.
- Advise clients who wear soft contact lenses to administer brimonidine with lenses removed. Delay insertion of the lens at least 15 min after administration to prevent absorption of medication into the lens. Qpcc

INTERACTIONS

Antihypertensive medications can intensify hypotension caused by brimonidine.
CLIENT EDUCATION: Inform the provider if taking any antihypertensive medications.

MAOIs can decrease effects of brimonidine and cause hypertensive crisis.
CLIENT EDUCATION: Inform the provider if taking MAOIs.

NURSING ADMINISTRATION

- Review proper method of administering eye drops and minimizing systemic effects.
- Monitor blood pressure for hypotension or hypertension.

Prostaglandin analogs

SELECT PROTOTYPE MEDICATION: Latanoprost

OTHER MEDICATIONS
- Travoprost
- Bimatoprost

PURPOSE

EXPECTED PHARMACOLOGICAL ACTION
Latanoprost reduces IOP by increasing aqueous humor outflow through relaxation of ciliary muscle.

THERAPEUTIC USES
These agents are topical first-line medications for clients who have POAG and ocular hypertension. (13.1

COMPLICATIONS

Bulging of ocular blood vessels

CLIENT EDUCATION: Inform clients about the possibility of this effect.

Increased pigmentation

Permanent increased brown pigmentation of the iris, usually occurring in individuals with a brown tint to the iris (can also cause pigmentation of lids, lashes)

CLIENT EDUCATION: This change is permanent but does not progress further after medication is discontinued.

Stinging, burning, reddened conjunctiva

CLIENT EDUCATION: Do not rub the eyes.

13.1 Second-line topical medications for glaucoma

Direct-acting cholinergic (muscarinic) agonist

PROTOTYPE: Pilocarpine

PURPOSE
• Second-line treatment for POAG; lowers IOP indirectly through ciliary contraction
• Also used to treat closed-angle glaucoma

WARNINGS
• Pregnancy: Safety not established
• Lactation: Use lowest effective dose if the benefits to the client outweigh the risk to the newborn.

ADVERSE EFFECTS
• Retinal detachment
• Parasympathetic effects (bradycardia, increase in saliva, sweating, flushing, pupil constriction)
• Decreased visual acuity
• Miosis
• Blurred vision
• Hypotension
• Bronchospasm

Carbonic anhydrase inhibitor

PROTOTYPE: Dorzolamide
Also available in combination with timolol

PURPOSE
• Second-line treatment for POAG, which decreases aqueous humor production
• Timolol/dorzolamide combination produces increased effect of both medications.

WARNINGS
• Pregnancy: Avoid use, especially during the first trimester.
• Lactation: Avoid use.

ADVERSE EFFECTS
• Localized allergic reactions in up to 15%
• Blurred vision, dryness, photophobia
• Can absorb into soft contacts
• Ocular stinging, conjunctivitis, and lid reaction
• Bitter taste

Blurred vision

CLIENT EDUCATION: Report to the provider.

Migraine

Rare adverse effect

CLIENT EDUCATION: Report to the provider.

CONTRAINDICATIONS/PRECAUTIONS

Warnings
• Pregnancy: Safety not established
• Lactation: Use lowest effective dose if the benefits to the client outweigh the risk to the newborn.

Osmotic agents

SELECT PROTOTYPE MEDICATION: Mannitol

PURPOSE

EXPECTED PHARMACOLOGICAL ACTION: Osmotic agents decrease intraocular pressure by making the plasma hypertonic, thus drawing fluid from the anterior chamber of the eye.

THERAPEUTIC USES: These agents treat the rapid progression of closed-angle glaucoma to prevent blindness.

COMPLICATIONS

Adverse effects include headache, nausea, vomiting, edema, and fluid and electrolyte imbalance.

CONTRAINDICATIONS/PRECAUTIONS

Warnings
• Pregnancy: Safety not established
• Lactation: Safety not established

Carbonic anhydrase inhibitor (systemic)

SELECT PROTOTYPE MEDICATION: Acetazolamide

OTHER MEDICATIONS: Methazolamide

PURPOSE

EXPECTED PHARMACOLOGICAL ACTION: Reduces production of aqueous humor by causing diuresis through renal effects

---

THERAPEUTIC USES
- Quickly lower IOP in clients for whom other medications have been ineffective.
- Acetazolamide, a nonantimicrobial sulfonamide, can be used as an emergency medication prior to surgery for acute angle-closure glaucoma and as a second-line medication for treatment of POAG.
- Acetazolamide can also be used to treat acute altitude sickness, seizures, and heart failure (as a diuretic).

COMPLICATIONS

Severe allergic reactions

Severe allergic reactions (anaphylaxis)

CLIENT EDUCATION: Monitor for effects and notify provider.

Serious blood disorders

Rare serious blood disorders (bone marrow depression)

CLIENT EDUCATION: Recognize and immediately report effects.

Gastrointestinal effects

Gastrointestinal (GI) effects (nausea, diarrhea)

NURSING ACTIONS: Report GI adverse effects and weight loss to provider.

Electrolyte depletion (sodium and potassium), dehydration, altered liver function

NURSING ACTIONS: Prepare clients for the need to obtain regular laboratory testing. Weigh daily, monitor for postural hypotension, and increase fluid intake to 2 to 3 L/day, unless contraindicated.

Generalized flu-like manifestations

Headache, fever, body aches malaise

CLIENT EDUCATION: Monitor for possible reactions.

Central nervous system disturbances

Paresthesias of extremities, fatigue, sleepiness, rarely seizures

NURSING ACTIONS
- Educate client about possible reactions.
- Medication can be discontinued.

Glucose disturbances

In clients who have diabetes mellitus

CLIENT EDUCATION: If diabetic, closely monitor blood glucose and watch for indications of hypo- or hyperglycemia.

Nephrolithiasis

CLIENT EDUCATION: Report manifestations of stones to the provider (flank pain).

CONTRAINDICATIONS/PRECAUTIONS

Warnings
- Pregnancy: Avoid use during the first trimester.

INTERACTIONS

Serious effects (metabolic acidosis) can occur in clients using high-dose aspirin.
NURSING ACTIONS: Question clients about aspirin use, and notify the provider.

Acetazolamide can increase the risk of toxic effects of quinidine.
CLIENT EDUCATION: Notify the provider of concurrent use and watch for indications of toxicity (decreased heart rate).

Acetazolamide can decrease blood levels of lithium.
CLIENT EDUCATION: If taking lithium, watch for increased indications of mania. Monitor lithium levels regularly.

Acetazolamide can increase osteomalacia, an adverse effect of phenytoin.
CLIENT EDUCATION: If taking phenytoin, watch for bone pain or weakness and report manifestations to the provider.

Sodium bicarbonate increases the risk of kidney stones.
NURSING ACTIONS: Question clients about the use of sodium bicarbonate and other over-the-counter antacids

NURSING ADMINISTRATION

Acetazolamide is available orally as a tablet or a capsule. It is also available for parenteral administration.

NURSING EVALUATION OF MEDICATION EFFECTIVENESS

Depending on therapeutic intent, effectiveness can be evidenced by the following.
- Reduced IOP
- Safe self-administration of medication
- Prevention or minimization of systemic effects

Ear disorders

Acute otitis media

- This condition occurs most often in young children.
- A bacterial or a viral infection causes a buildup of fluid in the middle ear (middle ear effusion).
- The major indication is acute onset of pain. Objective findings include erythema, bulging of the tympanic membrane, and fever. Diagnosis is confirmed when there is acute onset of manifestations, middle-ear effusion, and middle-ear inflammation.
- Treatment for bacterial infection, especially in infants and young children, is an antibiotic. Treatment for viral infection involves managing manifestations (promote comfort, reduce fever).

Because of the increase in antibiotic-resistant bacteria, the current trend is to administer medications for pain relief (acetaminophen, ibuprofen), observe children over age 2 for 48 to 72 hr, and prescribe antibiotics if the condition does not resolve or worsens over several days.

- Medications for treating otitis media
  - Oral penicillins
  - Other antimicrobials, oral or parenteral
  - Pain medication
- Incidence of acute otitis media in infants and children can be reduced by yearly influenza immunization and immunization with pneumococcal conjugate vaccine.

Otitis externa

- This condition, also known as swimmer's ear, is caused by a bacterial infection of the external auditory canal.
- Any object that abrades or leaves moisture in the canal facilitates colonization of bacteria and the onset of otitis externa.
- Manifestations include acute onset of pain, especially with movement of the pinna, itching, diminished hearing, and purulent discharge.
- Treatment usually resolves infection within 10 days.
- Otitis externa is usually treated with acetic acid solution or topical antimicrobial/anti-inflammatory combination. If severe, systemic medications can be used.

Antimicrobials

SELECT PROTOTYPE MEDICATION: Amoxicillin

OTHER MEDICATION: Amoxicillin/clavulanate PO

Antibiotics used to treat acute otitis media in clients who have a type II penicillin allergy (mild) or penicillin-resistant otitis media
- Ceftriaxone IM, IV (severe illness)
- Cefdinir PO
- Cefuroxime PO, IM, IV
- Cefpodoxime PO

Antibiotics used to treat acute otitis media in clients who have a type I penicillin allergy (severe)
- Azithromycin PO, IV (severe allergy)
- Clarithromycin PO, IV (severe allergy)

PURPOSE

EXPECTED PHARMACOLOGICAL ACTION
Eradication of infection

THERAPEUTIC USES
Used to treat otitis media and various other bacterial infections throughout the body

COMPLICATIONS

Possible allergic reaction

Most common risk when taking penicillin

NURSING ACTIONS
- Question the client and family regarding the presence of penicillin or other antibiotic allergy.
- The client might need alternative medication.
- A skin test can be used to test for sensitivity.

GI upset

Usually less with amoxicillin than with ampicillin

NURSING ACTIONS: Educate family to inform the provider of severe diarrhea, especially in an infant or young child.

Suprainfection

With other microbes (oral candidiasis)

NURSING ACTIONS: Report indications of new infection to the provider.

CONTRAINDICATIONS/PRECAUTIONS

- **Warnings**
  - Pregnancy: Safe for use
  - Lactation: Safe for use
- Amoxicillin is contraindicated for clients who have an allergy to penicillin.
- Use amoxicillin with caution in clients who have an allergy to cephalosporins due to possibility of cross-sensitivity.
- Use cautiously in infants younger than 3 months of age due to immature renal system and increased risk for toxicity.

NURSING ADMINISTRATION

Amoxicillin is usually prescribed 2–3 times daily PO.

CLIENT EDUCATION
- Take amoxicillin with food to minimize GI upset.
- Take the full course of antibiotics as prescribed.
- If taking hormonal contraception to prevent pregnancy, use a backup birth control method (condom) while taking antibiotics.

NURSING EVALUATION OF MEDICATION EFFECTIVENESS

Depending on therapeutic intent, effectiveness can be evidenced by:
- Reduction of manifestations (fever, earache)
- Absence of infection
- Absence of recurrence of infection

Fluoroquinolone antibiotic plus steroid medication

SELECT PROTOTYPE MEDICATION: Ciprofloxacin plus hydrocortisone otic drops

OTHER MEDICATIONS
- Acetic acid 2% solution otic drops
- Ciprofloxacin plus dexamethasone otic drops
- Ofloxacin otic drops

PURPOSE

EXPECTED PHARMACOLOGICAL ACTION
The bactericidal effect of ciprofloxacin and anti-inflammatory effect of hydrocortisone should decrease pain, edema, and erythema in the ear canal.

THERAPEUTIC USES
Topical medications to treat otitis externa

COMPLICATIONS

CNS effects

Dizziness, lightheadedness, tremors, restlessness, convulsions

CLIENT EDUCATION: Inform the provider if any of these occur.

Rash

NURSING ACTIONS: Question the client/family about allergies to fluoroquinolone antibiotics or to steroids (dexamethasone or cortisone).

NURSING ADMINISTRATION

- Review the method for instilling otic drops.
- Warm the medication by gently rolling the container between hands before instilling drops. Cold drops can cause dizziness. Gently shake medication that is in suspension form.
- Place the client on the unaffected side.
- Keep clients in a side-lying position for 5 min with the affected ear up after instilling drops. Place a small piece of cotton in the ear. Avoid packing it tightly. Remove cotton after 15 min.

CLIENT EDUCATION
- Take the full course of medication.
- Movement of the tragus or pinna can be very painful when instilling otic drops.
- Prevent otic medications from being placed in the eye or ingested orally. Qs
- Prevent otitis externa by:
  - Keeping foreign bodies (cotton swabs), out of the ear canal, and avoiding the use of manual measures to remove cerumen.
  - Drying the ear canal after bathing or swimming, using a towel, and tilting the head to promote drainage
  - Avoiding the use of earplugs, except for swimming or if needed in a loud environment to prevent hearing loss

NURSING EVALUATION OF MEDICATION EFFECTIVENESS

Depending on therapeutic intent, effectiveness can be evidenced by the following.
- Subsiding of manifestations
- Use of measures to prevent reinfection

Application Exercises

1. A nurse is teaching a client who has a new prescription for timolol how to insert eye drops. The nurse should instruct the client to press on which of the following areas to prevent systemic absorption of the medication?

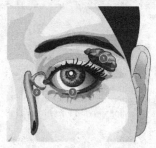

    A. 1

    B. 2

    C. 3

2. A nurse is teaching a client who has a new prescription for brimonidine ophthalmic drops and wears soft contact lenses. Which of the following instructions should the nurse include in the teaching?

    A. "This medication can stain your contacts."

    B. "You will need a new contact prescription while using this medication."

    C. "This medication can absorb into your contacts."

    D. "You will need to wear glasses while taking this medication."

3. A nurse is preparing to administer amoxicillin for the first time to a client who has otitis media. Which of the following questions should the nurse ask the client prior to administration?

    A. "Did you have any grapefruit with your breakfast?"

    B. "Are you allergic to eggs?"

    C. "Have you ever had an allergic reaction to penicillin?"

    D. "Do you have glaucoma?"

4. A nurse in a provider's office is instructing a guardian of a toddler how to administer ear drops. Which of the following instructions should the nurse include? (Select all that apply).

    A. "Place the child on the unaffected side when you are ready to administer the medication."

    B. "Warm the medication by gently rolling it between your hands for a few minutes."

    C. "Gently shake medication that is in suspension form."

    D. "Keep the child on their side for 5 minutes after instillation of the ear drops."

    E. "Tightly pack the ear with cotton after instillation of the ear drops."

Active Learning Scenario

A nurse in a provider's office is teaching a client who has a prescription for ciprofloxacin/hydrocortisone about the medication and how to prevent otitis externa. Use the ATI Active Learning Template: Medication to complete this item.

THERAPEUTIC USES: Identify two therapeutic effects of the medication.

COMPLICATIONS: Identify two potential adverse effects.

CLIENT EDUCATION: Identify two actions to prevent otitis externa.

Active Learning Scenario Key

THERAPEUTIC USES: The bactericidal effects of ciprofloxacin and the anti-inflammatory effect of hydrocortisone decrease pain, edema, and erythema in the ear.

COMPLICATIONS
- Rash
- Dizziness, lightheadedness, tremors, restlessness, and convulsions

CLIENT EDUCATION
- Keep foreign bodies out of ear canal.
- Avoid manual measures to remove cerumen.
- Dry ear canal after bathing or swimming using a towel.
- Avoid use of ear plugs except for swimming.

Ⓝ *NCLEX® Connection: Pharmacological and Parenteral Therapies, Medication Administration*

Application Exercises Key

1. B. **CORRECT:** When taking actions and instructing a client about how to insert eye drops, the nurse should inform the client to place gentle pressure on the nasolacrimal duct which blocks the lacrimal punctum and prevents systemic absorption of the medication.

Ⓝ *NCLEX® Connection: Pharmacological and Parenteral Therapies, Medication Administration*

2. C. **CORRECT:** When taking actions and teaching a client about their new prescription for brimonidine eye drops, the nurse should instruct the client that these drops can be absorbed into soft contact lenses. The client should remove their contacts then instill the medication and wait at least 15 min before putting the contacts back in.

Ⓝ *NCLEX® Connection: Pharmacological and Parenteral Therapies, Medication Administration*

3. C. **CORRECT:** The nurse should plan to generate solutions for a client taking amoxicillin for the first time by determining if the client has any previous allergies to penicillin medications. The administration of amoxicillin is contraindicated for clients who have an allergy to penicillin.

Ⓝ *NCLEX® Connection: Pharmacological and Parenteral Therapies, Medication Administration*

4. A. **CORRECT:** When taking actions and instructing the guardian of a toddler about how to administer ear drops, the nurse should tell the guardian to have the child lie on the unaffected side to allow access to the affected ear and to promote drainage of the medication by gravity into the ear.
B, C, D. **CORRECT:** The nurse should instruct the guardian to warm the medication by rolling it between their hands, and to gently shake medication that is in suspension form to evenly disperse the medication.
E. The nurse should inform the guardians not to pack the child's ear tightly with cotton after instillation of drops because this action may prevent the movement of ear secretions.

Ⓝ *NCLEX® Connection: Pharmacological and Parenteral Therapies, Medication Administration*

UNIT 2   MEDICATIONS AFFECTING THE NERVOUS SYSTEM

CHAPTER 14   *Miscellaneous Central Nervous System Medications*

Neuromuscular blocking agents have various uses, including causing muscle relaxation during general anesthesia, control of seizures during electroconvulsive therapy, suppression of gag reflex during endotracheal intubation and suppression of spontaneous respiratory movements during mechanical ventilation. Medications include succinylcholine and vecuronium.

Muscle relaxants and antispasmodic agents can affect both the central and peripheral nervous systems. These agents are used for spasticity related to muscle injury, cerebral palsy, spinal cord injury, and multiple sclerosis. Agents include diazepam, baclofen, and dantrolene. Bethanechol, a muscarinic agonist, is used for urinary retention. Oxybutynin, a muscarinic antagonist, is used for neurogenic bladder.

Neuromuscular blocking agents

SELECT PROTOTYPE MEDICATION
- **Depolarizing** neuromuscular blockers: Succinylcholine
- **Nondepolarizing** neuromuscular blockers: Pancuronium

OTHER MEDICATIONS: Nondepolarizing neuromuscular blockers
- Atracurium
- Cisatracurium
- Rocuronium
- Vecuronium

PURPOSE

EXPECTED PHARMACOLOGICAL ACTION
Nondepolarizing neuromuscular blocking agents block acetylcholine (ACh) at the neuromuscular junction, resulting in muscle relaxation and hypotension. They do not cross the blood-brain barrier, so complete paralysis is achieved without loss of consciousness or decreased pain sensation. Depolarizing neuromuscular blockers (succinylcholine) bind to the nicotinic receptors on the motor end–plate and remain bound preventing the end-plate from repolarizing.

Succinylcholine
- Mimics ACh by binding with cholinergic receptors at the neuromuscular junction. This agent fills the cholinergic receptors, preventing ACh from binding with them, and causes sustained depolarization of the muscle, resulting in muscle paralysis.
- Short duration of action because of degradation by the plasma enzyme pseudocholinesterase.

Pancuronium, atracurium, vecuronium
- Block ACh from binding with cholinergic receptors at the motor end plate. Muscle paralysis occurs because of inhibited nerve depolarization and skeletal muscle contraction.
- Reversal agent: neostigmine

THERAPEUTIC USES
- Neuromuscular blocking agents are used as adjuncts to general anesthesia to promote muscle relaxation.
- These agents are used to control spontaneous respiratory movements in clients receiving mechanical ventilation.
- These agents are used as seizure control during electroconvulsive therapy.
- Neuromuscular blocking agents are used during endotracheal intubation and endoscopy.

COMPLICATIONS

Respiratory arrest

From paralyzed respiratory muscles

NURSING ACTIONS
- Maintain continuous cardiac and respiratory monitoring.
- Have equipment ready for resuscitation and mechanical ventilation.
- Monitor for return of respiratory function when medication is discontinued.
- Administer a cholinesterase inhibitor, neostigmine, to reverse the action of nondepolarizing neuromuscular blocking agents as needed.

ATRACURIUM

Hypotension

Due to histamine release

NURSING ACTIONS: Monitor for decreased blood pressure. Administer antihistamine if indicated.

SUCCINYLCHOLINE

Prolonged apnea

Low pseudocholinesterase activity can lead to prolonged apnea.

NURSING ACTIONS
- Test blood or administer a small test dose for clients suspected of having low levels of pseudocholinesterase.
- Withhold medication if pseudocholinesterase activity is low.

Malignant hyperthermia

Manifestations include muscle rigidity accompanied by increased temperature, as high as 43° C (109.4° F). Other manifestations include cardiac dysrhythmias, unstable b/p, electrolyte imbalances, and metabolic acidosis.

NURSING ACTIONS
- Monitor vital signs.
- Stop succinylcholine and other anesthetics.
- Administer oxygen at 100%.
- Initiate cooling measures including administration of iced 0.9% sodium chloride, applying a cooling blanket, and placing ice bags in groin and other areas.
- Administer dantrolene to decrease metabolic activity of skeletal muscle.

Muscle pain

After 12 to 24 hr postoperative, clients can experience muscle pain in the upper body and back.

NURSING ACTIONS: Notify the provider to consider short-term use of muscle relaxant.

CLIENT EDUCATION: This response is not unusual and eventually will subside.

Hyperkalemia

NURSING ACTIONS
- Monitor potassium levels.
- Observe for manifestations of hyperkalemia.
- Do not use succinylcholine for clients who have severe burns, multiple trauma, or upper motor neuron injury.

CONTRAINDICATIONS/PRECAUTIONS

- **Warnings**
  - Pregnancy: Safety not established
  - Lactation: Safety not established
- Succinylcholine is contraindicated in clients who have risk of hyperkalemia (major trauma, severe burns).
- Use cautiously in clients who have myasthenia gravis, respiratory dysfunction, or fluid and electrolyte imbalances.

Note that neuromuscular blocker medications are not anesthetics and therefore have no effect on hearing, thinking, or ability to feel pain.

INTERACTIONS

Concurrent use with general anesthetics (common during surgery) can cause extreme neuromuscular blockade.
NURSING ACTIONS: Reduce dosage of neuromuscular blocker to prevent this effect.

Aminoglycosides and tetracyclines can increase the effects of neuromuscular blockade.
NURSING ACTIONS: Take complete medication history of clients who are to receive neuromuscular blockade. Monitor for prolonged neuromuscular blockage.

14.1 Case study

Scenario introduction
Candy is an RN in the operating room caring for Mr. Rook who is scheduled for an appendectomy and will receive succinylcholine. Dr. Matty is the anesthesiologist for the procedure.

Scene 1
Candy: "Hello Mr. Rook, I understand this is not the first time you have had surgery performed. Have you ever experienced any difficulties during surgery before?"
Mr. Rook: "No, my brother did though."

Scene 2
Candy: "Do you know what type of difficulties he encountered?"
Mr. Rook: "Not really. I just remember they gave him some medicine and he was okay."

Scene 3
Dr. Matty: "We will need to monitor Mr. Rook very carefully. It sounds as though he may be at an increased risk for developing malignant hyperthermia."
Candy: "I will report any manifestations to you immediately."

Scenario conclusion
During surgery, Mr. Rook suddenly develops rigidity and a rise in body temperature. Candy reports these changes to Dr. Matty immediately. When safe, Mr. Rook is transferred to PACU.

Case study exercises

1. Candy, the nurse in the operating room caring for Mr. Rook who received a dose of succinylcholine, reports their findings to Dr. Matty immediately. Candy should expect a prescription for which of the following medications?

   A. Neostigmine

   B. Naloxone

   C. Dantrolene

   D. Vecuronium

2. A nurse in the PACU is caring for Mr. Rook, who is experiencing malignant hyperthermia. Which of the following actions should the nurse take? (Select all that apply).

   A. Place a cooling blanket on the client.

   B. Administer oxygen at 100%.

   C. Administer cold 0.9% sodium chloride.

   D. Administer potassium chloride IV.

   E. Monitor core body temperature.

Neostigmine and other cholinesterase inhibitors increase the effects of depolarizing neuromuscular blockers (succinylcholine).

NURSING ACTIONS: Monitor clients during neuromuscular blockade reversal after surgery.

NURSING ADMINISTRATION

- Clients must receive continuous cardiac and respiratory monitoring during therapy. Qs
- Monitor clients following administration of a neuromuscular blocker for respiratory depression. Have life support equipment available.
- Continue to carefully monitor for return of respiratory function.
- Have a cholinesterase inhibitor available to reverse nondepolarizing neuromuscular blocking agents.

NURSING EVALUATION OF MEDICATION EFFECTIVENESS

Depending on therapeutic intent, effectiveness can be evidenced by the following.
- Muscle relaxation during surgery
- No spontaneous respiratory movements in clients receiving mechanical ventilation
- Absence of seizures in clients receiving electroconvulsive therapy
- Successful endotracheal intubation

Muscle relaxants and antispasmodics

SELECT PROTOTYPE MEDICATION
- **Centrally acting muscle relaxants:** Diazepam
- **Peripherally acting muscle relaxants:** Dantrolene

OTHER MEDICATIONS: Centrally acting muscle relaxants
- Baclofen
- Cyclobenzaprine
- Tizanidine

PURPOSE

Diazepam

EXPECTED PHARMACOLOGICAL ACTION: Acts in the CNS by mimicking the actions of GABA at receptors in the spinal cord and brain to produce sedative effects and depress spasticity of muscles

THERAPEUTIC USES
- Muscle spasm related to muscle injury and spasticity
- Anxiety and panic disorders
- Insomnia
- Status epilepticus
- Alcohol withdrawal
- Anesthesia induction

Cyclobenzaprine, tizanidine

EXPECTED PHARMACOLOGICAL ACTION: Act in the CNS to enhance GABA and produce sedative effects and depress spasticity of muscles. They have no direct muscle relaxant action and so do not decrease muscle strength.

THERAPEUTIC USES: Relief of muscle spasm related to muscle injury

Baclofen

EXPECTED PHARMACOLOGICAL ACTION: Acts in the CNS to enhance GABA, produce sedative effects, and depress hyperactive spasticity of muscles. There are no direct effects on skeletal muscles.

THERAPEUTIC USES: Relief of spasticity related to cerebral palsy, spinal cord injury, and multiple sclerosis

Dantrolene

EXPECTED PHARMACOLOGICAL ACTION: A peripherally acting muscle relaxant that acts directly on spastic muscles and inhibits muscle contraction by preventing release of calcium in skeletal muscles

THERAPEUTIC USES
- Relief of spasticity related to cerebral palsy, spinal cord injury, and multiple sclerosis
- Treatment of malignant hyperthermia

COMPLICATIONS

CNS depression

Sleepiness, lightheadedness, fatigue

NURSING ACTIONS
- Start at low doses.
- Can occur with all muscle relaxants and antispasmodic medications

CLIENT EDUCATION
- Observe for potential adverse effects.
- Avoid hazardous activities (driving) and concurrent use of other CNS depressants, including alcohol.

DIAZEPAM, CYCLOBENZAPRINE, TIZANIDINE

Hepatic toxicity with tizanidine

Anorexia, nausea, vomiting, abdominal pain, jaundice

NURSING ACTIONS
- Obtain baseline liver function and perform periodic follow-up liver function tests.
- Observe for indications of toxicity and notify the provider if they occur.
- Start at a low dose and use only as long as is necessary.

Physical dependence from chronic long-term use

CLIENT EDUCATION: Do not discontinue the medication abruptly.

BACLOFEN

Nausea, constipation, urinary retention

NURSING ACTIONS: Monitor I&O.

CLIENT EDUCATION
- Monitor for adverse effects and notify the provider if they occur.
- Take with meals to reduce gastric upset.
- Increase intake of high-fiber foods.

Seizures

NURSING ACTIONS: Monitor for seizure activity.

CLIENT EDUCATION: Monitor for adverse effects and notify the provider if they occur.

DANTROLENE

Hepatic toxicity

Anorexia, nausea, vomiting, abdominal pain, jaundice

NURSING ACTIONS
- Obtain baseline liver function studies and perform periodic follow-up liver function tests.
- Observe for indications of toxicity and notify the provider if they occur.
- Start at low doses and use only as long as is necessary.

Muscle weakness

Treatment may cause a significant decrease in strength, reducing client's overall function.

NURSING ACTIONS: Monitor for increased skeletal weakness.

CONTRAINDICATIONS/PRECAUTIONS

Warnings
- Pregnancy
  - Diazepam: Contraindicated due to increased risk of fetal malformations
  - Baclofen: Safety not established
  - Dantrolene: Use only if the benefits to the client outweigh the risks to the fetus.
- Lactation
  - Baclofen: Safety not established
  - Diazepam and dantrolene: Contraindicated

Diazepam: Controlled Substance (Schedule IV)

Use these medications cautiously in clients who have impaired liver and renal function.

INTERACTIONS

CNS depressants (alcohol, opioids, antihistamines) have additive CNS depressant effects.
CLIENT EDUCATION: Avoid concurrent use.

NURSING ADMINISTRATION

Provide assistance as needed in self-administration of medication and performance of ADLs. Qᴘᴄᴄ

CLIENT EDUCATION
- Take medications as prescribed.
- Do not stop taking the medication abruptly to avoid withdrawal reaction.
- Avoid CNS depressants while using these medications.

NURSING EVALUATION OF MEDICATION EFFECTIVENESS

Depending on therapeutic intent, effectiveness can be evidenced by the following.
- Absence of muscle rigidity and spasms, good range of motion
- Absence of pain
- Increased ability to perform ADLs

Muscarinic agonists

SELECT PROTOTYPE MEDICATION: Bethanechol

OTHER MEDICATIONS
- Cevimeline
- Pilocarpine
- Acetylcholine

PURPOSE

EXPECTED PHARMACOLOGICAL ACTION: Stimulation of muscarine receptors of the GU tract, thereby causing relaxation of the trigone and sphincter muscles and contraction of the detrusor muscle to increase bladder pressure and excretion of urine

THERAPEUTIC USES
- Nonobstructive urinary retention, usually postoperatively or postpartum
- On an investigational basis to treat gastroesophageal reflux

COMPLICATIONS

Extreme muscarinic stimulation (Poisoning) can result in increased gastric acid secretion, abdominal cramps, diarrhea, sweating, tearing, urinary urgency, bradycardia and hypotension; bronchoconstriction causing exacerbation of asthma, dysrhythmias in clients who have hyperthyroidism.
NURSING ACTIONS: Administer on an empty stomach to reduce effects.

CLIENT EDUCATION: Report adverse effects if they occur. Monitor for bradycardia and hypotension.

CONTRAINDICATIONS/PRECAUTIONS

Contraindicated in clients who have urinary or gastrointestinal obstruction, urinary bladder weakness, peptic ulcer disease, coronary insufficiency, asthma and hyperthyroidism

NURSING ADMINISTRATION

- Administer by oral route, 1 hr before or 2 hr after meals to minimize nausea and vomiting.
- Monitor I&O.

NURSING EVALUATION OF MEDICATION EFFECTIVENESS

Depending on therapeutic intent, effectiveness can be evidenced by relief of urinary retention.

Muscarinic antagonists

SELECT PROTOTYPE MEDICATION: M_3 receptor selective: oxybutynin

OTHER MEDICATIONS
- **M_3 receptor selective:** Darifenacin, solifenacin
- **Nonselective:** Tolterodine, fesoterodine, trospium

PURPOSE

EXPECTED PHARMACOLOGICAL ACTION: Inhibit muscarinic receptors of the detrusor muscle of the bladder, which prevents contractions of the bladder and the urge to void

THERAPEUTIC USES: Overactive bladder

COMPLICATIONS

Anticholinergic effects

Constipation, dry mouth, blurred vision, photophobia, dry eyes, tachycardia, anhidrosis

CLIENT EDUCATION: Increase dietary fiber, consume 2 to 3 L/day fluid from beverage and food sources, sip fluids, and avoid driving or other hazardous activities if vision is impaired.

CNS, cardiovascular effects

CNS effects: hallucinations, confusion, insomnia, nervousness

Cardiovascular effects: prolonged QT interval, tachycardia

NURSING ACTIONS
- Avoid use in older adult clients.
- Monitor ECG.

CLIENT EDUCATION: Report manifestations to the provider. Discontinue medication.

CONTRAINDICATIONS/PRECAUTIONS

- Contraindicated in clients who have glaucoma, myasthenia gravis, paralytic ileus, GI or GU obstruction, or urinary retention
- Use cautiously in children and older adults.
- Use cautiously in clients who have gastroesophageal reflux disease, heart failure, or kidney or liver impairment.

INTERACTIONS

Antihistamines, tricyclic antidepressants, or phenothiazines used concurrently can result in extreme muscarinic blockage.

NURSING ACTIONS: Concurrent use is not recommended.

NURSING ADMINISTRATION

Oral formulations are available as syrup, immediate-release (IR) tablets, and also extended-release (ER) tablets, which minimize anticholinergic effects. Qpcc

CLIENT EDUCATION
- Swallow ER tablets whole and avoid chewing or crushing the tablets. The shell of ER tablets will be eliminated whole in the stool.
- The transdermal patch is administered two times per week. Apply to dry skin of the hip, abdomen, or buttock and to rotate sites.

NURSING EVALUATION OF MEDICATION EFFECTIVENESS

Depending on therapeutic intent, effectiveness can be evidenced by a decrease in urinary urgency and frequency, nocturia, and urge incontinence.

Application Exercises

1. A nurse is teaching a client who has a new prescription for baclofen to treat muscle spasms. Which of the following statements by the client indicates an understanding of the teaching? (Select all that apply.)

   A. "I will stop taking this medication right away if I develop dizziness."

   B. "I know the doctor will gradually increase my dose of this medication for a while."

   C. "I should increase fiber to prevent constipation from this medication."

   D. "I won't be able to drink alcohol while I'm taking this medication."

   E. "I should take this medication on an empty stomach each morning."

2. A nurse is assessing a client who has been taking bethanechol to treat urinary retention. The nurse should identify that which of the following findings can be a manifestation of muscarinic poisoning?

   A. Dry mouth

   B. Hypertension

   C. Excessive perspiration

   D. Fecal impaction

3. A nurse is reviewing the medical record of a client who reports urinary incontinence and asks about a prescription for oxybutynin. The nurse should identify that oxybutynin is contraindicated in the presence of which of the following client's conditions?

   A. Bursitis

   B. Sinusitis

   C. Depression

   D. Glaucoma

Active Learning Scenario

A nurse manager in a surgical center is reviewing nursing responsibilities regarding administration of succinylcholine. Use the ATI Active Learning Template: Medication to complete this item.

THERAPEUTIC USES: Identify two common indications for use.

MEDICATION ADMINISTRATION: Identify two nursing responsibilities regarding the use of succinylcholine.

Application Exercises Key

1. B. **CORRECT:** When evaluating outcomes for client teaching, the nurse should identify client understanding when the clients states they will begin on a low dose, and the dose is increased gradually to prevent CNS depression.
   C, D. **CORRECT:** The nurse should identify client understanding when the client acknowledges they should increase fluids and fiber to reduce the risk for constipation and that due to the fact that the intake of alcohol and other CNS depressants can exacerbate the CNS depressant effects of baclofen, they should avoid CNS depressants while taking baclofen.
   E. The client should take baclofen with meals to reduce gastric upset.

   (N) NCLEX® Connection: Pharmacological and Parenteral Therapies, Medication Administration

2. C. **CORRECT:** The nurse should analyze cues from the client's assessment findings and determine that diaphoresis can be a manifestation of muscarinic poisoning.

   (N) NCLEX® Connection: Pharmacological and Parenteral Therapies, Adverse Effects/Contraindications/Side Effects/Interactions

3. D. **CORRECT:** The nurse should analyze cues from the client's medical record and identify that oxybutynin is an anticholinergic and can increase intraocular pressure. It is contraindicated for clients who have glaucoma.

   (N) NCLEX® Connection: Pharmacological and Parenteral Therapies, Adverse Effects/Contraindications/Side Effects/Interactions

Active Learning Scenario Key

Using the Active Learning Template: Medication

THERAPEUTIC USES
- Endotracheal intubation
- Electroconvulsive therapy
- Endoscopy
- Adjunct to mechanical ventilation
- Muscle relaxation during surgery

MEDICATION ADMINISTRATION
- Clients must receive continuous cardiac and respiratory monitoring during therapy.
- Monitor clients following administration of a neuromuscular blocker for respiratory depression and have life support equipment available.
- Continue to carefully monitor for return of respiratory function.
- Succinylcholine is contraindicated for clients at risk for hyperkalemia (trauma, severe burns).

(N) NCLEX® Connection: Pharmacological and Parenteral Therapies, Adverse Effects/Contraindications/Side Effects/Interactions

Case Study Exercises Key

1. C. **CORRECT:** Candy should plan to generate solutions to address the client's new manifestations by identifying that muscle rigidity and a sudden rise in temperature are manifestations of malignant hyperthermia. They should expect a prescription for dantrolene which acts on skeletal muscles to reduce metabolic activity and treat malignant hyperthermia.

   (N) NCLEX® Connection: Pharmacological and Parenteral Therapies, Expected Actions/Outcomes

2. A, B, C, E. **CORRECT:** The nurse should take actions to address Mr. Rook's malignant hyperthermia by applying a cooling blanket and ice to the axilla and groin, administering oxygen at 100% to treat decreasing oxygen saturation, decrease body temperature by administering iced IV fluids, and monitoring core body temperature to prevent hypothermia and to determine progress with treatment measures.

   (N) NCLEX® Connection: Pharmacological and Parenteral Therapies, Parenteral/Intravenous Therapies

UNIT 2   MEDICATIONS AFFECTING THE NERVOUS SYSTEM

CHAPTER 15 *Sedative-Hypnotics*

Anxiolytics are CNS depressants that induce a sense of calm and decrease anxiety. Hypnotics are CNS depressants that induce sleep.

The three types of sedative-hypnotics are benzodiazepines, barbiturates, and benzodiazepine-like medications. The most commonly used are benzodiazepines and benzodiazepine-like medications because barbiturates cause tolerance and dependence, have multiple interactions, and are powerful respiratory depressants.

IV anesthetics usually are administered during induction of general anesthesia. Most have a quick onset of action and short duration. These medications can be non-opioids or opioids.

Benzodiazepines

SELECT PROTOTYPE MEDICATION: Diazepam

OTHER MEDICATIONS
- Alprazolam
- Lorazepam
- Midazolam
- Temazepam
- Triazolam
- Clonazepam
- Oxazepam
- Chlordiazepoxide
- Clorazepate

PURPOSE

EXPECTED PHARMACOLOGICAL ACTION: Enhance the action of gamma-aminobutyric acid (GABA) in the CNS.

THERAPEUTIC USES ⓆEBP
- Anxiety disorders (alprazolam, chlordiazepoxide, diazepam, lorazepam, oxazepam)
- Seizure disorders (clonazepam, diazepam, lorazepam, clorazepate)
- Insomnia (triazolam, temazepam)
- Muscle spasm (diazepam)
- Alcohol withdrawal (chlordiazepoxide, diazepam, lorazepam, oxazepam)
- Panic disorder (clonazepam)
- Induction of anesthesia/preoperative sedation (diazepam, midazolam, lorazepam)

COMPLICATIONS

CNS depression

Lightheadedness, drowsiness, incoordination

CLIENT EDUCATION
- Observe for manifestations, and notify the provider if they occur.
- Avoid hazardous activities (driving or operating heavy equipment/machinery).

Paradoxical response

Manifestations including insomnia, excitation, euphoria, anxiety, and rage can be seen when administered to treat anxiety.

CLIENT EDUCATION: Observe for manifestations. If manifestations occur, notify the provider and stop the medication.

Nausea, vomiting, anorexia

NURSING ACTIONS: Clients can take with food.

Respiratory depression

Especially with IV administration

NURSING ACTIONS
- Monitor vital signs.
- Have resuscitation equipment available.

Physical dependence

- Withdrawal following short-term therapy manifests as anxiety, insomnia, tremors, dizziness, and sweating.
- Withdrawal following long-term therapy manifests as delirium, paranoia, panic, hypertension, muscle twitches, and seizures.

NURSING ACTIONS: Discontinue medication slowly by tapering dose over weeks to months. Warn clients against sudden cessation of medication. Monitor clients for 3 weeks after discontinuation for indications of withdrawal or recurrence of original symptoms.

Acute toxicity

- Oral: drowsiness, lethargy, confusion
- IV: respiratory depression, cardiac arrest, and profound hypertension.

NURSING ACTIONS
- Oral: Gastric lavage can be used, followed by the administration of activated charcoal or saline cathartics.
- IV: Administer flumazenil to counteract sedation and reverse adverse effects.
- Monitor vital signs, maintain patent airway, and provide fluids to maintain blood pressure.
- Have resuscitation equipment available.

TEMAZEPAM, TRIAZOLAM

Anterograde amnesia and sleep-related behaviors

Sleep driving, sleep eating, impaired recall of events after dosing

CLIENT EDUCATION: Observe for manifestations, and notify the provider if they occur.

CONTRAINDICATIONS/PRECAUTIONS

- **Warnings**
  - Pregnancy
    - Avoid use during pregnancy. Benzodiazepines cross the placenta and have teratogenic effects and can result in neonatal withdrawal syndrome.
    - Diazepam: Increased risk of congenital malformation (cleft lip, inguinal hernia, cardiac anomalies)
    - Triazolam and temazepam: Contraindicated
  - Lactation
    - Triazolam and temazepam: Contraindicated
    - Diazepam: Contraindicated
- Contraindicated in clients who have sleep apnea, respiratory depression, and organic brain disease
- Use cautiously in clients who have a history of substance use disorder, liver dysfunction, and kidney failure.
- Older adults can require decreased dosages. Precautions should be taken when administering benzodiazepines to older adult clients because memory difficulties can result. Ⓒ

INTERACTIONS

CNS depressants (alcohol, barbiturates, and opioids) cause additive CNS depressant effects with concurrent use.
NURSING ACTIONS
- CNS depressants can be hazardous when used in combination with other CNS depressants. Combined toxicity can cause profound respiratory arrest, coma, and death.
- Take complete medication history to identify concurrent use of other CNS depressants.

CLIENT EDUCATION: Avoid alcohol and other CNS depressants.

NURSING ADMINISTRATION

- Ensure proper route of administration.
  - All agents can be given by oral route.
  - IV administration is acceptable with diazepam, midazolam, and lorazepam.
  - Lorazepam is the agent of choice for IM injection.

- When discontinuing benzodiazepines, taper dose over several weeks.
- Administer medication with meals. Advise clients to swallow sustained-release tablets and to avoid chewing or crushing the tablet.
- For insomnia, take 15 to 20 minutes before bedtime. Limit continuous use to 7 to 10 days. Teach client nonpharmacologic strategies to facilitate sleep. Ⓠᴘᴄᴄ

CLIENT EDUCATION
- Take the medication as prescribed and to avoid abrupt discontinuation of treatment to prevent manifestations of medication withdrawal. Ⓠs
- Be aware of possible development of dependency during and after treatment, and notify the provider if manifestations occur.

NURSING EVALUATION OF MEDICATION EFFECTIVENESS

Depending on therapeutic intent, effectiveness can be evidenced by improvement of well-being as evidenced by absence of panic attacks, decrease or absence of anxiety, normal sleep pattern, absence of seizures, absence of withdrawal manifestations from alcohol, and relaxation of muscles.

Nonbenzodiazepines

SELECT PROTOTYPE MEDICATION: Zolpidem

OTHER MEDICATIONS
- Zaleplon
- Eszopiclone

PURPOSE

EXPECTED PHARMACOLOGICAL ACTION: Enhance the action of GABA in the CNS. This results in prolonged sleep duration and decreased awakenings. These medications do not function as antianxiety, muscle relaxant, or antiepileptic agents. There is a low risk of tolerance, substance use disorder, and dependence.

THERAPEUTIC USES: Short-term management of insomnia

COMPLICATIONS

Daytime sleepiness and lightheadedness, headache

NURSING ACTIONS: Administer medication at bedtime.

CLIENT EDUCATION
- Take medication allowing for at least 8 hr of sleep.
- More rapid absorption occurs when the medication is taken when the stomach is empty.

CONTRAINDICATIONS/PRECAUTIONS

- **Warnings**
  - Pregnancy: Can increase risk of respiratory depression in neonates after birth
  - Lactation: Safety not established
- Neonatal flaccidity and withdrawal can occur in infants born to mothers taking nonbenzodiazepine medications.
- Produce sleep-related complex behaviors similar to the benzodiazepines.
- Use cautiously in older adult clients and in clients who have impaired kidney, liver, or respiratory function. ⓠ

INTERACTIONS

CNS depressants (alcohol, barbiturates, opioids) cause additive CNS depression.
CLIENT EDUCATION: Avoid alcohol and other CNS depressants.

NURSING ADMINISTRATION

Administer all agents by oral or sublingual route.

CLIENT EDUCATION: Take the medication just before bedtime.

NURSING EVALUATION OF MEDICATION EFFECTIVENESS

Depending on therapeutic intent, effectiveness can be evidenced by effective sleep pattern.

Melatonin agonist

SELECT PROTOTYPE MEDICATION: Ramelteon

PURPOSE

EXPECTED PHARMACOLOGICAL ACTION: Activation of melatonin receptors

THERAPEUTIC USES: Management of chronic insomnia when falling asleep is difficult. This will not help with maintenance of sleep. Long term use is permitted.

COMPLICATIONS

Sleepiness, dizziness, fatigue

NURSING ACTIONS: Ramelteon is generally well tolerated. Instruct clients to notify the provider if manifestations occur.

CLIENT EDUCATION: Avoid activities (driving) if manifestations occur.

Hormonal effects

Amenorrhea, decreased libido, infertility, and galactorrhea caused by increased levels of prolactin and reduced levels of testosterone.

CLIENT EDUCATION: Notify the provider if manifestations occur. Medication can be discontinued.

CONTRAINDICATIONS/PRECAUTIONS

- **Warnings**
  - Pregnancy: Use only if the benefit to the client outweighs the risks to the fetus.
- Lactation: Contraindicated
- Contraindicated in severe forms of liver disease, depression, apnea, and COPD
- Use cautiously in clients who have moderate liver disease and older adults. ⓒ

INTERACTIONS

High-fat meals can prolong absorption of ramelteon.
NURSING ACTIONS
- Avoid high-fat meals before taking the medication.
- Take medication on an empty stomach for rapid onset.

Concurrent use of fluvoxamine can increase levels of ramelteon.
NURSING ACTIONS: Avoid concurrent use.

CNS depressants (opioids, alcohol) can cause additive CNS depression.
NURSING ACTIONS: Avoid concurrent use.

NURSING ADMINISTRATION

Administer by oral route.

CLIENT EDUCATION
- Take medication 30 min prior to bedtime.
- Take medication on an empty stomach, and avoid high-fat foods before taking ramelteon.
- Avoid dangerous activities (driving and operating heavy machinery).
- The purpose of ramelteon is to induce sleep; it is not prescribed for sleep maintenance.

NURSING EVALUATION OF MEDICATION EFFECTIVENESS

Depending on therapeutic intent, effectiveness can be evidenced by improvement in sleep patterns.

Intravenous anesthetics

Intravenous non-opioid agents

SELECT PROTOTYPE MEDICATIONS
- **Barbiturates:** Pentobarbital sodium, methohexital sodium
- **Benzodiazepines** (used for preoperative sedation): Midazolam, diazepam, lorazepam
- **Other medications:** Propofol, ketamine

Intravenous opioid agents

SELECT PROTOTYPE MEDICATION: Fentanyl

OTHER MEDICATIONS
- Alfentanil
- Sufentanil
- Morphine sulfate

PURPOSE

EXPECTED PHARMACOLOGICAL ACTION: Loss of consciousness and elimination of response to painful stimuli

THERAPEUTIC USES
- Induction and maintenance of anesthesia
- Moderate (conscious) sedation (usually an IV non-opioid agent combined with an opioid agent)
- Intubation and mechanical ventilation

COMPLICATIONS

Respiratory and cardiovascular depression with high risk for hypotension

NURSING ACTIONS
- Provide continuous monitoring of vital signs and ECG.
- Maintain mechanical ventilation during procedure.
- Have equipment ready for resuscitation. Qs

PROPOFOL

Bacterial infection

NURSING ACTIONS
- Use opened vials within 6 hr.
- Monitor for indications of infection (fever, malaise) after surgery.

KETAMINE

Psychological reactions

- Hallucinations, mental confusion
- Children less than 15 years of age and adults older than 65 years of age at a decreased risk

---

15.1 Case study

Scenario introduction

Terry is a nurse in a provider's office taking care of Cameron who has come for a 3-month follow-up.

Scene 1

Terry: "Hello, Cameron. How have you been doing since we last saw you here in the office?"

Cameron: "My headaches are much better since I started on that blood pressure medicine."

Terry: "That is wonderful. Anything new that has been bothering you?"

Scene 2

Cameron: "I just don't seem to be able to sleep at night."

Terry: "Do you fall asleep but wake up frequently?"

Cameron: "No, sometimes I just lay there for what seems like hours trying to fall asleep. Sometimes I just give up and get up and read a book or something."

Terry: "This is something we will discuss with Dr. Smith."

Scene 3

Cameron: "That would be great. I know I would be able to exercise more like the doctor wants me to do if I just wasn't so tired all the time."

Terry: "There are several suggestions I have for you to help with this. We can discuss them while we wait for the doctor to arrive."

Scenario Conclusion

Terry offers a number of suggestions to assist Mr. Shaffer with his inability to fall asleep. Dr. Smith gives Cameron a prescription for zolpidem 5 mg PO daily at bedtime.

Case study exercises

1. Terry is teaching Cameron about his new prescription for zolpidem. Which of the following instructions should they include?

   A. "Limit your alcohol intake while taking this medication."

   B. "Take the medication 1 hr before you plan to go to sleep."

   C. "Allow at least 7 hr for sleep when taking zolpidem."

   D. "To increase the effectiveness of zolpidem, take it with a bedtime snack."

2. Terry is evaluating the teaching of Cameron regarding their new prescription for zolpidem. Which of the following statements by Cameron indicates an understanding?

   A. "I will stop taking the medication if it does not help within 2 weeks."

   B. "I may experience some sleepiness during the daytime."

   C. "I can take zolpidem without worrying about becoming dependent on it."

   D. "I should drink some chamomile tea with this medication at bedtime."

NURSING ACTIONS
- Avoid use in clients who have a history of mental illness.
- Maintain a quiet, low-stimulus environment during recovery.
- Give diazepam or midazolam prior to ketamine to reduce the risk of an adverse reaction.

CONTRAINDICATIONS/PRECAUTIONS

- **Warnings**
  - Pregnancy: Midazolam is contraindicated.
  - Lactation: Midazolam is contraindicated.
- Ketamine is a Schedule III drug because of its potential for misuse.
- Avoid use in clients who have a history of mental illness.
- Use cautiously in clients who have respiratory and cardiovascular disease.
- Midazolam is contraindicated in clients who have glaucoma. Precautions should be taken in children, older adults, and clients who have kidney or hepatic failure, status asthmaticus, or alcohol intoxication.

INTERACTIONS

Additive CNS depression
- Created by CNS depressants (alcohol, barbiturates, opioids)
- NURSING ACTIONS
  - Clients can require lower dose.
  - Provide continuous monitoring of vital signs and ECG.
  - Have equipment ready for resuscitation.

Additive CNS stimulation
- Created by CNS stimulants (amphetamines, cocaine)
- NURSING ACTIONS
  - Clients can require higher doses.
  - Provide continuous monitoring of vital signs and ECG.
  - Have equipment ready for resuscitation.

NURSING ADMINISTRATION

- For moderate (conscious) sedation or for neonatal anesthesia, administer slowly over 2 min.
- Monitor carefully during and after moderate sedation or anesthesia for respiratory arrest or hypotension.
- Inject propofol into large vein to decrease pain at injection site.

CLIENT EDUCATION: Arrange for a ride home following outpatient procedure. Qpcc

NURSING EVALUATION OF MEDICATION EFFECTIVENESS

Depending on therapeutic intent, effectiveness can be evidenced by:
- Surgical procedure occurring with loss of consciousness and elimination of pain
- Postoperative recovery as demonstrated by the following.
  - Vital signs return to baseline.
  - Client is oriented to time, place, and person.
  - Bowel sounds return.
  - Voiding occurs within 8 hr.
  - Nausea and vomiting are controlled.

Active Learning Scenario

A nurse manager is preparing an educational session to review client use of benzodiazepines for the nurses on their unit. Use the ATI Active Learning Template: Medication to complete this item.

THERAPEUTIC USES: Identify five therapeutic uses for benzodiazepines.

CONTRAINDICATIONS/PRECAUTIONS: Identify four contraindications for taking benzodiazepines.

Case Study Exercises Key

1. C. **CORRECT:** When taking actions and teaching the client about taking zolpidem, Terry should instruct Cameron to allow a full night of 7 to 8 hours of time in bed before morning activity.

   Ⓝ *NCLEX® Connection: Pharmacological and Parenteral Therapies, Medication Administration*

2. B. **CORRECT:** When evaluating outcomes of teaching effectiveness, Terry should identify that Cameron understood the teaching by stating that they could experience daytime sleepiness when taking zolpidem. Terry should further instruct Cameron to avoid driving or other activities requiring alertness until they know fully how they will react to the medication.

   Ⓝ *NCLEX® Connection: Pharmacological and Parenteral Therapies, Medication Administration*

Application Exercises

1. A nurse is teaching a client who has insomnia, about their new prescription for temazepam. The nurse should inform the client that which of the following manifestations can be adverse effects of temazepam? (Select all that apply.)

   A. Incoordination

   B. Hypertension

   C. Pruritus

   D. Sleep driving

   E. Amnesia

2. A nurse is teaching a client who has a new prescription for ramelteon. The nurse should instruct the client to avoid which of the following foods at the time of medication administration?

   A. Baked potato

   B. Fried chicken

   C. Whole-grain bread

   D. Citrus fruits

3. A nurse is caring for a client who is to undergo a surgical procedure. Which of the following preexisting conditions can be a contraindication for the use of ketamine as an intravenous anesthetic?

   A. Peptic ulcer disease

   B. Breast cancer

   C. Diabetes mellitus

   D. Schizophrenia

Application Exercises Key

1. **A, D, E. CORRECT:** When taking actions and teaching a client about potential adverse effects of temazepam, the nurse should include the following information. Due to CNS depression, incoordination can be an adverse effect. Sleep driving (driving after taking the medication without memory of doing so) can be an adverse effect as well as retrograde amnesia, the inability to remember the events that occurred after taking the medication.

   Ⓝ *NCLEX® Connection: Pharmacological and Parenteral Therapies, Adverse Effects/Contraindications/Side Effects/Interactions*

2. **B. CORRECT:** When taking actions and teaching a client about foods to avoid when taking ramelteon, the nurse should tell the client that high-fat foods (such as fried chicken) prolong the absorption of ramelteon. The client should not eat high-fat foods with or just before taking ramelteon.

   Ⓝ *NCLEX® Connection: Pharmacological and Parenteral Therapies, Adverse Effects/Contraindications/Side Effects/Interactions*

3. **D. CORRECT:** The nurse should analyze the cues from the client's history and determine that a history of schizophrenia can be a contraindication to receiving ketamine because it can produce psychological effects (hallucinations).

   Ⓝ *NCLEX® Connection: Pharmacological and Parenteral Therapies, Adverse Effects/Contraindications/Side Effects/Interactions*

Active Learning Scenario Key

Using the ATI Active Learning Template: Medication

THERAPEUTIC USES
- Anxiety disorders
- Seizure disorders
- Insomnia
- Muscle spasms
- Alcohol withdrawal
- Panic disorder
- Induction of anesthesia

CONTRAINDICATIONS/PRECAUTIONS
- Pregnancy: Benzodiazepines are Pregnancy Risk Category D (a high risk to the fetus).
- Sleep apnea
- Respiratory depression
- Organic brain disease
- Lactation
- Cautious use in clients who have a history of substance use disorders, liver dysfunction, and kidney failure.

Ⓝ *NCLEX® Connection: Pharmacological and Parenteral Therapies, Medication Administration*

When reviewing the following chapters, keep in mind the relevant topics and tasks of the NCLEX outline, in particular:

Pharmacological and Parenteral Therapies

ADVERSE EFFECTS/CONTRAINDICATIONS/SIDE EFFECTS/ INTERACTIONS: Provide information to the client on common side effects/adverse effects/potential interactions of medications, and inform the client of when to notify the primary health care provider.

EXPECTED ACTIONS/OUTCOMES
Use clinical decision–making/critical thinking when addressing expected effects/outcomes of medications.

Evaluate client response to medication.

MEDICATION ADMINISTRATION: Educate the client on medication self–administration procedures.

UNIT 3 MEDICATIONS AFFECTING THE
RESPIRATORY SYSTEM

CHAPTER 16 *Airflow Disorders*

Asthma is a chronic inflammatory disorder of the airways. It is an intermittent and reversible airflow obstruction that affects the bronchioles. The obstruction occurs either by inflammation or airway hyper-responsiveness leading to bronchoconstriction.

Medication management usually addresses both inflammation and bronchoconstriction. These same medications can also be used to treat the manifestations of chronic obstructive pulmonary disease (COPD).

Medications include bronchodilator agents (beta$_2$-adrenergic agonists), methylxanthines, inhaled anticholinergics, and anti-inflammatory agents (glucocorticoids, mast cell stabilizers, and leukotriene modifiers).

Bronchodilators can further be broken down into short-acting beta$_2$ agonists (SABAs), which are adrenergics or sympathomimetics used for acute symptom relief and long-acting beta$_2$ agonists (LABAs), which are adrenergics or sympathomimetics used for long-term management.

SABAs

- Albuterol
- Ephedrine
- Epinephrine
- Levalbuterol
- Metaproterenol
- Terbutaline

LABAs

- Aformoterol
- Formoterol
- Idacaterol

Beta$_2$-adrenergic agonists

SELECT PROTOTYPE MEDICATION
- Albuterol (inhaled short-acting)
- Salmeterol (inhaled long-acting)

OTHER MEDICATIONS
- Formoterol
- Levalbuterol
- Salmeterol
- Terbutaline

PURPOSE

EXPECTED PHARMACOLOGICAL ACTION

Beta$_2$-adrenergic agonists act by selectively activating the beta$_2$ receptors in the bronchial smooth muscle, resulting in bronchodilation. As a result of this:
- Bronchospasm is relieved.
- Histamine release is inhibited.
- Ciliary motility is increased.

THERAPEUTIC USES

Albuterol, levalbuterol

ROUTE
- Inhaled, short-acting
- Oral, long-acting (albuterol)

THERAPEUTIC USES
- Inhaled, short-acting prevention of asthma episode (exercise-induced)
- Inhaled, short-acting treatment for bronchospasm and asthma
- Oral, long-acting, long-term control of asthma

Formoterol, salmeterol

ROUTE: Inhaled, long-acting

THERAPEUTIC USES: Long-term control of asthma

Terbutaline

ROUTE: Oral, long-acting

THERAPEUTIC USES: Long-term control of asthma

COMPLICATIONS

Tachycardia, angina

Oral agents can cause tachycardia and angina due to activation of alpha$_1$ receptors in the heart.

NURSING ACTIONS: Dosage might need to be reduced.

CLIENT EDUCATION
- Observe for chest, jaw, or arm pain or palpitations, and notify the provider if they occur.
- Check pulse and report an increase of greater than 20 to 30/min.
- Avoid caffeine.

Tremors

Caused by activation of beta$_2$ receptors in skeletal muscle

NURSING ACTIONS
- Tremors usually resolve with continued medication use.
- Dosage might need to be reduced.

CONTRAINDICATIONS/PRECAUTIONS

- **Warnings**
  - Pregnancy: Safety not established
  - Lactation: Safety not established
- Contraindicated in clients who have tachydysrhythmia
- Use cautiously in clients who have diabetes mellitus, hyperthyroidism, heart disease, hypertension, and angina.

INTERACTIONS

Use of beta-adrenergic blockers can negate effects of both medications.
NURSING ACTIONS: Beta-adrenergic blockers should not be used concurrently.

MAOIs and tricyclic antidepressants can increase the risk of tachycardia and angina.
CLIENT EDUCATION: Report changes in heart rate and chest pain.

NURSING ADMINISTRATION

- When a client has prescriptions for an inhaled beta$_2$ agonist and an inhaled glucocorticoid, advise the client to inhale the beta$_2$ agonist before inhaling the glucocorticoid. The beta$_2$ agonist promotes bronchodilation and enhances absorption of the glucocorticoid.
- Formoterol and salmeterol are long-acting beta$_2$ agonist inhalers. These inhalers are used every 12 hr for long-term control and are not used to abort an asthma attack, or exacerbation. These long-acting agents are not used alone but are prescribed in combination with an inhaled glucocorticoid.
- A short-acting beta$_2$ agonist is used to treat an acute episode.

CLIENT EDUCATION
- Follow manufacturer's instructions for use of metered-dose inhaler (MDI), dry-powder inhaler (DPI), and nebulizer.
- Do not exceed prescribed dosages.
- Know the dosage schedule (if the medication is to be taken on a fixed or as-needed schedule).
- Observe for indications of an impending asthma episode, and keep a log of the frequency and intensity of exacerbations.
- Notify the provider if there is an increase in the frequency and intensity of asthma exacerbations.

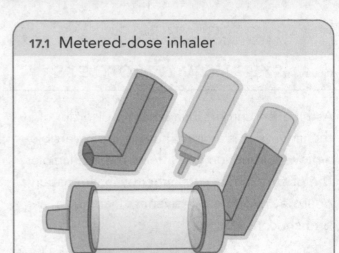

17.1 Metered-dose inhaler

NURSING EVALUATION OF MEDICATION EFFECTIVENESS

Depending on therapeutic intent, effectiveness is evidenced by:
- Long-term control of asthma
- Prevention of exercise-induced asthma
- Resolution of asthma exacerbations as evidenced by absence of shortness of breath, clear breath sounds, absence of wheezing, and return of respiratory rate to baseline

Methylxanthines

SELECT PROTOTYPE MEDICATION: Theophylline

PURPOSE

EXPECTED PHARMACOLOGICAL ACTION
- Relaxation of bronchial smooth muscle, resulting in bronchodilation
- Once the first-line medication for asthma, now used infrequently because newer medications are safer and more effective

THERAPEUTIC USES: Oral theophylline is used for long-term control of chronic asthma or COPD.

ROUTE OF ADMINISTRATION: Oral or IV (emergency use only)

COMPLICATIONS

Mild toxicity reaction can include GI distress and restlessness.

More severe reactions can occur with higher therapeutic levels and can include **dysrhythmias** and **seizures**.

NURSING ACTIONS
- Monitor theophylline blood levels to keep within therapeutic range (5 to 15 mcg/mL). Adverse effects are unlikely to occur at levels less than 20 mcg/mL.
- If manifestations occur, stop the medication. Activated charcoal is used to decrease absorption, lidocaine is used to treat dysrhythmias, and diazepam is used to control seizures.

CLIENT EDUCATION: Periodic monitoring of blood levels is needed. Report nausea, diarrhea, or restlessness, which are indicative of toxicity.

CONTRAINDICATIONS/PRECAUTIONS

- **Warnings**
  - Pregnancy: Safety not established
  - Lactation: Safe for use
- Use cautiously in clients who have heart disease, hypertension, liver and kidney dysfunction, and diabetes mellitus.
- Use cautiously in children and older adults. ⓒ

INTERACTIONS

Caffeine: Caffeine increases CNS and cardiac adverse effects of theophylline. Caffeine can increase theophylline levels.

CLIENT EDUCATION: Avoid consuming caffeinated beverages (coffee, caffeinated sodas, energy drinks).

Phenobarbital, phenytoin, and rifampin decrease theophylline levels.
NURSING ACTIONS: When theophylline is used concurrently with these medications, increase the dosage of theophylline.

Cimetidine, ciprofloxacin, and other fluoroquinolone antibiotics increase theophylline levels.
NURSING ACTIONS: When theophylline is used concurrently with these medications, decrease the dosage of theophylline.

NURSING ADMINISTRATION

CLIENT EDUCATION
- Take the medication as prescribed. If a dose is missed, the following dose should not be doubled.
- Do not chew or crush sustained-release preparations. These medications should be swallowed whole.

NURSING EVALUATION OF MEDICATION EFFECTIVENESS

Depending on therapeutic intent, effectiveness is evidenced by long-term control of asthma and COPD.

Inhaled anticholinergics

SELECT PROTOTYPE MEDICATION: Ipratropium (inhaled short-acting); Tiotropium (inhaled long-acting)

PURPOSE

EXPECTED PHARMACOLOGICAL ACTION: Block muscarinic receptors of the bronchi, resulting in bronchodilation

THERAPEUTIC USES
- Relieve bronchospasm associated with COPD
- Allergen-induced and exercise-induced bronchospasm
- Ipratropium is FDA approved only for bronchospasm associated with COPD, though is often used off-label for asthma and is part of the evidence-based guidelines for asthma management.

ROUTE OF ADMINISTRATION: Inhalation

COMPLICATIONS

Local anticholinergic effects

Dry mouth, hoarseness

CLIENT EDUCATION: Sip fluids and suck on sugar-free hard candies to control dry mouth.

CONTRAINDICATIONS/PRECAUTIONS

- **Warnings**
  - Pregnancy: Safety has not been established.
  - Lactation: Safety has not been established.
- Combination of ipratropium/albuterol is contraindicated in clients who have an allergy to soy or peanuts because the medication preparations can contain soy lecithin.
- Use cautiously in clients who have narrow-angle glaucoma and benign prostatic hyperplasia (due to anticholinergic effects).

NURSING ADMINISTRATION

Usual adult dosage is 2 puffs. Instruct clients to wait the length of time directed between puffs.

CLIENT EDUCATION
- Rinse the mouth after inhalation to decrease unpleasant taste.
- If two inhaled medications are prescribed, wait at least 5 min between medications.
- Do not swallow tiotropium capsules. An inhalation device is used for administration of the capsule.

NURSING EVALUATION OF MEDICATION EFFECTIVENESS

Depending on therapeutic intent, effectiveness is evidenced by the following.

- Control of bronchospasm in clients who have COPD
- Prevention of allergen-induced and exercise-induced bronchospasm

Glucocorticoids

SELECT PROTOTYPE MEDICATIONS

- Inhalation: beclomethasone
- Oral: prednisone

OTHER MEDICATIONS

- Inhalation
  - Budesonide
  - Budesonide and formoterol
  - Fluticasone and salmeterol
  - Fluticasone
  - Mometasone and formoterol
- Oral: prednisolone
- IV
  - Hydrocortisone
  - Methylprednisolone

PURPOSE

EXPECTED PHARMACOLOGICAL ACTION

- Prevent inflammation, suppress airway mucus production, and promote responsiveness of beta$_2$ receptors in the bronchial tree
- Reduction in airway mucosa edema

> The use of glucocorticoids does not provide immediate effects, but rather promotes decreased frequency and severity of exacerbations and acute attacks.

THERAPEUTIC USES

- Short-term IV agents are used for status asthmaticus.
- Inhaled agents are used for long-term prophylaxis of asthma.
- Short-term oral therapy is used to treat manifestations following an acute asthma episode.
- Long-term oral therapy is used to treat chronic, severe asthma.
- Promote lung maturity and decrease respiratory distress in fetuses at risk for preterm birth.

COMPLICATIONS

BECLOMETHASONE

Difficulty speaking, hoarseness, and candidiasis

CLIENT EDUCATION

- Rinse mouth or gargle with water after use.
- Monitor for redness, sores, or white patches and report to provider if they occur. Treat candidiasis with nystatin oral suspension.
- Use a spacer with inhaler.

PREDNISONE

Prednisone when used for 10 days or more can result in the following.

Suppression of adrenal gland function

A decrease in the ability of the adrenal cortex to produce glucocorticoids (can occur with inhaled agents and oral agents)

NURSING ACTIONS

- Administer oral glucocorticoid on an alternate-day dosing schedule.
- Monitor blood glucose levels.
- Taper the dose. Do not stop abruptly.

Bone loss

Can occur with inhaled agents and oral agents

NURSING ACTIONS

- Use the lowest dose possible to control manifestations.
- Oral medications should be given on an alternate-day dosing schedule.

CLIENT EDUCATION

- Perform weight-bearing exercises.
- Consume a diet with sufficient calcium and vitamin D intake.

Hyperglycemia and glycosuria

NURSING ACTIONS

- Clients who have diabetes should have their blood glucose monitored.
- Clients might need an increase in insulin dosage.

Myopathy

As evidenced by muscle weakness

NURSING ACTIONS: Medication dosage should be decreased.

CLIENT EDUCATION: Report indications of muscle weakness.

Peptic ulcer disease

NURSING ACTIONS: Administer with food or meals.

CLIENT EDUCATION
- Avoid NSAIDs.
- Report black, tarry stools. Check stool for occult blood periodically.

Infection

CLIENT EDUCATION
- Notify the provider if early manifestations of infection occur (sore throat, weakness, malaise).
- Avoid large crowds if possible.
- Practice proper hand hygiene.

Disturbances of fluid and electrolytes

Fluid retention as evidenced by weight gain, and edema and hypokalemia as evidenced by muscle weakness

CLIENT EDUCATION: Observe for manifestations and report to the provider.

Additional adverse effects

- Increased appetite and weight gain
- Trouble sleeping/insomnia

CONTRAINDICATIONS/PRECAUTIONS

- **Warnings**
  - Pregnancy: Budesonide and prednisone use during pregnancy has not been established.
  - Lactation: Avoid chronic use.
- Contraindicated in clients who have received a live virus vaccine and those who have systemic fungal infections.
- Use cautiously in children and in clients who have diabetes mellitus, hypertension, heart failure, peptic ulcer disease, osteoporosis, and/or kidney dysfunction.

INTERACTIONS

Prednisone

Concurrent use of potassium-depleting diuretics increases the risk of hypokalemia.
NURSING ACTIONS: Monitor potassium level and administer supplements as needed.

Concurrent use of NSAIDs increases the risk of GI ulceration.
CLIENT EDUCATION: Avoid use of NSAIDs. If GI distress occurs, notify the provider.

Concurrent use of glucocorticoids and hypoglycemic agents (oral and insulin) counteract the effects.
CLIENT EDUCATION: Notify the provider if hyperglycemia occurs. Increased dosage might be needed of insulin or oral hypoglycemics.

NURSING ADMINISTRATION

- Administer using an MDI device, DPI, or nebulizer.
- Glucocorticoid MDIs using chlorofluorocarbons (CFCs) as a propellant are being withdrawn from the market. The new devices using hydrofluoroalkane (HFA) no longer require a spacer to increase drug delivery.
- Oral glucocorticoids are used short-term, 3 to 10 days following an acute asthma exacerbation.
- If the client is on long-term oral therapy, additional dosages of oral glucocorticoids are required in times of stress (infection, trauma).
- Clients who discontinue oral glucocorticoid medications or switch from oral to inhaled agents require additional doses of oral or IV glucocorticoids during periods of stress.

CLIENT EDUCATION
- Use glucocorticoid inhalers on a regular, fixed schedule for long-term therapy of asthma. Glucocorticoids are not to be used to treat an acute episode.
- When a client is prescribed an inhaled beta$_2$ agonist and an inhaled glucocorticoid, inhale the beta$_2$ agonist before inhaling the glucocorticoid. The beta$_2$ agonist promotes bronchodilation and enhances absorption of the glucocorticoid.

NURSING EVALUATION OF MEDICATION EFFECTIVENESS

Depending on therapeutic intent, effectiveness is evidenced by the following.
- Long-term control of asthma
- Resolution of acute exacerbation as demonstrated by absence of shortness of breath, clear breath sounds, absence of wheezing, and return of respiratory rate to baseline

Leukotriene modifiers

SELECT PROTOTYPE MEDICATION: Zafirlukast

OTHER MEDICATIONS: Zileuton

PURPOSE

EXPECTED PHARMACOLOGICAL ACTION: Leukotriene modifiers suppress the effects of leukotrienes, thereby reducing inflammation, bronchoconstriction, airway edema, and mucus production.

THERAPEUTIC USES: Long-term therapy of asthma in adults and children, and to prevent exercise-induced bronchospasm
- Montelukast is used in children as young as 12 months of age.
- Zafirlukast is used in children age 5 years and up.
- Zileuton is used in adolescents and adults.

ROUTE OF ADMINISTRATION: Oral

COMPLICATIONS

Depression, suicidal ideation

More common with montelukast

NURSING ACTIONS: Monitor for behavior changes and report to provider.

Liver injury with use of zileuton and zafirlukast

NURSING ACTIONS: Obtain baseline liver function tests and monitor periodically.

CLIENT EDUCATION
- Monitor for indications of liver damage (nausea, anorexia, abdominal pain).
- Notify the provider if manifestations occur.

CONTRAINDICATIONS/PRECAUTIONS

- **Warnings**
  - Pregnancy: Safety established as safer than zileutron; inhaled glucocorticoids preferred choice of treatment
  - Lactation: Safety not established
- Use cautiously in clients who have liver dysfunction.

INTERACTIONS

Zileuton and zafirlukast inhibit metabolism of warfarin, leading to increased warfarin levels.
NURSING ACTIONS: Monitor prothrombin time (PT) and INR levels.

CLIENT EDUCATION: Observe for indications of bleeding and to notify the provider.

Zileuton and zafirlukast inhibit metabolism of theophylline, leading to increased theophylline levels.
NURSING ACTIONS: Monitor theophylline levels.

CLIENT EDUCATION: Observe for manifestations of theophylline toxicity (nausea, vomiting, seizures), and notify the provider.

Montelukast used concurrently with phenytoin can inhibit effects of montelukast.
CLIENT EDUCATION: Observe for therapeutic effects of montelukast.

NURSING ADMINISTRATION

- Zileuton is given orally and undergoes rapid absorption, both with and without food.
- Zafirlukast is advised to be taken 1 hr before or 2 hr after meals.

CLIENT EDUCATION
- Take zileuton as prescribed, 1 hr before or after a meal.
- Avoid taking zafirlukast with food.
- Take montelukast once daily at bedtime. For exercise-induced bronchospasm, take 2 hr before exercise. If taking daily montelukast, do not take an additional dose for exercise-induced bronchospasm.

NURSING EVALUATION OF MEDICATION EFFECTIVENESS

Depending on therapeutic intent, effectiveness is evidenced by long-term control of asthma.

Application Exercises

1. A nurse is providing instructions to a client who has a new prescription for oral albuterol. Which of the following instructions should the nurse include?

    A. "You can take this medication to abort an acute asthma attack."

    B. "Tremors are an adverse effect of this medication."

    C. "Prolonged use of this medication can cause hyperglycemia."

    D. "This medication can slow skeletal growth rate."

2. A nurse is teaching a client who has a new prescription for beclomethasone by inhaler. Which of the following instructions should the nurse include?

    A. "Rinse your mouth after each use of this medication."

    B. "Limit fluid intake while taking this medication."

    C. "Increase your intake of vitamin B$_{12}$ while taking this medication."

    D. "You can take the medication as needed."

3. A nurse is providing instructions to a client who has a new prescription for albuterol and beclomethasone inhalers for the control of asthma. Which of the following instructions should the nurse include in the teaching?

    A. Take the albuterol at the same time each day.

    B. Administer the albuterol inhaler prior to using the beclomethasone inhaler.

    C. Use beclomethasone if experiencing an acute episode.

    D. Avoid shaking the beclomethasone before use.

4. A nurse is teaching a client who has a prescription for long-term use of oral prednisone for treatment of chronic asthma. The nurse should instruct the client to monitor for which of the following manifestations as an adverse effect of this medication?

    A. Weight gain

    B. Nervousness

    C. Bradycardia

    D. Constipation

Application Exercises Key

1. B. **CORRECT:** When taking actions, the nurse should instruct the client that tremors can occur due to excessive stimulation of beta$_2$ receptors of skeletal muscles.

Ⓝ *NCLEX® Connection: Pharmacological and Parenteral Therapies, Medication Administration*

2. A. **CORRECT:** When taking actions, the nurse should instruct the client to rinse their mouth after each use to reduce the risk of oral fungal infections.

Ⓝ *NCLEX® Connection: Pharmacological and Parenteral Therapies, Medication Administration*

3. B. **CORRECT:** When taking actions, the nurse should instruct the client that when prescribed an inhaled beta$_2$-agonist (albuterol) and an inhaled glucocorticoid (beclomethasone), take the beta$_2$-agonist first. The beta$_2$-agonist promotes bronchodilation and enhances absorption of the glucocorticoid.

Ⓝ *NCLEX® Connection: Pharmacological and Parenteral Therapies, Medication Administration*

4. A. **CORRECT:** When taking actions, the nurse should instruct the client that weight gain and fluid retention are adverse effects of oral prednisone due to the effect of sodium and water retention.

Ⓝ *NCLEX® Connection: Pharmacological and Parenteral Therapies, Adverse Effects/Contraindications/Side Effects/Interactions*

Active Learning Scenario

A nurse is instructing a client who has a new prescription for albuterol PO. What should the nurse include in the teaching? Use the ATI Active Learning Template: Medication to complete this item.

THERAPEUTIC USES

COMPLICATIONS: List two adverse effects.

Active Learning Scenario Key

Using the ATI Active Learning Template: Medication

THERAPEUTIC USES: Beta$_2$-adrenergic agonists act by selectively activating the beta$_2$-receptors in the bronchial smooth muscle, resulting in bronchodilation. They also suppress histamine release and promote ciliary motility.

COMPLICATIONS
- Oral agents can cause tachycardia and angina due to activation of alpha$_1$ receptors in the heart.
- Activation of beta$_2$ receptors in skeletal muscle causes tremors.

Ⓝ *NCLEX® Connection: Pharmacological Therapies, Expected Actions/Outcomes*

CHAPTER 17 # Upper Respiratory Disorders

The medications in this section work on the CNS, nasal passages, or other parts of the respiratory system to treat the effects of allergic or nonallergic rhinitis or coughs from the common cold, influenza, and other disorders.

Antihistamines, often prescribed for allergic rhinitis, are also used to treat nausea, motion sickness, allergic reactions, and insomnia.

Medications in this section are frequently combined for increased effectiveness. For example, an antitussive is combined with an expectorant to reduce a cough.

Antitussives: Opioids

SELECT PROTOTYPE MEDICATION: Hydrocodone

OTHER MEDICATION: Codeine

PURPOSE

EXPECTED PHARMACOLOGICAL ACTION: Suppresses cough through its action on the central nervous system to increase cough threshold

THERAPEUTIC USES: Used for chronic nonproductive cough to decrease the frequency and intensity

COMPLICATIONS

CNS effects

Dizziness, lightheadedness, drowsiness, respiratory depression

NURSING ACTIONS
- Obtain baseline vital signs.
- Monitor clients when ambulating.
- Observe for manifestations of respiratory depression (respirations less than 12/min). Stimulate the client to breathe if respiratory depression occurs. It can be necessary to stop the medication and administer naloxone. Qs

CLIENT EDUCATION
- Change position slowly and lie down if feeling lightheaded.
- Avoid activities that require alertness (driving, operating heavy machinery) while taking codeine.

GI distress (nausea, vomiting, constipation)

CLIENT EDUCATION
- Take oral codeine with food.
- Increase fluids and dietary fiber.

Opioid use disorder

NURSING ACTIONS: Use for a short duration.

CLIENT EDUCATION: Opioids have a potential for abuse.

CONTRAINDICATIONS/PRECAUTIONS

- **Warnings**
  - Pregnancy
    - Codeine: Use with caution, and can cause respiratory depression to newborn.
    - Hydrocodone: Safety not established
  - Lactation
    - Codeine: Contraindicated
    - Hydrocodone: Use only if maternal benefit justifies potential risk to infant.
- Codeine used alone is in the Schedule II class of the Controlled Substances Act. Codeine that is mixed with other antitussives is classified as Schedule V.
- Contraindicated in clients who have respiratory depression, acute asthma, head trauma, liver and renal dysfunction, and acute alcohol use disorder.
- Use cautiously in children, older adults, and clients who have a history of substance use disorder. G

NURSING ADMINISTRATION

CLIENT EDUCATION
- Avoid activities that require alertness, (driving, operating heavy machinery) while taking codeine.
- Change positions slowly and lie down if feeling dizzy.
- Avoid alcohol and other CNS depressants while taking codeine.

Antitussives: Non-opioids

SELECT PROTOTYPE MEDICATION: Dextromethorphan (found in many different products for cough)

OTHER MEDICATIONS
- Benzonatate
- Diphenhydramine

PURPOSE

EXPECTED PHARMACOLOGICAL ACTION: Dextromethorphan suppresses cough through its action on the CNS. Although not an opioid, it is derived from opioids.

THERAPEUTIC USES
- Cough suppression
- Can reduce pain when combined with an opioid

COMPLICATIONS

- This medication has few adverse effects.
- Some mild nausea, dizziness, and sedation can occur.
- There is some potential for abuse as the medication can instill euphoria in high doses.

CONTRAINDICATIONS/PRECAUTIONS

- **Warnings**
  - Pregnancy
    - Dextromethorphan: Safe to use
    - Diphenhydramine: Safety not established
  - Lactation
    - Dextromethorphan: Use with caution.
    - Diphenhydramine: Contraindicated

INTERACTIONS

Can cause high fever when used within 2 weeks of MAOI antidepressants

NURSING ADMINISTRATION

- Some formulations contain alcohol and/or sucrose.
- Available forms include capsules, lozenges (for clients older than 12 years), liquids, and syrups.

NURSING EVALUATION OF MEDICATION EFFECTIVENESS

Depending on therapeutic intent, effectiveness is evidenced by absence or decreased episodes of coughing.

Expectorants

SELECT PROTOTYPE MEDICATION: Guaifenesin

Guaifenesin is an expectorant and has mucolytic properties, so clients should take this medication with a full glass of water.

PURPOSE

EXPECTED PHARMACOLOGICAL ACTION: Guaifenesin promotes increased cough production by increasing and thinning mucous secretions. These actions allow clients to decrease chest congestion by coughing out secretions.

THERAPEUTIC USES: Although guaifenesin is available as an expectorant alone, it is often combined with antitussives (either opioid or non-opioid) or a decongestant for treating manifestations of colds, allergic or nonallergic rhinitis, or for cough caused by lower respiratory disorders.

COMPLICATIONS

GI upset

CLIENT EDUCATION: Take with food if GI upset occurs.

Drowsiness, dizziness

CLIENT EDUCATION: Do not take prior to driving or activities that require alertness, if these reactions occur.

Allergic reaction (rash)

CLIENT EDUCATION: Stop taking guaifenesin and obtain medical care if rash or other manifestations of allergy occur.

CONTRAINDICATIONS/PRECAUTIONS

- **Warning**: Guaifenesin
  - Pregnancy: Safety not established
  - Lactation: Safety not established
- Caution should be taken regarding clients who have asthma because guaifenesin can cause bronchospasm.
- Advise clients who are breastfeeding to talk to the provider before taking medications containing guaifenesin.
- Depending on the formulation and medication combinations, preparations containing guaifenesin might be contraindicated for children.

NURSING ADMINISTRATION

- This medication is available in tablets (which should not be crushed) and capsules, which can be opened to sprinkle on foods.
- Report a cough lasting longer than 1 week to the provider.

CLIENT EDUCATION
- Take doses of guaifenesin with a full glass of water and continue optimal fluid intake throughout therapy.
- Read over-the-counter labels carefully to discover what medications have been combined in the preparation used. Guaifenesin is frequently combined with other medications (antitussives, decongestants) as a liquid or syrup (for example, guaifenesin is combined with the sympathomimetic decongestant, pseudoephedrine).

NURSING EVALUATION OF MEDICATION EFFECTIVENESS

Depending on therapeutic intent, effectiveness is evidenced by the following.
- Cough is more productive, and mucous is easier to expectorate.
- Chest congestion is decreased.

Mucolytics

SELECT PROTOTYPE MEDICATION: Acetylcysteine

OTHER MEDICATION: Hypertonic saline

PURPOSE

EXPECTED PHARMACOLOGICAL ACTION: Mucolytics thin and enhance the flow of secretions in the respiratory passages.

THERAPEUTIC USES
- Mucolytics are used in clients who have acute and chronic pulmonary disorders exacerbated by large amounts of secretions.
- Mucolytics are used in clients who have cystic fibrosis.
- Acetylcysteine is the antidote for acetaminophen poisoning.

COMPLICATIONS

Aspiration and bronchospasm when administered orally

NURSING ACTIONS: Monitor clients for manifestations of aspiration and bronchospasm. Stop medication immediately and notify the provider.

Dizziness, drowsiness, hypotension, tachycardia

NURSING ACTIONS: Monitor vital signs. Advise client to change positions slowly and avoid activities that require alertness.

Hepatotoxicity

NURSING ACTIONS: Monitor liver function tests.

CONTRAINDICATIONS/PRECAUTIONS

- **Warnings**
  - Pregnancy: Safety not established
  - Lactation: Safety not established
- This medication should not be used in clients who are hypersensitive to acetylcysteine.
- Use cautiously in clients who have hypothyroidism, CNS depression, renal, liver disease, and seizure disorders.
- Due to the potential for bronchospasm, acetylcysteine should be used cautiously in clients who have asthma.

NURSING ADMINISTRATION

- Acetylcysteine is administered by inhalation to liquefy nasal and bronchial secretions and facilitate coughing.
- The medication is administered orally or IV for acetaminophen toxicity.
- Be prepared to suction clients if aspiration occurs with oral administration.
- Monitor liver function tests, PT, BUN, creatinine, glucose, electrolytes and acetaminophen levels in clients who have acetaminophen toxicity.

CLIENT EDUCATION: Acetylcysteine has an odor that smells like rotten eggs.

NURSING EVALUATION OF MEDICATION EFFECTIVENESS

Depending on therapeutic intent, effectiveness is evidenced by improvement of manifestations as demonstrated by regular respiratory rate, clear lung sounds, and increased ease of expectoration.

Decongestants

SELECT PROTOTYPE MEDICATION: Phenylephrine

OTHER MEDICATIONS
- Ephedrine
- Naphazoline
- Pseudoephedrine

PURPOSE

EXPECTED PHARMACOLOGICAL ACTION: Sympathomimetic decongestants stimulate alpha$_1$-adrenergic receptors, causing reduction in the inflammation of the nasal membranes.

THERAPEUTIC USES
- This medication can be used to treat allergic or nonallergic rhinitis by relieving nasal stuffiness.
- Acts as a decongestant for clients who have sinusitis and the common cold

COMPLICATIONS

Rebound congestion

Secondary to prolonged use of topical agents

NURSING ACTIONS: Taper use and discontinue medication using one nostril at a time.

CLIENT EDUCATION: Use for short-term therapy, no more than 3 to 5 days.

CNS stimulation

Agitation, nervousness, uneasiness

NURSING ACTIONS
- CNS stimulation is rare with the use of topical agents.
- Stop medication if manifestations of CNS stimulation occur.

CLIENT EDUCATION: Observe and report manifestations of CNS stimulation.

Vasoconstriction

CLIENT EDUCATION: For clients who have hypertension, cerebrovascular disease, dysrhythmias, and coronary artery disease, avoid using these medications.

CONTRAINDICATIONS/PRECAUTIONS

- **Warnings**
  - Pregnancy: Phenylephrine, pseudoephedrine: Safety not established
  - Lactation: Phenylephrine, pseudoephedrine: Safety not established
- These medications are contraindicated in clients who have closed-angle glaucoma. Qs
- Use cautiously in clients who have coronary artery disease, hypertension, cerebrovascular disease, and dysrhythmias.

NURSING ADMINISTRATION

- When administering nasal drops, instruct clients to be in the lateral, head-low position to increase the desired effect and to prevent swallowing the medication.
- Drops are preferred for children because they can be administered precisely, and toxicity can be prevented.
- When nasal spray preparations are prescribed, teach clients regarding their proper use.
- Pseudoephedrine and ephedrine can produce effects similar to amphetamine and are easily converted into amphetamine. These medications are available without a prescription. However, they must be purchased with identification.

CLIENT EDUCATION
- Be aware of the differences between topical and oral agents.
  - Topical agents are usually more effective and work faster.
  - Topical agents have a shorter duration.
  - Vasoconstriction and CNS stimulation are uncommon with topical agents, but are a concern with oral agents.
  - Oral agents do not lead to rebound congestion.
- Use topical decongestants for no longer than 3 to 5 days to avoid rebound congestion.
- Do not exceed recommended doses.

NURSING EVALUATION OF MEDICATION EFFECTIVENESS

Depending on therapeutic intent, effectiveness is evidenced by improvement of manifestations (relief of congestion, increased ease of breathing).

Antihistamines

SELECT PROTOTYPE MEDICATIONS

1st generation H₁ antagonists
- Diphenhydramine
- Promethazine
- Dimenhydrinate

2nd generation H₁ antagonists
- Loratadine
- Cetirizine
- Fexofenadine
- Desloratadine

Intranasal antihistamines
- Azelastine
- Olopatadine

PURPOSE

EXPECTED PHARMACOLOGICAL ACTION: Antihistamine action is on the H_1 receptors, which results in the blocking of histamine release in the small blood vessels, capillaries, and nerves during allergic reactions. These medications relieve itching, sneezing, and rhinorrhea, but do not relieve nasal congestion. First generation antihistamines produce anticholinergic effects and drowsiness.

THERAPEUTIC USES
- Mild allergic reactions (seasonal allergic rhinitis, urticaria, mild transfusion reaction)
- Anaphylaxis (hypotension, acute laryngeal edema, bronchospasm)
- Motion sickness
- Insomnia
- Often used in combination with sympathomimetics to provide a nasal decongestant effect

COMPLICATIONS

Sedation

Common with 1st generation H_1 antagonists

CLIENT EDUCATION
- Take the medication at night to minimize daytime sedative effect.
- Avoid activities that require alertness (driving, operating heavy machinery).
- Avoid consumption of alcohol, and other CNS depressant medications (barbiturates, benzodiazepines, opioids).

Anticholinergic effects

- Dry mouth, constipation
- More common with 1st generation agents

CLIENT EDUCATION: Take sips of water, suck on sugarless candies, and maintain 2 to 3 L of water each day from food and beverage sources.

Gastrointestinal discomfort

Nausea, vomiting, constipation

CLIENT EDUCATION: Take antihistamine with meals.

Acute toxicity, excitation, hallucinations, incoordination, and seizures in children

Flushed face, high fever, tachycardia, dry mouth, urinary retention, pupil dilation

NURSING ACTIONS
- Administer activated charcoal and cathartic to decrease absorption of antihistamine.
- Administer acetaminophen for fever.
- Apply ice packs or sponge baths.

CLIENT EDUCATION: Notify the provider if effects occur.

Respiratory depression and local tissue injury at intravenous site

Promethazine

NURSING ACTIONS
- Monitor client for manifestations of respiratory distress, and have resuscitation equipment available.
- IM administration is the preferred route. If unavailable, administer through a large-bore IV in concentrations of 25 mg/mL or less.
- Monitor for manifestations of extravasation, and advise clients to report any pain or burning sensations.

CONTRAINDICATIONS/PRECAUTIONS

- **Warnings**
  - Pregnancy
    - Loratadine: Safety not established
    - Fexofenadine: Use only if the benefit to the client outweighs the risks to the fetus.
    - Promethazine: Avoid chronic use.
  - Lactation
    - Loratadine and fexofenadine: Safe
    - Promethazine: Safety not established
- Promethazine is contraindicated in clients who have cardiac dysrhythmias, hepatic diseases, and those on MAOI therapy. Promethazine is also contraindicated in clients under 2 years of age.
- Use cautiously in children and older adults (impact of adverse effects, especially respiratory depression). Ⓖ
- Use cautiously in clients who have asthma, seizure disorder, cardiac disease, renal disease, urinary retention, open-angle glaucoma, hypertension, and prostate hypertrophy (impact of anticholinergic medications).

INTERACTIONS

CNS depressants/alcohol cause additive CNS depression.
CLIENT EDUCATION: Avoid alcohol and medications causing CNS depression (opioids, barbiturates, and benzodiazepines).

NURSING ADMINISTRATION

CLIENT EDUCATION: If taking 1st generation medications, be aware of sedating effects.

NURSING EVALUATION OF MEDICATION EFFECTIVENESS

Depending on therapeutic intent, effectiveness is evidenced by the following.
- Improvement of allergic reaction (absence of rhinitis, urticaria)
- Relief of motion sickness (decreased nausea and vomiting)

Nasal glucocorticoids

SELECT PROTOTYPE MEDICATION: Mometasone

OTHER MEDICATIONS
- Fluticasone
- Triamcinolone
- Budesonide

PURPOSE

EXPECTED PHARMACOLOGICAL ACTION: Nasal glucocorticoids decrease inflammation associated with allergic rhinitis. They are the first line of treatment for nasal congestion. By decreasing nasal congestion, they also help with sinusitis in addition to allergic rhinitis.

THERAPEUTIC USE: To reduce the effects of allergic rhinitis including sneezing, nasal itching, runny nose

COMPLICATIONS

Sore throat, nosebleed, headache, burning in the nose

NURSING ACTIONS: Contact provider if adverse effects occur.

CONTRAINDICATIONS/PRECAUTIONS

- **Warnings**
  - Pregnancy
    - Safety not established.
    - Prolonged use or high dosages can lead to complications.
  - Lactation: Safety not established

CLIENT EDUCATION
- A metered-dose spray device is used to administer the medication.
- Administer dose daily, not just when manifestations occur.
- If having seasonal allergic rhinitis, it can take 7 days or more to get the maximum relief.
- If having perennial allergic rhinitis, it can take as long as 21 days to get the maximum relief.
- Clear blocked nasal passages with a topical decongestant prior to glucocorticoid administration.

Active Learning Scenario

A nurse in a provider's office is providing teaching for a client who has a new prescription for guaifenesin. Use the ATI Active Learning Template: Medication to complete this item.

COMPLICATIONS: Identify two adverse effects of this medication.

EVALUATION OF MEDICATION EFFECTIVENESS: Identify two findings that indicate that the medication is effective.

Application Exercises

1. A nurse is teaching a client who has a new prescription for dextromethorphan to suppress a cough. The nurse should instruct the client to monitor for which of the following manifestations as an adverse effect of this medication?

    A. Diarrhea

    B. Anxiety

    C. Sedation

    D. Palpitations

2. A nurse is teaching the family of a child who has cystic fibrosis and a new prescription for acetylcysteine. Which of the following information should the nurse include in the instructions?

    A. "Expect this medication to suppress your child's cough."

    B. "Expect this medication to smell like rotten eggs."

    C. "Expect this medication to cause euphoria."

    D. "Expect this medication to turn your child's urine orange."

3. A nurse is caring for a client who has been taking phenylephrine nasal drops for the past 10 days for sinusitis. The nurse should assess the client for which of the following manifestations as an adverse effect of this medication?

    A. Sedation

    B. Nasal congestion

    C. Productive cough

    D. Constipation

4. A nurse is teaching a client who has a new prescription for diphenhydramine for allergic rhinitis. The nurse should instruct the client to monitor for which of the following manifestations as an adverse effect of this medication? (Select all that apply.)

    A. Dry mouth

    B. Nonproductive cough

    C. Skin rash

    D. Drowsiness

    E. Urinary retention

5. A nurse is teaching a client about the use of fluticasone to treat perennial rhinitis. Which of the following statements by the client indicates an understanding of the teaching?

    A. "I should use the spray every 4 hours while I am awake."

    B. "It can take as long as 3 weeks before the medication takes a maximum effect."

    C. "This medication can also be used to treat motion sickness."

    D. "I can use this medication when my nasal passages are blocked."

Application Exercises Key

1. C. **CORRECT:** The nurse should take actions and instruct the client that dextromethorphan can cause sedation. Advise the client to avoid activities that require alertness

    Ⓝ *NCLEX® Connection: Pharmacological and Parenteral Therapies, Adverse Effects/Contraindications/Side Effects/Interactions*

2. B. **CORRECT:** The nurse should take actions and instruct the client that acetylcysteine has a sulfur content that causes a rotten-egg odor.

    Ⓝ *NCLEX® Connection: Pharmacological and Parenteral Therapies, Medication Administration*

3. B. **CORRECT:** The nurse should plan to generate solutions to assess the client for potential adverse reactions. When used for over 5 days, rebound nasal congestion can occur when taking nasal sympathomimetic medications (phenylephrine).

    Ⓝ *NCLEX® Connection: Pharmacological and Parenteral Therapies, Adverse Effects/Contraindications/Side Effects/Interactions*

4. A, D, E. **CORRECT:** When taking actions, the nurse should instruct the client to monitor for a dry mouth and urinary retention due to the anticholinergic effects of diphenhydramine. The client should also monitor for drowsiness. The medication may be taken at night for this reason.

    Ⓝ *NCLEX® Connection: Pharmacological and Parenteral Therapies, Adverse Effects/Contraindications/Side Effects/Interactions*

5. B. **CORRECT:** When evaluating client education, the nurse should identify the client has understood the teaching when stating that the maximum benefits can take up to 3 weeks.

    Ⓝ *NCLEX® Connection: Pharmacological and Parenteral Therapies, Medication Administration*

Active Learning Scenario Key

Using the ATI Active Learning Template: Medication

COMPLICATIONS
- GI upset
- Drowsiness
- Dizziness
- Rash

EVALUATION OF MEDICATION EFFECTIVENESS
- Cough is more productive, and mucous is easier to expectorate.
- Chest congestion is decreased.

Ⓝ *NCLEX® Connection: Pharmacological and Parenteral Therapies, Medication Administration*

NCLEX® Connections

When reviewing the following chapters, keep in mind the relevant topics and tasks of the NCLEX outline, in particular:

Pharmacological and Parenteral Therapies

ADVERSE EFFECTS/CONTRAINDICATIONS/SIDE EFFECTS/INTERACTIONS

Notify the primary health care provider of side effects, adverse effects, and contraindications of medications and parenteral therapy.

Provide information to the client on common side effects/adverse effects/potential interactions of medications, and inform the client of when to notify the primary health care provider.

DOSAGE CALCULATIONS: Use clinical decision–making/critical thinking when calculating dosages.

EXPECTED ACTIONS/OUTCOMES

Evaluate client response to medication.

Evaluate the client's use of medications over time.

MEDICATION ADMINISTRATION

Titrate dosage of medication based on assessment and ordered parameters.

Educate client on medication self-administration procedures.

Review pertinent data prior to medication administration.

Reduction of Risk Potential

LABORATORY VALUES: Notify primary health care provider about laboratory test results.

CHAPTER 18

Medications Affecting Urinary Output

Indications for medications that affect urinary output include management of blood pressure; excretion of edematous fluid related to heart failure and kidney and liver disease; and prevention of kidney failure.

Medications include high-ceiling loop diuretics, thiazide diuretics, potassium-sparing diuretics, and osmotic diuretics.

High-ceiling loop diuretics

SELECT PROTOTYPE MEDICATION: Furosemide

OTHER MEDICATIONS
- Ethacrynic acid
- Bumetanide
- Torsemide

PURPOSE

EXPECTED PHARMACOLOGICAL ACTION
High-ceiling loop diuretics work in the loop of Henle.
- Block reabsorption of sodium and chloride and prevent reabsorption of water
- Causes extensive diuresis even with severe renal impairment

THERAPEUTIC USES
High-ceiling loop diuretics are used when there is an emergent need for rapid mobilization of fluid.
- Pulmonary edema caused by heart failure
- Conditions not responsive to other diuretics (edema caused by liver, cardiac, or kidney disease)
- Hypertension (torsemide)

UNLABELED USE: Hypercalcemia

ROUTE OF ADMINISTRATION: Oral, IV, IM

COMPLICATIONS

Dehydration, hypovolemia, electrolyte imbalances (hyponatremia, hypochloremia, hypokalemia, hypomagnesemia, hypocalcemia)

NURSING ACTIONS
- Assess/monitor for manifestations of dehydration: dry mouth, increased thirst, oliguria, and lethargy; report findings to the provider.
- Monitor electrolytes.
- If headache or chest, calf, or pelvic pain occur, notify the provider. This can indicate thrombosis or embolism.
- Minimize the risk for dehydration by starting clients on low doses and monitoring daily weights.

Hypotension

NURSING ACTIONS
- Monitor blood pressure.
- Advise clients to avoid sudden changes of position and arise slowly from lying down or sitting.

CLIENT EDUCATION: Monitor for manifestations of postural hypotension (lightheadedness, dizziness). If these occur, sit or lie down.

Ototoxicity

Transient with furosemide and irreversible with ethacrynic acid

NURSING ACTIONS: Avoid use with other ototoxic medications (aminoglycoside antibiotics [gentamicin]).

CLIENT EDUCATION: Notify the provider of tinnitus, which can indicate ototoxicity.

Hypokalemia

K+ less than 3.5 mEq/L

NURSING ACTIONS
- Monitor cardiac status and potassium levels.
- Report a decrease in potassium level (K+ less than 3.5 mEq/L).
- Monitor blood glucose, uric acid, calcium, magnesium, and lipid levels For clients also taking digoxin, monitor digoxin levels closely.
- Report levels outside of the expected reference range.

CLIENT EDUCATION
- Teach client to observe and report manifestations of low magnesium levels (weakness, muscle twitching, tremors).
- Teach clients to consume high-potassium foods (bananas, potatoes, dried fruits, nuts, spinach, citrus fruit).
- Teach clients to observe and report manifestations of hypokalemia (nausea, vomiting, fatigue, leg cramps, and general weakness).

Other adverse effects

Hyperglycemia, hyperuricemia, hypocalcemia, hypomagnesemia decrease in HDL cholesterol levels, increase in LDL cholesterol levels, increase in triglycerides level

NURSING ACTIONS: Monitor laboratory values and report levels outside the expected reference range

CONTRAINDICATIONS/PRECAUTIONS

- **Warnings**
  - Pregnancy: Furosemide safety not established
  - Lactation: Furosemide safety not established
- Contraindicated in clients who have anuria (no urine output)
- Use cautiously in clients who have severe liver disease, diabetes mellitus, dehydration, electrolyte depletion, and gout. Use cautiously in clients taking digoxin, lithium, ototoxic medications, NSAIDs, or antihypertensives.
- Administration to clients who have hypoproteinemia can result in ototoxicity.

INTERACTIONS

Digoxin toxicity (ventricular dysrhythmias) can occur in the presence of hypokalemia.
NURSING ACTIONS
- Monitor cardiac status and potassium and digoxin levels.
- Potassium-sparing diuretics often are used in conjunction with loop diuretics to reduce the risk of hypokalemia.
- Administer potassium supplements as prescribed by the provider.

Concurrent use of antihypertensives can have additive hypotensive effect.
NURSING ACTIONS: Monitor blood pressure.

Lithium carbonate blood levels can increase, which can lead to toxicity, if hyponatremia occurs due to the loop diuretic.
NURSING ACTIONS: Monitor lithium levels. Adjust dosage if needed.

NSAIDs decrease blood flow to the kidneys, which reduces the diuretic effect.
NURSING ACTIONS: Watch for a decrease in the effectiveness of the diuretic (a decrease in urine output).

NURSING ADMINISTRATION

- Obtain baseline data, including orthostatic blood pressure, weight, electrolytes, and location and extent of edema.
- Weigh clients at the same time each day with same amount of clothing and bed linen (if using a bed scale), usually upon awakening.
- Monitor blood pressure and I&O.
- Avoid administering the medication late in the day to prevent nocturia. Usual dosing time is 0800 and 1400.
- Administer furosemide orally, IM, IV bolus dose, or continuous IV infusion. Administer IV bolus doses at 20 mg/min or slower to avoid abrupt hypotension and hypovolemia.
- If potassium level drops below 3.5 mEq/L, monitor the ECG, and notify the provider because the client might require a potassium supplement.
- Initiate fall precautions for older adult clients taking diuretics.
- Monitor for pain in the chest, calves or pelvis and notify provider if these occur.

CLIENT EDUCATION
- If the medication is used for hypertension, self-monitor blood pressure and weight by keeping a log.
- Get up slowly to minimize postural hypotension and monitor blood pressure, and assess for hypovolemia. If faintness or dizziness occurs, instruct clients to sit or lie down.
- Report significant weight loss, lightheadedness, dizziness, GI distress, or general weakness to the provider. These can indicate hypokalemia or hypovolemia.
- Consume foods high in potassium.
- For clients who have diabetes, monitor for elevated blood glucose levels.
- Observe for manifestations of low magnesium levels (weakness, muscle twitching, tremors).
- Observe for manifestations of low calcium levels (muscle twitching, muscle cramps, tingling in hands and feet).
- Report manifestations of ototoxicity (vertigo, ringing, buzzing, or sense of fullness in the ears).

NURSING EVALUATION OF MEDICATION EFFECTIVENESS

Depending on therapeutic intent, effectiveness is evidenced by the following.
- Decrease in pulmonary or peripheral edema
- Weight loss
- Decrease in blood pressure
- Increase in urine output
- Decrease in calcium level

Thiazide diuretics

SELECT PROTOTYPE MEDICATION: Hydrochlorothiazide

OTHER MEDICATIONS
- Chlorothiazide
- Methyclothiazide
- Thiazide-type diuretics
  - Indapamide
  - Chlorthalidone
  - Metolazone

PURPOSE

EXPECTED PHARMACOLOGICAL ACTION
- Thiazide diuretics work in the early distal convoluted tubule.
- Blocks the reabsorption of sodium and chloride and prevents the reabsorption of water at this site
- Promotes diuresis when renal function is not impaired

THERAPEUTIC USES
- Thiazide diuretics are often the medication of first choice for essential hypertension.
- These medications are used for edema of mild to moderate heart failure and liver and kidney disease.
- Thiazide diuretics often are used in combination with antihypertensive agents for blood pressure control.
- These medications are used to reduce urine production in clients who have diabetes insipidus.
- These medications promote reabsorption of calcium and can reduce the risk for postmenopausal osteoporosis.

COMPLICATIONS

Dehydration and hyponatremia

NURSING ACTIONS
- Assess and monitor clients for manifestations of dehydration (dry mouth, increased thirst, minimal urine output, weight loss).
- Monitor electrolytes and weight.
- Report urine output less than 30 mL/hr. Stop medication and notify the provider.

Hypokalemia and hypochloremia

NURSING ACTIONS
- Monitor cardiac status and K+ levels, especially if taking digoxin.
- Report a decrease in K+ level (less than 3.5 mEq/L).

CLIENT EDUCATION
- Consume foods high in potassium.
- Recognize manifestations of hypokalemia (nausea/vomiting, general weakness, fatigue, leg cramps).

Hyperglycemia

NURSING ACTIONS: Monitor for an increase in blood glucose levels.

Hyperuricemia, hypomagnesemia, increased lipids

NURSING ACTIONS: Monitor uric acid, magnesium, total, HDL, LDL cholesterol levels, and triglycerides.

CLIENT EDUCATION: Observe for manifestations of low magnesium levels (weakness, muscle twitching, tremors).

CONTRAINDICATIONS/PRECAUTIONS

- **Warnings**
  - Pregnancy: Use thiazide diuretics with caution because of the risk of jaundice or thrombocytopenia in the newborn.
  - Lactation: Thiazide diuretics are contraindicated.
- Contraindicated in clients who have renal impairment
- Use cautiously in clients who have cardiovascular disease, diabetes mellitus, hypokalemia, hyperlipidemia, hypomagnesemia, and gout. Use cautiously in clients taking digoxin, lithium, or antihypertensives.

INTERACTIONS

- Medication and food interactions are the same as for loop diuretic medication.
- Thiazide diuretics cause no risk of hearing loss and can be combined with ototoxic medications.

NURSING ADMINISTRATIONS

- Chlorothiazide is administered orally and IV; all others are given orally.
- Obtain baseline data, including orthostatic blood pressure, weight, electrolytes, and location and extent of edema.
- Monitor potassium levels.
- Alternate-day dosing can decrease electrolyte imbalances.
- Weigh clients at the same time each day with same amount of clothing and bed linen (if using a bed scale), usually upon awakening.
- Monitor blood pressure and I&O.
- If potassium level drops below 3.5 mEq/L, monitor the ECG, and notify the provider because the client might require a potassium supplement.
- Advise clients to get up slowly to minimize postural hypotension, monitor blood pressure, and assess for hypovolemia. If faintness or dizziness occurs, instruct clients to sit or lie down.

CLIENT EDUCATION
- Take the medication first thing in the morning; if twice-a-day dosing is prescribed, be sure the second dose is taken by 1400 to prevent nocturia. Weigh self at the same time each day wearing the same amount of clothing and notify provider for a weight gain of more than 3 pounds in one day.
- Consume foods high in potassium and maintain adequate fluid intake (1,500 mL/day, unless contraindicated).
- If GI upset occurs, take the medication with or after meals.

- If the medication is used for hypertension, self-monitor blood pressure and weight by keeping a log.
- Report significant weight loss, lightheadedness, dizziness, GI distress, or general weakness to the provider. These can indicate hypokalemia or hypovolemia.
- If with diabetes, monitor for elevated blood glucose levels.
- Observe for manifestations of low magnesium levels (weakness, muscle twitching, tremors).

NURSING EVALUATION OF MEDICATION EFFECTIVENESS

Depending on therapeutic intent, effectiveness is evidenced by the following.
- Decrease in blood pressure
- Decrease in edema
- Increase in urine output
- Reduced urine output in diabetes insipidus
- Preserved bone integrity in postmenopausal clients.

Potassium-sparing diuretics

SELECT PROTOTYPE MEDICATION: Spironolactone

OTHER MEDICATIONS
- Triamterene
- Amiloride

PURPOSE

EXPECTED PHARMACOLOGICAL ACTION
Potassium-sparing diuretics block the action of aldosterone (sodium and water retention), which results in potassium retention and the excretion of sodium and water.

THERAPEUTIC USES
- Potassium-sparing diuretics are combined with other diuretics (loop and thiazide diuretics) for potassium-sparing effects to treat hypertension and edema.
- Administered for heart failure.
- Potassium-sparing diuretics block actions of aldosterone in primary hyperaldosteronism by retaining potassium and increasing sodium excretion, causing an opposite effect of the action of aldosterone in the distal nephrons.
- Therapeutic effects can take 48 to 72 hr.

ROUTE OF ADMINISTRATION: Oral

COMPLICATIONS

Hyperkalemia

NURSING ACTIONS
- Monitor potassium level. Initiate cardiac monitoring for blood potassium greater than 5 mEq/L.

- Monitor electrolytes and for manifestations of hyperkalemia (weakness, fatigue, dyspnea, and dysrhythmias).
- Treat hyperkalemia by discontinuing medication and restricting potassium in the diet. If needed, administer a potassium-excreting diuretic, or administer glucose and insulin IV to drive potassium back into the cell.
- Do not administer potassium supplements or other potassium-sparing diuretics in conjunction with spironolactone.
- Caution is recommended when administered with angiotensin-converting enzyme (ACE) inhibitors, angiotensin receptor blockers, and direct renin inhibitors because these can cause elevated potassium levels.

Endocrine effects

- Deepened voice
- Impotence
- Irregularities of menstrual cycle
- Gynecomastia
- Hirsutism

CLIENT EDUCATION
- Observe for adverse effects.
- Notify the provider if these responses occur.
- Avoid salt substitutes which contain potassium chloride.

Drowsiness, metabolic acidosis

NURSING ACTIONS: Monitor for metabolic acidosis (drowsiness, and restlessness).

CLIENT EDUCATION: Avoid activities that require alertness until effects of medication are known.

CONTRAINDICATIONS/PRECAUTIONS

- **Warnings**
  - Pregnancy: Exposure is associated with fetal harm; wear gloves when handling medication.
  - Lactation: Safety has not been established.
- Do not administer to clients who have hyperkalemia or are taking potassium supplements or another potassium sparing diuretic.
- Do not administer to clients who have severe kidney failure and anuria.
- Use with caution in clients who have kidney or liver disease, electrolyte imbalances, or metabolic acidosis.

INTERACTIONS

Concurrent use of ACE inhibitors, angiotensin receptor blockers, and direct renin inhibitors increases the risk of hyperkalemia.
NURSING ACTIONS: Monitor the client's K+ levels. Notify the provider if K+ is greater than 5.0 mEq/L. Avoid concurrent use.

Concurrent use of potassium supplements, salt substitutes, and another potassium sparing diuretic increases the risk of hyperkalemia.
NURSING ACTIONS: Avoid concurrent use.

NURSING ADMINISTRATION

- Obtain baseline data.
- Weigh clients at the same time each day with same amount of clothing and bed linen (if using a bed scale), usually upon awakening.
- Monitor blood pressure and I&O.
- Monitor ECG periodically.
- Monitor potassium levels.

18.1 Case study

Scenario introduction

Tracy is a nurse on the medical unit caring for Mr. Toll, a recent admission who has gained 7 pounds in the past 4 days and is reporting shortness of breath.

Scene 1

Tracy: "Your provider has written a prescription for you to receive furosemide IV for your peripheral edema."

Mr. Toll: "What will that do for me?"

Tracy: "Furosemide will cause you to urinate more frequently to help you get rid of the extra fluid you have in your feet and legs."

Scene 2

Mr. Toll: "I think this medication in my IV is making me dizzy."

Tracy: "Yes, that is one of the adverse effects of furosemide. That is why I recommended that you use your call light and ask for assistance when getting out of bed."

Mr. Toll: "Yes, I will definitely do that from now on."

Scene 3

Tracy: "While I am here, is this a good time for me to provide you with some information about taking furosemide?"

Mr. Toll: "Yeah, now is good for me."

Scenario conclusion

Tracy teaches Mr. Toll about furosemide, its potential adverse effects, and precautions they should take while taking this medication. Mr. Toll verbalizes an understanding.

Case study exercises

1. Tracy is developing the plan of care for Mr. Toll. Which of the following interventions should the nurse include in the plan of care? (Select all that apply.)

   A. Assess for tinnitus.

   B. Report urine output 50 mL/hr.

   C. Monitor blood potassium levels.

   D. Initiate fall precautions.

   E. Recommend increasing protein intake.

2. Tracy is reviewing the laboratory results from Mr. Toll. Which of the following electrolyte imbalances should she monitor for?

   A. Hypocalcemia

   B. Hypermagnesemia

   C. Hypophosphatemia

   D. Hyperkalemia

CLIENT EDUCATION

- Avoid salt substitutes that contain potassium and reduce intake of potassium-rich foods (oranges, bananas, potatoes, dates).
- Self-monitor blood pressure.
- Keep a log of blood pressure and weight.
- Triamterene can turn urine a bluish color.
- Report cramps, diarrhea, thirst, altered menstruation, or deepened voice.
- Avoid activities that require alertness until effects of medication are known.

NURSING EVALUATION OF MEDICATION EFFECTIVENESS

Depending on therapeutic intent, effectiveness is evidenced by the following.

- Maintenance of expected potassium levels: 3.5 to 5.0 mEq/L
- Weight loss
- Decrease in blood pressure and edema

Osmotic diuretics

SELECT PROTOTYPE MEDICATION: Mannitol

PURPOSE

EXPECTED PHARMACOLOGICAL ACTION

Osmotic diuretics reduce intracranial pressure and intraocular pressure by raising serum osmolality and drawing fluid back into the vascular and extravascular space.

THERAPEUTIC USES

- Prevents kidney failure in specific situations (hypovolemic shock and severe hypotension) because mannitol is not reabsorbed and remains in the nephron, drawing off water, thus preserving urine flow and preventing kidney failure
- Decreases intracranial pressure (ICP) caused by cerebral edema by drawing off fluid from the brain into the bloodstream
- Decreases intraocular pressure by drawing ocular fluid into the bloodstream
- Promotes sodium retention and water excretion in clients who have hyponatremia and fluid volume excess
- Administered for the oliguria phase of acute kidney injury

COMPLICATIONS

Heart failure, pulmonary edema
NURSING ACTIONS: If manifestations of heart failure develop (dyspnea, weakness, fatigue, distended neck veins, and/or weight gain), stop the medication immediately, and notify the provider.

Rebound increased intracranial pressure
NURSING ACTIONS: Monitor for increased ICP (change in level of consciousness, change in pupils, headache, nausea, and vomiting).

Fluid and electrolyte imbalances, metabolic acidosis
NURSING ACTIONS: Monitor laboratory values. Monitor for manifestations of metabolic acidosis (drowsiness and restlessness).

CONTRAINDICATIONS/PRECAUTIONS

- This medication is contraindicated in clients who have active intracranial bleed, anuria, severe pulmonary edema, severe dehydration, and renal failure.
- Use extreme caution in clients who have heart failure, are pregnant or breast feeding, or have renal insufficiency and electrolyte imbalances.
- **Warnings**
  - Pregnancy: Safety has not been established.
  - Lactation: Safety has not been established.

INTERACTIONS

Lithium excretion through the kidneys is increased.
NURSING ACTIONS: Monitor lithium levels.

Increased risk for hypokalemia with cardiac glycosides.
NURSING ACTIONS: Monitor potassium and ECG.

NURSING ADMINISTRATION

- Administer mannitol by continuous IV infusion.
- To prevent administering microscopic crystals, use a filter needle when drawing from the vial and a filter in the IV tubing.
- Monitor daily weight, I&O, and blood electrolytes.
- Monitor for manifestations of dehydration, and increased edema.
- Obtain baseline data, including orthostatic blood pressure, weight, electrolytes, and location and extent of edema.
- Weigh clients at the same time each day with same amount of clothing and bed linen (if using a bed scale), usually upon awakening.
- Monitor blood pressure.
- If potassium level drops below 3.5 mEq/L, monitor the ECG, and notify the provider because the client might require a potassium supplement.
- Monitor for increased ICP (change in level of consciousness, change in pupils, headache, nausea, and vomiting).
- Monitor for metabolic acidosis (drowsiness and restlessness).

CLIENT EDUCATION
- Get up slowly to minimize postural hypotension, monitor blood pressure, and assess for hypovolemia. If faintness or dizziness occurs, sit or lie down.
- Report significant weight loss, lightheadedness, dizziness, GI distress, or general weakness to the provider. These can indicate hypokalemia or hypovolemia.

NURSING EVALUATION OF MEDICATION EFFECTIVENESS

Depending on therapeutic intent, effectiveness is evidenced by the following.
- Normal kidney function as demonstrated by:
  - Urine output of at least 30 mL/hr
  - Blood creatinine 0.6 to 1.3 mg/dL for males and 0.5 to 1.1 mg/dL for females
  - BUN levels 10 to 20 mg/dL
- Decrease in intracranial pressure
- Decrease in intraocular pressure

COMPLEMENTARY THERAPIES

- Taking ginkgo biloba with a thiazide diuretic can cause hypertension.
- Hypokalemia can occur after taking antihypertensives and consuming licorice.

Active Learning Scenario

A charge nurse is reviewing the use of loop diuretics with a group of nurses. Use the ATI Active Learning Template: Medication to complete this item.

THERAPEUTIC USES: Identify two.

COMPLICATIONS: Describe three adverse effects.

NURSING INTERVENTIONS: Describe two interventions for each of the three adverse effects.

Application Exercises

1. A nurse is providing information to a client who has a new prescription for hydrochlorothiazide. Which of the following information should the nurse include?

   A. Take the medication with food.

   B. Plan to take the medication at bedtime.

   C. Expect increased swelling of the ankles.

   D. Fluid intake should be limited in the morning.

2. A nurse is monitoring a client who is receiving spironolactone. Which of the following findings should the nurse report to the provider?

   A. Blood sodium 144 mEq/L

   B. Urine output 120 mL in 4 hr

   C. Blood potassium 5.2 mEq/L

   D. Blood pressure 140/82 mm Hg

Case Study Exercises Key

1. A, C, D. **CORRECT:** The nurse should plan to generate solutions to include in Mr. Toll's plan of care. An adverse effect of furosemide is ototoxicity. Manifestations of tinnitus should be reported to the provider. A decrease in blood potassium levels is an adverse effect of furosemide, and the provider should be notified. The nurse should initiate fall precautions due to dizziness which Mr. Toll reported. He should also be encouraged to use the call light for assistance when getting out of bed.

   Ⓝ *NCLEX® Connection: Pharmacological and Parenteral Therapies, Parenteral/Intravenous Therapies*

2. A. **CORRECT:** Tracy should plan to generate solutions by monitoring for potential electrolyte imbalances. When observing for hypocalcemia, she should monitor for manifestations including muscle twitching, muscle cramps, and tingling in the hands and feet.

   Ⓝ *NCLEX® Connection: Pharmacological and Parenteral Therapies, Parenteral/Intravenous Therapies*

Application Exercises Key

1. A. **CORRECT:** When taking actions the nurse should instruct the client to take hydrochlorothiazide with or after meals to prevent gastrointestinal upset.

   Ⓝ *NCLEX® Connection: Pharmacological and Parenteral Therapies, Medication Administration*

2. C. **CORRECT:** When evaluating outcomes, the nurse should identify that a potassium level of 5.2 mEq/L indicates hyperkalemia. Because spironolactone causes potassium retention, the nurse should withhold the medication and notify the provider.

   Ⓝ *NCLEX® Connection: Pharmacological and Parenteral Therapies, Adverse Effects/Contraindications/Side Effects/Interactions*

Active Learning Scenario Key

Using the ATI Active Learning Template: Medication

THERAPEUTIC USES
- Used when there is an emergent need for rapid mobilization of fluid
- Pulmonary edema caused by heart failure
- Liver, cardiac, or kidney disease
- Hypertension
- Unlabeled use: Hypercalcemia

COMPLICATIONS
- Dehydration
- Hypotension
- Ototoxicity
- Hypokalemia

NURSING INTERVENTIONS
- Dehydration: Assess for dry mouth, increased thirst, low urine output, and weight loss.
- Hypotension: Monitor orthostatic blood pressure and pulse; monitor for manifestations of postural hypotension.
- Ototoxicity: Assess for tinnitus; avoid administering ototoxic medications.
- Hypokalemia: Monitor laboratory values; offer potassium-rich foods; assess for general weakness, nausea, and vomiting.

Ⓝ *NCLEX® Connection: Pharmacological and Parenteral Therapies, Medication Administration*

CHAPTER 19 **Medications Affecting Blood Pressure**

Blood pressure is controlled in a variety of ways with many medications that are used alone or in combination. Guidelines for pharmacological management of hypertension are found in The Eighth Report of the Joint National Committee on Prevention, Detection, Evaluation, and Treatment of High Blood Pressure released in 2013 by the U.S. Department of Health and Human Services.

Angiotensin-converting enzyme inhibitors

SELECT PROTOTYPE MEDICATION: Captopril

OTHER MEDICATIONS
- Enalapril
- Enalaprilat
- Fosinopril
- Lisinopril
- Ramipril
- Moexipril
- Benazepril
- Quinapril
- Trandolapril
- Perindopril

PURPOSE

EXPECTED PHARMACOLOGICAL ACTION: Angiotensin-converting enzyme (ACE) inhibitors reduce production of angiotensin II by blocking the conversion of angiotensin I to angiotensin II and increasing levels of bradykinin, leading to the following.
- Vasodilation (mostly arteriole)
- Excretion of sodium and water, and retention of potassium by actions in the kidneys
- Reduction in pathological changes in the blood vessels and heart that result from the presence of angiotensin II and aldosterone

THERAPEUTIC USES
- Hypertension
- Heart failure
- Myocardial infarction (to decrease mortality and to decrease risk of heart failure and left ventricular dysfunction)
- Diabetic and nondiabetic nephropathy
- For clients at high risk for a cardiovascular event, ramipril is used to prevent MI, stroke, or death.

COMPLICATIONS

First-dose orthostatic hypotension

NURSING ACTIONS
- If the client is already taking a diuretic, stop the medication temporarily for 2 to 3 days prior to the start of an ACE inhibitor.
- Taking another type of antihypertensive medication increases the hypotensive effects of an ACE inhibitor.
- Start treatment with a low dosage of the medication.
- Monitor blood pressure for several hours after initiation of treatment. Qs
- If hypotension occurs, place client in supine position or intravenous fluid may be indicated.

CLIENT EDUCATION: Change positions slowly and lie down if feeling dizzy, lightheaded, or faint.

Cough

Related to inhibition of kinase II (alternative name for ACE), which results in increase in bradykinin

CLIENT EDUCATION: Inform clients of the possibility of experiencing a dry cough and to notify the provider. Discontinue the medication.

Hyperkalemia

NURSING ACTIONS
- Monitor potassium levels to maintain a level within the expected reference range of 3.5 to 5 mEq/L.
- Advise clients to avoid the use of salt substitutes containing potassium.
- Monitor for manifestations of hyperkalemia (numbness and tingling) and paresthesia in hands and feet.

Rash and dysgeusia (altered taste)

CLIENT EDUCATION
- Inform the provider if these effects occur.
- Adverse effects will stop with discontinuation of the medication.

Angioedema

Swelling of the tongue and oral pharynx

NURSING ACTIONS
- Treat severe effects with subcutaneous injection of epinephrine.
- Discontinue medication.

Neutropenia

Rare but serious complication of captopril

NURSING ACTIONS
- Monitor WBC counts every 2 weeks for 3 months, then periodically.
- This condition is reversible when detected early.
- Inform clients to notify the provider at the first indications of infection (fever, sore throat). Discontinue medication.

CONTRAINDICATIONS/PRECAUTIONS

- **Warnings**
  - Pregnancy: ACE inhibitors are contraindicated.
  - Lactation: ACE inhibitors are contraindicated.
- Contraindicated in clients who have a history of allergy to or angioedema from ACE inhibitors, in bilateral renal artery stenosis, or in clients who have a single kidney.
- Use cautiously in clients who have kidney impairment and collagen vascular disease because they are at greater risk for developing neutropenia. Closely monitor these clients for manifestations of infection.

INTERACTIONS

Diuretics can contribute to first-dose hypotension.
CLIENT EDUCATION: Temporarily stop taking diuretics 2 to 3 days before the start of therapy with an ACE inhibitor.

Antihypertensive medications can have an additive hypotensive effect.
CLIENT EDUCATION: Dosage of medication might need to be adjusted if ACE inhibitors are added to the treatment regimen.

Potassium supplements and potassium-sparing diuretics increase the risk of hyperkalemia.
CLIENT EDUCATION: Only take potassium supplements if prescribed. Avoid salt substitutes that contain potassium.

ACE inhibitors can increase levels of lithium.
NURSING ACTIONS: Monitor lithium levels to avoid toxicity.

Use of NSAIDs can decrease the antihypertensive effect of ACE inhibitors.
NURSING ACTIONS: Avoid concurrent use.

NURSING ADMINISTRATION

Administer ACE inhibitors orally except enalaprilat, which is the only ACE inhibitor for IV use. **Q**EBP

CLIENT EDUCATION
- The medication is prescribed as a single formulation or in combination with hydrochlorothiazide (a thiazide diuretic).
- Blood pressure is monitored after the first dose for at least 2 hr to detect hypotension.
- Take captopril and moexipril at least 1 hr before meals. Other ACE inhibitors are taken with or without food.

- Notify the provider if cough, rash, dysgeusia (altered taste), or indications of infection occur.
- Rise slowly from sitting.
- Avoid activities that require alertness until effects are known.

Angiotensin II receptor blockers

SELECT PROTOTYPE MEDICATION: Losartan

OTHER MEDICATIONS
- Irbesartan
- Candesartan
- Olmesartan
- Telmisartan
- Azilsartan
- Valsartan

PURPOSE

EXPECTED PHARMACOLOGICAL ACTION: These medications block the action of angiotensin II in the body. This results in the following.
- Vasodilation (arterioles and veins)
- Excretion of sodium and water (by decreasing release of aldosterone)

THERAPEUTIC USES
- Hypertension
- Heart failure (valsartan and candesartan)
- Stroke prevention (losartan)
- Delay progression of diabetic nephropathy (irbesartan and losartan)
- Protect against MI, stroke, and death from cardiac causes in individuals unable to tolerate ACE inhibitors (telmisartan)
- Reduce mortality following an acute myocardial infarction (valsartan)
- Slow the development of diabetic retinopathy (losartan)

COMPLICATIONS

The major difference between angiotensin II receptor blockers (ARBs) and ACE inhibitors is that ARBs block the actions of angiotensin II and ACE inhibitors block the formation of angiotensin II. In contrast to ACEI, ARBs do not cause hyperkalemia and have much lower risk of a cough.

Angioedema

NURSING ACTIONS
- Treat severe effects with subcutaneous injection of epinephrine.
- Discontinue medication.

CLIENT EDUCATION: Observe for manifestations (skin wheals, swelling of tongue and pharynx) and notify the provider immediately.

Fetal injury

CLIENT EDUCATION: If a client is of childbearing age, use contraception while on this medication.

Hypotension

NURSING ACTIONS: Monitor blood pressure. Advise clients to rise slowly from a sitting position.

Dizziness, lightheadedness

CLIENT EDUCATION: Avoid activities that require alertness until effects are known.

CONTRAINDICATIONS/PRECAUTIONS

- **Warnings**
  - Pregnancy: ARBs are contraindicated.
  - Lactation: ARBs are contraindicated.
  - Reproductive: If the client is of childbearing age, use contraception while taking this medication due to the risk of fetal injury. These medications are contraindicated in clients who have bilateral renal stenosis or in a single remaining kidney because of the risk for kidney injury.
- These medications are contraindicated in clients who have bilateral renal stenosis or in a single remaining kidney because of the risk for kidney injury.
- Use cautiously in clients who experienced angioedema with an ACE inhibitor.

INTERACTIONS

Antihypertensive medications can have an additive effect when used with ARBs.
NURSING ACTIONS: Adjust dosage of medication if ARBs are added to the treatment regimen.

Increased risk for lithium toxicity
NURSING ACTIONS: Monitor lithium levels and adjust dosage.

NURSING ADMINISTRATION

- Administer medications by oral route. Q EBP
- Take ARBs with or without food.

CLIENT EDUCATION
- Medication is prescribed as a single formulation or in combination with hydrochlorothiazide.
- If taken for heart failure, monitor weight and edema.

Aldosterone antagonists

SELECT PROTOTYPE MEDICATION: Eplerenone

OTHER MEDICATION: Spironolactone

PURPOSE

EXPECTED PHARMACOLOGICAL ACTION: Aldosterone antagonists reduce blood volume by blocking aldosterone receptors in the kidney, thus promoting excretion of sodium and water and retention of potassium.

THERAPEUTIC USES
- Hypertension
- Heart failure
- Premenstrual syndrome
- Polycystic ovary syndrome
- Acne in young females
- Primary hyperaldosteronism

COMPLICATIONS

Hyperkalemia, hyponatremia

NURSING ACTIONS: Monitor blood potassium and sodium levels periodically. Do no combine with potassium-sparing diuretics.

CLIENT EDUCATION
- Do not use potassium supplements or salt substitutes containing potassium.
- Monitor and report manifestations of hyperkalemia (paresthesia and tingling of hands and feet).
- Do not drink grapefruit juice when taking eplerenone because this medication requires CYP3A4 isoenzyme to be metabolized. If the isoenzyme production is inhibited when consuming grapefruit juice, then there is risk for hyperkalemia.

Flu-like manifestations

Fatigue, headache, diarrhea, abdominal pain, cough

CLIENT EDUCATION: Report severe manifestations to provider.

Endocrine changes

Gynecomastia, menstrual irregularities, deepening of the voice, hirsutism, impotence

CLIENT EDUCATION: Report severe manifestations to the provider.

Dizziness, fatigue

CLIENT EDUCATION: Avoid activities that require alertness until reaction is known.

CONTRAINDICATIONS/PRECAUTIONS

- **Warnings**
  - Pregnancy
    - Eplerenone use only if necessary, during pregnancy.
    - Spironolactone safety not established.
  - Lactation: Spironolactone safety not established.
- Contraindicated in clients who have high potassium levels, kidney impairment, hepatic disease, or type 2 diabetes mellitus with microalbuminuria. Qs
- Use cautiously in clients who have liver impairment.

INTERACTIONS

Verapamil, ACE inhibitors, ARBs, erythromycin, potassium-sparing diuretics, NSAIDs, or ketoconazole can increase risk of hyperkalemia.
NURSING ACTIONS: Monitor blood potassium more frequently if client must take these medication concurrently.

CLIENT EDUCATION: Monitor for manifestations of hyperkalemia.

Lithium toxicity can occur if it is taken concurrently.
NURSING ACTIONS: Monitor clients on lithium more frequently for lithium toxicity.

Salt substitutes with potassium can increase the risk of hyperkalemia.
CLIENT EDUCATION: Avoid using salt substitutes that contain potassium.

Concurrent use with diuretics increases the risk for orthostatic hypotension.
NURSING ACTIONS: Monitor blood pressure.

NURSING ADMINISTRATION

- Administer orally with or without food. QEBP
- Do not administer with potassium supplements.

Direct renin inhibitors

SELECT PROTOTYPE MEDICATION: Aliskiren

PURPOSE

EXPECTED PHARMACOLOGICAL ACTION: Binds with renin to inhibit production of angiotensin I, thus decreasing production of both angiotensin II and aldosterone.

THERAPEUTIC USE: Relieves hypertension when used alone or with another antihypertensive medication.

COMPLICATIONS

Angioedema, rash, and cough

Angioedema is swelling of the pharynx, tongue, glottis

CLIENT EDUCATION: Monitor for rash and angioedema. Stop medication and notify provider, or call 911 for severe manifestations.

Hyperkalemia

NURSING ACTIONS: Monitor blood potassium periodically during treatment. Do no combine with potassium-sparing diuretics.

CLIENT EDUCATION:
- Do not use potassium supplements or salt substitutes containing potassium.
- Monitor and report manifestations of hyperkalemia (paresthesias of hands and feet).

Diarrhea

- Dose-related
- Seen most often in females and older adult clients

NURSING ACTIONS: Monitor for dehydration, especially in older adults. C

CLIENT EDUCATION: Notify the provider for severe diarrhea.

Hypotension

NURSING ACTIONS: Monitor blood pressure. Advise clients to rise slowly from sitting.

CLIENT EDUCATION: Avoid activities that require alertness until effects are known.

CONTRAINDICATIONS/PRECAUTIONS

Warnings
- Pregnancy: Aliskiren is contraindicated during the second and third trimester of pregnancy. It should be discontinued when pregnancy occurs.
- Advise clients of childbearing age to use contraception and discontinue medication if pregnancy occurs.
- Contraindicated in clients who have hyperkalemia.
- Use cautiously in older adults and clients who have asthma, other respiratory disorders, history of angioedema, diabetes mellitus, renal stenosis, hypotension, or kidney or hepatic disease.

INTERACTIONS

Decreases blood levels of furosemide.
NURSING ACTIONS: Possible need to increase furosemide dosage.

Increases effect of other antihypertensive medications.
NURSING ACTIONS: Monitor blood pressure for hypotension when combinations are used.

Atorvastatin and ketoconazole increase levels of aliskiren.
NURSING ACTIONS: Monitor for hypotension if used concurrently.

High-fat foods reduce absorption.
CLIENT EDUCATION: Do not take medication with foods high in fat.

Increased hyperkalemia with ACE inhibitors, potassium supplements, or potassium-sparing diuretics.
NURSING ACTIONS: Monitor potassium levels and for manifestations of hyperkalemia. Avoid concurrent use.

NURSING ADMINISTRATION

- High-fat meals interfere with absorption. Instruct clients to take at the same time daily away but to avoid high-fat foods at the time of administration. Q EBP
- Available alone or in combination tablets with a variety of other antihypertensives (hydrochlorothiazide, a diuretic; valsartan, an ARB).

Calcium channel blockers

SELECT PROTOTYPE MEDICATIONS
- Nifedipine
- Verapamil
- Diltiazem

OTHER MEDICATIONS
- Amlodipine
- Felodipine
- Nicardipine
- Isradipine
- Nislodipine

PURPOSE

EXPECTED PHARMACOLOGICAL ACTION

Nifedipine

- Blocking of calcium channels in blood vessels leads to vasodilation of vascular smooth muscle (peripheral arterioles) and arteries/arterioles of the heart.
- Nifedipine acts primarily on arterioles. Veins are not significantly affected.

Verapamil, diltiazem

- Blocking of calcium channels in blood vessels leads to vasodilation of peripheral arterioles and arteries/arterioles of the heart.
- Blocking of calcium channels in the myocardium, SA node, and AV node leads to a decreased force of contraction, decreased heart rate, and slowing of the rate of conduction through the AV node.
- These medications act on arterioles and the heart at therapeutic doses.
- Veins are not significantly affected.

19.1 Therapeutic uses	NIFEDIPINE	AMLODIPINE	NICARDIPINE	FELODIPINE	VERAPAMIL, DILTIAZEM
Angina pectoris	✓	✓	✓		✓
Hypertension	✓	✓	✓	✓	✓
Cardiac dysrhythmias (atrial fibrillation, atrial flutter, SVT)					✓

COMPLICATIONS

NIFEDIPINE

Reflex tachycardia

NURSING ACTIONS
- Monitor clients for an increased heart rate.
- Administer a beta blocker (metoprolol) to counteract tachycardia.

Acute toxicity

NURSING ACTIONS
- With excessive doses, the heart, in addition to blood vessels, is affected.
- Monitor vital signs and ECG. Provide gastric lavage and cathartic if indicated.
- Administer medications (norepinephrine, calcium, isoproterenol, lidocaine, and IV fluids).
- Have equipment for cardioversion and cardiac pacer available.

Orthostatic hypotension and peripheral edema

NURSING ACTIONS
- Monitor blood pressure, edema, and daily weight.
- A diuretic can be prescribed to control edema.

CLIENT EDUCATION
- Observe for swelling in the lower extremities, and notify the provider if it occurs.
- Monitor for manifestations of postural hypotension (lightheadedness, dizziness). If these occur, sit or lie down. Can be minimized by getting up slowly.

VERAPAMIL, DILTIAZEM

Orthostatic hypotension and peripheral edema

NURSING ACTIONS
- Monitor blood pressure, edema, and daily weight.
- Instruct clients to observe for swelling in the lower extremities and notify the provider if it occurs.
- A diuretic can be prescribed to control edema.
- Instruct clients about the manifestations of postural hypotension (lightheadedness, dizziness). If these occur, advise clients to sit or lie down. Can be minimized by getting up slowly.

Constipation (primarily verapamil)

CLIENT EDUCATION: Increase intake of high fiber food and oral fluids, if not restricted.

Suppression of cardiac function

Bradycardia, heart failure

NURSING ACTIONS: Monitor ECG, pulse rate, and rhythm.

CLIENT EDUCATION: Observe for suppression of cardiac function (slow pulse, activity intolerance), and notify provider if these occur. Discontinue medication if needed.

Dysrhythmias

QRS complex is widened and QT interval is prolonged.

NURSING ACTIONS: Monitor vital signs and ECG.

Acute toxicity

Resulting in hypotension, bradycardia, AV block, and ventricular tachydysrhythmias

NURSING ACTIONS
- Monitor vital signs and ECG. Gastric lavage and cathartic can be indicated.
- Administer medications (norepinephrine, calcium, isoproterenol, lidocaine, and IV fluids).
- Have equipment for cardioversion and cardiac pacer available.

CONTRAINDICATIONS/PRECAUTIONS

- **Warnings**
  - Pregnancy
    - Verapamil safety has not been established.
    - Use nifedipine only if the benefit to the client outweighs the risks to the fetus.
  - Lactation
    - Verapamil safety has not been established
    - Use nifedipine only if the benefit to the client outweighs the risks to the fetus.
- Nifedipine is contraindicated in clients who are in cardiogenic shock.
- Use nifedipine with caution in clients who have acute MI, unstable angina, aortic stenosis, hypotension, sick sinus syndrome, and second- or third-degree AV block.
- Verapamil is contraindicated in clients who have hypotension, heart block, digoxin toxicity, severe heart failure, and during lactation.
- Use cautiously in older adults and clients who have kidney or liver disorders, mild to moderate heart failure, or GERD. Ⓒ

INTERACTIONS

NIFEDIPINE

Beta blockers (metoprolol) are used to decrease reflex tachycardia.
NURSING ACTIONS: Monitor for excessive slowing of heart rate.

Cimetidine, famotidine, and grapefruit juice can lead to toxicity.
NURSING ACTIONS
- Monitor for indications of toxicity (decrease in blood pressure, increase in heart rate, and flushing).
- Advise clients to avoid drinking grapefruit juice.
- Avoid concurrent use with cimetidine and famotidine.

VERAPAMIL, DILTIAZEM

Verapamil can increase digoxin levels, increasing the risk of digoxin toxicity. Digoxin can cause an additive effect and intensify AV conduction suppression.
NURSING ACTIONS
- Monitor digoxin levels to maintain therapeutic range.
- Monitor vital signs for bradycardia and for manifestations of AV block (a reduced ventricular rate).

Concurrent use of beta blockers can lead to heart failure, AV block, and bradycardia.
NURSING ACTIONS
- Allow several hours between administration of IV verapamil and beta blockers.
- Monitor ECG and heart rate.

Consuming grapefruit juice and verapamil or diltiazem can lead to toxicity.
NURSING ACTIONS:
- Monitor for indications of toxicity (decrease in blood pressure, decrease in heart rate, and AV block).
- Advise clients to avoid drinking grapefruit juice.

NURSING ADMINISTRATION

- For IV administration of verapamil, administer injections slowly over a period of 2 to 3 min. Ⓠᴇʙᴘ
- Teach clients to monitor blood pressure and heart rate, as well as keep a blood pressure record. Withhold medication and notify provider for pulse less than 50/min and systolic blood pressure less than 90 mm Hg.

CLIENT EDUCATION
- Do not chew or crush sustained-release tablets.
- If with angina, record pain frequency, intensity, duration, and location. Notify the provider if attacks increase in frequency, intensity, and/or duration.
- Change positions slowly and avoid activities that require alertness until effects are known.

Alpha adrenergic blockers /sympatholytics

SELECT PROTOTYPE MEDICATION: Prazosin

OTHER MEDICATIONS
- Doxazosin
- Terazosin

PURPOSE

EXPECTED PHARMACOLOGICAL ACTION
Selective $alpha_1$ blockade results in the following.
- Venous and arterial dilation
- Smooth muscle relaxation of the prostatic capsule and bladder neck

THERAPEUTIC USES

- Primary hypertension.
- Doxazosin and terazosin are used to decrease manifestations of benign prostatic hyperplasia (BPH), which include urgency, frequency, and dysuria.

COMPLICATIONS

First-dose orthostatic hypotension

NURSING ACTIONS
- Start treatment with low dosage of medication.
- First dose often is given at night.
- Monitor blood pressure for 2 to 6 hr after initiation of treatment.

CLIENT EDUCATION
- Avoid activities requiring mental alertness for the first 12 to 24 hr.
- Change positions slowly and lie down if feeling dizzy, lightheaded, or faint.

CONTRAINDICATIONS/PRECAUTIONS

- **Warnings**
  - Pregnancy: Safety for has not been established.
  - Lactation: Safety has not been established.
- Contraindicated in clients who have hypotension.
- Use cautiously clients who have angina pectoris or renal insufficiency, and in older adults. Ⓒ

INTERACTIONS

Antihypertensive medications can have an additive hypotensive effect.
CLIENT EDUCATION
- Observe for indications of hypotension (dizziness, lightheadedness, faintness).
- Lie down if these manifestations occur, and change positions slowly.

NURSING ADMINISTRATION

CLIENT EDUCATION
- The medication can be taken with food.
- Take the initial dose at bedtime to decrease "first-dose" hypotensive effect.
- Perform safety measures to minimize effects of orthostatic hypotension/dizziness.

Centrally acting alpha₂ agonists

SELECT PROTOTYPE MEDICATION: Clonidine

OTHER MEDICATIONS
- Guanfacine
- Methyldopa

PURPOSE

EXPECTED PHARMACOLOGICAL ACTION
These medications act within the CNS to decrease sympathetic outflow resulting in decreased stimulation of the adrenergic receptors (both alpha and beta receptors) of the heart and peripheral vascular system.
- Decrease in sympathetic outflow to the myocardium results in bradycardia and decreased cardiac output (CO)
- Decrease in sympathetic outflow to the peripheral vasculature results in vasodilation, which leads to decreased blood pressure

THERAPEUTIC USES
- Primary hypertension (administered alone, with a diuretic, or with another antihypertensive agent)
- Severe cancer pain (administered parenterally by epidural infusion)
- Management of ADHD

INVESTIGATIONAL USE
- Migraine headache
- Flushing from menopause
- Management of Tourette syndrome
- Management of withdrawal from alcohol, tobacco, and opioids

COMPLICATIONS

Drowsiness and sedation

NURSING ACTIONS: Drowsiness will diminish as use of medication continues.

CLIENT EDUCATION: Avoid activities that require mental alertness until manifestations subside.

Dry mouth

CLIENT EDUCATION
- Be compliant with medication regimen.
- Dry mouth usually resolves in 2 to 4 weeks.
- Chew gum or suck on hard candy, and take small amounts of water or ice chips.

Rebound hypertension if abruptly discontinued

NURSING ACTIONS: Discontinue clonidine gradually over 2 to 4 days.

CLIENT EDUCATION: Do not discontinue treatment without consulting the provider.

CONTRAINDICATIONS/PRECAUTIONS

- **Warnings**
  - Pregnancy
    - Clonidine safety has not been established.
    - Methyldopa safe for use during pregnancy.
  - Lactation
    - Clonidine safety has not been established.
    - Methyldopa safe for lactation
- Avoid use of transdermal patch on affected skin in scleroderma and systemic lupus erythematosus.
- Contraindicated in clients who have a bleeding disorder or are on anticoagulants.
- Use cautiously in clients who have had a stroke, asthma, COPD, recent MI, diabetes mellitus, major depressive disorder, or chronic kidney disease.

INTERACTIONS

Antihypertensive medications can have an additive hypotensive effect.
CLIENT EDUCATION
- Observe for manifestations of hypotension (dizziness, lightheadedness, faintness).
- Lie down if feeling dizzy, lightheaded, or faint, and change positions slowly.

Concurrent use of prazosin, MAOIs, and tricyclic antidepressants can counteract the antihypertensive effect of clonidine.
NURSING ACTIONS: Monitor clients for therapeutic effect. Monitor blood pressure. Do not use concurrently.

Additive CNS depression can occur with concurrent use of other CNS depressants (alcohol).
CLIENT EDUCATION: Be aware of additive CNS depression with alcohol, and avoid use.

NURSING ADMINISTRATION

- Administer medication by oral, epidural, and transdermal routes (clonidine only).
- Medication is usually administered twice a day in divided doses. Take larger dose at bedtime to decrease the occurrence of daytime sleepiness. QEBP
- Transdermal patches are applied every seven days. Advise clients to apply patch on hairless, intact skin on torso or upper arm.

Beta adrenergic blockers (sympatholytics)

SELECT PROTOTYPE MEDICATIONS

Cardioselective: Beta₁ (affects only the heart)
- Metoprolol
- Atenolol
- Esmolol

Nonselective: Beta₁ and beta₂ (affecting both the heart and lungs)
- Propranolol
- Nadolol

Alpha and beta blockers
- Carvedilol
- Labetalol

PURPOSE

EXPECTED PHARMACOLOGICAL ACTION
- In cardiac conditions, the primary effects of beta-adrenergic blockers are a result of beta₁ adrenergic blockade in the myocardium and in the electrical conduction system of the heart.
- Decreased heart rate (negative chronotropic [rate] action).
- Decreased myocardial contractility (negative inotropic [force] action); decreases cardiac output.
- Decreased rate of conduction through the AV node (negative dromotropic action).
- Alpha blockade adds vasodilation (carvedilol and labetalol).
- Reduces release of renin which decreases angiotensin II and causes vasodilation and promotes excretion of sodium and water.

THERAPEUTIC USES
- Primary hypertension (exact mechanism unknown: long-term use causes reduction in peripheral vascular resistance).
- Angina, tachydysrhythmias, heart failure, and myocardial infarction.
- Suppresses reflex tachycardia due to vasodilators. Other uses can include treatment of hyperthyroidism, migraine headache, pheochromocytoma, and glaucoma.

COMPLICATIONS

BETA₁ BLOCKADE: METOPROLOL, PROPRANOLOL

Bradycardia

NURSING ACTIONS
- Monitor pulse. If below 50/min, hold medication and notify the provider.
- Use cautiously in clients who have diabetes mellitus. This medication can mask tachycardia, an early manifestation of low blood glucose. Advise clients to monitor blood glucose to detect hypoglycemia.

Decreased cardiac output

NURSING ACTIONS
- Use cautiously with clients who have heart failure. Doses are started very low and titrated to the desired level.
- Advise clients to observe for manifestations of worsening heart failure (shortness of breath, edema, weight gain, fatigue).
- Notify the provider if manifestations occur.

AV block

NURSING ACTIONS: Obtain a baseline ECG and monitor.

Orthostatic hypotension

CLIENT EDUCATION
- Sit or lie down if experiencing dizziness or faintness.
- Avoid sudden changes of position and rise slowly.

Rebound myocardium excitation

NURSING ACTIONS
- The myocardium becomes sensitized to catecholamines with long-term use of beta blockers.
- Discontinue use of beta blockers over 1 to 2 weeks.

CLIENT EDUCATION: Do not stop taking beta blockers abruptly, but follow the provider's instructions.

BETA$_2$ BLOCKADE: PROPRANOLOL

Bronchoconstriction

NURSING ACTIONS
- Avoid in clients who have asthma.
- Clients who have asthma should receive a beta$_1$ selective agent.

Glycogenolysis is inhibited

NURSING ACTIONS
- Clients who have diabetes mellitus are at increased risk for harm from hypoglycemia because the process of converting glycogen into glucose is impaired. Risk is further increased by beta blockade of tachycardia, a manifestation of hypoglycemia.
- Clients who have diabetes mellitus receive a beta$_1$ selective agent.

CONTRAINDICATIONS/PRECAUTIONS

- **Warnings**
  ○ Pregnancy: Use metoprolol, propranolol, and labetalol with caution because it can cross the placenta.
  ○ Lactation
    ▪ Propranolol: Appears in breast milk and bottle-feeding with formula is recommended.
    ▪ Metoprolol: Safety has not been established.
    ▪ Labetalol: Safe for lactation.
- Contraindicated in clients who have AV block and sinus bradycardia. Qs

- Nonselective beta-adrenergic blockers are contraindicated in clients who have asthma, bronchospasm, and heart failure.
- Use cardioselective beta-adrenergic blockers cautiously in clients who have asthma.
- In general, use beta-adrenergic blockers cautiously in clients who have myasthenia gravis, hypotension, peripheral vascular disease, diabetes mellitus, depression, in older adults and those who have a history of severe allergies. ©

INTERACTIONS

BETA$_1$ BLOCKADE: METOPROLOL, PROPRANOLOL

Calcium channel blockers (CCB) verapamil and diltiazem intensify the effects of beta blockers
- Decreased heart rate
- Decreased myocardial contractility
- Decreased rate of conduction through the AV node
- NURSING ACTIONS
  ○ Monitor ECG and blood pressure.
  ○ Monitor clients closely if taking a CCB and beta blocker concurrently. Reduce dose if needed.

Concurrent use of antihypertensive medications with beta blockers can intensify the hypotensive effect of both medications.
NURSING ACTIONS: Monitor for a drop in blood pressure.

BETA$_2$ BLOCKADE: PROPRANOLOL

Propranolol use can mask the hypoglycemic effect of insulin and prevent the breakdown of fat in response to hypoglycemia.
NURSING ACTIONS: Monitor blood glucose levels.

NURSING ADMINISTRATION

- Administer medications orally, usually once or twice a day.
- Atenolol, metoprolol, labetalol, and propranolol can be administered by the IV route.
- Take with food to increase absorption.

CLIENT EDUCATION
- Do not discontinue medication without consulting the provider.
- Avoid sudden changes in position to prevent occurrence of orthostatic hypotension.
- Do not crush or chew extended-release tablets.
- Self-monitor heart rate and blood pressure at home on a daily basis.

NURSING EVALUATION OF MEDICATION EFFECTIVENESS

Depending on therapeutic intent, effectiveness is evidenced by the following.
- Absence of chest pain
- Absence of cardiac dysrhythmias
- Normotensive blood pressure readings
- Control of heart failure manifestations

Medications for hypertensive crisis

SELECT PROTOTYPE MEDICATION: Nitroprusside (centrally-acting vasodilator)

OTHER MEDICATIONS
- Nitroglycerin (vasodilator)
- Nicardipine (calcium channel blocker)
- Clevidipine (calcium channel blocker)
- Enalaprilat (ACE inhibitor)
- Esmolol (beta blocker)
- Labetalol (beta blocker)

PURPOSE

EXPECTED PHARMACOLOGICAL ACTION: Direct vasodilation of arteries and veins resulting in rapid reduction of blood pressure (decreased preload and afterload)

THERAPEUTIC USES: Hypertensive crisis

COMPLICATIONS

Excessive hypotension

NURSING ACTIONS
- Administer medication slowly because rapid administration will cause blood pressure to go down rapidly.
- Monitor blood pressure and ECG continuously.
- Keep client supine during administration. QEBP

Cyanide poisoning/thiocyanate toxicity

- Headache and drowsiness, and can lead to cardiac arrest
- Nitroprusside only

NURSING ACTIONS
- Clients who have liver dysfunction are at increased risk.
- Risk of cyanide poisoning is reduced by administering medication for no longer than 3 days, and at a rate of 5 mcg/kg/min or less. Avoid prolonged use of nitroprusside.
- Manifestations include weakness, disorientation and delirium. Administer thiosulfate to reverse effects.
- Monitor plasma levels if used for more than 3 days. Level should be maintained at less than 10 mg/dL.
- Discontinue medication if cyanide toxicity occurs.

Bradycardia, tachycardia, ECG changes

NURSING ACTIONS: Monitor ECG for changes

CONTRAINDICATIONS/PRECAUTIONS

- **Warnings**
  - Pregnancy: Nitroprusside safety has not been established.
  - Lactation: Nitroprusside safety has not been established.
- Contraindicated in clients who have heart failure with reduced peripheral vascular resistance, or an AV shunt. Ⓖ
- Use cautiously in clients who have liver and kidney disease, hypothyroidism, hypovolemia, or fluid and electrolyte imbalances, and in older adults.

INTERACTIONS

Do not administer nitroprusside in the same infusion as any other medication.

NURSING ADMINISTRATION

- Prepare medication by adding to diluent for IV infusion.
- Note color of solution. Solution can be light brown in color. Discard solution of any other color. QEBP
- Protect IV container and tubing from light.
- Discard medication after 24 hr.
- Monitor vital signs and ECG continuously.

NURSING EVALUATION OF MEDICATION EFFECTIVENESS

Depending on therapeutic intent, effectiveness is evidenced by the following.
- Decrease in blood pressure and maintenance of normotensive blood pressure.
- Improvement of heart failure (ability to perform activities of daily living, improved breath sounds, and absence of edema).

Application Exercises

1. A nurse is caring for a client who has a new prescription for captopril for hypertension. The nurse should monitor the client for which of the following as an adverse effect of this medication?

   A. Hypokalemia

   B. Hypernatremia

   C. Neutropenia

   D. Bradycardia

2. A nurse is planning to administer a first dose of captopril to a client who has hypertension. Which of the following medications can intensify first dose hypotension? (Select all that apply.)

   A. Simvastatin

   B. Hydrochlorothiazide

   C. Phenytoin

   D. Clonidine

   E. Aliskiren

3. A nurse is teaching a client who has a new prescription for verapamil to control hypertension. Which of the following instructions should the nurse include?

   A. Increase the amount of fiber in the diet.

   B. Drink grapefruit juice daily to increase vitamin C intake.

   C. Decrease the amount of calcium in the diet.

   D. Withhold food for 1 hr after the medication is taken.

4. A nurse is reviewing the medical record of a client who asks about using propranolol to treat hypertension. The nurse should recognize which of the following conditions is a contraindication for taking propranolol?

   A. Asthma

   B. Glaucoma

   C. Hypertension

   D. Tachycardia

5. A nurse is caring for a client who is receiving IV nitroprusside for hypertensive crisis. Which of the following conditions should the nurse monitor as an adverse effect of this medication?

   A. Intestinal ileus

   B. Neutropenia

   C. Delirium

   D. Hyperthermia

Active Learning Scenario

A nurse in an outpatient facility is teaching a client who has a new prescription for aliskiren to treat hypertension. What should the nurse teach the client about this medication? Use the ATI Active Learning Template: Medication to complete this item.

THERAPEUTIC USES: Identify the therapeutic use for aliskiren.

COMPLICATIONS: List two adverse effects of this medication.

NURSING INTERVENTIONS: Describe one test to monitor.

CLIENT EDUCATION: Identify two teaching points.

Active Learning Scenario Key

Using the ATI Active Learning Template: Medication

THERAPEUTIC USES: Aliskiren binds with renin to inhibit production of angiotensin I, thus decreasing production of both angiotensin II and aldosterone. Aliskiren is used solely for treating hypertension alone or in combination with other antihypertensives.

COMPLICATIONS
- Diarrhea: dose-related, occurs most frequently in females and older adult clients
- Risk for angioedema and rash caused by allergy to the medication
- Hyperkalemia
- Hypotension

NURSING INTERVENTIONS: Monitor blood electrolytes, paying close attention to potassium levels, because the client is at risk for hyperkalemia. This is especially important when the client takes ACE inhibitors concurrently, because these medications also raise potassium levels.

CLIENT EDUCATION
- Do not take aliskiren with foods high in fat, which decreases absorption of the medication.
- Do not take potassium supplements or salt substitutes containing potassium.
- Clients should not take aliskiren during pregnancy.
- If a rash or angioedema occurs, discontinue aliskiren and notify the provider.
- Call 911 if severe manifestations of allergy are present.

(N) *NCLEX® Connection: Pharmacological and Parenteral Therapies, Medication Administration*

Application Exercises Key

1. C. **CORRECT:** The nurse should analyze the findings and determine that the priority hypothesis is that the client is at risk for developing neutropenia which can be a serious adverse effect for clients taking an ACE inhibitor. Monitor the client's CBC and teach the client to report indications of infection to the provider.

(N) *NCLEX® Connection: Pharmacological and Parenteral Therapies, Adverse Effects/Contraindications/Side Effects/Interactions*

2. B. **CORRECT:** The nurse should plan to generate solutions to identify the medications that can affect the client's first-time taking captopril. These can include the following medications. Hydrochlorothiazide, a thiazide diuretic, is often used to treat hypertension. Diuretics can intensify first-dose orthostatic hypotension caused by captopril and can continue to interact with antihypertensive medications to cause hypotension. Monitor clients carefully for hypotension, especially after the first dose of captopril and keep the client safe from injury.
   D. **CORRECT:** Clonidine, a centrally acting alpha2 agonist, is an antihypertensive medication that can interact with captopril to intensify first-dose orthostatic hypotension.
   E. **CORRECT:** Aliskiren, a direct renin inhibitor, is an antihypertensive medication that can interact with captopril to intensify its first-dose orthostatic hypotension.

(N) *NCLEX® Connection: Pharmacological and Parenteral Therapies, Adverse Effects/Contraindications/Side Effects/Interactions*

3. A. **CORRECT:** When taking actions, the nurse should instruct the client that increasing dietary fiber intake can help prevent constipation, an adverse effect of verapamil.

(N) *NCLEX® Connection: Pharmacological and Parenteral Therapies, Medication Administration*

4. A. **CORRECT:** The nurse should analyze the cues from the client's medical record and determine that propranolol is a nonselective beta-adrenergic blocker that blocks both beta1 and beta2 receptors. Blockade of beta2 receptors in the lungs causes bronchoconstriction, so it is contraindicated in clients who have asthma.

(N) *NCLEX® Connection: Pharmacological and Parenteral Therapies, Adverse Effects/Contraindications/Side Effects/Interactions*

5. C. **CORRECT:** The nurse should analyze the findings and determine that the client is at risk for developing delirium. This and other mental status changes can occur in thiocyanate toxicity when IV nitroprusside is infused at a high dosage. The nurse should monitor thiocyanate level during therapy to remain below 10 mg/dL.

(N) *NCLEX® Connection: Pharmacological and Parenteral Therapies, Parenteral/Intravenous Therapies*

UNIT 4   MEDICATIONS AFFECTING THE
          CARDIOVASCULAR SYSTEM

CHAPTER 20 *Cardiac Glycosides*
            and Heart Failure

Heart failure results from inadequate pumping of the heart muscle with manifestations caused by the heart's inability to meet the circulation needs of the whole body. Decreased tissue perfusion results in fatigue, shortness of breath, weakness, and activity intolerance.

Heart failure causes a reduction in cardiac output (CO) and affects heart rate, stroke volume (SV), preload, and afterload. There are two types of heart failure: left-sided (with pulmonary manifestations [dyspnea, cough, and oliguria]) and right-sided (systemic congestion with peripheral edema, jugular vein distention, weight gain).

Diuretics, ACE inhibitors, angiotensin II receptor blockers (ARBs), and beta-adrenergic blockers are the medications of choice for treatment of heart failure. Cardiac glycosides are indicated if these medications are unable to control manifestations.

Cardiac glycosides

SELECT PROTOTYPE MEDICATION: Digoxin

PURPOSE

EXPECTED PHARMACOLOGICAL ACTION

Positive inotropic effect: increased force of myocardial contraction
• Increased force and efficiency of myocardial contraction improves the heart's effectiveness as a pump, improving stroke volume and cardiac output.

Negative chronotropic effect: decreased heart rate
• At therapeutic levels, digoxin slows the rate of sinoatrial (SA) node depolarization and the rate of impulses through the conduction system of the heart.
• A decreased heart rate gives the ventricles more time to fill with blood coming from the atria, which leads to increased SV and increased CO.

THERAPEUTIC USES

As a second-line medication
• Treatment of heart failure. Use with caution in female clients, due to the increased risk of life shortening events.
• Dysrhythmias (atrial fibrillation)
• Can reduce manifestations, but does not prolong life

COMPLICATIONS

Dysrhythmias, cardiotoxicity

• Dysrhythmias caused by interfering with the electrical conduction in the myocardium)
• Cardiotoxicity leading to bradycardia
• Conditions that increase the risk of developing digoxin-induced dysrhythmias include hypokalemia, increased blood digoxin levels, and heart disease. Older adult clients are particularly at risk. Ⓖ

NURSING ACTIONS
• Monitor blood levels of K+ to maintain a level between 3.5 to 5.0 mEq/L.
• Monitor digoxin level. Optimal therapeutic level 0.5–0.8 ng/mL. Obtain blood specimen at least 6-8 after the last dose, preferably just before the next scheduled dose.
• Therapeutic blood levels can vary between conditions and clients. Consider manifestations and digoxin level when toxicity is suspected.
• Dosages should be based on blood levels and client response to medication.

CLIENT EDUCATION
• Report manifestations of hypokalemia (nausea/vomiting, general weakness). Potassium supplements can be prescribed if clients are concurrently taking a potassium-depleting diuretic. If diuretic therapy causes potassium levels to fall, a potassium-sparing diuretic (such as spironolactone) can be prescribed.
• Consume high-potassium foods (green leafy vegetables, bananas, potatoes).
• Monitor pulse rate and recognize and report changes (irregular rate with early or extra beats). Teach client to monitor apical pulse.

GI effects

Include anorexia (usually the first manifestation of toxicity), nausea, vomiting, and abdominal pain

CLIENT EDUCATION: Monitor for these effects and report to the provider if they occur.

CNS effects

Include fatigue, weakness, vision changes (blurred vision, yellow-green or white halos around objects)

CLIENT EDUCATION: Monitor for these effects and report to the provider if they occur.

CONTRAINDICATIONS/PRECAUTIONS

- **Warnings**
  - Pregnancy: Digoxin safety is not established
  - Lactation: Use digoxin with caution; enters breast milk
- Contraindicated in clients who have disturbances in ventricular rhythm, including ventricular fibrillation, ventricular tachycardia, and second- and third-degree heart block.
- Use cautiously in clients who have hypokalemia, partial AV block, advanced heart failure, and impaired kidney function.

INTERACTIONS

Thiazide diuretics (hydrochlorothiazide) and loop diuretics (furosemide) can lead to hypokalemia, which increases the risk of developing dysrhythmias.
NURSING ACTIONS

- Monitor and maintain K+ level between 3.5 and 5.0 mEq/L.
- Treat hypokalemia with potassium supplements or a potassium-sparing diuretic.

ACE inhibitors and ARBs increase the risk of hyperkalemia, which can lead to decreased therapeutic effects of digoxin.
NURSING ACTIONS

- Use cautiously if these medications are used with potassium supplements or a potassium-sparing diuretic.
- Maintain K+ level between 3.5 to 5.0 mEq/L.

Sympathomimetic medications (dopamine) complement the inotropic action of digoxin and increase the rate and force of heart muscle contraction. These medications can increase the risk of tachydysrhythmias.
NURSING ACTIONS: Monitor ECG. Instruct clients to measure pulse rate and report palpitations.

Quinidine increases the risk of digoxin toxicity when used concurrently by displacing digoxin from its binding site and reducing kidney excretion.
NURSING ACTIONS: Avoid concurrent use.

Verapamil increases plasma levels of digoxin.
NURSING ACTIONS: If used concurrently, decrease digoxin dose. Concurrent use is usually avoided because of verapamil cardiosuppression action counteracting the action of digoxin.

Antacids decrease absorption of digoxin and can decrease its effectiveness.
NURSING ACTIONS: Advise clients to talk to the provider before taking any antacids.

NURSING ADMINISTRATION

- Check pulse rate and rhythm before administration of digoxin and record. Notify the provider if heart rate is less than 60/min in an adult, less than 70/min in children, and less than 90/min in infants.
- Administer digoxin at the same time daily.
- Evaluate manifestations and the client's digoxin level when toxicity is suspected.

- Avoid taking OTC medications to prevent adverse effects and medication interactions.
- Instruct clients to observe for indications of digoxin toxicity (fatigue, weakness, vision changes, GI effects), and to notify the provider if they occur.
- If administering IV digoxin, infuse over at least 5 min, (10 to 15 min in clients who have pulmonary edema) and monitor client for dysrhythmias. Q EBP

CLIENT EDUCATION

- Monitor pulses for rate and rhythm, and notify prescriber if changes occur.
- Take the medication as prescribed. If a dose is missed, the next dose should not be doubled. Q EBP

MANAGEMENT OF DIGOXIN TOXICITY

- Stop digoxin and potassium-wasting diuretics immediately.
- Monitor K+ levels. For levels less than 3.5 mEq/L, administer potassium IV infusion or by mouth. Do not give any further K+ if the level is greater than 5.0 mEq/L or AV block is present.
- Treat dysrhythmias with phenytoin or lidocaine.
- Treat bradycardia with atropine.
- For excessive toxicity, activated charcoal, cholestyramine, or digoxin immune Fab can be used to bind digoxin and prevent absorption.

NURSING EVALUATION OF MEDICATION EFFECTIVENESS

Depending on therapeutic intent, effectiveness is evidenced by the following.

- Control of heart failure
- Absence of cardiac dysrhythmias

Adrenergic agonists

SELECT PROTOTYPE MEDICATION: Catecholamines

- Epinephrine
- Dopamine
- Dobutamine
- Isoproterenol
- Norepinephrine

OTHER MEDICATIONS: Noncatecholamines

- Albuterol
- Ephedrine

PURPOSE

SITE/RESPONSE

Alpha₁ receptors

- Activation of receptors in arterioles of skin, viscera and mucous membranes, and veins leads to vasoconstriction.
- Mydriasis (dilation of pupil)

Beta$_1$ receptors

- Heart stimulation leads to increased heart rate, increased myocardial contractility, and increased rate of conduction through the AV node, thus improving cardiac performance in heart failure.
- Activation of receptors in the kidney lead to the release of renin.

Beta$_2$ receptors

- Activation of receptors in the arterioles of the heart, lungs, and skeletal muscles leads to vasodilation.
- Bronchial stimulation leads to bronchodilation.
- Activation of receptors in uterine smooth muscle causes relaxation, thus delaying preterm labor.
- Activation of receptors in the liver and skeletal muscle causes glycogenolysis, which raises blood glucose.

Dopamine receptors

Activation of receptors in the kidney cause the renal blood vessels to dilate. This increases renal perfusion and reduces the risk of renal failure.

MEDICATIONS

Epinephrine

Alpha$_1$ receptors
- PHARMACOLOGICAL ACTION: Vasoconstriction
- THERAPEUTIC USE
  - Anaphylactic shock
  - Slows absorption of local anesthetics
  - Manages superficial bleeding
  - Decreased congestion of nasal mucosa
  - Increased blood pressure

Beta$_1$ receptors
- PHARMACOLOGICAL ACTION
  - Increased heart rate
  - Increased myocardial contractility
  - Increased rate of conduction through the AV node
  - Increased cardiac output
  - Improved tissue perfusion
- THERAPEUTIC USE: Treatment of AV block, heart failure, shock, and cardiac arrest

Beta$_2$ receptors
- PHARMACOLOGICAL ACTION: Bronchodilation
- THERAPEUTIC USE: Asthma

Dopamine

Low dose: Dopamine receptor
- PHARMACOLOGICAL ACTION: Renal blood vessel dilation
- THERAPEUTIC USE
  - Shock
  - Heart failure
  - Acute kidney injury

Moderate dose: Beta$_1$ receptor
- PHARMACOLOGICAL ACTION
  - Renal blood vessel dilation
  - Increased heart rate
  - Increased myocardial contractility
  - Increased rate of conduction through the AV node
- THERAPEUTIC USE
  - Shock
  - Heart failure

High dose: Dopamine, beta$_1$, alpha$_1$ receptors
- PHARMACOLOGICAL ACTION
  - Renal blood vessel constriction
  - Increased heart rate
  - Increased myocardial contractility
  - Increased rate of conduction through the AV node
  - Vasoconstriction (viscera, skin, mucous membranes)
  - Mydriasis
- THERAPEUTIC USE
  - Shock
  - Heart failure

Dobutamine

Beta$_1$
- PHARMACOLOGICAL ACTION
  - Increased heart rate
  - Increased myocardial contractility and cardiac output
  - Increased rate of conduction through the AV node
- THERAPEUTIC USE: Heart failure

COMPLICATIONS

Hypertensive crisis

Hypertensive crisis due to activation of alpha$_1$ receptors in the blood vessels can lead to cerebral hemorrhage.

NURSING ACTIONS
- Provide for continuous cardiac and blood pressure monitoring.
- Report changes in vital signs to the provider.

Cardiac complications

Dysrhythmias due to activation of beta$_1$ receptors in the heart. Beta$_1$ receptor activation also increases the workload of the heart and increases oxygen demand, leading to the development of angina.

NURSING ACTIONS
- Monitor urine output.
- Provide for continuous cardiac monitoring.
- Monitor clients closely for dysrhythmias, change in heart rate, and chest pain.
- Notify the provider of dysrhythmias, increased heart rate, and chest pain. Treat per protocol.

Necrosis

Can occur from extravasation.

NURSING ACTIONS: If extravasation occurs, administer phentolamine, an alpha blocker to counteract alpha mediated vasoconstriction.

DOPAMINE

Cardiac complications

Beta₁ receptor activation in the heart can cause dysrhythmias. Beta₁ receptor activation also increases the workload of the heart and increases oxygen demand, leading to development of angina.

NURSING ACTIONS
- Provide for continuous cardiac monitoring.
- Monitor clients closely for dysrhythmias, change in heart rate, and chest pain.
- Notify the provider of dysrhythmias, increased heart rate, and chest pain. Treat per protocol.
- Monitor urine output.

Necrosis

Can occur from extravasation of high doses of dopamine

NURSING ACTIONS
- Monitor IV site carefully. Infuse through central IV line if possible. Qs
- Discontinue infusion at first indication of irritation.
- If extravasation occurs, administer phentolamine, an alpha blocker to counteract alpha mediated vasoconstriction.
- Phentolamine should be administered subcutaneously in the extravasation area.

DOBUTAMINE

Increased heart rate

NURSING ACTIONS
- Provide continuous cardiac monitoring.
- Report changes in vital signs to the provider.

CONTRAINDICATIONS/PRECAUTIONS

- **Warnings**
  ○ Pregnancy
    ▪ Dopamine/dobutamine: Safety not established.
    ▪ Epinephrine: Use only if the benefit to the client outweighs the risks to the fetus.
  ○ Lactation
    ▪ Dopamine/dobutamine: Safety not established.
    ▪ Epinephrine: High doses can decrease milk production; low dose considered safe.
- Dopamine is contraindicated in clients who have tachydysrhythmias and ventricular fibrillation.
- Use dopamine and dobutamine cautiously in clients who have hypovolemia, angina, history of myocardial infarction, hypertension, and diabetes.
- Older adult clients have an increased susceptibility to adverse effects. Ⓖ
- Epinephrine should be used with caution in clients who have hyperthyroidism, angina, cardiac dysrhythmias, and hypertension.

INTERACTIONS

MAOIs prevent inactivation of epinephrine and therefore prolong the effects of epinephrine. MAOIs used with dobutamine and dopamine can cause cardiotoxicity.
NURSING ACTIONS: Avoid use of MAOIs in clients receiving epinephrine, dopamine, and dobutamine.

Tricyclic antidepressants block uptake of epinephrine, dopamine, and dobutamine, which will prolong and intensify effects of epinephrine.
NURSING ACTIONS: Clients taking these medications concurrently might need a lowered dosage of epinephrine, dopamine, and dobutamine.

General anesthetics can cause the heart to become hypersensitive to the effects of epinephrine, dopamine, and dobutamine, leading to dysrhythmias.
NURSING ACTIONS
- Perform continuous ECG monitoring.
- Notify the provider of evidence of chest pain, dysrhythmias, and increased heart rate.

Alpha adrenergic blocking agents (phentolamine) block action at alpha receptors.
NURSING ACTIONS: Phentolamine can be used to treat epinephrine toxicity and extravasation of epinephrine, and dopamine. QEBP

Beta adrenergic blocking agents (propranolol) block action at beta receptors.
NURSING ACTIONS: Use propranolol to treat chest pain and dysrhythmias.

Diuretics promote beneficial effects of dopamine.
NURSING ACTIONS: Monitor for therapeutic effects.

NURSING ADMINISTRATION

- These medications must be administered IV by continuous infusion. QEBP
- Use an IV pump to control infusion.
- Dosage is titrated based on blood pressure response.
- Assess/monitor for chest pain. Notify the provider if chest pain occurs.
- Monitor urine output frequently for indications of decreased kidney perfusion.
- Monitor ECG and blood pressure continuously and notify provider of indications of tachycardia or dysrhythmias.
- Monitor perfusion to extremities.
- Monitor cardiac output, pulmonary capillary wedge pressure, central venous pressure.
- Monitor clients who have diabetes for hyperglycemia while taking epinephrine, isoproterenol, or albuterol.

NURSING EVALUATION OF MEDICATION EFFECTIVENESS

Depending on therapeutic intent, effectiveness is evidenced by improved perfusion as evidenced by urine output of greater than or equal to 30 mL/hr (with adequate kidney function), improved mental status, and systolic blood pressure maintained at greater than or equal to 90 mm Hg.

Angiotensin receptor neprilysin inhibitor (ARNI)

SELECT PROTOTYPE MEDICATION: Sacubitril/Valsartan

PURPOSE

Inhibitor of the renin angiotensin–aldosterone system

THERAPEUTIC USE

Approved for patients who have Class II–IV heart failure and reduced ejection fraction to replace an ACE inhibitor or ARB.

COMPLICATIONS

Adverse effects include angioedema, hyperkalemia, hypotension, cough, dizziness, renal failure.

CONTRAINDICATIONS/PRECAUTIONS

Warnings
- ○ Pregnancy: Avoid use during pregnancy because it can cause harm to fetus.
- ○ Lactation: Avoid use while breastfeeding.
- • Avoid use in clients who have severe hepatic impairment.

INTERACTIONS

Clients taking this medication should not use it with an ACE inhibitor or an ARB, potassium sparing diuretics, NSAIDs or lithium. This medication should not be taken by clients with diabetes who are taking aliskiren.

NURSING ADMINISTRATION

- • Available as an oral tablet.
- • Monitor renal function and potassium.

NURSING EVALUATION OF MEDICATION EFFECTIVENESS

- • Control of heart failure

Application Exercises

1. A nurse is caring for a client who has a new prescription for digoxin and takes multiple other medications. The nurse should identify that concurrent use of which of the following medications increases the client's risk for developing digoxin toxicity?

   A. Phenytoin

   B. Verapamil

   C. Warfarin

   D. Aluminum hydroxide

2. A nurse is teaching a client who has a new prescription for digoxin. The nurse should instruct the client to monitor and report which of the following adverse effects that is a manifestation digoxin toxicity? (Select all that apply.)

   A. Headache

   B. Constipation

   C. Anorexia

   D. Rash

   E. Blurred vision

3. A nurse is reviewing laboratory results of electrolytes for four clients who take digoxin. Which of the following electrolyte values increases a client's risk for digoxin toxicity?

   A. Calcium 9.2 mg/dL

   B. Calcium 10.3 mg/dL

   C. Potassium 3.4 mEq/L

   D. Potassium 4.8 mEq/L

4. A nurse is teaching a client who has a new prescription for digoxin to treat heart failure. Which of the following instructions should the nurse include in the teaching?

   A. Contact provider if heart rate is less than 60/min.

   B. Check pulse rate for 30 seconds and multiply result by 2.

   C. Increase intake of sodium.

   D. Take with food if nausea occurs.

5. A nurse is administering a low dose dopamine infusion to a client who has severe heart failure. Which of the following findings is an expected effect of this medication?

   A. Lowered heart rate

   B. Increased urine output

   C. Decreased conduction through the AV node

   D. Vasoconstriction of renal blood vessels

Application Exercises Key

1. B. **CORRECT:** The nurse should analyze the findings and determine that the priority hypothesis is that the client is at risk for a medication interaction which could lead to digoxin toxicity. Verapamil, a calcium-channel blocker, can increase digoxin levels. If these medications are given concurrently, the digoxin dosage may need to be decreased, and the nurse should monitor digoxin levels carefully.

   Ⓝ *NCLEX® Connection: Pharmacological and Parenteral Therapies, Adverse Effects/Contraindications/Side Effects/Interactions*

2. A, C, E. **CORRECT:** When taking actions, the nurse should teach the client that headaches, GI disturbances, such as anorexia, and visual changes, such as blurred and yellow-tinged vision, are manifestations of digoxin toxicity. The client should be instructed to notify the provider if these manifestations occur.

   Ⓝ *NCLEX® Connection: Pharmacological and Parenteral Therapies, Adverse Effects/Contraindications/Side Effects/Interactions*

3. C. **CORRECT:** The nurse should analyze the cues from the client's laboratory results and determine that a potassium level of 3.4 mEq/L is below the expected reference range and increases a client's risk for developing digoxin toxicity. Low potassium can cause fatal dysrhythmias, especially in older clients who take digoxin.

   Ⓝ *NCLEX® Connection: Pharmacological and Parenteral Therapies, Adverse Effects/Contraindications/Side Effects/Interactions*

4. A. **CORRECT:** When taking actions, the nurse should teach the client to contact the provider for a heart rate less than 60/min prior to taking the medication.

   Ⓝ *NCLEX® Connection: Pharmacological and Parenteral Therapies, Adverse Effects/Contraindications/Side Effects/Interactions*

5. B. **CORRECT:** When evaluating outcomes the nurse should identify that dopamine increases urinary output because of increased renal perfusion. This occurs due to the activation of the dopamine receptors in the kidneys when dopamine is administered at low doses. An increase in urinary output indicates the client's condition is improving.

   Ⓝ *NCLEX® Connection: Pharmacological and Parenteral Therapies, Parenteral/Intravenous Therapies*

Active Learning Scenario

A nurse is caring for a client who has heart failure and a new prescription for digoxin 0.125 mg PO daily. What should the nurse teach the client about this medication? Use the ATI Active Learning Template: Medication to complete this item.

THERAPEUTIC USES

COMPLICATIONS: Identify two adverse effects.

NURSING INTERVENTIONS: Describe two diagnostic tests to monitor.

CLIENT EDUCATION: Include three teaching points.

Active Learning Scenario Key

Using the ATI Active Learning Template: Medication

THERAPEUTIC USES: Digoxin improves the heart's pumping effectiveness and increases cardiac output and stroke volume. It decreases heart rate by slowing depolarization through the SA node, thus allowing more time for the ventricles to fill with blood. Due to these effects, digoxin is used to treat heart failure, atrial fibrillation, and some other tachydysrhythmias.

COMPLICATIONS: The client should monitor for manifestations of digoxin toxicity, which include GI effects (nausea, vomiting, diarrhea), CNS effects (fatigue, weakness), visual effects (yellow-tinged vision, halos around lights, diplopia), heart rate less than 60/min in adults, or skipped beats when checking the pulse.

NURSING INTERVENTIONS
- Monitor digoxin blood levels periodically during treatment. The expected reference range is 0.5 to 0.8 ng/mL.
- Monitor blood potassium levels because hypokalemia can cause cardiac dysrhythmias, especially in older adult clients. Monitoring ECG is also important to check for dysrhythmias.

CLIENT EDUCATION
- Take oral digoxin at the same time each day. Do not skip a dose or take more than the prescribed dose each day.
- Monitor for manifestations of toxicity.
- Report any new prescriptions and to contact provider before taking OTC medications, because digoxin interacts with many other substances.

Ⓝ *NCLEX® Connection: Pharmacological and Parenteral Therapies, Medication Administration*

CHAPTER 21 ## *Angina and Antilipemic Agents*

Anginal pain often manifests as a sudden pain beneath the sternum radiating to the left shoulder, arm, and jaw. It is a result of inadequate supply of oxygen to meet the myocardial demand. Pharmacological management is aimed at prevention of myocardial ischemia, pain, myocardial infarction, and death.

Anginal pain is managed with organic nitrates, beta-adrenergic blocking agents, calcium channel blockers, and ranolazine. Clients who have chronic stable angina should concurrently take an antiplatelet agent (aspirin or clopidogrel), a cholesterol-lowering agent, and an ACE inhibitor to prevent myocardial infarction and death.

Antilipemic agents work in different ways to help lower low-density lipoprotein (LDL) cholesterol levels, raise high-density lipoprotein (HDL) cholesterol levels, and possibly decrease very low-density lipoprotein (VLDL) levels. These medications should be used along with lifestyle modifications (regular activity, diet, weight control).

Prior to starting these medications, the client should have lab work including baseline levels of total cholesterol, LDL cholesterol, HDL cholesterol, and triglycerides. These blood values should be monitored periodically throughout the course of therapy. In addition, baseline liver and kidney function tests should be obtained and monitored periodically.

Medications are not considered first-line therapy for coronary artery disease and should only be used if lifestyle changes do not reduce the LDL cholesterol to an acceptable level.

Medication classifications include HMG-CoA reductase inhibitors (statins), cholesterol absorption inhibitors, bile-acid sequestrants, fibrates, and monoclonal antibodies.

Angina

Organic nitrates

SELECT PROTOTYPE MEDICATION: Nitroglycerin (NTG)
- Oral extended–release capsules
- Sublingual tablet
- Translingual spray
- Topical ointment
- Transdermal patch
- Intravenous

OTHER MEDICATIONS
- Isosorbide dinitrate (sublingual)
- Isosorbide mononitrate (oral)

PURPOSE

EXPECTED PHARMACOLOGICAL ACTION
- In chronic stable exertional angina, nitroglycerin dilates veins and decreases venous return (preload), which decreases cardiac oxygen demand.
- In variant (Prinzmetal's or vasospastic) angina, nitroglycerin prevents or reduces coronary artery spasm, thus increasing oxygen supply. Oxygen demand is not decreased.

THERAPEUTIC USES
- Treatment of acute angina attack
- Prophylaxis of chronic stable angina or variant angina

COMPLICATIONS

Headache

CLIENT EDUCATION
- Use aspirin or acetaminophen to relieve pain.
- Notify the provider if headache does not resolve in a few weeks. Dosage can be reduced.

Orthostatic hypotension

CLIENT EDUCATION
- Sit or lie down if experiencing dizziness or faintness.
- Avoid sudden changes of position and rise slowly.
- Lie down with feet elevated to promote venous return and increase blood pressure.

Reflex tachycardia

NURSING ACTIONS

- Monitor vital signs.
- Administer a beta blocker (metoprolol) if needed or a calcium channel blocker (verapamil) which can prevent sympathetic cardiac stimulation, resulting in a decreased cardiac oxygen demand by direct suppression of the heart.

Tolerance

NURSING ACTIONS

- Use lowest dose needed to achieve effect.
- Long-acting preparations should be used on an intermittent schedule that allows at least 8 drug-free hours every day. This action reduces the risk of tolerance.

CONTRAINDICATIONS/PRECAUTIONS

- **Warnings**
  - Pregnancy: Use nitroglycerin with caution; can affect maternal and fetal circulation.
  - Lactation: Nitroglycerin safety has not been established.
- This medication is contraindicated in clients who have hypersensitivity to nitrates.
- Nitroglycerin is contraindicated in clients who have severe anemia, closed-angle glaucoma, and traumatic head injury because the medication can increase intracranial pressure.
- Use cautiously in clients taking antihypertensive medications, and clients who have hyperthyroidism or kidney or liver dysfunction.
- Inhibitors of phosphodiesterase type 5 (PDES5) for erectile dysfunction administered with nitroglycerin can intensify the nitroglycerin-induced vasodilation and result in life threatening hypotension.

INTERACTIONS

Use of alcohol can contribute to the hypotensive effect of nitroglycerin.
CLIENT EDUCATION: Avoid use of alcohol.

Antihypertensive medications (beta blockers, calcium channel blockers, and diuretics) can contribute to hypotensive effect.
NURSING ACTIONS: Use nitroglycerin cautiously in clients receiving these medications.

NURSING ADMINISTRATION

Sublingual tablet and translingual spray

TYPES

- Rapid onset
- Short duration

USE

- Treat acute attack
- Prophylaxis of acute attack when exertion is anticipated

NURSING ACTIONS

- Use this rapid-acting nitrate at the first indication of chest pain. Do not wait until pain is severe. Qs
- Use prior to activity that is known to cause chest pain (climbing a flight of stairs).

For sublingual tablet

- Place the tablet under the tongue and allow it to dissolve.
- Store tablets in original bottles, and in a cool, dark place.
- Spray translingual spray against oral mucosa and do not inhale.

Sustained-release oral capsules

TYPES

- Slow onset
- Long duration

USE: Long-term prophylaxis against anginal attacks

NURSING ACTIONS

- Swallow capsules without crushing or chewing. To reduce the risk of tolerance, oral tablets should be taken only once or twice daily.
- Take capsules on an empty stomach with at least 8 oz of water.

Transdermal

TYPES

- Slow onset
- Long duration

USE: Long-term prophylaxis against anginal attacks

NURSING ACTIONS

- To ensure appropriate dose, patches should not be cut.
- Place the patch on a hairless area of skin (chest, back, or abdomen) and rotate sites to prevent skin irritation.
- Remove old patch, wash skin with soap and water, and dry thoroughly before applying new patch.
- Remove the patch at night to reduce the risk of developing tolerance to nitroglycerin. Be medication-free between 10 and 12 hr/day. QEBP

Topical ointment

TYPES

- Slow onset
- Long duration

USE: Long-term prophylaxis against anginal attacks

NURSING ACTIONS

- Remove the prior dose before a new dose is applied. Measure specific dose with applicator paper and spread over 2.5 to 3.5 inches of the paper.
- Apply to a clean, hairless area of the body, and cover with clear plastic wrap.
- Follow same guidelines for site selection as for transdermal patch.
- Avoid touching ointment with the hands.

Intravenous

USE

- Control of angina not responding to other medications.
- Control of hypertension during the perioperative period create controlled hypotension during surgery.
- Heart failure resulting from acute MI.

NURSING ACTIONS

- Administer with IV tubing supplied by manufacturer using a glass IV bottle.
- Administer continuously due to short duration of action.
- Start at a slow rate, usually 5 mcg/min, and titrate gradually until desired response is achieved or for a maximum of 2 mcg/minute.
- Provide continuous cardiac and blood pressure monitoring during administration.

TREATMENT OF ANGINAL ATTACK USING SUBLINGUAL TABLETS OR TRANSLINGUAL SPRAY

- Stop activity. Sit or lie down. ○EBP
- Immediately put one sublingual tablet under the tongue and let it dissolve. Rest for 5 min.
- If pain not relieved by first tablet, call 911, then take a second tablet.
- After another 5 min, take a third tablet if pain is still not relieved. Do not take more than three sublingual tablets.
- If using nitroglycerin translingual spray, one spray substitutes for one sublingual tablet when treating an anginal attack.

CLIENT EDUCATION

- Do not stop taking long-acting nitroglycerin abruptly and follow the provider's instructions.
- If having angina, record pain frequency, intensity, duration, and location. Notify the provider if attacks increase in frequency, intensity, and/or duration.
- Do not crush or chew oral nitroglycerin or isosorbide tablets because sublingual nitroglycerin is ineffective if swallowed.

NURSING EVALUATION OF MEDICATION EFFECTIVENESS

Depending on therapeutic intent, effectiveness is evidenced by the following.
- Prevention and termination of acute anginal attacks
- Long-term management of stable angina
- Control of perioperative blood pressure
- Control of heart failure following acute MI

Antianginal agent

SELECT PROTOTYPE MEDICATION: Ranolazine

PURPOSE

EXPECTED PHARMACOLOGICAL ACTION
- Lowers cardiac oxygen demand and thereby improves exercise tolerance and decreases pain.
- Myocardial energy use is more efficient due to the decreased accumulation of sodium and calcium in the myocardial cells.

THERAPEUTIC USES: Chronic stable angina in combination with amlodipine, a beta adrenergic blocker, or an organic nitrate

COMPLICATIONS

QT prolongation

Can increase the risk for torsades de pointes

NURSING ACTIONS
- Monitor ECG. Do not use in clients who have a prolonged QT or are taking other medications that prolong QT. Caution is taken if the client is subjected to multiple medication interactions.

CLIENT EDUCATION: Report palpitations, chest pain, or dyspnea.

Elevated blood pressure

NURSING ACTIONS
- Monitor blood pressure.
- If the client has severe kidney impairment, monitor the client's blood pressure closely because ranolazine can raise the blood pressure by 15 mm Hg.

CONTRAINDICATIONS/PRECAUTIONS

- **Warnings**
  - Pregnancy: Use ranolazine only if the benefit to the client outweighs the risks to the fetus.
  - Lactation: Ranolazine contraindicated
- Ranolazine is contraindicated in clients who have QT prolongation or in clients taking other medications that can result in QT prolongation, and clients who have hepatic impairment, ventricular tachycardia, ventricular dysrhythmias, and hypokalemia.
- Use cautiously in older adult clients and in clients who have hypotension or kidney impairment. Ⓖ

INTERACTIONS

Inhibitors of CYP3A4 can increase levels of ranolazine and lead to torsades de pointes.
Agents include grapefruit juice, HIV protease inhibitors, macrolide antibiotics, azole antifungals, and some calcium channel blocker medications.

NURSING ACTIONS: Avoid concurrent use.

Quinidine and sotalol can further prolong QT interval.
NURSING ACTIONS: Avoid concurrent use.

Concurrent use of digoxin and simvastatin increases blood levels of digoxin and simvastatin.
NURSING ACTIONS: Monitor digoxin level.

CLIENT EDUCATION: Report muscle weakness.

NURSING ADMINISTRATION

- Administer as an extended release oral tablet, twice daily with or without food. Do not crush or chew tablet. ⓠEBP
- Obtain baseline and monitor ECG for QT prolongation.
- Obtain baseline and monitor digoxin level with concurrent use.
- Can take concurrently with other antianginal medications (nitroglycerin).
- Monitor blood pressure and pulse periodically.
- Amlodipine is the only calcium channel blocker that can be used with ranolazine because it does not inhibit CYP3A4.

CLIENT EDUCATION: Ranolazine is not indicated for the treatment of an acute anginal attack.

NURSING EVALUATION OF MEDICATION EFFECTIVENESS

Depending on therapeutic intent, effectiveness can be evidenced by the following.
- Prevention of acute anginal attacks
- Long-term management of stable angina

Antilipemic Agents

HMG-CoA reductase inhibitors (statins)

SELECT PROTOTYPE MEDICATION: Atorvastatin
- Simvastatin
- Lovastatin
- Pravastatin
- Rosuvastatin
- Fluvastatin
- Pitavastatin

COMBINATION MEDICATIONS: Simvastatin and ezetimibe

PURPOSE

EXPECTED PHARMACOLOGICAL ACTIONS
- Decrease manufacture of LDL and VLDL cholesterol
- Lowers triglycerides in some clients
- Increase manufacture of HDL
- Other beneficial effects include promotion of vasodilation, decrease in plaque site inflammation, thromboembolism, and risk of atrial fibrillation.

THERAPEUTIC USES
- Primary hypercholesterolemia
- Prevention of coronary events (primary and secondary)
- Protection against myocardial infarction (MI) and stroke for clients who have diabetes mellitus
- Increasing levels of HDL in clients who have primary hypercholesterolemia
- Primary prevention in clients who have normal LDL

COMPLICATIONS

HEPATOTOXICITY

Evidenced by increase in aspartate transaminase (AST)

NURSING ACTIONS
- Obtain baseline liver function.
- Monitor liver function tests after 12 weeks and then every 6 months.
- Medication might be discontinued if liver function tests are above the expected reference range.

CLIENT EDUCATION
- Observe for indications of liver dysfunction (anorexia, vomiting, nausea, jaundice), and notify the provider if manifestations occur.
- Avoid alcohol.

MYOPATHY

- Evidenced by muscle aches, pain, and tenderness
- Can progress to myositis or rhabdomyolysis
- Increased risk for older adult clients and clients who are frail, have a small body frame, or have hypothyroidism.

NURSING ACTIONS
- Obtain baseline creatine kinase (CK) level.
- Monitor CK levels periodically while on treatment.
- Medication might be discontinued if CK levels are elevated.

CLIENT EDUCATION: Report muscle aches, pain, and tenderness.

CONTRAINDICATIONS/PRECAUTIONS

- **Warnings**
  - Pregnancy: HMG–CoA reductase inhibitors (statins) contraindicated.
  - Lactation: HMG–CoA reductase inhibitors (statins) contraindicated.
  - Reproductive: Use effective contraception during HMG–CoA reductase inhibitors (statins) therapy. Notify provider immediately if pregnancy is planned or suspected.
- Contraindicated in clients who have a liver disorder.
- For clients of Asian descent, rosuvastatin should be avoided or prescribed in a smaller dose than for other clients.
- Use cautiously in clients who have previously had liver disease. Dosage of several statins (lovastatin, pitavastatin, pravastatin, rosuvastatin, and simvastatin) should be reduced for clients who have severe kidney impairment.

INTERACTIONS

Fibrates (gemfibrozil, fenofibrate) and ezetimibe increase the risk of myopathy and liver and kidney injury.

NURSING ACTIONS
- Obtain baseline CK level.
- Monitor CK levels, liver enzymes, and kidney function periodically during treatment.
- Medication might be discontinued if CK levels are elevated.

CLIENT EDUCATION: Report muscle aches and pain.

Medications that suppress CYP3A4 (erythromycin, ketoconazole), along with HIV protease inhibitors, amiodarone, and cyclosporine can increase levels of some statins when taken concurrently.

NURSING ACTIONS
- Avoid concurrent use with atorvastatin, lovastatin, and simvastatin.
- Dosage of statin might need to be decreased.

CLIENT EDUCATION: Inform the provider of all medications currently taken.

Grapefruit juice suppresses CYP3A4 and can increase levels of some statins.

NURSING ACTIONS: Avoid concurrent use with atorvastatin, lovastatin, and simvastatin.

NURSING ADMINISTRATION

- Administer statins via oral route.
- Administer lovastatin with evening meal. Other statins can be taken without food, but evening dosing is best because most cholesterol is synthesized during the night. Q EBP

CLIENT EDUCATION: It is important to obtain baseline cholesterol, HDL, LDL, and triglyceride levels, as well as liver and kidney function tests, and monitor periodically during treatment.

Cholesterol absorption inhibitor

Select Prototype Medication: Ezetimibe

PURPOSE

EXPECTED PHARMACOLOGICAL ACTION
Ezetimibe inhibits reabsorption of cholesterol secreted in bile and absorption of cholesterol from food.

THERAPEUTIC USES
- Clients who have modified diets can use this medication as an adjunct to lower LDL cholesterol, total cholesterol, and apolipoprotein B.
- Medication can be used alone or in combination with a statin medication.

COMPLICATIONS

HEPATITIS

NURSING ACTIONS
- Obtain baseline liver function.
- Medication might be discontinued if liver function tests are greater than the expected reference range.

CLIENT EDUCATION
- Observe for liver dysfunction (anorexia, vomiting, nausea, jaundice) and notify the provider if effects occur.
- Avoid alcohol.

MYOPATHY

NURSING ACTIONS
- Obtain baseline CK level.
- Monitor CK levels periodically while on treatment.
- Medication might be discontinued if CK levels are elevated.

CLIENT EDUCATION: Notify the provider if manifestations (muscle aches and pains) occur.

CONTRAINDICATIONS/PRECAUTIONS

- **Warnings**
  - Pregnancy: Ezetimibe contraindicated
  - Lactation: Ezetimibe contraindicated
  - Reproductive: Notify provider immediately if pregnancy is suspected or planned.
- Contraindicated in clients who have active moderate-to-severe liver disorders, especially those taking a statin concurrently.
- Use caution in clients who have mild liver disorders. Q s

INTERACTIONS

Bile acid sequestrants (cholestyramine) interfere with absorption.
NURSING ACTIONS: Take ezetimibe 2 hr before or 4 hr after taking bile sequestrants.

Statins (atorvastatin) can increase the risk of liver dysfunction and myopathy.
NURSING ACTIONS
- Obtain baseline liver function tests and monitor periodically.
- Medication might be discontinued if CK levels are elevated.

CLIENT EDUCATION
- Observe for indications of liver damage (anorexia, vomiting, nausea). The provider should be notified, and the medication will most likely be discontinued.
- Notify the provider of manifestations (muscle aches and pains).

Concurrent use with fibrates (gemfibrozil) increases the risk of cholelithiasis and myopathy.
NURSING ACTIONS: Ezetimibe is not recommended for use with fibrates.

Levels of ezetimibe can be increased with concurrent use of cyclosporine.
NURSING ACTIONS: Monitor for adverse effects (liver damage, myopathy).

NURSING ADMINISTRATION

Clients can take this medication in a fixed-dose combination with simvastatin.

CLIENT EDUCATION
- It is important to obtain baseline cholesterol, HDL, LDL, and triglyceride levels, as well as liver and kidney function tests, and monitor periodically during treatment.
- Follow a low-fat, low-cholesterol diet and become involved in a regular exercise regimen. Qpcc

Bile-acid sequestrants

SELECT PROTOTYPE MEDICATION: Colesevelam

OTHER MEDICATION: Colestipol

PURPOSE

EXPECTED PHARMACOLOGICAL ACTION: Decrease in LDL cholesterol

THERAPEUTIC USE: May be used alone or as an adjunct with an HMG-CoA reductase inhibitor (atorvastatin) and with dietary measures to lower cholesterol levels.

COMPLICATIONS

CONSTIPATION

CLIENT EDUCATION: Increase the intake of high-fiber food and oral fluids, if not restricted.

CONTRAINDICATIONS/PRECAUTIONS

- **Warnings**
  - Pregnancy: Colesevelam safety has not been established.
  - Lactation: Colesevelam safety has not been established.
  - Reproductive: Do not use colesevelam with oral contraceptives; notify provider if pregnancy is planned or suspected.
- Colesevelam is contraindicated in clients who have bowel obstruction or pancreatitis caused by high triglycerides.
- Use cautiously in clients who have dysphagia or gastrointestinal disorders. Ⓒ

INTERACTIONS

Bile-acid sequestrants interfere with absorption of many medications, including levothyroxine; second-generation sulfonylureas (glipizide); phenytoin; fat-soluble vitamins (A, D, E, K); and oral contraceptives. They also form insoluble complexes with thiazide diuretics, digoxin, and warfarin.

CLIENT EDUCATION

- Take medications that interact with bile-acid sequestrants 1 hr before or 4 hr after
- Inform the provider of all medications currently taken.

NURSING ADMINISTRATION

- Colesevelam is taken orally in tablet form. It should be taken with food and 8 oz of water, and not concurrently with other medications. Qebp
- Colestipol is supplied as oral tablet that should not be crushed or chewed. Give 30 min before a meal.
- Colestipol is also supplied in a powder formulation.

CLIENT EDUCATION
- Increase dietary fiber and fluids and take a mild laxative if needed for constipation.
- Use an adequate amount of fluid (4 to 8 oz) to dissolve the medication. This will prevent irritation or impaction of the esophagus.

Fibrates

Select Prototype Medication: Gemfibrozil

Other Medications: Fenofibrate

PURPOSE

EXPECTED PHARMACOLOGICAL ACTION
- Decrease in triglyceride levels (increase in VLDL excretion for clients unable to lower triglyceride levels with lifestyle modification or other antilipemic medications)
- Increase in HDL levels by promoting production of precursors to HDLs

THERAPEUTIC USES
- Reduction of plasma triglycerides (VLDL)
- Increased levels of HDL

COMPLICATIONS

GI DISTRESS

Usually mild and self-limiting

GALLSTONES

CLIENT EDUCATION
- Observe for indications of gallbladder disease (right upper quadrant pain, fat intolerance, bloating).
- Notify the provider if manifestations occur.

MYOPATHY (MUSCLE TENDERNESS, PAIN)

- Obtain baseline CK level.
- Monitor CK levels periodically during treatment.
- Monitor for muscle aches, weakness, pain, and tenderness, and notify the provider if adverse effects occur.
- Stop medication if CK levels are elevated.

HEPATOTOXICITY

NURSING ACTIONS
- Obtain baseline liver function tests and monitor periodically.
- Stop medication if liver function tests are elevated.

CONTRAINDICATIONS/PRECAUTIONS

- **Warnings**
  - Pregnancy: Gemfibrozil safety not established
  - Lactation: Gemfibrozil safety not established
  - Reproductive: Gemfibrozil: Notify provider if pregnancy is planned or suspected.
- Contraindicated in clients who have liver disorders, severe kidney dysfunction, and gallbladder disease

INTERACTIONS

With concurrent use, warfarin increases the risk of bleeding.
NURSING ACTIONS: Obtain baseline prothrombin time (PT) and INR and perform periodic monitoring.

CLIENT EDUCATION: Report indications of bleeding (bruising, bleeding gums), and notify the provider if these occur.

Statins increase the risk of myopathy.
NURSING ACTIONS: Avoid using concurrently.

NURSING ADMINISTRATION

Administer via oral route.

CLIENT EDUCATION: Take medication 30 min prior to breakfast or dinner. ◯EBP

Monoclonal Antibodies

SELECT PROTOTYPE MEDICATION: Alirocumab

OTHER MEDICATIONS: Evolocumab

PURPOSE

EXPECTED PHARMACOLOGICAL ACTION: Decreases LDL by binding to low density lipoprotein receptors.

THERAPEUTIC USES: Used as an adjunct to dietary modifications in clients who have elevated LDL cholesterol.

COMPLICATIONS

HYPERSENSITIVITY REACTION

CLIENT EDUCATION: Report rash, vasculitis, urticaria

LOCAL INJECTION SITE REACTION

CLIENT EDUCATION: Rotate injection sites, and avoid areas of inflammation, rash, or injured skin.

CONTRAINDICATIONS/PRECAUTIONS

- **Warnings**
  - Pregnancy: Use alirocumab with caution; can cross the placenta.
  - Lactation: Use alirocumab with caution with lactation
  - Reproductive: Alirocumab: Notify provider if pregnancy is planned or suspected.
- History of hypersensitivity to medication

INTERACTIONS

No significant drug interactions with these medications

NURSING ADMINISTRATION

Administer via subcutaneous route.

1. A nurse is teaching a client who has a new prescription for nitroglycerin transdermal patch for angina pectoris. Which of the following instructions should the nurse include?

   A. Remove the patch for at least 10 hr daily.

   B. Cut each patch in half if angina attacks are under control.

   C. Take off the nitroglycerin patch for 30 min if a headache occurs.

   D. Apply a new patch every 48 hr.

2. A nurse is teaching a client who has angina how to use nitroglycerin transdermal ointment. The nurse should include which of the following instructions?

   A. "Remove the prior dose before applying a new dose."

   B. "Rub the ointment directly into your skin until it is no longer visible."

   C. "Cover the applied ointment with a clean gauze pad."

   D. "Apply the ointment to the same skin area each time."

3. A nurse is teaching a client who has angina pectoris and is learning how to treat acute anginal attacks. The client asks, "What is my next step if I take one nitroglycerin tablet, wait 5 minutes, but still have anginal pain?" Which of the following responses should the nurse make?

   A. "Take two more sublingual tablets at the same time."

   B. "Call for emergency medical assistance."

   C. "Take a sustained-release nitroglycerin capsule."

   D. "Wait another 5 minutes then take a second sublingual tablet."

4. A nurse is taking a medication history from a client who has angina and is to begin taking ranolazine. The nurse should report which of the following medications in the client's history that can interact with ranolazine? (Select all that apply.)

   A. Digoxin

   B. Simvastatin

   C. Verapamil

   D. Amlodipine

   E. Nitroglycerin transdermal patch

5. A nurse is teaching a client who is starting simvastatin. Which of the following information should the nurse include?

   A. Take this medication in the evening.

   B. Change position slowly when rising from a chair.

   C. Maintain a steady intake of green leafy vegetables.

   D. Consume no more than 1 L/day of fluid.

6. A nurse is assessing a client who is taking gemfibrozil. Which of the following findings should the nurse identify as an adverse effect of this medication?

   A. Mental status changes

   B. Tremor

   C. Diarrhea

   D. Pneumonia

Active Learning Scenario

A nurse is caring for a client who has elevated total cholesterol, LDL, and triglycerides, and has a new prescription for atorvastatin once daily. The client has type 2 diabetes mellitus and hypertension. What should the nurse instruct the client about atorvastatin? Use the ATI Active Learning Template: Medication to complete this item.

THERAPEUTIC USES:
Identify for atorvastatin.

COMPLICATIONS: Identify two adverse effects.

NURSING INTERVENTIONS: Describe three two tests to monitor.

CLIENT EDUCATION: Include two education points.

Application Exercises Key

1. A. **CORRECT:** When taking actions, the nurse should instruct the client to prevent tolerance to nitroglycerin, the client should remove the patch for 10 to 12 hr during each 24-hr period.

   Ⓝ *NCLEX® Connection: Pharmacological and Parenteral Therapies, Medication Administration*

2. A. **CORRECT:** When taking actions, the nurse should teach the client to remove the prior dose before applying a new dose to prevent toxicity.

   Ⓝ *NCLEX® Connection: Pharmacological Therapies, Medication Administration*

3. B. **CORRECT:** When taking actions, the nurse should inform the client that the next step is to call 911 and then take a second sublingual tablet. If the first tablet does not work, the client might be having a myocardial infarction. The client can take a third tablet if the second one has not relieved the pain after waiting an additional 5 minutes.

   Ⓝ *NCLEX® Connection: Pharmacological and Parenteral Therapies, Medication Administration*

4. A. **CORRECT:** The nurse should analyze the cues from the client's medication history and determine that ranolazine should not be given concurrently with digoxin because it can increase blood levels of digoxin, increasing the risk of developing digoxin toxicity can result.
   B. **CORRECT:** Ranolazine increases blood levels of simvastatin, so liver toxicity can result when administered concurrently.
   C. **CORRECT:** Verapamil is an inhibitor of CYP3A4, which can increase levels of ranolazine and lead to the dysrhythmia torsades de pointes when administered concurrently.

   Ⓝ *NCLEX® Connection: Pharmacological and Parenteral Therapies, Adverse Effects/Contraindications/Side Effects/Interactions*

5. A. **CORRECT:** When taking actions, the nurse should teach the client to take simvastatin in the evening because nighttime is when the most cholesterol is synthesized in the body. Taking statin medications in the evening increases medication effectiveness.

   Ⓝ *NCLEX® Connection: Pharmacological Therapies, Medication Administration*

6. C. **CORRECT:** The nurse should analyze the cues from the client's manifestations and determine that diarrhea, nausea, flatulence, and abdominal pain can be GI adverse effects of this medication.

   Ⓝ *NCLEX® Connection: Pharmacological and Parenteral Therapies, Adverse Effects/Contraindications/Side Effects/Interactions*

Active Learning Scenario Key

Using the ATI Active Learning Template: Medication

THERAPEUTIC USES: Atorvastatin decreases LDL and triglycerides and elevates HDL. It reduces the risk for cardiovascular events (myocardial infarction) and also provides secondary prevention in clients who have had a cardiovascular event. In clients who have diabetes mellitus and hypertension, atorvastatin can reduce mortality by controlling cholesterol levels.

COMPLICATIONS:
- Muscle pain/tenderness (myopathy)
- Liver toxicity with findings (jaundice, upper abdominal pain, anorexia, and nausea)

NURSING INTERVENTIONS: Monitor baseline and periodic cholesterol levels (including LDL, HDL, and triglycerides), creatine kinase levels for myopathy, and liver function tests for liver toxicity.

CLIENT EDUCATION
- Perform additional ways to help decrease cholesterol and improve health (exercise, low-fat diet, weight control, and smoking cessation).
- Take atorvastatin in the evening without regard to meals. (Antilipemic agents are given in the evening because cholesterol is mostly synthesized during the night.)

Ⓝ *NCLEX® Connection: Pharmacological Therapies, Medication Administration*

UNIT 4 MEDICATIONS AFFECTING THE
CARDIOVASCULAR SYSTEM

CHAPTER 22 *Medications
Affecting
Cardiac Rhythm*

Medications affecting cardiac rhythm act by altering cardiac electrophysiologic function in order to treat or prevent dysrhythmias.

Electrophysiological changes can include prolonging the AV node; increasing or reducing conduction speed; altering ectopic pacemakers and SA node; reducing myocardial excitability; lengthening effective refractory period; and stimulating the autonomic nervous system.

There are four main classification groups of antidysrhythmics: sodium channel blockers, beta-adrenergic blockers, potassium channel blockers, and calcium channel blockers.

Toxicity is major concern for antidysrhythmic medications. Medication toxicity can lead to increased cardiac dysrhythmias.

Antidysrhythmic medications

CLASS I MEDICATIONS

Sodium channel blockers slow cardiac conduction velocity They are divided into three groups: IA, IB, and IC.

Class IA

SELECT PROTOTYPE MEDICATION: Quinidine

OTHER MEDICATIONS: Disopyramide

Class IB

SELECT PROTOTYPE MEDICATION: Lidocaine (IV)

OTHER MEDICATIONS
- Mexiletine
- Phenytoin

Class IC

SELECT PROTOTYPE MEDICATION: Propafenone (oral)

OTHER MEDICATIONS: Flecainide

CLASS II MEDICATIONS

Beta-adrenergic blockers prevent sympathetic nervous system stimulation of the heart.

SELECT PROTOTYPE MEDICATION: Propranolol (oral, IV)

OTHER MEDICATIONS
- Esmolol
- Acebutolol

CLASS III MEDICATIONS

Potassium channel blockers prolong the action potential and refractory period of the cardiac cycle.

SELECT PROTOTYPE MEDICATION: Amiodarone (oral, IV)

OTHER MEDICATIONS
- Sotalol
- Ibutilide
- Dofetilide
- Dronedarone

CLASS IV MEDICATIONS

Calcium channel blockers prolongs cardiac conduction, depresses depolarization and decreases oxygen demand of the heart.

SELECT PROTOTYPE MEDICATION: Verapamil (oral, IV)

OTHER MEDICATIONS: Diltiazem

OTHER MEDICATIONS

- Adenosine (IV)
- Digoxin (oral, IV)

PURPOSE

Class IA

EXPECTED PHARMACOLOGICAL ACTION
- Slow impulse conductions in the atria, ventricles, and His–Purkinje system
- Delay repolarization

THERAPEUTIC USES
Long-term suppression of the following dysrhythmias:
- Supraventricular tachycardia (SVT)
- Ventricular tachycardia
- Atrial flutter
- Atrial fibrillation

Class IB

EXPECTED PHARMACOLOGICAL ACTION
In the atria, ventricles, and His–Purkinje system:
- Decrease electrical conduction
- Decrease automaticity
- Increase rate of repolarization

THERAPEUTIC USE: Short-term use only for ventricular dysrhythmias

Class IC

EXPECTED PHARMACOLOGICAL ACTION
- Decrease conduction velocity in atria, ventricles, and His-Purkinje system
- Delay ventricular repolarization

THERAPEUTIC USE: SVT

Class II

EXPECTED PHARMACOLOGICAL ACTION
- Decrease heart rate
- Decrease automaticity through the SA node, decrease velocity of conduction through the AV node, decrease myocardial contractility
- Decrease atrial ectopic stimulation

THERAPEUTIC USES
- Atrial fibrillation
- Atrial flutter
- Paroxysmal SVT
- Hypertension
- Angina
- PVCs
- Severe recurrent ventricular tachycardia
- Exercise-induced tachydysrhythmias
- Paroxysmal atrial tachycardia

Class III

EXPECTED PHARMACOLOGICAL ACTION
- Delays repolarization
- Prolongs action potential
- Reduced automaticity in the SA node
- Reduced contractility and conduction in the AV node, ventricles, and His-Purkinje system
- Dilates coronary blood vessels

THERAPEUTIC USES
- Conversion of atrial fibrillation: oral route
- Recurrent ventricular fibrillation
- Recurrent ventricular tachycardia
- Atrial flutter using dronedarone, sotalol (which is also a beta blocker), dofetilide, and ibutilide.

Class IV calcium channel blockers, verapamil, diltiazem

EXPECTED PHARMACOLOGICAL ACTION
- Decrease force of contraction
- Decrease heart rate
- Slow rate of conduction through the SA and AV nodes
- Effects of calcium channel blockers are the same effects as beta blockers, because beta blockers also promote calcium channel blockage in the heart.

THERAPEUTIC USES
- Control ventricular rate in atrial fibrillation and flutter
- SVT
- Hypertension
- Angina pectoris

OTHER ANTIDYSRHYTHMIC MEDICATIONS

Adenosine

EXPECTED PHARMACOLOGICAL ACTION: Decrease electrical conduction through AV node and decrease automaticity in the SA node.

THERAPEUTIC USES
- Paroxysmal SVT
- Wolff-Parkinson-White syndrome

Digoxin

EXPECTED PHARMACOLOGICAL ACTION
- Decrease electrical conduction through AV node and decrease automaticity in the SA node.
- Increase myocardial contraction

THERAPEUTIC USES: Heart failure, atrial fibrillation and flutter, paroxysmal SVT

COMPLICATIONS

QUINIDINE (SODIUM CHANNEL BLOCKER, CLASS IA)

Diarrhea

Other GI manifestations. Can be intense and lead to discontinuation of the medication.

NURSING ACTIONS
- Manifestations resolve with discontinuation of medication.
- Administer with food to reduce gastric upset.

Cinchonism

Tinnitus, headache, nausea, vertigo, disturbed vision

NURSING ACTIONS: Can develop after one dose. Monitor for manifestations and notify provider if they occur.

Cardiotoxicity

Widening of the QRS by more than 50%, increasing of the QT interval, and prolonging of the PR interval are indications of procainamide cardiotoxicity.

NURSING ACTIONS
- Monitor medication levels (therapeutic quinidine level is 2 to 5 mcg/mL).
- Monitor for other manifestations of toxicity (confusion, drowsiness, vomiting).
- Monitor vital signs and ECG.
- If dysrhythmia occurs, hold medication, and contact the provider.

Hypotension

NURSING ACTIONS: Monitor blood pressure. Might need to withhold medication for hypotension.

LIDOCAINE (SODIUM CHANNEL BLOCKER, CLASS IB)

CNS effects

Drowsiness, altered mental status, paresthesias, seizures

NURSING ACTIONS
- Carefully monitor clients and notify the provider if manifestations occur.
- Administer phenytoin to control seizure activity.

Respiratory arrest

NURSING ACTIONS
- Monitor vital signs and ECG.
- Ensure resuscitation equipment ready at bedside. Qs

PROPAFENONE (SODIUM CHANNEL BLOCKER, CLASS IC)

Bradycardia, heart failure, dizziness, weakness, hypotension, bronchospasm

NURSING ACTIONS:
- Monitor heart rate, blood pressure. Monitor for chest pain, dyspnea, crackles, weight gain, and edema.
- Exacerbation of existing dysrhythmias and new dysrhythmias can occur with all Class IC medications.

PROPRANOLOL (BETA BLOCKER)

Hypotension, bradycardia, heart failure, AV block, sinus arrest, fatigue, bronchospasm in clients who have asthma

NURSING ACTIONS
- Monitor blood pressure and heart rate. Monitor for chest pain, dyspnea, crackles, weight gain, or edema. Check apical pulse prior to dosage.
- Monitor breathing and for evidence of bronchospasm.
- Notify provider for pulse rate less than 50/min, or other prescribed rate.

AMIODARONE (POTASSIUM CHANNEL BLOCKER)

Pulmonary toxicity

NURSING ACTIONS
- Obtain baseline chest x-ray and pulmonary function tests.
- Continue to monitor pulmonary function through course of therapy.
- Notify the provider if effects occur.

CLIENT EDUCATION: Observe for dyspnea, cough, and chest pain.

Sinus bradycardia and AV block

Can lead to heart failure

NURSING ACTIONS
- Monitor blood pressure and ECG.
- Monitor for indications of heart failure (dyspnea, cough, chest pain, neck vein distention, crackles) and notify the provider if they occur.
- If AV block occurs, medication should be discontinued. Insert a pacemaker if indicated.
- Discontinue medication if indicated.

Visual disturbances

Photophobia, blurred vision, can lead to blindness

CLIENT EDUCATION: Report visual disturbances.

Other effects

Can include liver and thyroid dysfunction, GI disturbances, CNS effects, photosensitivity, and blue–gray discoloration to skin

NURSING ACTIONS
- Obtain baseline liver and thyroid function and monitor periodically.
- Advise clients to avoid sun lamps, and wear sunscreen and protective clothing.
- Advise clients to observe for manifestations, and report to the provider if they occur.

Phlebitis with IV administration

NURSING ACTIONS: Use of central venous catheter is indicated. Qs

Hypotension, bradycardia, AV block

NURSING ACTIONS: Monitor cardiac status and blood pressure.

VERAPAMIL (CALCIUM CHANNEL BLOCKER)

Bradycardia, hypotension, heart failure, AV block, constipation, peripheral edema

NURSING ACTIONS
- Monitor ECG and blood pressure. Treat severe hypotension with IV fluid therapy, modified Trendelenburg position, or IV calcium gluconate.
- Reduce dose in clients who have a history of heart failure. Increase fiber and fluids as prescribed. Monitor for chest pain, dyspnea, crackles, weight gain, or edema. Check apical pulse prior to dosage.
- Notify provider for pulse rate less than 50/min, or other prescribed rate.

OTHER ANTIDYSRHYTHMIC MEDICATIONS

Sinus bradycardia, hypotension, dyspnea, vasodilation

Sinus bradycardia (decreased conduction through AV node), hypotension, dyspnea (bronchoconstriction), and flushing of face (vasodilation) can occur as complications of adenosine.

NURSING ACTIONS
- Monitor ECG. Effects usually last 1 min or less
- Administered IV bolus.
- Monitor for manifestations, and notify the provider if they occur.

Bradycardia, hypotension, cardiotoxicity, GI disturbances, fatigue, visual disturbances

Can occur as complications of digoxin

NURSING ACTIONS
- Monitor apical heart rate. Hold dose for heart rate less than 60/min.
- Monitor digoxin level. Optimal therapeutic level is 0.8 to 2.0 ng/mL.
- Monitor for indications of digoxin toxicity: anorexia, nausea, vomiting, visual disturbances, dysrhythmias
- Monitor potassium level. Hypokalemia increases risk for toxicity; keep potassium level between 3.5 and 5.0 mEq/L. The dose may need to be decreased for clients who have renal impairment.

CONTRAINDICATIONS/PRECAUTIONS

Quinidine

- **Warnings**
  - Pregnancy: Can cause fetal harm. Use only if benefits outweigh the risks.
  - Lactation: Safety not established
- Contraindicated in clients who have hypersensitivity to procaine complete heart block, atypical ventricular tachycardia, and systemic lupus erythematosus.
- Use cautiously in clients who have partial AV block, myasthenia gravis, liver or kidney disorders, heart failure, and digoxin toxicity.

Lidocaine

- **Warnings**
  - Pregnancy: Use only if the potential benefit justifies the potential risk to the fetus
  - Lactation: Use only if the potential benefit justifies the potential risk to the fetus
- Contraindicated in clients who have Stokes-Adams syndrome, Wolff-Parkinson-White syndrome, and severe heart block.
- Use cautiously in clients who have liver and kidney dysfunction, second-degree heart block, sinus bradycardia, and heart failure.

Propafenone

- **Warnings**
  - Pregnancy: Can cause fetal harm. Use only if benefits outweigh the risks.
  - Lactation: Safety not established
- Contraindicated in clients who have AV block, severe heart failure, severe hypotension, and cardiogenic shock.
- Use cautiously in older adult clients and clients who have heart failure, liver or kidney dysfunction, and chronic respiratory disorders (asthma).
- When treating cardiac dysrhythmias, propafenone is reserved for use after other safer medications are tried first.

Propranolol

- **Warnings**
  - Pregnancy: Crosses the placenta and can cause fetal/neonatal bradycardia, hypotension, hypoglycemia, or respiratory depression. Can also decrease blood supply to the placenta. Can increase the risk for premature birth or infant death, can cause intrauterine growth retardation and can increase risk of cardiac and pulmonary complications in the infant during the neonatal time frame.
  - Lactation: Appears in breast milk. Use formula if propranolol must be taken.
- Contraindicated in clients who have greater than first-degree AV block, heart failure, and bradycardia.
- Use cautiously in clients who have Wolff-Parkinson-White syndrome; diabetes mellitus; or liver, thyroid, or respiratory dysfunction (asthma).

Amiodarone

- **Warnings**
  - Pregnancy: Crosses the placental barrier and can harm the developing fetus (cardiac, thyroid, neurodevelopmental, neurological and growth adverse effects)
  - Lactation: Can be found in breast milk causing harm to neonate. Avoid breastfeeding.
- Contraindicated in newborns, infants, and clients who have AV block and bradycardia.
- Use cautiously in clients who have liver, thyroid, or respiratory dysfunction; heart failure; and fluid and electrolyte imbalances.

Verapamil

- **Warnings**
  - Pregnancy: Safety not established
  - Lactation: Safety not established
  - Contraindicated in clients who have greater than first-degree AV block (unless they have a working pacemaker), severe heart failure, and severe hypotension.
- IV form is contraindicated in ventricular tachycardia and for clients taking beta blockers.
- Use cautiously in clients who have liver or kidney dysfunction, heart failure, hypotension, or are taking digoxin or beta blockers.

Adenosine

- **Warnings**
  - Pregnancy: Safety not established
  - Lactation: Safety not established
- Contraindicated in clients who have second- and third-degree heart block, AV block, atrial flutter, and atrial fibrillation.
- Use cautiously in older adults and clients who have asthma.

Digoxin

- **Warnings**
  - Pregnancy: No adverse effects to the fetus.
  - Lactation: Can be found in breast milk. Use with caution.
- Contraindicated in clients who have ventricular tachycardia or ventricular fibrillation not caused by heart failure.
- Use cautiously in clients who have AV block, bradycardia, kidney disease, hypothyroidism, and cardiomyopathy.

INTERACTIONS

Quinidine

Antidysrhythmics have additive effects and can increase the risk for toxicity.
NURSING ACTIONS
- Monitor heart rate and rhythm.
- Notify the provider of change or start of new dysrhythmia.

Beta blockers and cimetidine can increase quinidine effects.
NURSING ACTIONS: Avoid concurrent use. Monitor ECG and blood pressure. Reduce dose if needed.

Antihypertensives have an additive hypotensive effect.
NURSING ACTIONS: Monitor blood pressure and notify the provider if there is a significant decrease.

Lidocaine

Cimetidine, beta blockers, and phenytoin can decrease metabolism of lidocaine, increasing risk of toxicity.
NURSING ACTIONS
- Monitor client for CNS depression (sedation, irritability, seizures).
- Monitor lidocaine level. Reduce dosage.

Propafenone

Propafenone can slow medication metabolism and cause an increase in the levels of digoxin, oral anticoagulants, and propranolol.
NURSING ACTIONS
- Monitor for medication toxicity.
- Monitor coagulation.

Quinidine and amiodarone increase risk of propafenone toxicity.
NURSING ACTIONS: Do not use concurrently.

Grapefruit juice can reduce propafenone metabolism and cause toxicity.
CLIENT EDUCATION: Avoid grapefruit juice.

Propranolol

Verapamil and diltiazem have additive cardiosuppression effects.
NURSING ACTIONS: Monitor ECG, heart rate, and blood pressure.

Propranolol use can mask the hypoglycemic effect of insulin and prevent the breakdown of fat in response to hypoglycemia.
NURSING ACTIONS: Use with caution. Monitor blood glucose levels.

Amiodarone

Amiodarone can increase plasma levels of quinidine, procainamide, digoxin, diltiazem, and warfarin.
NURSING ACTIONS: Lower dosages of these medications. Monitor ECG.

Cholestyramine, St. John's wort, and rifampin decreases levels of amiodarone.
NURSING ACTIONS: Monitor for therapeutic effects.

Diuretics, other antidysrhythmics, and antibiotics (erythromycin, azithromycin) can increase the risk of dysrhythmias
NURSING ACTIONS: Use cautiously with clients taking these medications.

Concurrent use of beta blockers, verapamil, and diltiazem can lead to bradycardia.
NURSING ACTIONS: Monitor clients closely.

Amiodarone can increase digoxin level.
NURSING ACTIONS: Monitor digoxin level. Monitor heart rate.

Consuming grapefruit juice can lead to toxicity.
CLIENT EDUCATION: Avoid grapefruit juice. Qs

Verapamil

Concurrent use of atenolol, esmolol, or propranolol can cause additive effects of both medications.
NURSING ACTIONS: Monitor ECG. Reduce dosages if needed.

Verapamil can potentiate carbamazepine and digoxin. Increased risk for heart block with concurrent use with digoxin.
NURSING ACTIONS: Monitor medication levels, heart rate, and ECG.

Beta blockers can cause heart failure, AV block, and bradycardia.
NURSING ACTIONS: Monitor heart rate and ECG; monitor for heart failure. Use caution.

Grapefruit juice can reduce verapamil metabolism and cause toxicity.
CLIENT EDUCATION: Avoid grapefruit juice.

Adenosine

Methylxanthines, such as theophylline and caffeine, block receptors for adenosine and therefore prevent therapeutic effect.
NURSING ACTIONS: Avoid concurrent use.

Theophylline and aminophylline decrease the effect of adenosine.
NURSING ACTIONS: Clients who have asthma and take theophylline and aminophylline may need larger doses of adenosine

Cellular uptake of dipyridamole is blocked, leading to intensification of effects of adenosine.
NURSING ACTIONS: Monitor for indications of excessive dosage, and notify the provider if these occur.

Digoxin

Amiodarone, quinidine, verapamil, diltiazem, propafenone, and flecainide are antidysrhythmics, which increase digoxin levels.
NURSING ACTIONS: Monitor for medication level and for toxicity. Reduce medication dosage if needed.

Corticosteroids, diuretics, thiazides, and amphotericin B can cause decreased potassium level.
NURSING ACTIONS: Monitor potassium and monitor medication levels for toxicity.

Antacids and metoclopramide can decrease digoxin absorption.
NURSING ACTIONS
- Monitor blood levels and effective response.
- Give dosages at wide intervals.

NURSING ADMINISTRATION

Quinidine

CLIENT EDUCATION: Take medications as prescribed.

Lidocaine

NURSING ACTIONS
- IV administration is usually started with a loading dose, which is weight-based, followed by a maintenance dose of 1 to 4 mg/min.
- Adjust the rate according to cardiac response.
- Usually used for no more than 24 hr.
- Never administer lidocaine preparation that contains epinephrine (usually in lidocaine used for local anesthesia). Severe hypertension or dysrhythmias can occur. Qs
- Monitor blood pressure, cardiac rhythm, and CNS effects (drowsiness, confusion, paresthesias, seizures, respiratory arrest).

Propafenone

NURSING ACTIONS
- Monitor ECG during treatment.
- Monitor for bradycardia and hypotension. Monitor for dizziness or weakness.

CLIENT EDUCATION: Take medication with food.

Propranolol

NURSING ACTIONS: Administer IV propranolol no faster than 1 mg/min.

CLIENT EDUCATION
- Check pulse daily and notify provider for pulse rate less than 50/min, or another prescribed rate.
- Change positions slowly. If dizziness occurs, lie flat until dizziness subsides

Amiodarone

NURSING ACTIONS
- Amiodarone is highly toxic. Monitor closely for adverse effects (lung injury, visual impairment).
- Obtain a baseline ECG, eye examination, and chest x-ray, along with potassium and magnesium levels and tests for thyroid, pulmonary, and liver function
- Provide clients with written information regarding potential toxicities.

CLIENT EDUCATION: Adverse effects can continue for weeks or months after the medication is discontinued.

Verapamil

NURSING ACTIONS
- The initial dose of verapamil should be administered IV and then followed with oral medication for long-term use.
- Monitor heart rate before doses and notify provider for HR less than 50/min. Verapamil can cause orthostatic hypotension.

CLIENT EDUCATION
- Change positions slowly. If dizziness occurs, lie flat until dizziness subsides.
- Avoid activities that require alertness until effects are known.
- Notify the provider for peripheral edema, chest pain, or shortness of breath.

Adenosine

NURSING ACTIONS
- Adenosine has a very short half-life, so adverse reactions are mild and last for less than 1 min.
- Administration should be by IV bolus, flushed with saline following administration. QEBP
- Administer an IV bolus through an IV line close to the heart because the half-life is approximately 1.5 to 10 seconds.

Digoxin

CLIENT EDUCATION
- Take apical pulse for 1 min before taking a dose. If the heart rate is less than 60/min, the client should hold the dose and notify the provider.
- Eat a high-potassium diet.

NURSING EVALUATION OF MEDICATION EFFECTIVENESS

Depending on therapeutic intent, effectiveness is evidenced by the following.
- Improvement of manifestations (chest pain, shortness of breath, bradycardia, or tachycardia)
- Absence of dysrhythmias
- Return to baseline ECG, heart rate, and regular rhythm

Active Learning Scenario

A nurse is preparing to provide teaching to a client who has a new prescription for verapamil for recurrent supraventricular tachycardia. What should the nurse teach the client about this medication? Use the ATI Active Learning Template: Medication to complete this item.

THERAPEUTIC USES

COMPLICATIONS: Identify three adverse effects.

NURSING INTERVENTIONS: Describe three, including diagnostic tests the nurse should monitor.

Application Exercises

1. A nurse is assessing a client who has taken quinidine to treat dysrhythmias for the last 12 months. The nurse should assess the client for which of the following manifestations as an adverse effect of this medication? (Select all that apply.)
   - A. Hypertension
   - B. Widened QRS complex
   - C. Narrowed QT interval
   - D. Tinnitus
   - E. Diarrhea

2. A nurse is assessing a client who is taking amiodarone to treat atrial fibrillation. Which of the following findings can be an indication of amiodarone toxicity?
   - A. Light yellow urine
   - B. Report of tinnitus
   - C. Productive cough
   - D. Blue-gray skin discoloration

3. A nurse is caring for a client who received IV verapamil to treat supraventricular tachycardia (SVT). The client's pulse rate is now 98/min, and the blood pressure is 74/44 mm Hg. The nurse should expect a prescription for which of the following IV medications?
   - A. Calcium gluconate
   - B. Sodium bicarbonate
   - C. Potassium chloride
   - D. Magnesium sulfate

4. A nurse is assessing a client who is taking digoxin to treat heart failure. Which of the following findings is a manifestation of digoxin toxicity?
   - A. Bruising
   - B. Report of metallic taste
   - C. Muscle pain
   - D. Report of anorexia

5. A nurse is preparing to administer propranolol to a client who has a dysrhythmia. Which of the following actions should the nurse plan to take?
   - A. Hold propranolol for an apical pulse greater than 100/min.
   - B. Administer propranolol to increase the client's blood pressure.
   - C. Assist the client when sitting up or standing after taking this medication.
   - D. Check for hypokalemia frequently due to the risk for propranolol toxicity.

Active Learning Scenario Key

Using the ATI Active Learning Template: Medication

THERAPEUTIC USES: Verapamil is a calcium channel blocker and a class IV antidysrhythmic medication that decreases heart rate, slows conduction through both the SA and AV nodes, and decreases force of contraction of the heart. It is used to treat supraventricular tachycardia (SVT).

COMPLICATIONS

- Bradycardia
- Hypotension
- Heart failure
- Constipation

NURSING INTERVENTIONS

- Monitor both kidney and liver function because the medication dosage might need to be lowered if either kidney or liver impairment are present.
- Monitor blood pressure and pulse.
- Monitor periodic ECG testing for dysrhythmias and for improvement of SVT.
- Assess for manifestations of heart failure, such as dyspnea and crackles in the lungs.
- Question the client about dizziness, which can occur due to hypotension.
- Teach the client to move slowly from lying to sitting or standing and to avoid driving or operating heavy machinery until effects of verapamil are known.

Ⓝ *NCLEX® Connection: Pharmacological and Parenteral Therapies, Medication Administration*

Application Exercises Key

1. B. **CORRECT:** When taking actions, the nurse should assess the client for manifestations of potential adverse effects of this medication. On the ECG, quinidine can cause a widened QRS complex, which is a manifestation of cardiotoxicity if the QRS complex becomes widened by more than 50% of the expected reference range.
   D. **CORRECT:** It can cause cinchonism which is characterized by tinnitus, headache, nausea, vertigo, and disturbed vision.
   E. **CORRECT:** The nurse should assess the client for diarrhea as an adverse effect of quinidine. It can be intense and lead to discontinuation of the medication.

Ⓝ *NCLEX® Connection: Pharmacological and Parenteral Therapies, Adverse Effects/Contraindications/Side Effects/Interactions*

2. C. **CORRECT:** The nurse should analyze the cues from the client's manifestations and determine that a productive cough can indicate pulmonary toxicity or heart failure. The nurse should assess for cough, chest pain, and shortness of breath.

Ⓝ *NCLEX® Connection: Pharmacological and Parenteral Therapies, Adverse Effects/Contraindications/Side Effects/Interactions*

3. A. **CORRECT:** The nurse should plan to generate solutions to address the client's hypotension which includes the administration of calcium gluconate, given slowly via IV. The calcium counteracts vasodilation caused by verapamil. Other measures to increase blood pressure can include IV fluid therapy and placing the client in a modified Trendelenburg position.

Ⓝ *NCLEX® Connection: Pharmacological and Parenteral Therapies, Expected Actions/Outcomes*

4. D. **CORRECT:** The nurse should analyze the cues from the client's manifestations and determine that anorexia, blurred vision, stomach pain, and diarrhea are manifestations of digoxin toxicity.

Ⓝ *NCLEX® Connection: Pharmacological and Parenteral Therapies, Adverse Effects/Contraindications/Side Effects/Interactions*

5. C. **CORRECT:** The nurse should plan to generate solutions to address the client's potential orthostatic hypotension following administration of propranolol which includes assessing for dizziness during ambulation or when moving to a standing or sitting position.

Ⓝ *NCLEX® Connection: Pharmacological and Parenteral Therapies, Medication Administration*

When reviewing the following chapters, keep in mind the relevant topics and tasks of the NCLEX outline, in particular:

Pharmacological and Parenteral Therapies

ADVERSE EFFECTS/CONTRAINDICATIONS/SIDE EFFECTS/INTERACTIONS

Evaluate and document the client's response to actions taken to counteract side effects and adverse effects of medications and parenteral therapy.

Assess the client for actual or potential side effects and adverse effects of medications.

DOSAGE CALCULATIONS: Perform calculations needed for medication administration.

MEDICATION ADMINISTRATION

Administer and document medications given by parenteral routes.

Evaluate appropriateness and accuracy of medication order for client.

EXPECTED ACTIONS/OUTCOMES: Use clinical decision making/critical thinking when addressing expected effects/outcomes of medications.

PARENTERAL/INTRAVENOUS THERAPIES: Apply knowledge and concepts of mathematics/nursing procedures/psychomotor skills when caring for a client receiving intravenous and parenteral therapy.

CHAPTER 23
Medications Affecting Coagulation

Pharmaceutical agents that modify coagulation are used to prevent clot formation or break apart an existing clot. These medications work in the blood to alter the clotting cascade, prevent platelet aggregation, or dissolve a clot. All carry a significant risk of bleeding.

The goal of medications that alter coagulation is to increase circulation and perfusion, decrease pain, and prevent further tissue damage.

The groups of medications used include oral and parenteral anticoagulants, antiplatelet medications, and thrombolytic agents. Anticoagulant medications include heparins, vitamin K antagonists, direct thrombin inhibitors, and direct factor Xa inhibitors.

Anticoagulants

Heparins

SELECT PROTOTYPE MEDICATION: Heparin (unfractionated)

Low molecular weight (LMW) heparins

SELECT PROTOTYPE MEDICATION: Enoxaparin

OTHER MEDICATIONS: Dalteparin

Activated factor Xa inhibitor

SELECT PROTOTYPE MEDICATION: Fondaparinux

PURPOSE

EXPECTED PHARMACOLOGICAL ACTION
Heparin prevents clotting by activating antithrombin, thus indirectly inactivating both thrombin and factor Xa. This inhibits fibrin formation. LMW heparins and activated factor Xa inhibitors only inactivate factor Xa.

THERAPEUTIC USES

Heparin
- Conditions necessitating prompt anticoagulant activity (evolving stroke, pulmonary embolism [PE], massive deep-vein thrombosis)
- An adjunct for clients having open heart surgery or dialysis
- Low-dose therapy for prophylaxis against postoperative venous thrombosis (for example, hip/knee or abdominal surgery)
- Treatment of disseminated intravascular coagulation

Low molecular weight heparins
- Prevent deep-vein thrombosis (DVT) in clients who are postoperative.
- Treat DVT and PE.
- Prevent complications in angina, non-Q wave MI, and ST elevation MI.

Activated factor Xa inhibitor (fondaparinux)
- Prevent DVT and PE in postoperative clients.
- Treat acute DVT or PE in conjunction with warfarin.

COMPLICATIONS

Heparin

Toxicity
NURSING ACTIONS
- Administer protamine, which binds with heparin and forms a heparin-protamine complex that has no anticoagulant properties.
- Protamine should be administered slowly IV, no faster than 20 mg/min or 50 mg in 10 min.
- Do not exceed 100 mg in a 2-hr period. Administer carefully to prevent protamine toxicity.

Hemorrhage secondary to heparin toxicity or other factors
Hemorrhage can occur if medication administration leads to high activated partial thromboplastin time. Other risk factors include client history of bleeding disorder or taking antiplatelet medications concurrently.

NURSING ACTIONS
- Monitor vital signs.
- Advise clients to observe for bleeding: increased heart rate, decreased blood pressure, bruising, petechiae, hematomas, black tarry stools.
- Monitor activated partial thromboplastin time (aPTT). Keep value at 1.5 to 2 times the baseline. Ⓠ EBP
- If hemorrhage occurs, stop heparin administration. Check for toxicity and follow treatment protocols, and discontinue other medications that affect coagulation as indicated.

Epidural or spinal hematoma

- The risk for hematoma at the puncture site for spinal or epidural medication administration is increased while taking heparin.
- Factors that further increase risk include taking other anticoagulants or antiplatelet medications, history of spinal problems or surgery, or use of an indwelling epidural catheter.

NURSING ACTIONS: Monitor carefully for neurologic changes, which could indicate hematoma development.

Heparin-induced thrombocytopenia

Evidenced by low platelet count and increased development of thrombi: mediated by antibody development (white clot syndrome)

NURSING ACTIONS

- Monitor platelet count periodically throughout treatment, especially in the first month.
- Stop heparin if platelet count is less than 100,000/mm³. Nonheparin anticoagulants (lepirudin, argatroban), can be used as a substitute if anticoagulation is still needed.

Hypersensitivity reactions (chills, fever, urticaria)

NURSING ACTIONS: Administer a small test dose prior to the administration of heparin.

Enoxaparin

Hemorrhage

NURSING ACTIONS

- Monitor vital signs.
- Monitor platelet count.

CLIENT EDUCATION

- Observe for bleeding: increased heart rate, decreased blood pressure, bruising, petechiae, hematomas, black tarry stools.
- Avoid aspirin.

Neurologic damage from hematoma formed during spinal or epidural anesthesia

NURSING ACTIONS: In clients who have spinal or epidural anesthesia: Assess insertion site for indications of hematoma formation (redness, swelling). Monitor sensation and movement of lower extremities. Notify provider of abnormal findings.

Heparin-induced (immune mediated) thrombocytopenia

NURSING ACTIONS: Monitor platelets. Discontinue medication for platelet count less than 100,000/mm³.

Toxicity

NURSING ACTIONS

- Administer protamine (heparin antagonist)
- Protamine should be administered slowly IV, no faster than 20 mg/min or 50 mg in 10 min.

Fondaparinux

Hemorrhage

NURSING ACTIONS

- Monitor vital signs.
- Monitor platelet count.

CLIENT EDUCATION

- Observe for bleeding: increased heart rate, decreased blood pressure, bruising, petechiae, hematomas, black tarry stools.
- Avoid aspirin.

Neurologic damage from hematoma formed during spinal or epidural anesthesia

NURSING ACTIONS: In clients who have spinal or epidural anesthesia: Assess insertion site for indications of hematoma formation (redness or swelling). Monitor sensation and movement of lower extremities. Notify provider of abnormal findings.

Decreased platelet count

NURSING ACTIONS: Monitor platelets. Discontinue medication for platelet count less than 100,000/mm³.

CONTRAINDICATIONS/PRECAUTIONS

- **Warnings**
  - Pregnancy
    - Heparin: Use with caution.
    - LMW heparins: Safety not established. Caution with clients who have prosthetic heart valves.
    - Fondaparinux: Use only if needed.
  - Lactation
    - Heparin: Use with caution.
    - LMW heparins and fondaparinux: Safety not established.
- Contraindicated in clients who have low platelet counts (thrombocytopenia) or uncontrollable bleeding. Qs
- These medications should not be used during or following surgeries of the eye(s), brain, or spinal cord; lumbar puncture; or regional anesthesia.
- Use cautiously in clients who have hemophilia, increased capillary permeability, dissecting aneurysm, peptic ulcer disease, severe hypertension, hepatic or kidney disease, or threatened abortion.
- Heparin and LMW heparins are used during pregnancy, if anticoagulation is desired. For clients who are pregnant and have heparin-induced thrombocytopenia, argatroban can be prescribed instead.

INTERACTIONS

Antiplatelet agents (aspirin, NSAIDs, and other anticoagulants) can increase risk for bleeding. Resveratrol and saw palmetto can also have antiplatelet effects.
NURSING ACTIONS

- Avoid concurrent use when possible.
- Monitor carefully for evidence of bleeding.
- Take precautionary measures to avoid injury (limit venipunctures and injections).

Garlic, ginger, glucosamine or ginkgo biloba can increase the risk of bleeding.
CLIENT EDUCATION: This medication has an increased risk for bleeding and to monitor for bleeding.

NURSING ADMINISTRATION

These medications cannot be absorbed by the intestinal tract and must be given via subcutaneous injection or IV infusion.

Heparin Q EBP

- Obtain baseline vital signs.
- Obtain baseline and monitor aPTT, platelet count, and hematocrit levels.
- Read label carefully. Heparin is dispensed in units and in a variety of concentrations.
- Check dosages with another nurse before administration.
- Use an infusion pump for continuous IV administration.
  - Monitor rate of infusion every 30 to 60 min. Qs
  - Monitor aPTT every 4 to 6 hr until appropriate dose is determined, then monitor daily.
- Administer deep subcutaneous injections in the abdomen, ensuring a distance of 2 inches from the umbilicus. Do not aspirate.
  - Use a 20- to 22-gauge needle to withdraw medication from the vial. Then, change the needle to a smaller needle (25- or 31-gauge, 3/8 to 5/8 inches long).
  - Apply gentle pressure for 1 to 2 min after the injection. Rotate and record injection sites.
- Advise clients to use an electric razor for shaving and to brush with a soft toothbrush.

CLIENT EDUCATION
- Monitor for indications of bleeding: bruising, gums bleeding, abdominal pain, nose bleeds, coffee-ground emesis, and tarry stools.
- Avoid the use of over-the-counter (OTC) NSAIDs, aspirin, or medications containing salicylates.

Enoxaparin/fondaparinux

- Monitoring is not required. These medications are acceptable for home use.
- Provide instruction regarding self-administration. Medications can be available in prefilled syringes.
- Prefilled syringes are available in various dosages for subcutaneous injection. Do not expel the air bubble in the syringe unless adjustments must be made to the dose.
- For subcutaneous injections when a prefilled syringe is not available, use a 20- to 22-gauge needle to withdraw medication from the vial. Then, change to a small needle (25- to 31-gauge, 3/8 to 5/8 inches long). Deep subcutaneous injections should be administered in the abdomen, ensuring a distance of 2 inches from the umbilicus. Do not aspirate.
- Rotate sites between right and left anterolateral and posterolateral abdominal walls at least 2 inches from umbilicus. Pinch up an area of skin, inject at a 90° angle, and insert needle completely. Do not aspirate. Inject entire contents of syringe. Q EBP
- Do not rub the site for 1 to 2 min after the injection. Rotate and record injection sites.

CLIENT EDUCATION
- Monitor for indications of bleeding, (bruising, gums bleeding, abdominal pain, nose bleeds, coffee-ground emesis, and tarry stools).
- Avoid the use of OTC NSAIDs, aspirin, or medications containing salicylates.
- Use an electric razor for shaving and brush with a soft toothbrush.

NURSING EVALUATION OF MEDICATION EFFECTIVENESS

Depending on therapeutic intent, effectiveness can be evidenced by the following.

Heparin: aPTT levels of 60 to 80 seconds during treatment

Heparin, enoxaparin, and fondaparinux: No development or no further development of venous thrombi or emboli

Vitamin K inhibitors (Coumarins)

SELECT PROTOTYPE MEDICATION: Warfarin

PURPOSE

EXPECTED PHARMACOLOGICAL ACTION: Antagonizes vitamin K, thereby preventing the synthesis of four coagulation factors: factor VII, IX, X, and prothrombin.

THERAPEUTIC USES
- Prevention of venous thrombosis and PE.
- Prevention of thrombotic events for clients who have atrial fibrillation or prosthetic heart valves.
- Reduction of the risk for recurrent transient ischemic attacks or myocardial infarction.

COMPLICATIONS

Hemorrhage

NURSING ACTIONS
- Monitor vital signs.
- Advise clients to observe for bleeding (increased heart rate, decreased blood pressure, bruising, petechiae, hematomas, black tarry stools).
- Obtain baseline prothrombin time (PT) and monitor levels of PT and international normalized ratio (INR) periodically. In the case of warfarin toxicity, discontinue administration of warfarin, and administer vitamin K_1.

Hepatitis

NURSING ACTIONS: Monitor liver enzymes. Assess for jaundice.

Toxicity

NURSING ACTIONS
- Administer vitamin K₁ to promote synthesis of coagulation factors VII, IX, X, and prothrombin.
- Administer IV vitamin K₁ slowly and in a diluted solution to prevent anaphylactoid-type reaction. Qs
- Administer small doses of vitamin K₁ (2.5 mg PO, 0.5 to 1 mg IV) to prevent development of resistance to warfarin.
- If vitamin K₁ cannot control bleeding, administer fresh frozen plasma or whole blood.

CONTRAINDICATIONS/PRECAUTIONS

- **Warnings**
  - Pregnancy: Warfarin is contraindicated.
  - Lactation: Warfarin is safe. Monitor infant for bruising or bleeding.
  - Reproductive: Use warfarin with caution. Notify provider if pregnancy is planned.
- Contraindicated in clients who have low platelet counts (thrombocytopenia) or uncontrollable bleeding.
- Contraindicated during or following surgeries of the eye(s), brain, or spinal cord; lumbar puncture; or regional anesthesia.
- Contraindicated in clients who have vitamin K deficiencies, liver disorders, and alcohol use disorder due to the additive risk of bleeding.
- Use cautiously in clients who have hemophilia, dissecting aneurysm, peptic ulcer disease, severe hypertension, or threatened abortion.

INTERACTIONS

Concurrent use of heparin, aspirin, acetaminophen, glucocorticoids, sulfonamides, and parenteral cephalosporins increases effects of warfarin, which increases the risk for bleeding.
NURSING ACTIONS
- Avoid concurrent use if possible.
- If used concurrently, monitor carefully for indications of bleeding and increased PT, INR, and aPTT levels.
- Medication dosage should be adjusted accordingly.
CLIENT EDUCATION: Observe for inclusion of aspirin in OTC medications.

Concurrent use of phenobarbital, carbamazepine, phenytoin, oral contraceptives, and vitamin K decreases anticoagulant effects.
NURSING ACTIONS
- Avoid concurrent use if possible.
- If used concurrently, monitor carefully for reduced PT and INR levels.
- Medication dosage should be adjusted accordingly.

Foods high in vitamin K (dark green leafy vegetables [lettuce, cooked spinach], cabbage, broccoli, Brussels sprouts, mayonnaise, and canola and soybean oil) can decrease anticoagulant effects.
NURSING ACTIONS: Provide clients with a list of foods high in vitamin K.

CLIENT EDUCATION: Maintain a consistent intake of vitamin K to avoid sudden fluctuations that could affect the action of warfarin. If there is a need to increase consumption of these foods, discuss dosage increase with the provider. Qs

Resveratrol and saw palmetto increase the risk of bleeding through antiplatelet effects.

Coenzyme Q-10 (CoQ-10) can decrease warfarin effectiveness due to a similar structure to vitamin K.
CLIENT EDUCATION: Avoid taking these concurrently, or discuss with the provider.

Feverfew, garlic, ginger, glucosamine or ginkgo biloba can increase the risk of bleeding.
NURSING ACTIONS: Monitor for bleeding.

Multiple other medications interact with warfarin.
NURSING ACTIONS: Take a complete medication history for clients taking warfarin, and advise clients to inform the provider if any new medication is started.

NURSING ADMINISTRATION

- Administration is usually oral, once daily, and at the same time each day.
- Obtain baseline vital signs.
- Monitor PT levels (therapeutic level 18 to 24 seconds) and INR levels (therapeutic levels 2 to 3). INR levels are the most accurate. Hold dose and notify the provider if these levels exceed therapeutic ranges. QEBP
- Obtain baseline and monitor CBC, platelet count, and Hct levels.
- Be prepared to administer vitamin K₁ for warfarin toxicity.
- Plan for frequent PT monitoring for clients who are prescribed medications that interact with warfarin. The client is at greatest risk for harm when the interacting medication is being deleted or added. Frequent PT monitoring allows for dosage adjustments as necessary.
CLIENT EDUCATION
- Anticoagulant effects can take 8 to 12 hr, and full therapeutic effect is not achieved for 3 to 5 days. If in the hospital setting, continued heparin infusion is needed when starting oral warfarin.
- Anticoagulation effects can persist for up to 5 days following discontinuation of medication due to a long half-life.
- Avoid alcohol and OTC and nonprescription medications to prevent adverse effects and medication interactions (risk of bleeding).
- Prevent development of thrombi by avoiding sitting for prolonged periods of time, not wearing constricting clothing, and elevating and moving legs when sitting.
- Wear a medical alert bracelet indicating warfarin use.
- Record dosage, route, and time of warfarin administration on a daily basis. Report this information to the provider during follow ups.
- Use a soft-bristle toothbrush to prevent gum bleeding and an electric razor for shaving.
- Follow up with the provider for regular PT and INR monitoring, or monitor the INR at home. Qpcc

NURSING EVALUATION OF MEDICATION EFFECTIVENESS

Depending on therapeutic intent, effectiveness can be evidenced by the following.
- PT 1.5 to 2 times control
- INR of 2 to 3 for treatment of acute myocardial infarction, atrial fibrillation, venous thrombosis, or tissue heart valves
- INR of 2.5 to 2.5 for treatment of a PE.
- INR of 3 to 4.5 for mechanical heart valve or recurrent systemic embolism
- No development or no further development of venous thrombi

Direct thrombin inhibitors

SELECT PROTOTYPE MEDICATION: Dabigatran

OTHER MEDICATIONS
- **Hirudin analogs:** Bivalirudin, desirudin
- Argatroban

PURPOSE

EXPECTED PHARMACOLOGICAL ACTION: These medications work by binding with and inhibiting thrombin, thus preventing a thrombus from developing.

THERAPEUTIC USES
- **Dabigatran** prevents stroke or embolism in clients who have atrial fibrillation not caused by valvular heart disease. It is also used to treat and prevent DVT and PE.
- **Bivalirudin** is given concurrently with aspirin for clients who undergo percutaneous coronary angioplasty or intervention.
- **Argatroban** is used to prevent or treat thrombosis in clients who cannot take heparin due to heparin-induced thrombocytopenia.
- **Desirudin** is administered to clients having hip replacement surgery to prevent DVT.

COMPLICATIONS

Bleeding

NURSING ACTIONS
- Teach clients to report manifestations of bleeding to the provider.
- For severe bleeding, idarucizumab can be administered as an antidote. Dialysis or injections of recombinant factor VIIa can be used.
- Clients undergoing elective surgery should stop taking dabigatran before surgery.

GI effects

GI discomfort, nausea, vomiting, esophageal reflux, ulcer formation

NURSING ACTIONS
- Take dabigatran with food.
- The client might need a proton pump inhibitor (omeprazole) or an H_2 receptor antagonist (cimetidine) for these manifestations.

Other effects

- Bivalirudin can also cause back pain, nausea, hypotension, and headache.
- Desirudin can also cause injection-site mass, anemia, nausea, and deep thrombophlebitis.

CONTRAINDICATIONS/PRECAUTIONS

- **Warnings**
  - Pregnancy
    - Dabigatran: Safety not established.
    - Argatroban and bivalirudin: Use only if needed.
  - Lactation
    - Dabigatran: Use with caution.
    - Argatroban: Contraindicated.
    - Bivalirudin: Safety not established.
  - Reproductive: For dabigatran, notify provider if pregnancy is planned or suspected.
- Contraindicated in clients who have active bleeding or allergy to the medication. Qs
- Use cautiously in clients who have liver impairment or who are at risk for bleeding.
- Use dabigatran, bivalirudin, and desirudin cautiously in clients who have kidney impairment.

INTERACTIONS

Rifampin decreases levels of dabigatran.
NURSING ACTIONS: Use cautiously together, and watch for therapeutic effect.

Medications that inhibit P-glycoprotein (ketoconazole, verapamil, quinidine) can increase blood levels of dabigatran.
NURSING ACTIONS: Avoid administering these medications concurrently with dabigatran.

Other thrombolytics and anticoagulants can increase risk for bleeding with argatroban, desirudin, bivalirudin, or dabigatran.
NURSING ACTIONS: Monitor coagulation studies carefully with concurrent use.

Feverfew, garlic, ginger, glucosamine ginkgo biloba, resveratrol, or saw palmetto can increase the risk of bleeding.
CLIENT EDUCATION: This medication has an increased risk for bleeding; monitor for bleeding.

NURSING ADMINISTRATION

- Dabigatran is available in oral capsules that should be swallowed whole and can be taken with or without food. The container should be used within 30 days of opening. Discontinue other anticoagulants when starting dabigatran.
- Bivalirudin is administered IV by direct bolus or continuous infusion.
- Argatroban is administrated IV by continuous infusion. Before starting, discontinue heparin and check aPTT.
- Desirudin is administered by deep subcutaneous injection into the abdomen or thigh.

NURSING EVALUATION OF MEDICATION EFFECTIVENESS

Depending on therapeutic intent, effectiveness can be evidenced by prevention or reduction of thrombus formation.

Direct inhibitor of factor Xa

SELECT PROTOTYPE MEDICATION: Rivaroxaban

OTHER MEDICATIONS
- Apixaban
- Dabigatran

PURPOSE

EXPECTED PHARMACOLOGICAL ACTION: Provides anticoagulation selectively and directly by inhibiting factor Xa to prevent formation of thrombin.

THERAPEUTIC USES
- Stroke prevention for clients who have atrial fibrillation.
- Prevention of postoperative DVT or PE for clients having hip or knee replacement.
- Treatment of DVT or PE unrelated to orthopedic surgery.

COMPLICATIONS

Bleeding

GI, GU, cranial, retinal, or epidural bleeding following removal of epidural catheter

NURSING ACTIONS
- Teach the client to report bleeding, bruising, headache, or eye pain.
- Monitor hemoglobin and hematocrit.
- Wait at least 18 hr following last dose to remove an epidural catheter, and wait 6 hr after removal before starting rivaroxaban again. Qs
- For reversal, administer andexanet alfa (apixaban, rivaroxaban) or idarucizumab (dabigatran). Dialysis is ineffective in removing the medication from the bloodstream. Activated charcoal can be given to prevent further absorption.

Elevated liver enzymes and bilirubin

Liver enzymes: ALT, AST, and GGT

NURSING ACTIONS
- Monitor baseline and periodic liver function.
- Report elevated values to provider.

CONTRAINDICATIONS/PRECAUTIONS

- **Warnings**
  - Pregnancy: Use rivaroxaban only if the benefit to the client outweighs the risks to the fetus.
  - Lactation: Rivaroxaban is contraindicated.
  - Reproductive: For rivaroxaban, notify provider if pregnancy is planned or suspected.
- Contraindicated in clients who have previous allergy to rivaroxaban, or who have active bleeding, severe kidney impairment, or moderate to severe liver impairment.
- Use cautiously in clients taking anticoagulants, antiplatelet medications, or fibrinolytics, and clients who have mild liver or moderate kidney impairment.

INTERACTIONS

Itraconazole, ritonavir, or ketoconazole can increase blood levels of rivaroxaban. For clients who have renal impairment, amiodarone, quinidine, diltiazem, verapamil, ranolazine, and macrolide antibiotics can increase blood levels of rivaroxaban.
NURSING ACTIONS: Monitor carefully for bleeding if these medications are taken concurrently.

Rifampin, carbamazepine, phenytoin, and St. John's wort can decrease rivaroxaban levels.
NURSING ACTIONS: Monitor for therapeutic effect in clients who take medications concurrently.

Feverfew, garlic, ginger, glucosamine ginkgo biloba, resveratrol, or saw palmetto can increase the risk of bleeding.
CLIENT EDUCATION: This medication has an increased risk for bleeding; monitor for bleeding.

NURSING ADMINISTRATION

- Administer tablets orally, once daily, with or without food, and at the same time each day. QEBP
- For stroke and systemic embolism prevention, administer orally once daily with the evening meal.
- Monitor hemoglobin, hematocrit, and liver and kidney function periodically during treatment.

Antiplatelets

Antiplatelet/cyclooxygenase inhibitor

SELECT PROTOTYPE MEDICATION: Aspirin

Antiplatelet/glycoprotein inhibitors

SELECT PROTOTYPE MEDICATION: Abciximab

OTHER MEDICATIONS: Eptifibatide, tirofiban

Antiplatelet/ADP inhibitors

SELECT PROTOTYPE MEDICATIONS: Clopidogrel

OTHER MEDICATIONS: Ticagrelor

Antiplatelet/arterial vasodilator

SELECT PROTOTYPE MEDICATION: Dipyridamole

OTHER MEDICATIONS: Cilostazol

PURPOSE

EXPECTED PHARMACOLOGICAL ACTIONS
- Antiplatelets prevent platelets from clumping together by inhibiting enzymes and factors that normally lead to arterial clotting.
- Antiplatelet medications inhibit platelet aggregation at the onset of the clotting process. These medications alter bleeding time.

THERAPEUTIC USES
- Primary prevention of acute myocardial infarction
- Prevention of reinfarction in clients following an acute myocardial infarction
- Prevention of ischemic stroke or transient ischemic attack
- Acute coronary syndromes (abciximab, tirofiban, eptifibatide, clopidogrel)
- Intermittent claudication (cilostazol, pentoxifylline, dipyridamole)

ROUTES OF ADMINISTRATION
- Aspirin: Oral
- Abciximab: IV
- Clopidogrel: Oral
- Dipyridamole: Oral

COMPLICATIONS

Aspirin

GI effects (nausea, vomiting, dyspepsia)
NURSING ACTIONS: Concurrent use of a proton pump inhibitor (omeprazole) might decrease GI effects.
CLIENT EDUCATION: Use enteric-coated tablets and to take aspirin with food. ○EBP

Hemorrhagic stroke
CLIENT EDUCATION: Observe for weakness, dizziness, and headache, and notify the provider if effects occur.

Prolonged bleeding time, gastric bleed, thrombocytopenia
NURSING ACTIONS: Monitor bleeding time. Monitor for manifestations of gastric bleed (coffee-ground emesis or bloody, tarry stools). Monitor for bruising, petechiae, and bleeding gums.

Tinnitus, hearing loss
NURSING ACTIONS
- Monitor for hearing loss.
- If manifestations occur, withhold the dose and notify the provider.

Abciximab

Hypotension and bradycardia
NURSING ACTIONS: Monitor heart rate and blood pressure.

Prolonged bleeding time, gastric bleed, thrombocytopenia, bleed from cardiac catheterization site
NURSING ACTIONS
- Monitor bleeding time (risk of bleeding doubled).
- Monitor for gastric bleed (coffee-ground emesis or bloody, tarry stools).
- Monitor for bruising, petechiae, and bleeding gums Monitor for flank bruising (retroperitoneal bleed), and for blood in the urine, emesis, or stool.
- Apply pressure to the cardiac catheter access site.

Clopidogrel

Bleeding
Prolonged bleeding time, gastric bleed, thrombocytopenia
NURSING ACTIONS
- Monitor bleeding time.
- Monitor for gastric bleed (coffee-ground emesis or bloody, tarry stools).
- Monitor for bruising, petechiae, and bleeding gums.
- Apply pressure to cardiac catheter access.

GI effects (diarrhea, dyspepsia, pain)
CLIENT EDUCATION: Monitor for effects and notify the provider.

Dipyridamole

Dyspepsia, nausea, vomiting
NURSING ACTIONS
- Take with food.
- Do not crush or chew medication.
- Monitor hydration if GI upset occurs.

CONTRAINDICATIONS/PRECAUTIONS

Aspirin

- **Warnings**
  - Pregnancy: Use with caution. Avoid during the third trimester.
  - Lactation: Safety not established.
- Contraindicated in clients who have bleeding disorders and thrombocytopenia.
- Use cautiously in clients who have peptic ulcer disease and severe kidney or hepatic disorders. Do not give to children or adolescents who have fever or recent chickenpox.
- Use with caution in older adults. Ⓖ

Abciximab

- **Warnings**
  - Pregnancy: Safety not established.
  - Lactation: Contraindicated.
- Contraindications include clients who have thrombocytopenia, recent stroke, AV malformation, aneurysm, uncontrolled hypertension, and recent major surgery.

Clopidogrel

- **Warnings**
  - Pregnancy: Use only if needed.
  - Lactation: Contraindicated.
  - Reproductive: Notify provider if pregnancy is planned or suspected.
- Contraindications include clients who have thrombocytopenia, or history of bleeding due to peptic ulcer disease, and intracranial bleed.
- Use cautiously in clients who have peptic ulcer disease and severe kidney or hepatic disorders. Clients who are breastfeeding should not take this medication.

Dipyridamole

- **Warnings**
  - Pregnancy: Safety not established
  - Lactation: Contraindicated
- Contraindicated for clients who have bleeding disorders or retinal or cerebral bleeds.

INTERACTIONS

Aspirin

Feverfew, garlic, ginger, glucosamine ginkgo biloba, resveratrol, or saw palmetto can increase the risk of bleeding.
CLIENT EDUCATION: This medication has an increased risk for bleeding; monitor for bleeding.

Concurrent use of other medications that enhance bleeding (heparin, warfarin, thrombolytics, antiplatelets) increases risk for bleeding.
NURSING ACTIONS: If used concurrently, monitor carefully for indications of bleeding.

CLIENT EDUCATION: Avoid concurrent use.

Urine acidifiers (ammonium chloride) can increase aspirin levels.
NURSING ACTIONS: Monitor for aspirin toxicity (hearing loss, tinnitus).

Non-aspirin NSAIDS can reduce the antiplatelet effects of immediate-release aspirin.
NURSING ACTIONS: Take NSAIDS 2 hr after taking aspirin, if taking aspirin for cardioprotective effect.

Corticosteroids can increase aspirin excretion and decrease aspirin effects. These medications can increase risk for GI bleed.
NURSING ACTIONS
- Monitor for decreased aspirin effectiveness.
- Monitor for gastric bleed (coffee-ground emesis and tarry or bloody stools).

Caffeine can increase aspirin absorption.
NURSING ACTIONS: Monitor for toxicity.

Abciximab

Concurrent use of other medications that enhance bleeding (NSAIDs, heparin, warfarin, thrombolytics, antiplatelets) increases risk for bleeding.
NURSING ACTIONS: If used concurrently, monitor carefully for indications of bleeding.

CLIENT EDUCATION: Avoid concurrent use.

Clopidogrel

Concurrent use of other medications that enhance bleeding (NSAIDs, heparin, warfarin, thrombolytics, antiplatelets) increases risk for bleeding.
NURSING ACTIONS: If used concurrently, monitor carefully for indications of bleeding.

CLIENT EDUCATION: Avoid concurrent use.

Proton pump inhibitors or other medications that inhibit CYP2C19 (fluoxetine, fluconazole, etravirine, felbamate) decrease effectiveness.
NURSING ACTIONS: If needed for GI effects, pantoprazole interferes the least with platelet inhibition.

Dipyridamole

Concurrent use of anticoagulants increases risk for bleeding.
NURSING ACTIONS: Monitor PT and INR. Clients can require reduced dosage.

NURSING ADMINISTRATION

- Aspirin 325 mg should be taken during initial acute episode of myocardial infarction.
- Clopidogrel is sometimes prescribed concurrently with aspirin, which increases the risk for bleeding. Clopidogrel should be discontinued 5 to 7 days before an elective surgery.

CLIENT EDUCATION

- Prevention of strokes, myocardial infarctions, and reinfarction can be accomplished with low-dose aspirin (81 mg).
- Notify the provider regarding aspirin use. Qs

NURSING EVALUATION OF MEDICATION EFFECTIVENESS

Depending on therapeutic intent, effectiveness can be evidenced by absence of arterial thrombosis, adequate tissue perfusion, and blood flow without occurrence of abnormal bleeding.

Thrombolytic medications

SELECT PROTOTYPE MEDICATION: Alteplase, often called tPA (tissue plasminogen activator)

OTHER MEDICATIONS
- Tenecteplase
- Reteplase

PURPOSE

EXPECTED PHARMACOLOGICAL ACTION: Thrombolytic medications dissolve clots that have already formed. Clots are dissolved by conversion of plasminogen to plasmin, which destroys fibrinogen and other clotting factors.

THERAPEUTIC USES
- Treat acute myocardial infarction (all three medications).
- Treat massive PE (alteplase only).
- Treat acute ischemic stroke (alteplase only).
- Restore patency to central IV catheters (alteplase only).

ROUTE OF ADMINISTRATION: IV only

COMPLICATIONS

BLEEDING FOR ALL 3 FORMS

Serious risk of bleeding from different sites
- Internal bleeding: GI or GU tracts and cerebral bleeding
- Superficial bleeding: wounds, IV catheter sites

NURSING ACTIONS
- Limit venipunctures and injections.
- Apply pressure dressings to recent wounds.
- Monitor for changes in vital signs, alterations in level of consciousness, weakness, and indications of intracranial bleeding.
- Notify the provider if manifestations occur.
- Monitor aPTT and PT, Hgb, and Hct.
- The client might require blood product replacement.
- For severe bleeding, fibrinolysis following alteplase can be reversed by administration of aminocaproic acid IV.

CONTRAINDICATIONS/PRECAUTIONS

- **Warnings**
  - Pregnancy: Alteplase safety is not established.
  - Lactation: Alteplase safety is not established.
- Because of the additive risk for serious bleeding, use is contraindicated in clients who have the following. Qs
  - Any prior intracranial hemorrhage (hemorrhagic stroke)
  - Known structural cerebral lesion (arteriovenous malformation, neoplasm)
  - Active internal bleeding
  - Ischemic stroke within past 3 months other than the current episode (within prior 4.5 hr)
- Use cautiously in clients who have severe or uncontrolled hypertension, cerebral disorders (other than those contraindicated), bleeding within 2 to 4 weeks, concurrent anticoagulant use at therapeutic levels, major surgery or prolonged/traumatic CPR within prior 3 weeks, active peptic ulcer, or presence of vascular punctures that cannot be compressed, and in older adult clients.

INTERACTIONS

Concurrent use of other medications that enhance bleeding (NSAIDs, heparin, warfarin, thrombolytics, antiplatelets) increases risk for bleeding.

NURSING ACTIONS: If used concurrently, monitor the client carefully for indications of bleeding.

NURSING ADMINISTRATION

- Use of thrombolytic agents should take place as soon as possible after onset of manifestations (within 3 hr is best). QEBP
- Clients receiving a thrombolytic agent should be monitored in a setting that provides for close supervision and continuous monitoring during and after administration of the medication.
- Obtain the client's weight to calculate the dosage. Obtain baseline platelet counts, hemoglobin (Hgb), hematocrit (Hct), aPTT, PT, INR, and fibrinogen levels. Monitor periodically.
- Obtain baseline vital signs (heart rate, blood pressure), and monitor frequently per protocol.
- Nursing care includes continuous monitoring of hemodynamic status to assess for therapeutic and adverse effects of thrombolytic (relief of chest pain, indications of bleeding). Follow facility protocol.
- Provide for client safety per facility protocol.
- Ensure adequate IV access for administration of emergency medications and availability of emergency equipment.
- Do not mix any medications in an IV with thrombolytic agents.
- Minimize bruising or bleeding by limiting venipunctures and subcutaneous/IM injections. Hold direct pressure to injection site or ABG site for up to 30 min until oozing stops. Qs

- Discontinue thrombolytic therapy if life-threatening bleeding occurs. Treat blood loss with whole blood, packed red blood cells, and/or fresh frozen plasma. Ensure that IV aminocaproic acid is available for administration in the event of excessive fibrinolysis.
- Following thrombolytic therapy, administer heparin or aspirin as prescribed to decrease the risk of rethrombosis.
- Following thrombolytic therapy, administer beta blockers as prescribed to decrease myocardial oxygen consumption and to reduce the incidence and severity of reperfusion arrhythmias.
- Administer H_2 antagonists (cimetidine) or proton pump inhibitors (omeprazole) as prescribed to prevent GI bleeding.

NURSING EVALUATION OF MEDICATION EFFECTIVENESS

Depending on therapeutic intent, effectiveness can be evidenced by evidence of thrombus lysis and restoration of circulation (relief of chest pain, reduction of initial ST segment injury pattern as shown on ECG 60 to 90 min after start of therapy).

Active Learning Scenario

A nurse is teaching a client who has a new prescription for clopidogrel following a myocardial infarction. Use the ATI Active Learning Template: Medication to complete this item.

THERAPEUTIC USES: Identify the intended effect.

COMPLICATIONS: Identify two adverse effects for this medication.

NURSING INTERVENTIONS: Describe three, including one test the nurse should monitor periodically.

Application Exercises

1. A nurse is caring for a client who is receiving heparin by continuous IV infusion. The client begins vomiting blood. After the heparin has been stopped, which of the following medications should the nurse prepare to administer?
   A. Vitamin K_1
   B. Atropine
   C. Protamine
   D. Calcium gluconate

2. A nurse is planning to administer subcutaneous enoxaparin 40 mg using a prefilled syringe of enoxaparin 40 mg/0.4 mL to an adult client following hip arthroplasty. Which of the following actions should the nurse plan to take?
   A. Expel the air bubble from the prefilled syringe before injecting.
   B. Insert the needle completely into the client's tissue.
   C. Administer the injection in the client's thigh.
   D. Aspirate carefully after inserting the needle into the client's skin.

3. A nurse is caring for a client who has atrial fibrillation and a new prescription for dabigatran. Which of the following medications is prescribed concurrently to treat an adverse effect of dabigatran?
   A. Vitamin K_1
   B. Protamine
   C. Omeprazole
   D. Probenecid

4. A nurse is monitoring a client who takes aspirin daily. The nurse should identify which of the following manifestations as adverse effects of aspirin? (Select all that apply.)
   A. Hypertension
   B. Coffee-ground emesis
   C. Tinnitus
   D. Paresthesias of the extremities
   E. Nausea

5. A nurse is planning to administer IV alteplase to a client. Which of the following interventions should the nurse plan to take?
   A. Administer IM enoxaparin along with the alteplase dose.
   B. Obtain the client's weight.
   C. Administer aminocaproic acid IV prior to alteplase infusion.
   D. Prepare to administer alteplase within 8 hr of manifestation onset.

Application Exercises Key

1. C. **CORRECT:** The nurse should plan to generate solutions to address the client's vomiting of blood which includes the administration of protamine which reverses the anticoagulant effect of heparin.

   Ⓝ *NCLEX® Connection: Pharmacological and Parenteral Therapies, Parenteral/Intravenous Therapies*

2. B. **CORRECT:** The nurse should plan to generate solutions to address the client's need for enoxaparin subcutaneously which includes the need to inject the needle on the prefilled syringe completely when administering enoxaparin to administer the medication by deep subcutaneous injection.

   Ⓝ *NCLEX® Connection: Pharmacological and Parenteral Therapies, Medication Administration*

3. C. **CORRECT:** The nurse should plan to generate solutions to address the client's potential GI adverse effects from taking dabigatran which includes the concurrent administration of omeprazole or another proton pump inhibitor. Advise the client who has GI effects to take dabigatran with food.

   Ⓝ *NCLEX® Connection: Pharmacological and Parenteral Therapies, Medication Administration*

4. B, C, E. **CORRECT:** The nurse should analyze the cues from the client's manifestations and determine that dark stools or coffee-ground emesis can indicate GI bleeding, tinnitus and hearing loss, and nausea, vomiting, and abdominal pain can indicate adverse effects of aspirin therapy.

   Ⓝ *NCLEX® Connection: Pharmacological and Parenteral Therapies, Adverse Effects/Contraindications/Adverse Effects/Interactions*

5. B. **CORRECT:** When generating solutions to address the client's need for alteplase administration, which includes obtaining an accurate weight which is required to calculate the dosage for alteplase administration.

   Ⓝ *NCLEX® Connection: Pharmacological and Parenteral Therapies, Medication Administration*

Active Learning Scenario Key

Using the ATI Active Learning Template: Medication

THERAPEUTIC USES: Clopidogrel inhibits platelet aggregation and prolongs bleeding time. It is used to prevent myocardial infarction (MI) or stroke in clients who have already had an MI or stroke.

COMPLICATIONS: Like other platelet inhibitors, clopidogrel can cause bleeding due to thrombocytopenia. It can also cause GI effects (abdominal pain, nausea, diarrhea).

NURSING INTERVENTIONS
- The nurse should plan to monitor the platelet count periodically while the client takes clopidogrel.
- Teach the client to monitor for bleeding. The client should watch for black stools, coffee-ground emesis, blood in the urine, nose bleeds, unusual bruising, or petechiae. The client should inform the provider if these occur and about GI effects.
- The nurse should be aware of all medications the client is taking, because risk for bleeding increases if the medication is taken with anticoagulants or antiplatelet medications. Clopidogrel is sometimes administered concurrently with aspirin, and that increases the risk for bleeding. The medication should be discontinued 7 days before any elective surgery.

Ⓝ *NCLEX® Connection: Pharmacological and Parenteral Therapies, Medication Administration*

UNIT 5 MEDICATIONS AFFECTING THE HEMATOLOGIC SYSTEM

CHAPTER 24 *Growth Factors*

Blood cells and platelets are produced in the body by the biological process hematopoiesis. In the body, this process is naturally controlled by hormones, also known as hematopoietic growth factors.

THERAPEUTIC PURPOSES

Genetically engineered products are available for therapeutic purposes.
- Replacement of neutrophils and platelets after chemotherapy
- Hastening of bone marrow function after a bone marrow transplant
- Increase in red blood cell production for clients who have chronic kidney disease

HEMATOPOIETIC GROWTH FACTORS

There are three groups of hematopoietic growth factors.

ERYTHROPOIETIC GROWTH FACTORS: also known as erythropoiesis stimulating agents (ESAs)

Biological name: erythropoietin

LEUKOPOIETIC GROWTH FACTORS
- Biological names
  - Granulocyte colony stimulating factor
  - Granulocyte-macrophage colony-stimulating factor

Erythropoietic growth factors

SELECT PROTOTYPE MEDICATION: Epoetin alfa: erythropoietin

OTHER MEDICATIONS: Darbepoetin alfa: long-acting erythropoietin

PURPOSE

EXPECTED PHARMACOLOGICAL ACTION
Hematopoietic growth factors act on the bone marrow to increase production of red blood cells.

THERAPEUTIC USES

Epoetin alfa
- Anemia related to chronic kidney disease
- For clients who have anemia caused by chemotherapy (nonmyeloid cancers)
- To increase erythrocyte counts in clients who will undergo elective surgery
- For clients who have anemia caused by taking zidovudine for HIV/AIDS

Darbepoetin alfa: For clients who have chronic kidney disease and clients who have anemia caused by chemotherapy (nonmyeloid cancer)

COMPLICATIONS

Hypertension

Secondary to elevations in hematocrit level

NURSING ACTIONS: Monitor Hgb levels and blood pressure. If elevated, administer antihypertensive medications.

Risk for a thrombotic event

- Such as myocardial infarction or stroke if the client has an Hgb of 11 g/dL or higher, or an increase of more than 1 g/dL in 2 weeks.
- Seizures can also occur with a too-rapid rise in the blood counts.

NURSING ACTIONS
- Decrease dosage when these limits are reached. Therapy can be resumed when Hgb drops to acceptable level, but dosage should be reduced.
- Consider placing client on seizure precautions if rapid increase in Hgb or blood pressure occurs.

Deep-vein thrombosis

Increased risk in preoperative clients

NURSING ACTIONS: Prophylactic use of an anticoagulant might be needed for preoperative clients.

Headache and body aches

NURSING ACTIONS: Report headaches that are frequent or severe to the provider. Hypertension can be the cause.

CONTRAINDICATIONS/PRECAUTIONS

- **Warnings**
  - Pregnancy: Use epoetin alfa/erythropoietin only if the benefit to the client outweighs the risks to the fetus.
  - Lactation: Epoetin alfa/erythropoietin is safe for use while lactating.
- Contraindicated in clients who have uncontrolled hypertension.
- Contraindicated in clients who have some cancers due to possible increase in tumor growth.

NURSING ADMINISTRATION

- Obtain baseline blood pressure. In clients who have chronic kidney disease, control hypertension before the start of treatment. Q EBP
- Monitor blood pressure frequently, because adjustments in antihypertensive medication can also be required as treatment progresses.
- Administer by subcutaneous or IV bolus injection. Dosage is based on the client's weight.

- Do not agitate the vial of medication. Use each vial for one dose, and do not put the needle back into the vial when withdrawing the medication.
- Do not mix the medication with any other medication in the syringe.
- Dosing is usually three times per week, but can be once per week with some types of chemotherapy.
- Monitor iron levels, and implement measures to ensure an iron level that is within the expected reference range. RBC growth depends on adequate quantities of iron, folic acid, and vitamin B12. Without adequate levels of these, erythropoietin is significantly less effective.
- Monitor Hgb and Hct once weekly (darbepoetin) or at least twice per week (erythropoietin) until they reach the target range.
- Ensure that clients receive the FDA's Risk Evaluation and Mitigation Strategy medication guide that explains risks and benefits of ESAs. The medication guide also discusses ways clients can help minimize risks of the medication. Qᴘᴄᴄ
- The longer-acting forms are administered less frequently.

NURSING EVALUATION OF MEDICATION EFFECTIVENESS

Depending on therapeutic intent, effectiveness can be evidenced by Hgb level of 10 to 11 g/dL and maximum Hct of 33%.

Leukopoietic growth factors

SELECT PROTOTYPE MEDICATION: Filgrastim

OTHER MEDICATION: Pegfilgrastim

PURPOSE

EXPECTED PHARMACOLOGICAL ACTION: Leukopoietic growth factors stimulate the bone marrow to increase production of neutrophils.

THERAPEUTIC USES
- Decreases the risk of infection in clients who have neutropenia, from cancer and other conditions
- To build up numbers of hematopoietic stem cells prior to harvesting for autologous transplant

COMPLICATIONS

Elevation of plasma uric acid, lactate dehydrogenase, and alkaline phosphatase

NURSING ACTIONS: These increases are usually moderate and reverse spontaneously.

Bone pain

NURSING ACTIONS
- Monitor for bone pain, and notify the provider.
- Administer acetaminophen, or opioid analgesic if acetaminophen is not effective.

Leukocytosis

NURSING ACTIONS
- Monitor WBC two times per week during treatment.
- Decrease dose or interrupt treatment if WBC is greater than $100,000/mm^3$ or absolute neutrophil count exceeds $10,000/mm^3$.

Splenomegaly and risk of splenic rupture

With long-term use

NURSING ACTIONS: Evaluate reports of left upper quadrant abdominal pain or shoulder tip pain carefully, and report to provider.

CONTRAINDICATIONS/PRECAUTIONS

- **Warnings**
  - Pregnancy: Use filgrastim only if the benefit to the client outweighs the risks to the fetus.
  - Lactation: Use filgrastim with caution.
- Contraindicated in clients who are sensitive to Escherichia coli protein.
- Use cautiously in clients who have cancer of the bone marrow, sickle cell disease, or respiratory disease, in clients who are breastfeeding, and in children.

NURSING ADMINISTRATION

- Administer filgrastim via intermittent IV bolus, continuous IV, subcutaneous infusion, or subcutaneous injection.
- Do not agitate the vial of medication. Use each vial for one dose, and do not combine with other medications. Do not put the needle back into the vial when withdrawing the medication. Qᴇʙᴘ
- Monitor CBC two times per week.
- If the client will be administering subcutaneous filgrastim at home, provide thorough instruction on self-administration procedures.
- Administer pegfilgrastim by subcutaneous injection 24 hr after each round of chemotherapy. The client must then wait at least 14 days before starting the next round of chemotherapy.

NURSING EVALUATION OF MEDICATION EFFECTIVENESS

Depending on therapeutic intent, effectiveness can be evidenced by the following.
- Absence of infection
- WBC count and differential within expected reference ranges

Granulocyte-macrophage colony-stimulating factor

SELECT PROTOTYPE MEDICATION: Sargramostim

PURPOSE

EXPECTED PHARMACOLOGICAL ACTION: This medication acts on the bone marrow to increase production of WBCs (neutrophils, monocytes, macrophages, eosinophils).

THERAPEUTIC USES
- Hastens bone marrow function after bone marrow transplant
- Used in the treatment of failed bone marrow transplant
- Given to older adult clients who have acute myelogenous leukemia after induction of chemotherapy to accelerate neutrophil recovery and decrease incidence of life-threatening infections

COMPLICATIONS

Diarrhea, weakness, rash, malaise, and bone pain

NURSING ACTIONS
- Monitor for adverse effects, and notify the provider if they occur.
- Administer acetaminophen.

Leukocytosis, thrombocytosis

NURSING ACTIONS
- Monitor CBC two times per week during treatment.
- Reduce dose or interrupt treatment for absolute neutrophil count 20,000/mm³ or greater, WBC 50,000/mm³ or greater, or platelets 500,000/mm³ or greater.

CONTRAINDICATIONS/PRECAUTIONS

- **Warnings**
  ○ Pregnancy: Sargramostim safety not established.
  ○ Lactation: Sargramostim caution with lactation.
- Contraindicated in clients allergic to yeast and certain other products.
- Use cautiously in clients who have lung, cardiac, kidney, or hepatic disease; hypoxia; peripheral edema; or pleural or pericardial effusion.
- Use cautiously in clients who have cancer of the bone marrow.

NURSING ADMINISTRATION

- Obtain baseline CBC, differential, and platelet count. Monitor periodically during treatment. Q EBP
- When administered subcutaneously, reconstitute with sterile water. Mix contents gently, but do not shake vial.
- Administer by IV infusion, diluted and without an in-line membrane filter. Slow or discontinue infusion if client who has pre-existing heart failure or respiratory disorders experiences increase in dyspnea.

NURSING EVALUATION OF MEDICATION EFFECTIVENESS

Depending on therapeutic intent, effectiveness can be evidenced by the following.
- Absence of infection
- WBC and differential within expected reference ranges

Application Exercises

1. A nurse is monitoring a client who is receiving epoetin alfa for adverse effects. The nurse should identify which of the following findings as an adverse effect of this medication? (Select all that apply)
   A. Leukocytosis
   B. Hypertension
   C. Edema
   D. Blurred vision
   E. Headache

2. A nurse is assessing a client who has chronic neutropenia and has been receiving filgrastim. Which of the following actions should the nurse take to assess for an adverse effect of filgrastim?
   A. Assess for bone pain.
   B. Assess for right lower quadrant pain.
   C. Auscultate for crackles in the bases of the lungs.
   D. Auscultate the chest to listen for a heart murmur.

3. A nurse is preparing to administer filgrastim for the first time to a client who has just undergone a bone marrow transplant. Which of the following actions should the nurse take?
   A. Administer IM in a large muscle mass to prevent injury.
   B. Ensure that the medication is refrigerated until just prior to administration.
   C. Shake vial gently to mix well before withdrawing dose.
   D. Discard vial after removing one dose of the medication.

4. A nurse is reviewing the medical record of a client who has a new prescription for sargramostim. Which of the following findings should the nurse identify as a contraindication to administering the medication?
   A. Allergy to yeast
   B. Hypermagnesemia
   C. Hypotension
   D. Allergy to eggs

Application Exercises Key

1. **B, E. CORRECT:** The nurse should analyze the cues from the client's manifestations and determine that Hypertension and headache can be adverse effects of epoetin alfa that the nurse should monitor for throughout treatment.

   Ⓝ *NCLEX® Connection: Pharmacological and Parenteral Therapies, Adverse Effects/Contraindications/Side Effects/Interactions*

2. **A. CORRECT:** When taking actions to assess a client for potential adverse effects of filgrastim, the nurse should identify that bone pain is a dose-related adverse effect of filgrastim. It can be treated with acetaminophen and, if necessary, an opioid analgesic.

   Ⓝ *NCLEX® Connection: Pharmacological and Parenteral Therapies, Adverse Effects/Contraindications/Side Effects/Interactions*

3. **D. CORRECT:** When taking actions to administer filgrastim, the nurse should only withdraw one dose of the medication from the vial and the vial should then be discarded.

   Ⓝ *NCLEX® Connection: Pharmacological and Parenteral Therapies, Medication Administration*

4. **A. CORRECT:** The nurse should analyze the findings and determine that the priority hypothesis is that the client is at risk for an adverse reaction since a documented allergy to yeast is a contraindication for receiving sargramostim.

   Ⓝ *NCLEX® Connection: Pharmacological and Parenteral Therapies, Contraindications*

Active Learning Scenario

A nurse is teaching a client who has chronic kidney disease and a new prescription for subcutaneous epoetin alfa three times weekly. What should the nurse teach the client about this medication? Use the ATI Active Learning Template: Medication to complete this item.

THERAPEUTIC USES: Identify why epoetin alfa would benefit this client.

COMPLICATIONS: Identify two adverse effects the client should watch for.

NURSING INTERVENTIONS: Describe four, including two tests the nurse should monitor periodically.

Active Learning Scenario Key

Using the ATI Active Learning Template: Medication

THERAPEUTIC USES: Erythropoietin, a substance that stimulates bone marrow to produce red blood cells, is produced by the kidney. In clients who have chronic kidney disease, erythropoietin is no longer present and anemia results. Epoetin alfa stimulates production of red blood cells in these clients.

COMPLICATIONS
- Headaches and myalgia (body aches)
- Thrombotic events, such as myocardial infarction and stroke
- Hypertension (common, sometimes serious)
- A too-rapid increase (Hgb greater than 1 g/dL over 2 weeks, or Hgb greater than 10 g/dL) can worsen hypertension, increase risk of thrombosis, and cause seizures.

NURSING INTERVENTIONS
- Monitor baseline iron levels, CBC with differential, and platelet count.
- Monitor Hgb and Hct twice weekly until blood counts stabilize.
- Calculate dosages carefully. Both subcutaneous and IV epoetin alfa have dosages based on the client's weight. Do not shake the epoetin alfa vial, and discard vial after one dose is removed.
- Monitor blood pressure carefully, and report increases to the provider. Question the client about frequency and severity of headaches, which could be an indication of increasing blood pressure or a simple adverse effect.

Ⓝ *NCLEX® Connection: Pharmacological and Parenteral Therapies, Medication Administration*

UNIT 5   MEDICATIONS AFFECTING THE
HEMATOLOGIC SYSTEM

CHAPTER 25 *Blood and*
Blood Products

Blood and blood products are used to increase intravascular volume, replace clotting factors and components of blood, replace blood loss, and improve oxygen carrying capacity. Blood products include whole blood and components of blood (packed red blood cells, platelets, plasma, white blood cells, and albumin).

PURPOSE

Whole blood

EXPECTED PHARMACOLOGICAL ACTION: Increases circulating blood volume

THERAPEUTIC USES
- Replacement therapy for acute blood loss secondary to traumatic injuries or surgical procedures
- Volume expansion in clients who have extensive burn injury, dehydration, shock

TYPE OF REACTION
- Acute hemolytic reaction
- Febrile nonhemolytic reaction
- Anaphylactic reactions
- Mild allergic reactions
- Circulatory overload
- Hyperkalemia
- Transfusion-associated graft-versus-host disease
- Sepsis

Packed red blood cells (packed RBCs)

EXPECTED PHARMACOLOGICAL ACTION: Increases the number of RBCs

THERAPEUTIC USES
- Packed RBCs indicated in severe anemia (Hgb 6 to 10 g/dL)
- Hemoglobinopathies
- Medication-induced hemolytic anemia
- Erythroblastosis fetalis

TYPE OF REACTION
- Acute hemolytic reaction
- Febrile nonhemolytic reaction
- Anaphylactic reactions
- Mild allergic reactions
- Hyperkalemia
- Transfusion-associated graft-versus-host disease
- Sepsis

Platelet concentrate

EXPECTED PHARMACOLOGICAL ACTION: Increases platelet counts

THERAPEUTIC USES
- Platelets indicated in thrombocytopenia (aplastic anemia, chemotherapy-induced bone marrow suppression)
- Platelets indicated in active bleeding Platelets indicated in clients with a platelet count less than 10,000/mm3

TYPE OF REACTION
- Febrile nonhemolytic reaction
- Mild allergic reactions
- Sepsis

Fresh frozen plasma (FFP)

EXPECTED PHARMACOLOGICAL ACTION: Replaces coagulation factors

THERAPEUTIC USES
- Active bleeding or massive hemorrhage
- Extensive burns
- Shock
- Disseminated intravascular coagulation
- Antithrombin III deficiency
- Thrombotic thrombocytopenic purpura
- Reversal of anticoagulation effects of warfarin
- Replacement therapy for coagulation factors II, V, VII, IX, X, and XI

TYPE OF REACTION
- Acute hemolytic reaction
- Febrile nonhemolytic reaction
- Anaphylactic reactions
- Mild allergic reactions
- Circulatory overload
- Sepsis

Apheresed granulocytes

EXPECTED PHARMACOLOGICAL ACTION: Replaces neutrophils/granulocytes

THERAPEUTIC USES
- Severe neutropenia (absolute neutrophil count less than 500/mm3)
- Life-threatening bacterial/fungal infection not responding to antibiotic therapy
- Neonatal sepsis
- Neutrophil dysfunction

TYPE OF REACTION
- Acute hemolytic reaction
- Febrile nonhemolytic reaction
- Anaphylactic reactions
- Mild allergic reactions
- Circulatory overload
- Sepsis (infusion of contaminated products)

Blood typing and crossmatching

- When a client requires a blood product transfusion, the client's blood type must be determined to detect the presence of A and B antibodies; clients with both types have type O blood.
  - ABO typing is not required for autologous transfusions.
  - Transfusions of plasma products require ABO typing only.
- Testing for Rh antigens occurs next. If none are present the client is Rh-. If any are present, the client is Rh+.
- Crossmatching must be performed when a client requires transfusion of a blood product that contains RBCs. This occurs after ABO typing and Rh testing.
  - After obtaining a sample of the client's blood, some donor RBCs are mixed with the client's blood. If there is evidence the client's blood has antibodies that recognize the donor RBCs as foreign, it indicates that the transfusion would cause a hypersensitivity reaction and that the donor blood and client's blood are not compatible.

Albumin

EXPECTED PHARMACOLOGICAL ACTION: Expands circulating blood volume by exerting oncotic pressure

THERAPEUTIC USES
- Hypovolemia
- Hypoalbuminemia
- Burns
- Adult respiratory distress
- Cardiopulmonary bypass surgery
- Hemolytic disease of the newborn

TYPE OF REACTION: Risk for fluid volume excess (pulmonary edema)

COMPLICATIONS

Acute hemolytic reaction

Chills, fever, low back pain, tachycardia, tachypnea, hypotension

NURSING ACTIONS
- Prevent by using the following safety guidelines, or as guided by facility policy. Ensure client identity (using two nurses) and that Rh and ABO types are compatible.
- Assess vital signs at baseline and during the first 15 to 30 min. Stay with the client during that time. Continue to take vital signs at least hourly.
- Acute hemolytic reaction usually occurs during first 50 mL of infusion, but onset can be delayed.
- If manifestations occur, stop infusion immediately, keeping IV line open with 0.9% sodium chloride and new IV tubing. Notify the provider.

Febrile nonhemolytic reaction, fever, headache

- Occurs due to client antibodies against the donor's white blood cells.
- Findings include sudden chills, headache, flushing, anxiety, muscle pain, and an increasing temperature of at least 1° C (2° F) or more from baseline.

NURSING ACTIONS
- Observe for manifestations of a reaction and stop the transfusion if they occur, keeping the IV line open with 0.9% sodium chloride.
- Notify the provider immediately.
- Administer acetaminophen for fever.

Anaphylactic reactions

Anxiety, urticaria, wheezing, shock, cardiac arrest

NURSING ACTIONS
- If manifestations occur, stop the transfusion and notify the provider immediately, keeping the IV line open with 0.9% sodium chloride.
- Initiate CPR if necessary.
- Have epinephrine ready for IM or IV injection.

Mild allergic reactions (flushing, itching, urticaria)

NURSING ACTIONS
- Note that a client who has a history of allergic reaction to blood transfusion or has undergone a stem cell transplant might receive a prescription for washed (leukocyte-poor) red blood cells to prevent allergic reaction.
- If manifestations occur, stop the transfusion and notify the provider immediately, keeping the IV line open with 0.9% sodium chloride.
- If manifestations are very mild and there is no respiratory compromise, antihistamines can be prescribed, and the transfusion restarted slowly.

Circulatory overload

Cough, shortness of breath, crackles, hypertension, tachycardia, distended neck veins

NURSING ACTIONS
- Observe for manifestations of fluid volume excess.
- In older adults or clients at risk for overload, transfuse 1 unit of Packed RBCs over 2 to 4 hr, avoiding any concurrent fluid infusion into another IV site. Monitor vital signs every 15 min throughout transfusion. If possible, wait 2 hr between units of blood when multiple units have been prescribed.
- If manifestations occur, stop the transfusion, place the client in a sitting position with the legs down, and notify the provider.
- Administer diuretics and oxygen as appropriate.
- Monitor I&O.
- Prior to any transfusion, assess kidney, respiratory, and cardiovascular function for risk of overload.

Sepsis

Rapid onset of chills and fever, vomiting, diarrhea, hypotension, shock

NURSING ACTIONS

- Ensure IV access, and have equipment prepared prior to removing blood product from refrigeration.
- Inspect blood product for gas bubbles, discoloration, or cloudiness (which can indicate bacterial contamination) and return to blood bank if abnormalities are seen.
- Transfuse unit of blood within 4 hr after removal from refrigeration.
- Observe for sepsis during and following transfusion.
- Stop the transfusion and keep the line open with 0.9% sodium chloride.
- Notify the provider immediately if manifestations of sepsis occur.
- Obtain blood culture, send transfusion bag for analysis for possible contaminants, and treat sepsis with antibiotics, IV fluids, vasopressors, and steroids.

Hyperkalemia due to lysis of blood cells

Bradycardia, hypotension, irregular heartbeat, paresthesia of extremities, muscle twitching, potassium level 5.0 mEq/L or greater

NURSING ACTIONS

- Be aware that lysis of blood cells is more likely in products that were previously frozen or older than 1 week.
- Check potassium level before transfusion to obtain baseline.
- Notify the provider immediately for manifestations of hyperkalemia.

Transfusion-associated graft-versus-host disease

Rare, and occurring 1 to 2 weeks following transfusion

MANIFESTATIONS: Nausea, vomiting, weight loss, hepatitis, thrombocytopenia

NURSING ACTIONS

- Can be prevented by using irradiated blood products that contain decreased T-cells and cytokines.
- Teach clients to report manifestations to the provider.

CONTRAINDICATIONS/PRECAUTIONS

- Contraindicated in clients who have hypersensitivity reactions.
- Respect client cultural or religious values regarding blood transfusion. In some cases, infusing colloids and other plasma expanders can be acceptable when whole blood is not allowed. Qpcc

NURSING ADMINISTRATION

- Obtain baseline laboratory values: Hgb, Hct, platelet count, total protein, albumin levels, PT, PTT, fibrinogen, potassium, pH, and blood calcium.
- Prior to start of transfusion, assess laboratory values, and blood transfusion history, verify the prescription, and ensure that client has signed consent for transfusion.
- Assess for risk of fluid overload. A diuretic can be prescribed between units for clients at risk for fluid overload. Qs
- Obtain baseline vital signs before beginning transfusion. Stay with the client and monitor vital signs per facility policy for 15 to 30 min and then at least hourly until completed.
- Assess existing infusion site for patency or infection. Ensure that a 20-gauge or larger IV catheter is used to avoid hemolysis of blood cells.
- Obtain the blood product from the blood bank just before beginning transfusion (no more than 30 min between taking unit of Packed RBCs from blood bank refrigeration and beginning of transfusion). Ensure transfusion is complete at least 4 hr after product is taken from the blood bank refrigerator.
- Carefully perform all safety checks to ensure correct product is administered to the correct client. Qs
- Use only 0.9% sodium chloride solution to administer with blood products: prime IV and blood tubing with this solution. Use a blood filter for most blood products and either a Y-type or straight tubing set depending on facility policy. Change tubing after every 2 units to prevent bacterial sepsis.
- For platelet transfusion, use a specialized platelet filter with shorter tubing. Platelets stick onto the standard blood administration filter and to the longer tubing, so it is important to use a platelet filter.
- Document blood product type, blood bank number of product, total volume infused, time of start and completion of transfusion, vital signs, and any adverse effects, as well as actions taken.
- Observe universal precautions during handling and administration of blood products.
- Do not administer blood products with any other medications.

COMPLETE TRANSFUSION WITHIN SPECIFIED TIME QEBP
- **Whole blood, Packed RBCs:** about 250 mL/unit; infuse within 2 to 4 hr.
- **Platelet concentrate:** about 300 mL/unit; infuse within 15 to 30 min/unit.
- **FFP:** about 200 mL/unit; infuse over 30 to 60 min/unit.
- **White blood cells:** about 400 mL/unit; infuse over 45 min to 1 hr.
- **Albumin**
  - 5%: 250 to 500 mL bottle; infuse 1 to 10 mL/min.
  - 25%: 50 to 100 mL bottle; infuse 4 mL/min.

IF A BLOOD TRANSFUSION REACTION IS NOTED
- Stop the transfusion and notify the provider immediately. Qs

- Do not turn on IV fluids that are connected to the Y tubing because the remaining blood in the Y tubing will be infused and aggravate the client's reaction. Administer 0.9% sodium chloride through new tubing.
- Document start and completion times of transfusion, total volume of transfusion, and client response to the transfusion.
- Stay with the client and monitor vital signs and urinary output.
- Notify the blood bank, recheck the identification tag and numbers on the blood bag, and send the blood bag and IV tubing to the blood bank for analysis.
- Obtain a urine specimen and send to the laboratory to determine RBC hemolysis. Insert an indwelling catheter if hemolytic reaction is suspected to monitor urine output.
- Repeat type and cross match. Obtain CBC and bilirubin to determine hemolysis.
- Complete a transfusion log sheet, which includes complete record of baseline vital signs, ongoing monitoring, and client response to transfusion. Incorporate this in the medical record.

CONSIDERATIONS FOR OLDER ADULT CLIENTS Ⓒ
- Use caution to prevent overload of fluid. Transfuse whole blood or Packed RBCs slowly, over 2 to 4 hr. If possible, wait 2 hr between transfusion of multiple units.
- Take vital signs every 15 min throughout the procedure. Monitor for findings of fluid overload frequently during and after the transfusion.

FOR MASSIVE TRANSFUSION
Greater than or equal to replacement of total blood volume in 24 hr, about 10 units for an adult or 5 units in 4 hr
- Monitor platelets, PT, and aPTT every 5 units and replace as needed.
- Monitor potassium and calcium levels.
- Monitor ECG for changes associated with hypokalemia, hyperkalemia, or hypocalcemia.
- Warm blood using blood warmer to prevent hypothermia.

AUTOLOGOUS BLOOD TRANSFUSION
- Several weeks prior to elective surgery the client donates blood which can be used for that client after surgery.
- Weekly blood collection can be done if client has normal laboratory values. Iron supplements are prescribed.
- Fresh blood can be saved for up to 40 days, or blood can be frozen for up to 10 years before use for a client who has a rare blood type.
- Autologous transfusion prevents some blood reactions (such as acute hemolytic), but client is still at risk for circulatory overload and sepsis.

Active Learning Scenario

A nurse is preparing to transfuse a unit of packed red blood cells (PRBCs) to a client who has who has a GI bleed and Hgb 6.0 g/dL. Use the *ATI Active Learning Template: Therapeutic Procedure* to complete this item.

INDICATIONS: What assessment data would indicate to the nurse that transfusion of PRBCs is indicated in this client?

Active Learning Scenario Key

Using the ATI Active Learning Template: Therapeutic Procedure

INDICATIONS: A client who lost blood from a GI bleed can need a unit of Packed RBCs for a Hgb level below 10 g/dL especially if demonstrating manifestations of hypovolemia (increase in pulse and respiration rate; decrease in blood pressure; low oxygen saturation; cool and pale or cyanotic; increased capillary refill time; increased urinary output). If hypoxic, the client will exhibit decreased level of consciousness and confusion. Packed RBCs restore red blood cells and improve oxygenation. If the client has lost a large amount of fluid volume, whole blood, rather than Packed RBCs, can be indicated.

Ⓝ NCLEX® Connection: Pharmacological and Parenteral Therapies, Expected Actions/Outcomes

Application Exercises

1. A nurse is preparing to transfuse a unit of packed red blood cells (PRBCs) to a client who has severe anemia. Which of the following interventions can prevent an acute hemolytic reaction?

    A. Ensure that the client has a patent IV line before obtaining blood product from the refrigerator.

    B. Ask another nurse to confirm the correct client and blood product.

    C. Take a complete set of vital signs before beginning transfusion and periodically during the transfusion.

    D. Stay with the client for the first 15 to 30 min of the transfusion.

2. A nurse is assessing a client during transfusion of a unit of whole blood. The client develops a cough, shortness of breath, elevated blood pressure, and distended neck veins. The nurse should expect a prescription for which of the following medications?

    A. Epinephrine

    B. Lorazepam

    C. Furosemide

    D. Diphenhydramine

3. A nurse is preparing to administer fresh frozen plasma (FFP) to a client who has a coagulation factor deficiency. Which of the following actions should the nurse plan to take?

    A. Ensure the product is red in color.

    B. Allow the product to warm to room temperature prior to administration.

    C. Verify there is a signed consent form in the medical record.

    D. Monitor that the infusion time is not greater than 4 hr.

4. A nurse is preparing to administer a transfusion of 300 mL of pooled platelets to a client who has severe thrombocytopenia. The nurse should plan to administer the transfusion over which of the following time frames?

    A. Within 30 min/unit

    B. Within 60 min/unit

    C. Within 2 hr/unit

    D. Within 4 hr/unit

5. A nurse is transfusing a unit of packed red blood cells (PRBCs) to a client who has anemia due to chemotherapy. The client reports a sudden headache and chills. The client's temperature is 2° F higher than the baseline reading. In addition to notifying the provider, which of the following actions should the nurse take? (Select all that apply.)

    A. Stop the transfusion.

    B. Place the client in an upright position with feet down.

    C. Remove the blood bag and tubing from the IV catheter.

    D. Obtain a urine specimen.

    E. Infuse dextrose 5% in water through the IV.

Application Exercises Key

1. B. **CORRECT:** The nurse should plan to generate solutions to reduce the client's risk of developing a hemolytic reaction which includes identifying and matching the correct blood product with the correct client will prevent an acute hemolytic reaction from occurring because this reaction is caused by ABO or Rh incompatibility.

   Ⓝ *NCLEX® Connection: Pharmacological and Parenteral Therapies, Expected Actions/Outcomes*

2. A. Epinephrine can be prescribed for a client who has anaphylactic shock caused by a severe allergic reaction, but is not indicated for the manifestations assessed in this client.
   B. Lorazepam, a benzodiazepine, can be prescribed for a client who has severe anxiety, but it is not indicated for the manifestations assessed in this client.
   C. **CORRECT:** Furosemide, a loop diuretic, can be prescribed to relieve manifestations of circulatory overload.
   D. Diphenhydramine, a histamine blocker, can be prescribed to treat mild allergic reactions, but it is not indicated for the manifestations assessed in this client.

   Ⓝ *NCLEX® Connection: Pharmacological and Parenteral Therapies, Medication Administration*

3. C. **CORRECT:** The nurse should plan to generate solutions to address the client's need for the administration of FFP which includes verifying the client has signed an informed consent and that it is in the medical record.

   Ⓝ *NCLEX® Connection: Pharmacological and Parenteral Therapies, Expected Actions/Outcomes*

4. A. **CORRECT:** Platelets are fragile and should be administered quickly to reduce the risk of clumping. Administer the platelets within 15 to 30 min/unit.

   Ⓝ *NCLEX® Connection: Pharmacological and Parenteral Therapies, Parenteral/Intravenous Therapies*

5. A. **CORRECT:** Stop the transfusion for a rise in temperature of at least 0.5° C (1° F) from baseline and reports of chills and fever. The client can be having a hemolytic reaction to the blood or a febrile reaction.
   B. Place a client who has circulatory overload in the upright position with the feet down. This client's manifestations do not indicate circulatory overload.
   C. **CORRECT:** Avoid infusing more PRBCs into the client's vein, and remove the blood bag and tubing from the client's IV catheter.
   D. **CORRECT:** Obtaining a urine specimen to check for hemolysis is standard procedure when the client has a reaction to a blood transfusion.
   E. Only infuse 0.9% sodium chloride into the client's IV along with a transfusion of PRBCs. Infuse 0.9% sodium chloride until a new prescription is received.

   Ⓝ *NCLEX® Connection: Pharmacological and Parenteral Therapies, Adverse Effects/Contraindications/Side Effects/Interactions*

NCLEX® Connections

When reviewing the following chapters, keep in mind the relevant topics and tasks of the NCLEX outline, in particular:

Pharmacological and Parenteral Therapies

ADVERSE EFFECTS/CONTRAINDICATIONS/SIDE EFFECTS/INTERACTIONS

Document side effects and adverse effects of medications and parenteral therapy.

Identify a contraindication to the administration of a medication to the client.

Provide information to the client on common side effects/adverse effects/potential interactions of medications, and inform the client of when to notify the primary health care provider.

Evaluate and document the client's response to actions taken to counteract side effects and adverse effects of medications and parenteral therapy.

EXPECTED ACTIONS/OUTCOMES

Evaluate client response to medication.

Use clinical decision-making/critical thinking when addressing expected effects/outcomes of medications

PARENTERAL/INTRAVENOUS THERAPIES

Evaluate the client's response to intermittent parenteral fluid therapy.

Apply knowledge and concepts of mathematics/nursing procedures/psychomotor skills when caring for a client receiving intravenous and parenteral therapy.

MEDICATION ADMINISTRATION

Educate client about medications.

Educate client on medication self-administration procedures.

UNIT 6   MEDICATIONS AFFECTING THE
GASTROINTESTINAL SYSTEM AND NUTRITION

CHAPTER 26 *Peptic Ulcer Disease*

Pharmacological management of peptic ulcer disease addresses the imbalance between gastric mucosal defenses, including mucus and bicarbonate, and antagonistic factors (*H. pylori* infection, gastric acid, pepsin, smoking) and use of NSAIDs.

For clients who have *H. pylori*, antibiotics are used to eradicate the disease process. All of the other medications prescribed are used to promote healing of the GI tract.

Therapeutic management outcomes include reduction of manifestations, promotion of healing, prevention of complications, and prevention of recurrence.

Antibiotics

SELECT PROTOTYPE MEDICATIONS
- Amoxicillin
- Bismuth
- Clarithromycin
- Metronidazole
- Tetracycline
- Tinidazole

PURPOSE

EXPECTED PHARMACOLOGICAL ACTION: Eradication of *H. pylori* bacteria

THERAPEUTIC USES: Therapy should include combination of two or three antibiotics for 14 days to increase effectiveness and to minimize the development of medication resistance. Qpcc

NURSING ADMINISTRATION

Administer metronidazole with food to decrease gastric disturbances.

CLIENT EDUCATION
- Nausea and diarrhea are common adverse effects.
- Take the full course of prescribed medications.

Histamine₂-receptor antagonists

SELECT PROTOTYPE MEDICATION: Cimetidine

OTHER MEDICATIONS
- Famotidine
- Nizatidine: PO use only

PURPOSE

EXPECTED PHARMACOLOGICAL ACTION: Block H_2 receptors, which suppress secretion of gastric acid and lowers the concentration of hydrogen ions in the stomach

THERAPEUTIC USES
- Prescribed to prevent or treat gastric and duodenal ulcers, GERD, hypersecretory conditions (Zollinger-Ellison syndrome), heartburn, and acid indigestion
- Used in conjunction with antibiotics to treat ulcers caused by *H. pylori*

COMPLICATIONS

CIMETIDINE

Blocked androgen receptors

Resulting in decreased libido, gynecomastia, and impotence.

CLIENT EDUCATION: Adverse effects reverse when dosing stops.

CNS effects (lethargy, hallucinations, confusion, restlessness)

NURSING ACTIONS: These effects are seen more often in older adults who have kidney or liver dysfunction.

Constipation, diarrhea, nausea

NURSING ACTIONS: Report these effects to the provider.

CONTRAINDICATIONS/PRECAUTIONS

- **Warnings**
  - Pregnancy: Use with caution.
  - Lactation: Use with caution.
- Older adult clients are more likely to experience adverse CNS effects and can require a decreased dosage. Ⓖ
- H_2 receptor antagonists decrease gastric acidity, which promotes bacterial colonization of the stomach and the respiratory tract. Use cautiously in clients who are at a high risk for pneumonia, including clients who have chronic obstructive pulmonary disease (COPD).
- Dosages should be reduced in clients with moderate to severe kidney impairment.

INTERACTIONS

Cimetidine can inhibit medication-metabolizing enzymes and thus increase the levels of warfarin, phenytoin, theophylline, and lidocaine.

NURSING ACTIONS
- In clients taking warfarin, monitor for indications of bleeding.
- Monitor INR and PT levels, and adjust warfarin dosages accordingly. Q**EBP**
- In clients taking phenytoin, theophylline, and lidocaine, monitor blood levels and adjust dosages accordingly.

Concurrent use of antacids can decrease absorption of histamine2 receptor antagonists.

CLIENT EDUCATION: Do not take an antacid 1 hr before or after taking a histamine2-receptor antagonist.

Smoking can decrease the effectiveness of histamine2 receptor antagonists.

CLIENT EDUCATION: Stop smoking, or at least avoid smoking after the last dose of the day.

NURSING ADMINISTRATION

- Famotidine can be administered IV for acute situations.
- Clients should avoid smoking, which can delay healing.
- Availability of these medications OTC can discourage clients from seeking appropriate health care. Encourage clients to see a provider if manifestations persist.
- Treatment of peptic ulcer disease is usually started as an oral dose twice a day until the ulcer is healed, followed by a maintenance dose, which usually is taken once a day at bedtime.

CLIENT EDUCATION
- Notify the provider for any indication of obvious or occult GI bleeding (coffee-ground emesis).
- Avoid alcohol and foods that increase GI irritation, and limit use of aspirin or NSAIDs.
- Increase fiber and fluid intake to prevent or manage constipation.
- Several medications can be required several times a day. Adhere to the full treatment regimen to prevent recurrence. **SDoH**

Proton pump inhibitors

SELECT PROTOTYPE MEDICATION: Omeprazole

OTHER MEDICATIONS
- Pantoprazole
- Lansoprazole
- Dexlansoprazole
- Rabeprazole
- Esomeprazole

PURPOSE

EXPECTED PHARMACOLOGICAL ACTION: Block basal and stimulated acid production, and reduce gastric acid secretion by irreversibly inhibiting the enzyme that produces gastric acid

THERAPEUTIC USE
- Short-term therapy of gastric and duodenal ulcers, erosive esophagitis, and GERD. Treatment should be limited to 4 to 8 weeks.
- Approved for long-term therapy of hypersecretory conditions.
- Prevention of stress ulcers for at-risk clients experiencing acute events.

COMPLICATIONS

Pneumonia

CLIENT EDUCATION
- Observe for adverse effects.
- Monitor and report manifestations of a respiratory infection.

Osteoporosis and fractures

Decreased acid production can lead to decreased calcium absorption.

NURSING ACTIONS: Use the medication only for as long as needed and taper before

CLIENT EDUCATION: Increase vitamin D and calcium intake.

Rebound acid hypersecretion

CLIENT EDUCATION
- Take a low dose if possible and to taper slowly to discontinue.
- Take an antacid to manage the discomfort, which can persist for several months after stopping.

Hypomagnesemia

NURSING ACTIONS
- For long-term PPI therapy, obtain a baseline magnesium level and monitor throughout therapy.
- Administer oral magnesium supplements.

CLIENT EDUCATION: Advise clients to monitor and report manifestations of hypomagnesemia (tremors, muscle cramps, seizures).

Clostridium difficile–associated diarrhea

CLIENT EDUCATION: Report fever, diarrhea, abdominal cramping, or bloody stools immediately to the provider.

CONTRAINDICATIONS/PRECAUTIONS

- Pregnancy: Misoprostol is contraindicated.
- Lactation
  - Misoprostol: Contraindicated.
  - Omeprazole: Use only if the benefits outweigh the risks.
  - Pantoprazole: Contraindicated.
- Reproductive: Avoid pregnancy during therapy
- Contraindicated for clients hypersensitive to medication, taking rilpivirine, and during lactation.
- Use cautiously in children and with clients who have dysphagia or liver disease.
- These medications increase the risk for pneumonia. Use cautiously in clients at high risk for pneumonia, including clients who have COPD.

INTERACTIONS

Digoxin, methotrexate, diazepam, tacrolimus, antifungal agents and phenytoin levels can increase when used concurrently with omeprazole.

NURSING ACTIONS: Monitor digoxin and phenytoin levels carefully if prescribed concurrently.

Absorption of ketoconazole, itraconazole, and atazanavir is decreased when taken concurrently with proton pump inhibitors.

NURSING ACTIONS: Avoid concurrent use. If necessary to administer concurrently, separate medication administration by 2 to 12 hr.

The beneficial effects of clopidogrel can decrease with concurrent use.

NURSING ACTIONS: Monitor for thrombotic events.

NURSING ADMINISTRATION

- Do not crush, chew, or break sustained-release capsules.
- Do not open capsule and sprinkle contents over food to facilitate swallowing.
- Pantoprazole can be administered to clients intravenously. There can be irritation at the injection site leading to thrombophlebitis. Monitor the IV site for indications of inflammation (redness, swelling, local pain), and change the IV site if indicated.

CLIENT EDUCATION

- Take omeprazole once per day prior to eating in the morning.
- Active ulcers should be treated for 4 to 6 weeks.
- Notify the provider for any indication of obvious or occult GI bleeding (coffee-ground emesis).

Mucosal protectant

SELECT PROTOTYPE MEDICATION: Sucralfate

PURPOSE

EXPECTED PHARMACOLOGICAL ACTION

- The acidic environment of the stomach and duodenum changes sucralfate into a protective barrier that adheres to an ulcer. This protects the ulcer from further injury from acid and pepsin.
- This viscous substance can stick to the ulcer for up to 6 hr.

THERAPEUTIC USES: Treatment of acute duodenal ulcers and maintenance therapy.

COMPLICATIONS

There are no systemic effects because sucralfate is minimally absorbed and most of it is eliminated in the feces.

Constipation

CLIENT EDUCATION: To prevent constipation, increase dietary fiber and fluid intake.

CONTRAINDICATIONS/PRECAUTIONS

- **Warnings**
  - Pregnancy: Sucralfate is safe.
  - Lactation: Sucralfate is safe.
- Contraindicated in clients who are hypersensitive to the medication.
- Use cautiously in clients who have chronic kidney disease or diabetes mellitus.

INTERACTIONS

Sucralfate can interfere with the absorption of phenytoin, digoxin, warfarin, and ciprofloxacin.

NURSING ACTIONS: Maintain a 2-hr interval between these medications and sucralfate to minimize this interaction.

Antacids interfere with the effects of sucralfate.

NURSING ACTIONS: Take sucralfate 30 min before or after antacids.

NURSING ADMINISTRATION

CLIENT EDUCATION

- Take four times a day, 1 hr before meals, and again at bedtime.
- If needed, break or dissolve the medication in water, but do not crush or chew the tablet.
- Complete the course of treatment.

Antacids

SELECT PROTOTYPE MEDICATION: Aluminum hydroxide

OTHER MEDICATIONS
- Magnesium hydroxide
- Calcium carbonate

PURPOSE

EXPECTED PHARMACOLOGICAL ACTION
- Neutralize or reduce the acidity of gastric acid; can reduce pepsin activity if the pH is raised above 5.
- Mucosal protection can occur from stimulation of the production of prostaglandins.

THERAPEUTIC USES
- Treatment of peptic ulcer disease
- Prevention of stress-induced ulcers
- Relief of the manifestations of GERD

COMPLICATIONS

Constipation, diarrhea

Aluminum and calcium compounds: Constipation

Magnesium compounds: Diarrhea

CLIENT EDUCATION
- Alternate use of these compounds to offset intestinal effects and normalize bowel function, adjusting administration as needed to promote a normal bowel pattern. QEBP
- If a client has difficulty managing bowel function, recommend a combination product that contains aluminum hydroxide and magnesium hydroxide.

Fluid retention

Antacids containing sodium can result in fluid retention.

CLIENT EDUCATION: Avoid antacids that contain sodium if you have hypertension or heart failure.

Electrolyte imbalances

Aluminum compounds: Hypophosphatemia

Calcium compounds: Hypercalcemia

CLIENT EDUCATION: Report manifestations of hypercalcemia (constipation, anorexia, nausea, vomiting, confusion) to the provider.

Alkalosis

Risk increased with use of sodium compounds.

Toxicity, hypermagnesemia

Magnesium compounds can lead to toxicity and hypermagnesemia in clients who have impaired kidney function.

CLIENT EDUCATION
- If kidney function is impaired, avoid antacids that contain magnesium.
- Monitor for CNS depression.

CONTRAINDICATIONS/PRECAUTIONS
- Antacids should be used with caution in clients who have GI perforation or obstruction.
- Use cautiously in clients who have abdominal pain.

INTERACTIONS

Antacids decrease the absorption several medications, including famotidine and cimetidine.
CLIENT EDUCATION: Allow at least 1 hr time between taking antacids and these medications.

Aluminum compounds bind to warfarin, digoxin, and tetracycline interfering with absorption and reducing their effects.
CLIENT EDUCATION: Do not take other medications within 1 to 2 hr of taking aluminum compounds without provider approval.

NURSING ADMINISTRATION

Adherence is difficult for clients due to the frequency of administration. Medication can be administered seven times a day: 1 hr and 3 hr after meals, and again at bedtime. Encourage compliance by reinforcing the intended effect of the antacid (relief of pain, healing of ulcer). QPCC

CLIENT EDUCATION
- Chew tablets thoroughly and then drink at least 8 oz of water or milk.
- Shake liquid formulations to ensure even dispersion of the medication.
- Take all medications at least 1 hr before or after taking an antacid.

Prostaglandin E analog

SELECT PROTOTYPE MEDICATION: Misoprostol

PURPOSE

EXPECTED PHARMACOLOGICAL ACTION
Acts as an endogenous prostaglandin in the GI tract that decreases acid secretion, increases the secretion of bicarbonate and protective mucus, and promotes vasodilation to maintain submucosal blood flow. These actions serve to prevent gastric ulcers.

THERAPEUTIC USES
- Used in clients taking long-term NSAIDs to prevent gastric ulcers.
- Unlabeled use: Used in clients who are pregnant only to induce labor by causing cervical ripening or induce medical termination of pregnancy.

COMPLICATIONS

Diarrhea

With concurrent use of magnesium antacids

NURSING ACTION: Reduce dosage if needed.

CLIENT EDUCATION: Notify the provider of diarrhea or abdominal pain.

Dysmenorrhea, spotting

NURSING ACTIONS: The provider might discontinue the medication.

CLIENT EDUCATION: Notify the provider if dysmenorrhea and spotting occur.

CONTRAINDICATIONS/PRECAUTIONS

- **Warnings**
  - Pregnancy: Misoprostol is contraindicated.
  - Lactation: Misoprostol is contraindicated. The medication passes into breast milk and can cause severe diarrhea in the infant.
- Reproductive: Avoid pregnancy during therapy. Clients who could become pregnant must be warned verbally and in writing about the dangers of misoprostol. The client must have a negative blood pregnancy test 2 weeks before starting therapy, be able to adhere to contraceptive measures, and should start the medication on the second or third day of the menstrual cycle. Qs

NURSING ADMINISTRATION

Teach clients to take misoprostol with meals and at bedtime.

NURSING EVALUATION OF MEDICATION EFFECTIVENESS

Depending on therapeutic intent, effectiveness can be evidenced by the following.
- Reduced frequency or absence of GERD manifestations (heartburn, bloating, belching)
- Absence of GI bleeding
- Healing of gastric and duodenal ulcers
- No recurrence of ulcer

Application Exercises

1. A nurse is teaching a client about cimetidine. Which of the following are adverse effects of cimetidine? (Select all that apply.)
   - A. Increased libido
   - B. Insomnia
   - C. Enlargement of breast tissue
   - D. Confusion
   - E. Decreased sperm count

2. A nurse receives a new prescription for omeprazole for a client. After reviewing information in the drug guide, provide the therapeutic uses for this medication.

3. A nurse is teaching a client who takes phenytoin and has a new prescription for sucralfate tablets. Which of the following instructions should the nurse include?
   - A. Take an antacid with the sucralfate.
   - B. Take sucralfate with a glass of milk.
   - C. Allow a 2-hr interval between these medications.
   - D. Chew the sucralfate thoroughly before swallowing.

4. A nurse is teaching a client who will begin taking aluminum hydroxide. Which of the following information should the nurse include in the teaching?
   - A. "If constipation develops, switch to a calcium-based antacid."
   - B. "Take this medication 2 hours before or after other medications."
   - C. "This medication increases the risk for pneumonia."
   - D. "Have your magnesium level monitored while taking this medication."

5. A nurse is caring for four clients who have peptic ulcer disease. The nurse should identify misoprostol is contraindicated for which of the following clients?
   - A. A client who is pregnant
   - B. A client who has osteoarthritis
   - C. A client who has a kidney stone
   - D. A client who has a urinary tract infection

Active Learning Scenario

A nurse is caring for a client who has a prescription for calcium carbonate. Use the *ATI Active Learning Template: Medication* to complete this item.

THERAPEUTIC USES: Identify the therapeutic use of calcium carbonate.

CLIENT EDUCATION: Identify three instructions the nurse should include regarding taking this medication.

Active Learning Scenario Key

Using the ATI Active Learning Template: Medication

THERAPEUTIC USES: Calcium carbonate is an antacid that raises the pH of gastric contents, which reduces irritation of stomach mucosa, resulting in relief of pain.

CLIENT EDUCATION

- Shake liquid suspensions prior to taking each dose in order to disperse the medication.
- Take other medications at least 1 hr before or after taking aluminum hydroxide.
- Calcium carbonate can cause constipation. Notify the provider if it persists. You might need to alternate this antacid with one that is a magnesium compound and has diarrhea as an adverse effect.
- Report manifestations of hypercalcemia (constipation, anorexia, nausea, vomiting, confusion) to the provider.

Ⓝ *NCLEX® Connection: Pharmacological and Parenteral Therapies, Medication Administration*

Application Exercises Key

1. B. **CORRECT:** When taking actions, the nurse should instruct the client about potential adverse effects of cimetidine ch can include gynecomastia, confusion, and impotence.

   Ⓝ *NCLEX® Connection: Pharmacological and Parenteral Therapies, Medication Administration*

2. When taking actions, the nurse should identify the following therapeutic uses for omeprazole: Short-term therapy of gastric and duodenal ulcers, erosive esophagitis, and GERD. Treatment should be limited to 4 to 8 weeks. Approved for long-term therapy of hypersecretory conditions. Prevention of stress ulcers for at-risk clients experiencing acute events.

   Ⓝ *NCLEX® Connection: Pharmacological and Parenteral Therapies, Medication Administration*

3. A. Antacids can interfere with the effects of sucralfate, so the client should allow a 30 min interval between the sucralfate and the antacid.
   B. Sucralfate should be taken on an empty stomach, 1 hr before meals.
   C. **CORRECT:** Sucralfate can interfere with the absorption of phenytoin, so the client should allow a 2-hr interval between the sucralfate and phenytoin.
   D. The client should swallow the sucralfate whole.

   Ⓝ *NCLEX® Connection: Pharmacological and Parenteral Therapies, Medication Administration*

4. B. **CORRECT:** When taking actions, the nurse should instruct the client that antacids can alter the absorption of many medications. The client should ensure no other medications are taken within 1 to 2 hr of taking aluminum hydroxide.

   Ⓝ *NCLEX® Connection: Pharmacological and Parenteral Therapies, Medication Administration*

5. A. **CORRECT:** The nurse should analyze the cues from the client's history and determine that misoprostol can induce labor and is contraindicated in pregnancy.

   Ⓝ *NCLEX® Connection: Pharmacological and Parenteral Therapies, Adverse Effects/Contraindications/Side Effects/Interactions*

CHAPTER 27 *Gastrointestinal Disorders*

The medications in this section affect some aspect of the gastrointestinal tract to treat or prevent nausea, vomiting, motion sickness, diarrhea, or constipation; treat hiatal hernia by controlling reflux; and treat gastroesophageal reflux disease (GERD) by increasing gastric motility, protecting stomach lining, and inhibiting secretion of gastric acid.

Medications include antiemetics, laxatives, antidiarrheals, prokinetic agents, medications for irritable bowel syndrome (IBS), 5-aminosalicylates, probiotics, and medications for hiatal hernia.

Antiemetics

SELECT PROTOTYPE MEDICATIONS
- **Glucocorticoids:** Dexamethasone
- **Substance P/neurokinin₁ antagonists:** Aprepitant
- **Serotonin antagonists:** Ondansetron, granisetron
- **Dopamine antagonists:** Prochlorperazine, metoclopramide, promethazine
- **Cannabinoids:** Dronabinol
- **Anticholinergics:** Scopolamine
- **Antihistamines:** Dimenhydrinate, hydroxyzine
- **Benzodiazepines:** Lorazepam

PURPOSE

Glucocorticoids: dexamethasone

EXPECTED PHARMACOLOGICAL ACTION: The antiemetic mechanism is unknown.

THERAPEUTIC USES
- Usually used in combination with other antiemetics to treat chemotherapy-induced nausea and vomiting (CINV).
- Administer PO or IV.

Substance P/neurokinin₁ antagonists: aprepitant

EXPECTED PHARMACOLOGICAL ACTION: Inhibits substance P/neurokinin1 in the brain.

THERAPEUTIC USES
- For best results, it should be used in combination with a glucocorticoid and serotonin antagonist to prevent postoperative nausea, vomiting, and CINV.
- Extended duration of action makes it effective for immediate use and delayed response.
- Administer PO or IV.

Serotonin antagonist: ondansetron

EXPECTED PHARMACOLOGICAL ACTION: Prevents emesis by blocking the serotonin receptors in the chemoreceptor trigger zone (CTZ), and antagonizing the serotonin receptors on the afferent vagal neurons that travel from the upper GI tract to the CTZ.

THERAPEUTIC USES
- Prevents emesis related to chemotherapy, radiation therapy, and postoperative recovery.
- Off-label uses include treatment of nausea and vomiting related to pregnancy and childhood viral gastritis.
- Administer PO, IM, or IV.

Dopamine antagonists: prochlorperazine (a phenothiazine)

EXPECTED PHARMACOLOGICAL ACTION: Antiemetic effects result from blockade of dopamine receptors in the CTZ.

THERAPEUTIC USES
- Prevents emesis related to chemotherapy, toxins, and postoperative recovery.
- Administer PO, IM, rectal, or IV.

Cannabinoids: dronabinol

EXPECTED PHARMACOLOGICAL ACTION: Antiemetic mechanism is unknown.

THERAPEUTIC USES
- To control CINV and to increase appetite in clients who have AIDS. Reserved as second-line therapy for individuals who cannot take or was not responsive to other medications.
- Administer PO.

Anticholinergic: scopolamine

EXPECTED PHARMACOLOGICAL ACTION: Interferes with the transmission of nerve impulses traveling from the vestibular apparatus of the inner ear to the vomiting center (VC) in the brain.

THERAPEUTIC USES
- Prevention and treatment of motion sickness.
- Administer transdermally, PO, IV, or subcutaneously.

Antihistamines: dimenhydrinate

EXPECTED PHARMACOLOGICAL ACTION: Muscarinic and histaminergic receptors in nerve pathways that connect the inner ear and VC are blocked.

THERAPEUTIC USES
- Treats motion sickness.
- Administer PO, IM, or IV.

Benzodiazepines: lorazepam

EXPECTED PHARMACOLOGICAL ACTION: Depresses nerve function at multiple CNS sites.

THERAPEUTIC USES
- Used in combination with other medications to suppress CINV by causing sedation, anterograde amnesia, and emesis suppression.
- Administer PO, IM, or IV.

COMPLICATIONS

Glucocorticoids

The risk of adverse effects is reduced by taking lower dosages for short periods of time.

Adrenal insufficiency, infection, osteoporosis, glucose intolerance, peptic ulcer disease, sodium retention, and hypokalemia.
CLIENT EDUCATION
- To prevent adrenal insufficiency, additional dosing can be required during times of stress, and taper the dose before discontinuing.
- Monitor for and report manifestations of infection, hyperglycemia, edema, black, tarry stools, or low potassium (muscle cramping or weakness).

Substance P/neurokinin₁ antagonist: aprepitant

Fatigue, diarrhea, dizziness, possible liver damage
NURSING ACTIONS
- Treat headache with non-opioid analgesics.
- Monitor stool pattern.
- Monitor liver function tests periodically.
- Have the client change positions slowly.

Serotonin antagonist: ondansetron

Headache, diarrhea, dizziness
NURSING ACTIONS
- Treat headache with non-opioid analgesics.
- Monitor stool pattern.

Prolonged QT interval can lead to a serious dysrhythmia (torsades de pointes).
NURSING ACTIONS
- Monitor ECG in clients who have cardiac disorders or are taking other medications that can prolong the QT interval.
- Use with caution in clients with electrolyte abnormalities.

Dopamine antagonists: prochlorperazine

Extrapyramidal symptoms (EPSs)
NURSING ACTIONS: Administer an anticholinergic medication (diphenhydramine, benztropine) to treat EPSs.

CLIENT EDUCATION
- Possible adverse effects include restlessness, anxiety, and spasms of face and neck.
- Stop the medication and inform the provider if EPSs occur.

Hypotension
NURSING ACTIONS: Monitor clients receiving antihypertensive medications for low blood pressure.

CLIENT EDUCATION: Rise slowly from lying to standing to prevent dizziness and falls. Qs

Sedation
CLIENT EDUCATION: Avoid activities that require alertness, such as driving.

Anticholinergic effects: Dry mouth, urinary retention, constipation.
NURSING ACTIONS: Administer a stimulant laxative (senna) to counteract a decrease in bowel motility, or stool softeners (docusate sodium) to prevent constipation.

CLIENT EDUCATION
- Increase fluid intake.
- Increase physical activity by engaging in regular exercise.
- Suck on hard candy or chew gum to help relieve dry mouth.
- Void every 4 hr. Monitor I&O and palpate the lower abdomen area every 4 to 6 hr to check the bladder for fullness.

Cannabinoids: dronabinol

Potential for dissociation, dysphoria
NURSING ACTIONS: Avoid using in clients who have mental health disorders. For other clients, effects can be subjective.

Hypotension, tachycardia
NURSING ACTIONS: Use cautiously in clients who have cardiovascular disorders. Qs

Anticholinergics (scopolamine) and antihistamines (dimenhydrinate)

Sedation
CLIENT EDUCATION
- This medication can cause sedation.
- Avoid activities that require alertness (driving).

Anticholinergic effects
- Dry mouth, urinary retention, constipation
- Interscholastic adverse effects can be less intense with transdermal administration, than with PO or SQ.

NURSING ACTIONS: Administer a stimulant laxative (senna) to counteract a decrease in bowel motility, or stool softeners (docusate sodium) to prevent constipation.

CLIENT EDUCATION
- Increase fluid intake.
- Increase physical activity by engaging in regular exercise.
- Suck on hard candy or chew gum to help relieve dry mouth.
- Void every 4 hr. Monitor I&O and palpate the lower abdomen area every 4 to 6 hr to check the bladder for fullness.

Benzodiazepines

Sedation and complex sleep-related behaviors
CLIENT EDUCATION
- Avoid activities that require alertness (driving).
- Report behaviors (driving, eating, or making phone calls while asleep) to the provider.

Paradoxical effects
CLIENT EDUCATION: Report feelings of anxiety, rage, or increased excitement to the provider.

CONTRAINDICATIONS/PRECAUTIONS

- **Warnings**
  - Pregnancy
    - Ondansetron, metoclopramide, scopolamine: Safety not established.
    - Promethazine: Avoid chronic use during pregnancy.
  - Lactation
    - Ondansetron, metoclopramide, scopolamine: Safety not established.

Promethazine: Safety not established; can cause drowsiness in the infant.

- Ondansetron is contraindicated in clients who have long QT syndrome. **Qs**
- Use dopamine antagonists cautiously, if at all, with children and older adults due to the increased risk of extrapyramidal manifestations.
- Dopamine antagonists, antihistamines, and anticholinergic antiemetics should be used cautiously in clients who have urinary retention or obstruction, asthma, and narrow angle glaucoma.
- Aprepitant is contraindicated for clients taking pimozide or are breastfeeding. It should be used cautiously in children and in clients who have severe liver and kidney disease.
- Promethazine is contraindicated in children younger than 2 years old and should be used with extreme caution in older children. Respiratory depression from promethazine can be severe.
- Glucocorticoids are contraindicated in clients who have active, untreated infection, hypersensitivity. Avoid long-term use during lactation.
- Lorazepam is contraindicated for clients who have CNS depression, angle-closure glaucoma, severe hypotension, or uncontrolled, severe pain. Can cause fetal harm during the third trimester of pregnancy, and adverse effects to the breastfeeding infant.

INTERACTIONS

CNS depressants (opioids and alcohol) can intensify CNS depression of antiemetics.
CLIENT EDUCATION: Avoid sedatives, opioids, and alcohol when taking antiemetics.

Concurrent use of antihypertensives can intensify hypotensive effects of antiemetics.
NURSING ACTIONS: Provide assistance with ambulation as needed.

CLIENT EDUCATION: Sit or lie down if lightheadedness or dizziness occur. Avoid sudden changes in position by moving slowly from a lying to a sitting or standing position.

Concurrent use of anticholinergic medications (antihistamines) can intensify anticholinergic effects of antiemetics.
CLIENT EDUCATION: Sipping on fluids, use of laxatives, and voiding on a regular basis can reduce anticholinergic effects.

Aprepitant can decrease the effectiveness of warfarin and ethinyl estradiol and increase the levels of glucocorticoids. Many medications can alter the blood levels of aprepitant.
NURSING ACTIONS: Review the client's concurrent medications closely and space administration to avoid interaction. Instruct the client to talk to the provider before starting other medications.

NURSING ADMINISTRATION

- Antiemetics prevent or treat nausea and vomiting from various causes. Nursing assessment can identify the underlying related factors and verify that the appropriate medication is used.
- To prevent CINV, antiemetics are administered prior to chemotherapy as this is more effective than treating nausea that is already occurring. Combining three antiemetics is more effective than the use of a single antiemetic. **QEBP**

Aprepitant
- To prevent postoperative nausea and vomiting, administer a single dose within three hours of anesthesia induction.
- For CINV, administer one hour before chemotherapy. The client will take one dose daily the next two days.

Ondansetron
- Administer IV 1 hr before chemotherapy, or PO 1 hour before anesthesia to prevent nausea and vomiting
- For clients receiving radiation, administer PO three times a day.

Prochlorperazine: Obtain orthostatic blood pressure and pulse readings, respiratory rate, and ECG before therapy, and periodically. Monitor for Q- and T-wave changes.

Dronabinol: For appetite stimulation, administer before lunch and supper. For emesis prevention, administer every 4 hr as needed.

Scopolamine: To prevent motion sickness, apply transdermal patch behind the ear four hours before travel or take the tablet one hour before travel.

Lorazepam: Administer with food to prevent GI upset.
CLIENT EDUCATION
- When receiving a chemotherapy agent, the medication can cause CINV.
- When taking dexamethasone, do not suddenly stop the medication, but taper the dose. Do not receive a live vaccine while taking the medication. Carry an identification card to let emergency personnel know about the therapy.

NURSING EVALUATION OF MEDICATION EFFECTIVENESS

Depending on therapeutic intent, effectiveness can be evidenced by absence of nausea and vomiting.

Laxatives

SELECT PROTOTYPE MEDICATIONS
- Psyllium, methylcellulose
- Docusate sodium
- Bisacodyl
- Magnesium hydroxide

OTHER MEDICATIONS
- Senna
- Lactulose

PURPOSE

Bulk-forming laxatives: psyllium, methylcellulose

EXPECTED PHARMACOLOGICAL ACTION: Bulk-forming laxatives soften fecal mass and increase bulk, which is identical to the action of dietary fiber.

THERAPEUTIC USES
- For temporary treatment of constipation.
- Decrease diarrhea in clients who have diverticulosis and IBS.
- Control stool for clients who have an ileostomy or colostomy.

Surfactant laxatives: docusate sodium

EXPECTED PHARMACOLOGICAL ACTION: Surfactant laxatives lower surface tension of the stool to allow penetration of water. This softens the stool so it can be passed more easily.

THERAPEUTIC USES
- Treatment of constipation.
- Softening of fecal impaction.

Stimulant laxatives: bisacodyl, senna

EXPECTED PHARMACOLOGICAL ACTION: Stimulate intestinal peristalsis and increase the volume of water and electrolytes in the intestines.

THERAPEUTIC USES
- Bowel preparation prior to surgery or diagnostic tests (including colonoscopy).
- Short-term treatment of constipation caused by high-dose opioid use or slow intestinal transit.

Osmotic laxatives: magnesium hydroxide, lactulose

EXPECTED PHARMACOLOGICAL ACTION: Osmotic laxatives draw water into the intestine to increase the mass of stool, stretching musculature, which results in peristalsis.

THERAPEUTIC USES
- **Low dose:** Prevent painful elimination (clients who have episiotomy or hemorrhoids).
- **High dose:** Client preparation prior to surgery or diagnostic tests (a colonoscopy).
- Rapid evacuation of the bowel after ingestion of poisons or following anthelmintic therapy to rid the body of dead parasites.

COMPLICATIONS

GI irritation

CLIENT EDUCATION: Do not crush or chew enteric-coated tablets.

Rectal burning sensation, leading to proctitis

CLIENT EDUCATION: Do not use bisacodyl suppositories on a regular basis.

Toxic magnesium levels

Laxatives with magnesium salts (magnesium hydroxide) can lead to accumulation of toxic levels of magnesium.

NURSING ACTIONS: For clients experiencing impaired kidney function, read labels carefully and avoid laxatives that contain magnesium.

Sodium absorption and fluid retention

Laxatives with sodium salts (sodium phosphate) place clients at risk for sodium absorption and fluid retention.

NURSING ACTIONS: Monitor for fluid retention. Qs

Dehydration

Osmotic diuretics can cause dehydration.

NURSING ACTIONS
- Monitor I&O.
- Monitor/assess for manifestations of dehydration (poor skin turgor).

CLIENT EDUCATION: Increase water intake to at least 8 to 10 glasses of water per day.

Obstruction

Bulk-forming agents can cause obstruction of the esophagus or intestines.

NURSING ACTIONS: Administer with a full glass of water or juice. Avoid use if client has narrowing of the intestinal lumen.

CONTRAINDICATIONS/PRECAUTIONS

- **Warnings**
  - Pregnancy: Use docusate sodium, lactulose, and magnesium hydroxide with caution; safety not established.
  - Lactation: Use docusate sodium, lactulose, and magnesium hydroxide with caution; safety not established.
- Laxatives are contraindicated in clients who have fecal impaction, bowel obstruction, and acute surgical abdomen to prevent perforation. Qs
- Laxatives are contraindicated in clients who have nausea, cramping, and abdominal pain.
- Laxatives, except for bulk-forming laxatives, are contraindicated in clients who have ulcerative colitis and diverticulitis.

INTERACTIONS

Milk and antacids can destroy enteric coating of bisacodyl.

CLIENT EDUCATION: Take bisacodyl at least 1 hr apart from ingesting these substances.

NURSING ADMINISTRATION

- Obtain a complete history of laxative use, and provide teaching as appropriate. Qpcc
- Instruct clients to take bulk-forming and surfactant laxatives with 8 oz water.
- Administer bisacodyl at bedtime for results in 6 to 12 hr. Bisacodyl suppositories are effective within an hour.

CLIENT EDUCATION
- Chronic laxative use can lead to fluid and electrolyte imbalances.
- To promote defecation and resumption of normal bowel function, increase high-fiber foods (bran, fresh fruits and vegetables) in the daily diet and to increase amounts of fluids. Recommend at least 2 to 3 L/day from beverages and food sources.
- Use laxatives occasionally if needed, not routinely. It is not necessary for the bowels to move every day. Chronic laxative use can lead to fluid and electrolyte imbalances.
- Maintain a regular exercise regimen to improve bowel function.

NURSING EVALUATION OF MEDICATION EFFECTIVENESS

Depending on therapeutic intent, effectiveness can be evidenced by the following.
- Return to regular bowel function
- Evacuation of bowel in preparation for surgery or diagnostic tests

Antidiarrheals

SELECT PROTOTYPE MEDICATION: Diphenoxylate plus atropine

OTHER MEDICATIONS
- Loperamide
- Paregoric

PURPOSE

EXPECTED PHARMACOLOGICAL ACTION: Antidiarrheals activate opioid receptors in the GI tract to decrease intestinal motility and to increase the absorption of fluid and sodium in the intestine.

THERAPEUTIC USES
- Specific antidiarrheal agents can be used to treat the underlying cause of diarrhea. For example, antibiotics can be used to treat diarrhea caused by a bacterial infection.
- Nonspecific antidiarrheal agents minimize the manifestations of diarrhea (decrease in frequency and fluid content of stool).

COMPLICATIONS

- At recommended doses for diarrhea, diphenoxylate does not affect the CNS system.
- At high doses, clients can experience typical opioid effects, (euphoria or CNS depression). However, the addition of atropine, which has unpleasant adverse effects (blurred vision, dry mouth, urinary retention, constipation, tachycardia) in diphenoxylate discourages ingestion of doses higher than those prescribed.

CONTRAINDICATIONS/PRECAUTIONS

- **Warnings**
  - Pregnancy
    - Diphenoxylate plus atropine: Use with caution.
    - Loperamide: Safety not established.
  - Lactation
    - Diphenoxylate plus atropine: Use with caution.
    - Loperamide: Contraindicated.
- There is an increased risk of megacolon in clients who have inflammatory bowel disorders. This could lead to a serious complication (perforation of the bowel).
- Diphenoxylate is contraindicated in clients who have severe electrolyte imbalance or dehydration. It is a Schedule V agent under the Controlled Substances Act (CSA). Qs
- Paregoric is contraindicated in clients who have COPD. It is a Schedule III CSA agent.

INTERACTIONS

Alcohol and other CNS depressants can enhance CNS depression.

NURSING ADMINISTRATION

- Administer initial dose of diphenoxylate plus atropine 5 mg, and monitor client response, administering further medication as needed. The maximum dose 8 tabs/day.
- Loperamide is an analog of the opioid meperidine. This medication is not a controlled substance, and at high doses does not mimic morphine-like effects.
- Clients who have severe cases of diarrhea can be hospitalized for management of dehydration.
- Management of dehydration should include monitoring of weight, I&O, and vital signs. A hypotonic solution (0.45% sodium chloride) might be prescribed.

CLIENT EDUCATION

- If experiencing diarrhea, drink small amounts of clear liquids or a commercial oral electrolyte solution to maintain electrolyte balance for the first 24 hr. Qpcc
- Avoid drinking plain water to replace fluids because it does not contain necessary electrolytes that have been lost in the stool. **SDoH**
- Avoid caffeine. Caffeine exacerbates diarrhea by increasing GI motility.

NURSING EVALUATION OF MEDICATION EFFECTIVENESS

Depending on therapeutic intent, effectiveness can be evidenced by return of normal bowel pattern as evidenced by decrease in frequency and fluid volume of stool.

Prokinetic agents

- SELECT PROTOTYPE MEDICATION: Metoclopramide

PURPOSE

EXPECTED PHARMACOLOGICAL ACTION
- Metoclopramide controls nausea and vomiting by blocking dopamine and serotonin receptors in the CTZ which reduces the stimulus to empty the bowels.
- Metoclopramide augments action of acetylcholine, which causes an increase in upper GI motility, increasing peristalsis.

THERAPEUTIC USES
- The IV form is used for control of postoperative and chemotherapy-induced nausea and vomiting, as well as facilitation of small bowel intubation and examination of the GI tract.
- The oral form is used for diabetic gastroparesis (delayed stomach emptying with gas and bloating) and management of GERD through its ability to increase gastric motility.

COMPLICATIONS

Tardive dyskinesia

A complication of high-dose, long-term therapy.

CLIENT EDUCATION: Monitor for and immediately report repetitive involuntary movements.

Extrapyramidal symptoms

NURSING ACTIONS: Administer an antihistamine (diphenhydramine) to minimize EPSs.

CLIENT EDUCATION: Possible adverse effects include restlessness, anxiety, and spasms of the face and neck.

Sedation

CLIENT EDUCATION
- Medication has potential for sedation.
- Avoid activities that require alertness (driving).

Diarrhea

NURSING ACTIONS: Monitor bowel function and for indications of dehydration.

CONTRAINDICATIONS/PRECAUTIONS

- Contraindicated in clients who have GI perforation, GI bleeding, bowel obstruction, and hemorrhage.
- Contraindicated in clients who have a seizure disorder due to an increased risk of seizures.
- Use cautiously in children and older adults due to the increased risk for EPS.

INTERACTIONS

Concurrent use of alcohol and other CNS depressants increases the risk of seizures and sedation.

NURSING ACTIONS: Use cautiously with other CNS depressants.

CLIENT EDUCATION: Avoid the use of alcohol.

Opioids and anticholinergics decrease the effects of metoclopramide.

CLIENT EDUCATION: Avoid using opioids and medications with anticholinergic effects.

NURSING ADMINISTRATION

- Monitor for CNS depression and EPSs.
- The medication can be given orally or IV. If the IV dose 10 mg or less, it can be administered IVP undiluted over 2 min. If the dose is greater than 10 mg, it should be diluted and infused over 15 min. Dilute the medication in at least 50 mL dextrose 5% in water, sodium chloride, or lactated Ringer's. QEBP

NURSING EVALUATION OF MEDICATION EFFECTIVENESS

Depending on therapeutic intent, effectiveness can be evidenced by absence of nausea and vomiting.

Medications for irritable bowel syndrome with diarrhea (IBS-D)

SELECT PROTOTYPE MEDICATION: Alosetron

PURPOSE

EXPECTED PHARMACOLOGICAL ACTION: Selective blockade of 5-HT3 receptors, which innervate the viscera and result in increased firmness in stool and decrease in urgency and frequency of defecation.

THERAPEUTIC USES: Approved only for female clients who have severe IBS-D that has lasted more than 6 months and has been resistant to conventional management.

COMPLICATIONS

Constipation

Can result in GI toxicity (ischemic colitis, bowel obstruction, impaction, or perforation).

NURSING ACTIONS: Because of the potentially fatal outcome of GI toxicity, only clients who meet specific criteria and are willing to sign a treatment agreement can receive prescriptions for the medication. Qs

CLIENT EDUCATION: Watch for rectal bleeding, bloody diarrhea, or abdominal pain and report to the provider. Medication should be discontinued.

CONTRAINDICATIONS/PRECAUTIONS

Contraindicated for clients who have chronic constipation, history of bowel obstruction, Crohn's disease, ulcerative colitis, impaired intestinal circulation, diverticulitis, a history of toxic megacolon, GI perforation or adhesions, or thrombophlebitis.

INTERACTIONS

Medications that affect cytochrome P450 enzymes (phenobarbital) can alter levels of alosetron.
NURSING ACTIONS: Monitor the effectiveness of medication.

NURSING ADMINISTRATION

Alosetron can only be prescribed by providers enrolled in a special risk management program. The client must sign a Client–Physician Agreement discussing risks and benefits, and indications that the medication must be stopped.

CLIENT EDUCATION
- Manifestations should resolve within 1 to 4 weeks but will return 1 week after medication is discontinued.
- Dosage will start as once a day and can be increased to BID.

NURSING EVALUATION OF MEDICATION EFFECTIVENESS

Depending on therapeutic intent, effectiveness can be evidenced by relief of diarrhea, and decrease in urgency and frequency of defecation.

Medications for irritable bowel syndrome with constipation (IBS-C)

SELECT PROTOTYPE MEDICATION: Lubiprostone

PURPOSE

EXPECTED PHARMACOLOGICAL ACTION
Increases fluid secretion in the intestine to promote intestinal motility

THERAPEUTIC USES
- Irritable bowel syndrome with constipation in females
- Chronic constipation

COMPLICATIONS

Diarrhea

NURSING ACTIONS: Monitor frequency of stools. Notify the provider if severe diarrhea occurs.

Nausea

CLIENT EDUCATION: Take the medication with food.

CONTRAINDICATIONS/PRECAUTIONS

- **Warnings**
  - Pregnancy: Use lubiprostone only if the benefit to the client outweighs the risks to the fetus.
  - Lactation: Lubiprostone is unknown.
- Contraindicated for clients who have bowel obstruction

INTERACTIONS

No significant interactions

NURSING ADMINISTRATION

- Dosing for IBS-C is lower than for chronic idiopathic constipation or opioid-induced constipation.
- Oral dosage should be taken BID.

CLIENT EDUCATION: Take the medication with food to decrease nausea.

NURSING EVALUATION OF MEDICATION EFFECTIVENESS

Depending on therapeutic intent, effectiveness can be evidenced by relief of constipation.

Medications for inflammatory bowel disease

SELECT PROTOTYPE MEDICATION: Sulfasalazine

OTHER MEDICATIONS
- **5-aminosalicylates:** Mesalamine, sulfasalazine
- **Glucocorticoids:** Hydrocortisone, budesonide
- **Immunosuppressants:** Azathioprine
- **Immunomodulator:** Infliximab
- **Antibiotics:** Metronidazole

PURPOSE

EXPECTED PHARMACOLOGICAL ACTION: A 5-aminosalicylate that decreases inflammation by inhibiting prostaglandin synthesis

THERAPEUTIC USES
- Management of Crohn's disease.
- Relief of mild to moderate acute episodes of ulcerative colitis.

COMPLICATIONS

Blood disorders

Include agranulocytosis, hemolytic and macrocytic anemia

NURSING ACTIONS: Monitor complete blood count.

Nausea, fever, rash, arthralgia

NURSING ACTIONS: Notify the provider if adverse effects persist.

Contraindications/Precautions

- **Warnings**
  - Pregnancy
    - Sulfasalazine: Use with caution due to the risk of neural tube defects.
    - Infliximab: Use only if needed.
    - Mesalamine: Safety not established.
  - Lactation
    - Sulfasalazine: Safety not established.
    - Infliximab: Contraindicated.
    - Mesalamine: Use with caution; careful monitoring required.
  - Reproductive
    - Sulfasalazine: Can cause infertility in male clients.
    - Infliximab and mesalamine: Notify provider if pregnancy is planned or suspected.
- 5-aminosalicylates are contraindicated in clients who have sensitivity to sulfonamides, salicylates, or thiazide diuretics.
- Use cautiously in clients who have liver or kidney disease or blood dyscrasias.

INTERACTIONS

- Iron and antibiotics can alter the absorption of sulfasalazine.
- Mesalamine can decrease the absorption of some medications, including digoxin and oral antidiabetic medications.

NURSING ADMINISTRATION

- Administer with food or after meals.
- Ensure at least 1,200 to 1,500 mL of daily fluid intake to prevent crystalluria and calculi formation.
- Ensure that controlled-release and enteric-coated forms of the medications are not crushed or chewed.

NURSING EVALUATION OF MEDICATION EFFECTIVENESS

Depending on therapeutic intent, effectiveness can be evidenced by the following.
- Decreased bowel inflammation and relief of GI distress
- Return to normal bowel function

Probiotics: Dietary supplements

PURPOSE

EXPECTED PHARMACOLOGICAL ACTION: Various preparations of bacteria and yeast, which are normal flora of the intestine and colon, help to metabolize foods, promote nutrient absorption, and reduce colonization by pathogenic bacteria. They also can increase nonspecific cellular and humoral immunity.

THERAPEUTIC USE: Probiotics are used to treat the manifestations of IBS, ulcerative colitis, and Clostridium difficile-associated diarrhea and rotavirus diarrhea in children.

COMPLICATIONS

- Flatulence and bloating
- Infection has been reported among clients who are severely ill or immunocompromised after long-term antibiotic use.

INTERACTIONS

If antibiotics or antifungals are used concurrently, they should be administered at least 2 hr apart from probiotics. Q EBP

Medications for hiatal hernia

For complications and other information about these medications, refer to Chapter 26: Peptic Ulcer Disease.

PROTON PUMP INHIBITORS
- Omeprazole
- Esomeprazole
- Lansoprazole

ANTACIDS
- Aluminum hydroxide
- Sodium bicarbonate
- Calcium carbonate

PURPOSE

EXPECTED PHARMACOLOGICAL ACTION

Proton pump inhibitors block the final step of gastric acid production to prevent reflux in sliding hiatal hernia.

Antacids neutralize gastric acid to provide relief of manifestations (heartburn, belching, dysphagia).

NURSING EVALUATION OF MEDICATION

Reduced frequency of manifestations of hiatal hernia (heartburn, belching, and dysphagia).

Active Learning Scenario

A nurse is caring for a client who has a prescription for sulfasalazine. Use the *ATI Active Learning Template: Medication* to complete this item.

THERAPEUTIC USES: Identify two therapeutic uses for sulfasalazine.

COMPLICATIONS: Identify two blood disorders that occur as a complication with the use of sulfasalazine.

MEDICATION ADMINISTRATION: Identify how frequently the client should take the medication.

Application Exercises

1. A nurse is planning to administer ondansetron to a client. For which of the following adverse effects of ondansetron should the nurse monitor? (Select all that apply.)
   - A. Headache
   - B. Diarrhea
   - C. Shortened PR interval
   - D. Hyperglycemia
   - E. Prolonged QT interval

2. A nurse is caring for a client who received prochlorperazine 4 hr ago. The client reports spasms of the face. The nurse should expect a prescription for which of the following medications?
   - A. Fomepizole
   - B. Naloxone
   - C. Phytonadione
   - D. Diphenhydramine

3. A nurse is providing instructions about the use of laxatives to a client who has heart failure. The nurse should tell the client to avoid which of the following laxatives?
   - A. Psyllium
   - B. Bisacodyl
   - C. Polyethylene glycol
   - D. Sodium phosphate

4. A nurse is caring for a client who has diabetes and is experiencing nausea due to gastroparesis. The nurse should expect a prescription for which of the following medications?
   - A. Lubiprostone
   - B. Metoclopramide
   - C. Bisacodyl
   - D. Loperamide

5. A nurse is teaching a client about probiotic supplements. Which of the following information should the nurse include? (Select all that apply.)
   - A. "Probiotics are micro-organisms that are normally found in the GI tract."
   - B. "Probiotics are used to treat *Clostridium difficile*."
   - C. "Probiotics are used to treat benign prostatic hyperplasia."
   - D. "You can experience bloating while taking probiotic supplements."
   - E. "If you are prescribed an antibiotic, you should take it at the same time you take your probiotic supplement."

Active Learning Scenario Key

Using the ATI Active Learning Template: Medication

THERAPEUTIC USES: Crohn's disease and ulcerative colitis

COMPLICATIONS: Complications that occur with the use of sulfasalazine include agranulocytosis, and hemolytic and macrocytic anemia.

MEDICATION ADMINISTRATION: The client should take sulfasalazine four times per day in divided doses.

Ⓝ *NCLEX® Connection: Pharmacological and Parenteral Therapies, Medication Administration*

Application Exercises Key

1. A. **CORRECT:** Headaches are a common adverse effect of ondansetron.
   B. **CORRECT:** Diarrhea or constipation are both adverse effects of ondansetron.
   C. A shortened PR interval is not an adverse effect of ondansetron.
   D. Ondansetron does not affect blood glucose.
   E. **CORRECT:** A prolonged QT interval is a possible adverse effect of ondansetron that can lead to torsades de pointes, a serious dysrhythmia.

   Ⓝ *NCLEX® Connection: Pharmacological and Parenteral Therapies, Adverse Effects/Contraindications/Adverse Effects/Interactions*

2. D. **CORRECT:** When generating solutions, the nurse should identify that acute dystonia, evidenced by spasms of the muscles in the face, neck, and tongue. Is a potential adverse effect of prochlorperazine. The nurse should anticipate a prescription for diphenhydramine which is administered to suppress extrapyramidal effects of prochlorperazine.

   Ⓝ *NCLEX® Connection: Pharmacological and Parenteral Therapies, Expected Actions/Outcomes*

3. D. **CORRECT:** Absorption of sodium from sodium phosphate causes fluid retention which can exacerbate heart failure.

   Ⓝ *NCLEX® Connection: Pharmacological and Parenteral Therapies, Adverse Effects/Contraindications/Adverse Effects/Interactions*

4. B. **CORRECT:** Metoclopramide is a dopamine antagonist that is used to treat nausea and also increases gastric motility. It can relieve the bloating and nausea of diabetic gastroparesis.

   Ⓝ *NCLEX® Connection: Pharmacological and Parenteral Therapies, Adverse Effects/Contraindications/Adverse Effects/Interactions*

5. A. **CORRECT:** Probiotics consist of lactobacilli, bifidobacteria, and *Saccharomyces boulardii*, which are naturally found in the digestive tract.
   B. **CORRECT:** Probiotics are used to treat a number of GI conditions, including irritable bowel syndrome, diarrhea associated with *Clostridium difficile*, and ulcerative colitis.
   C. Saw palmetto is a supplement that clients might use to treat benign prostatic hyperplasia.
   D. **CORRECT:** Flatulence and bloating can be adverse effects of probiotic supplements.
   E. The client should take the probiotic supplement at least 2 hr after taking an antibiotic or antifungal medication. Antibiotics and antifungal medications destroy bacteria and yeast found in probiotic supplements.

   Ⓝ *NCLEX® Connection: Pharmacological and Parenteral Therapies, Medication Administration*

UNIT 6 MEDICATIONS AFFECTING THE
GASTROINTESTINAL SYSTEM AND NUTRITION

CHAPTER 28 *Vitamins and Minerals*

Vitamins and minerals have important roles in the body, including the production of red blood cells, building bones, making hormones, regulating body fluid volume, and supporting nerve cell function. Vitamin and mineral deficiencies can increase the risk for health problems (anemias, heart disease, cancers, and osteoporosis).

Supplements of vitamins and minerals can help prevent multiple health conditions.

Iron preparations

SELECT PROTOTYPE MEDICATIONS
- Oral: Ferrous sulfate
- Parenteral: Iron dextran

OTHER MEDICATIONS
- Oral: Ferrous gluconate, ferrous fumarate
- Parenteral: Ferumoxytol, iron sucrose, sodium-ferric gluconate complex (SFGC)

PURPOSE

EXPECTED PHARMACOLOGICAL ACTION: Iron preparations provide iron needed for RBC development and oxygen transport to cells. During times of increased growth (in growing children or during pregnancy) or when RBCs are in high demand (after blood loss), the need for iron can be greatly increased. Iron is poorly absorbed by the body, so relatively large amounts must be ingested orally to increase Hgb and Hct levels.

THERAPEUTIC USES
- Iron preparations are used to treat and prevent iron-deficiency anemia.
  - Ferumoxytol is limited to clients who have chronic kidney disease, regardless of dialysis or receiving erythropoietin. Ferumoxytol requires only two doses over 3 to 8 days compared with SFGC and iron sucrose, which require 3 to 10 doses over several weeks.
  - SFGC is used for clients who are undergoing long-term hemodialysis and are deficient in iron. It is always used along with erythropoietin.
  - Iron sucrose is used for clients who have chronic kidney disease, are receiving erythropoietin, and are hemodialysis- or peritoneal dialysis-dependent; and clients who have chronic kidney disease, are not receiving erythropoietin, and are not dialysis-dependent.

- Iron preparations are used to prevent iron deficiency anemia for clients who are at an increased risk (infants, children, and pregnant clients).
- Parenteral forms should only be used in clients who are unable to take oral medications, in which case the IV route is preferred.

COMPLICATIONS

GI distress (nausea, constipation, heartburn)

NURSING ACTIONS
- If intolerable, administer medication with food, but this greatly reduces absorption.
- Might need to reduce dosage.
- Monitor the client's bowel pattern and intervene as appropriate.

CLIENT EDUCATION: Stools can become black or dark green when taking an iron preparation. This usually resolves with continued use.

Teeth staining (liquid form)

CLIENT EDUCATION: Dilute liquid iron with water or juice, drink with a straw, and rinse mouth after swallowing.

Staining of skin and other tissues (IM injections)

IM doses are administered deep IM using Z-track technique. Avoid this route if possible.

NURSING ACTIONS
- Give IM doses deep IM using Z-track technique.
- Avoid this route if possible.

Anaphylaxis

- Risk with parenteral administration of iron dextran.
- Anaphylaxis is triggered by the dextran in iron dextran, not by the iron.
- Anaphylaxis is minimal with SFGC, iron sucrose, and ferumoxytol.
- IV route is safer than IM.

NURSING ACTIONS
- Administer a test dose and observe the client closely. No test dose is needed before administering ferumoxytol and iron sucrose.
- Administer slowly, and use manufacturer's recommendation for specific product.
- Be prepared with life-support equipment and epinephrine.

Hypotension

Can progress to circulatory collapse with parenteral administration

NURSING ACTIONS: Monitor vital signs when administering parenteral iron.

Fatal iron toxicity in children

Can occur when an overdose of iron (2 to 10 g) is ingested

NURSING ACTIONS
- Manifestations of toxicity include severe GI manifestations, shock, acidosis, and liver and heart failure. The chelating agent deferoxamine, given parenterally, is used to treat toxicity. Gastric lavage is used to remove iron from the stomach.
- Avoid using oral and parenteral iron concurrently.

CONTRAINDICATIONS/PRECAUTIONS

- **Warnings**
  - Pregnancy: Ferrous sulfate, iron dextran (PO) safe; parenteral safety not established.
  - Lactation: Ferrous sulfate, iron dextran (PO) safe; parenteral safety not established.
- Contraindicated for clients who have previous hypersensitivity to iron, anemias other than iron-deficiency anemia.
- Oral preparations should be used with caution in clients who have peptic ulcer disease, regional enteritis, ulcerative colitis, and severe liver disease.

Concurrent administration of antacids or tetracyclines reduces absorption of iron.
NURSING ACTIONS
- Avoid using antacids within 1 hr after administration of iron.
- Avoid administration of iron within 1 to 2 hr of tetracycline.
- Vitamin C increases absorption, but also increases incidence of GI complications.

Caffeine and dairy products can interfere with absorption.
NURSING ACTIONS: Avoid caffeine and dairy intake when taking medication.

Food reduces absorption but reduces gastric distress.
NURSING ACTIONS: Take with food at the start of therapy if gastric distress occurs.

NURSING ADMINISTRATION

CLIENT EDUCATION
- Take iron on an empty stomach (1 hr before meals) as stomach acid increases absorption.
- Take with food if GI adverse effects occur. This might increase adherence to therapy even though absorption is also decreased.
- Space doses at approximately equal intervals throughout day to most efficiently increase red blood cell production.
- Anticipate a harmless dark green or black color of stool.
- Dilute liquid iron with water or juice, drink with a straw, and rinse the mouth after swallowing.

- Increase water and fiber intake (unless contraindicated) and maintain an exercise program to counter the constipation effects.
- Therapy can last 1 to 2 months. Usually, dietary intake will be sufficient after Hgb has returned to a therapeutic level.
- Perform concurrent intake of appropriate quantities of foods high in iron (liver, egg yolks, muscle meats, yeast, grains, green leafy vegetables).

NURSING EVALUATION OF MEDICATION EFFECTIVENESS

Depending on therapeutic intent, effectiveness is evidenced by the following.
- Increased reticulocyte count is expected within 4 to 7 days after beginning iron therapy.
- Increase in hemoglobin of 2 g/dL is expected 1 month after beginning therapy.
- Fatigue and pallor (skin, mucous membranes) should subside, and the client reports increased energy level.

Vitamin B₁₂/Cyanocobalamin

SELECT PROTOTYPE MEDICATION: Vitamin B$_{12}$

OTHER MEDICATIONS: Intranasal cyanocobalamin

PURPOSE

EXPECTED PHARMACOLOGICAL ACTION
- Vitamin B$_{12}$ is necessary to convert folic acid from its inactive form to its active form. All cells rely on folic acid for DNA production.
- Vitamin B12 deficiency can result in megaloblastic (macrocytic) anemia and cause dysrhythmias and heart failure if not corrected. Vitamin B$_{12}$ is administered to prevent or correct deficiency. Damage to rapidly multiplying cells can affect the skin and mucous membranes, causing GI disturbances. Neurologic damage, which includes numbness and tingling of extremities and CNS damage caused by demyelination of neurons, can result from deficiency of this vitamin.
- Vitamin B$_{12}$ deficiency affects all blood cells produced in the bone marrow.
  - Loss of erythrocytes leads to heart failure, cerebral vascular insufficiency, and hypoxia.
  - Loss of leukocytes leads to infections.
  - Loss of thrombocytes leads to bleeding and hemorrhage.
- Loss of intrinsic factor within the cells of the stomach causes an inability to absorb vitamin B$_{12}$, making it necessary to administer parenteral or intranasal vitamin B$_{12}$ or high doses of oral B$_{12}$ for the rest of the client's life.

THERAPEUTIC USES
- Treatment of vitamin B$_{12}$ deficiency
- Megaloblastic (macrocytic) anemia related to vitamin B$_{12}$ deficiency

COMPLICATIONS

Hypokalemia

Secondary to the increased RBC production effects of vitamin B_{12}

NURSING ACTIONS
- Monitor potassium levels during the start of treatment.
- Observe clients for manifestations of potassium deficiency (muscle weakness, irregular cardiac rhythm).
- Clients might require potassium supplements.

GI distress (nausea, vomiting, dyspepsia, abdominal discomfort, diarrhea)

CONTRAINDICATIONS/PRECAUTIONS

- **Warnings**
  - Pregnancy: Cyanocobalamin (oral and nasal) safe; parenteral safety not established.
  - Lactation: Cyanocobalamin contraindicated (crosses breast milk).
- Moderate vitamin B_{12} deficiency can be managed with vitamin B_{12} alone.
- Severe vitamin B_{12} deficiency should be treated with vitamin B_{12} and folic acid.

INTERACTIONS

Masks manifestations of vitamin B_{12} deficiency with concurrent administration of folic acid
NURSING ACTIONS: Ensure clients receive adequate doses of vitamin B_{12} when using folic acid.

NURSING ADMINISTRATION

NURSING CARE
- Obtain baseline vitamin B_{12}, Hgb, Hct, RBC, reticulocyte counts, and folate levels. Monitor periodically.
- Monitor for manifestations of vitamin B_{12} deficiency (beefy red tongue, pallor, and neuropathy).
- Cyanocobalamin is administered intranasally, orally, IM, or subcutaneously. Injections are painful and usually reserved for clients who have significant reduced ability to absorb vitamin B_{12} (lack of intrinsic factor [pernicious anemia], enteritis, and partial removal of the stomach).
- Clients who have malabsorption syndrome can use intranasal or parenteral preparations.
- Intranasal cyanocobalamin should be administered 1 hr before or after eating hot foods, which can cause the medication to be removed from nasal passages without being absorbed, because of increased nasal secretions.

- Clients who have irreversible malabsorption syndrome (parietal cell atrophy or total gastrectomy) will need lifelong treatment, usually parenterally. If oral therapy is used, doses must be very high.
  - Encourage concurrent intake of quantities of foods high in vitamin B_{12} (dairy products).
  - Perform a Schilling test to determine vitamin B_{12} absorption in the gastrointestinal tract.
  - Measurement of plasma B_{12} levels helps determine the need for therapy.
  - Advise clients to adhere to prescribed laboratory tests. Monitor blood counts and vitamin B_{12} levels every 3 to 6 months.

NURSING EVALUATION OF MEDICATION EFFECTIVENESS

Depending on therapeutic intent, effectiveness can be evidenced by the following.
- Disappearance of megaloblasts (in 2 to 3 weeks)
- Increased reticulocyte count
- Increase in hematocrit
- Improvement of neurologic injury (absence of tingling sensation of hands and feet and numbness of extremities). Improvement can take months, and some clients never attain full recovery.

Folic Acid

SELECT PROTOTYPE MEDICATION: Folic acid

PURPOSE

EXPECTED PHARMACOLOGICAL ACTION: Folic acid is essential in the production of DNA and erythropoiesis (RBC, WBC, and platelets).

THERAPEUTIC USES
- Treatment of megaloblastic (macrocytic) anemia secondary to folic acid deficiency
- Prevention of neural tube defects that can occur early during pregnancy (thus needed for all females of child-bearing age who might become pregnant)
- Treatment of malabsorption syndrome (sprue)
- Supplement for alcohol use disorder (due to poor dietary intake of folic acid and injury to the liver)

CONTRAINDICATIONS/PRECAUTIONS

- **Warnings**
  - Pregnancy: Folic acid is safe.
  - Lactation: Use folic acid with caution.
- Avoid indiscriminate use of folic acid to reduce the risk of masking manifestations of vitamin B_{12} deficiency.

INTERACTIONS

Folic acid levels are decreased by methotrexate and sulfonamides.
NURSING ACTIONS: Avoid concurrent use of these medications.

Folic acid can decrease phenytoin blood levels because of increased metabolism.
NURSING ACTIONS: Monitor blood phenytoin levels.

NURSING ADMINISTRATION

NURSING CARE

- Assess for manifestations of megaloblastic anemia (pallor, easy fatigability, palpitations, paresthesia of hands or feet).
- Obtain baseline folic acid, Hgb and Hct levels, and RBC and reticulocyte counts. Monitor periodically.

CLIENT EDUCATION: If with folic acid deficiency, concurrently increase intake of food sources of folic acid (liver, green leafy vegetables, citrus fruits, and dried peas and beans). Monitor for risk factors indicating that folic acid therapy is needed (heavy alcohol use and child-bearing age).

NURSING EVALUATION OF MEDICATION EFFECTIVENESS

Depending on therapeutic intent, effectiveness is evidenced by the following.
- Folate level within expected reference range
- Return of RBC, reticulocyte count, and Hgb and Hct to levels within expected reference range
- Improvement of anemia findings (absence of pallor, dyspnea, easy fatigability)
- Absence of neural tube defects in newborns

Potassium supplements

SELECT PROTOTYPE MEDICATION: Potassium chloride

OTHER MEDICATION
- Potassium gluconate
- Potassium phosphate
- Potassium bicarbonate

PURPOSE

EXPECTED PHARMACOLOGICAL ACTION: Potassium is essential for conducting nerve impulses, maintaining electrical excitability of muscle, and regulation of acid/base balance.

THERAPEUTIC USES
- Treating hypokalemia (potassium less than 3.5 mEq/L).
- For clients receiving diuretics resulting in potassium loss (furosemide).
- For clients who have potassium loss due to excessive or prolonged vomiting, diarrhea, excessive use of laxatives, intestinal drainage, and GI fistula.

COMPLICATIONS

Local GI ulceration and GI distress

Nausea, vomiting, diarrhea, abdominal discomfort, and esophagitis with oral administration

CLIENT EDUCATION
- Take the medication with meals or at least 8 oz of water to minimize GI discomfort and prevent ulceration.
- Do not dissolve the tablet in the mouth because oral ulceration will develop.

Hyperkalemia (potassium more than 5.0 mEq/L)

NURSING ACTIONS
- Hyperkalemia rarely occurs with oral administration.
- Monitor clients receiving IV potassium for manifestations of hyperkalemia (bradycardia, ECG changes, vomiting, confusion, anxiety, dyspnea, weakness, numbness, and tingling).
- Severe hyperkalemia can require treatment (calcium salt, glucose and insulin, sodium bicarbonate, sodium polystyrene sulfonate, peritoneal dialysis, or hemodialysis).

CONTRAINDICATIONS/PRECAUTIONS

Contraindicated for clients who have severe kidney disease or hypoaldosteronism

INTERACTIONS

Concurrent use of potassium-sparing diuretics (spironolactone) or ACE inhibitors (lisinopril) increases the risk of hyperkalemia

NURSING ACTIONS
- Avoid concurrent use.
- Oxalates in spinach and rhubarb, and phytates in bran and whole grains, can decrease absorption.

NURSING ADMINISTRATION

ORAL FORMATIONS

- Mix powdered formulations in at least 90 mL to 240 mL (3 to 8 oz) of cold water or juice and drink slowly over 5 to 10 min.
- Effervescent tablets should be dissolved in 90 mL to 240 mL (3 to 8 oz) of cold water.

CLIENT EDUCATION
- Take potassium chloride with a meal or at least 8 oz of water to reduce the risk of adverse GI effects.
- Do not to crush or chew extended-release tablets.
- Notify the provider of any difficulty swallowing the pills. Medication can be supplied as a powder or a sustained-release tablet that is easier to tolerate.

IV ADMINISTRATION

- Never administer IV bolus. Rapid IV infusion can result in fatal hyperkalemia. Qs
- Use an IV infusion pump to control the infusion rate.
- Dilute potassium and give no more than 40 mEq/L of IV solution to prevent vein irritation.
- Infuse slowly, generally no faster than 10 mEq/hr.
- Cardiac monitoring is indicated for blood potassium levels outside of expected reference ranges. ECG changes (prolonged PR interval and peaked T-waves) can indicate potassium toxicity.
- Infuse potassium through a large bore needle. Assess the IV site for local irritation, phlebitis, and infiltration. Discontinue the IV immediately if infiltration occurs.
- Monitor I&O to ensure an adequate urine output of at least 30 mL/hr.

NURSING EVALUATION OF MEDICATION EFFECTIVENESS

Depending on therapeutic intent, effectiveness is evidenced by blood potassium level within the expected reference range (3.5 to 5.0 mEq/L).

Magnesium sulfate

SELECT PROTOTYPE MEDICATION
- Parenteral: Magnesium sulfate
- Oral: Magnesium hydroxide, magnesium oxide, magnesium citrate

> Magnesium hydroxide and magnesium oxide act as antacids when administered in a low dose, and all three act as laxatives.

PURPOSE

EXPECTED PHARMACOLOGICAL ACTION: Magnesium activates many intracellular enzymes, binds the messenger RNA to ribosomes, and plays a role in regulating skeletal muscle contractility and blood coagulation.

THERAPEUTIC USES
- Magnesium supplements are used for clients who have hypomagnesemia (magnesium level less than 1.3 mEq/L).
- Oral preparations of magnesium sulfate are used to prevent or treat low magnesium levels and as laxatives.
- Parenteral magnesium is used for clients who have severe hypomagnesemia.
- IV magnesium sulfate is used to stop preterm labor and as an anticonvulsant during labor and delivery.

COMPLICATIONS

Muscle weakness, flaccid paralysis, painful muscle contractions, suppression of AV conduction through the heart, respiratory depression

NURSING ACTIONS
- IV administration requires careful monitoring of cardiac and neuromuscular status.
- Monitor blood magnesium levels.
- Avoid administering with neuromuscular blocking agents, which can potentiate respiratory depression and apnea.
- Have IV calcium (calcium gluconate) available to reverse the effects of magnesium. Qs

Diarrhea

NURSING ACTIONS
- Monitor electrolyte levels for electrolyte loss from diarrhea.
- Monitor I&O and observe for manifestations of dehydration.

CONTRAINDICATIONS/PRECAUTIONS

- **Warnings**
  - Pregnancy
    - Magnesium sulfate: Avoid administering within 2 hr of delivery.
    - Magnesium salts (oral): Contraindicated; can be used for preterm labor.
  - Lactation: Magnesium sulfate present in breast milk; monitor for toxicity.
- Contraindicated in clients who have AV block, rectal bleeding, nausea, vomiting, and abdominal pain.
- Use cautiously with clients who have renal and/or cardiac disease.

INTERACTIONS

- Magnesium sulfate can decrease the absorption of tetracyclines and digoxin.
- Monitor the therapeutic effect to determine if absorption has been affected.

NURSING ADMINISTRATION

NURSING CARE
- Monitor blood magnesium, calcium, and phosphorus.
- Monitor blood pressure, heart rate, and respiratory rate when given intravenously.
- Assess for depressed or absent deep tendon reflexes as a manifestation of toxicity.
- Calcium gluconate is given for magnesium sulfate toxicity. Always have an injectable form of calcium gluconate available when administering magnesium sulfate by IV. Qs
- Teach clients about dietary sources of magnesium (whole-grain cereals, nuts, legumes, green leafy vegetables, bananas).

Active Learning Scenario

A nurse is educating a client about a new prescription for cyanocobalamin. What should the nurse include in the teaching? Use the *ATI Active Learning Template: Medication* to complete this item.

EXPECTED PHARMACOLOGICAL ACTION

CLIENT EDUCATION: Describe four teaching points for the client.

EVALUATION OF MEDICATION EFFECTIVENESS: Describe two nursing interventions.

Application Exercises

1. A nurse is teaching a client who has anemia and a new prescription for a liquid iron supplement. Which of the following information should the nurse include in the teaching? (Select all that apply.)

   A. "Add foods that are low in fiber to your diet."

   B. "Rinse your mouth after taking the medication."

   C. "Stools can be green or black in color."

   D. "Take the medication with a glass of milk."

   E. "Add red meat to your diet."

2. A nurse is evaluating a group of clients at a health fair to identify the need for folic acid therapy. Which of the following clients should the nurse refer to a provider for folic acid therapy? (Select all that apply.)

   A. 12-year-old child who has iron deficiency anemia

   B. 24-year-old female who has no health problems

   C. 44-year-old male who has hypertension

   D. 55–year-old female who has alcohol use disorder

   E. 35-year-old male who has type 2 diabetes mellitus

3. A nurse is caring for a client who is receiving IV potassium. The nurse should monitor the client for which of the following manifestations as an indication of hyperkalemia?

   A. Tachycardia

   B. Dyspnea

   C. Lethargy

   D. Increased thirst

4. A nurse is preparing to administer potassium chloride IV to a client who has hypokalemia. Which of the following actions should the nurse take? (Select all that apply.)

   A. Infuse medication through a large-bore needle.

   B. Monitor urine output to ensure at least 20 mL/hr.

   C. Administer medication via direct IV bolus.

   D. Implement cardiac monitoring.

   E. Administer the infusion using an IV pump.

5. A nurse is assessing a client who is receiving magnesium sulfate and notes the client has depressed deep tendon reflexes. The nurse should expect the need to administer which of the following medications?

   A. Potassium chloride

   B. Folic acid

   C. Calcium gluconate

   D. Cyanocobalamin

1. B, C, E. **CORRECT:** When taking actions, the nurse should teach the client that muscle meats are high in iron and recommended for clients to improve anemia when taken concurrently with iron supplements. Iron supplements can stain the teeth when taken in a liquid form, therefore the client should rinse orally after taking the medication. Dark green or black stools can occur when taking iron supplements.

   Ⓝ *NCLEX® Connection: Pharmacological and Parenteral Therapies, Medication Administration*

2. B, D. **CORRECT:** The nurse should analyze cues from the clients' history and follow up with referrals for the 24-year-old female who has no health problems (childbearing age) and the client who has alcohol use disorder (excess alcohol consumption leads to poor dietary intake of folic acid and injury to the liver) to a health care provider for folic acid therapy.

   Ⓝ *NCLEX® Connection: Pharmacological and Parenteral Therapies, Expected Actions/Outcomes*

3. B. **CORRECT:** The nurse should generate solutions to address the client's potential for hyperkalemia by monitoring the client for dyspnea as a manifestation of hyperkalemia.

   Ⓝ *NCLEX® Connection: Pharmacological and Parenteral Therapies, Medication Administration*

4. A, D, E. **CORRECT:** When taking actions, the nurse should identify that the focus of care is correct administration of the IV potassium chloride. The nurse should infuse potassium through a large-bore needle to prevent vein irritation, phlebitis, and infiltration. Implement cardiac monitoring to detect cardiac dysrhythmias in a client receiving IV potassium. It is important for the nurse to administer IV potassium using an infusion pump to prevent fatal hyperkalemia due to a rapid infusion rate.

   Ⓝ *NCLEX® Connection: Pharmacological and Parenteral Therapies, Parenteral/Intravenous Therapies*

5. C. **CORRECT:** The nurse should plan to generate solutions to address the client's magnesium toxicity as evidenced by depressed or absent deep tendon reflexes by anticipating the need to administer calcium gluconate.

   Ⓝ *NCLEX® Connection: Pharmacological and Parenteral Therapies, Adverse Effects/Contraindications/Side Effects/Interactions*

Using the ATI Active Learning Template: Medication

EXPECTED PHARMACOLOGICAL ACTION: Cyanocobalamin converts folic acid from an inactive form to an active form. It corrects megaloblastic anemia related to a deficiency of vitamin B_{12}.

CLIENT EDUCATION

- Review manifestations of hypokalemia.
- Discuss the use of potassium supplements, if prescribed.
- Discuss dietary sources of potassium.
- Consume foods high in vitamin B_{12}.
- Administer intranasal cyanocobalamin 1 hr before or after eating hot foods when nasal secretions are decreased.
- Periodic laboratory testing of Hgb, Hct, RBC, reticulocyte count, and folate levels is advised.

EVALUATION OF MEDICATION EFFECTIVENESS

- Review laboratory values for increased reticulocyte count and macrocytes and Hgb and Hct levels within the expected reference range.
- Assess for improvement of neurologic manifestations (numbness, tingling of hands and feet).

Ⓝ *NCLEX® Connection: Pharmacological and Parenteral Therapies, Medication Administration*

NCLEX® Connections

When reviewing the following chapters, keep in mind the relevant topics and tasks of the NCLEX outline, in particular:

Pharmacological and Parenteral Therapies

ADVERSE EFFECTS/CONTRAINDICATIONS/SIDE EFFECTS/INTERACTIONS

Document side effects and adverse effects of medications and parenteral therapy.

Identify a contraindication to the administration of a medication to the client.

Provide information to the client on common side effects/adverse effects/potential interactions of medications, and inform the client of when to notify the primary health care provider.

Notify the primary health care provider of side effects, adverse effects, and contraindications of medications and parenteral therapy.

MEDICATION ADMINISTRATION

Review pertinent data prior to medication administration.

Educate client about medications.

Administer and document medications given by parenteral routes.

PARENTERAL/INTRAVENOUS THERAPIES: Evaluate the client's response to intermittent parenteral fluid therapy.

CHAPTER 29 *Medications Affecting the Reproductive Tract*

Medications that affect the reproductive system include hormones that stimulate puberty (estrogen, progesterone, and testosterone), replace a hormonal deficiency, or prevent pregnancy (which includes oral contraceptives, the hormonal patch, ring, and injection).

Medications that are used to treat benign prostatic hyperplasia (BPH) include 5-alpha reductase inhibitors and alpha₁ adrenergic antagonists. Phosphodiesterase type 5 (PDE5) inhibitors are used to treat erectile dysfunction and BPH.

Estrogens

SELECT PROTOTYPE MEDICATIONS: Conjugated equine estrogens

OTHER MEDICATIONS
- Estradiol
- Estradiol hemihydrate

ROUTE OF ADMINISTRATION
- **Oral, transdermal, intravaginal, IM, and IV:** Transdermal therapy reduces incidents of nausea and vomiting. A smaller dose is prescribed, and there is a reduction of fluctuation of blood estrogen levels and a reduced risk of complications.
- **IV and IM:** Rare

PURPOSE

EXPECTED PHARMACOLOGICAL ACTION: Estrogens are hormones needed for growth and maturation of the female reproductive tract, development of secondary sex characteristics, and are active in the follicular phase of the menstrual cycle. Estrogens block bone resorption and reduce low-density lipoprotein (LDL) levels. At high levels, estrogens suppress the release of a follicle-stimulating hormone (FSH) needed for conception.

THERAPEUTIC USES
- Contraception, along with progestins
- Acne in young females
- Relief of moderate to severe postmenopausal manifestations (hot flashes, mood changes)
- Prevention of postmenopausal osteoporosis
- Treatment of dysfunctional uterine bleeding
- Treatment of prostate cancer, and hypogonadism
- Treatment of moderate to severe vulvar atrophy

COMPLICATIONS

Endometrial and ovarian cancers

When estrogen is used alone for postmenopausal therapy

NURSING ACTIONS: Administer progestins along with estrogen.

CLIENT EDUCATION
- Report persistent vaginal bleeding
- Schedule an endometrial biopsy every 2 years and pelvic exam yearly.

Potential risk for estrogen-dependent breast cancer

More often in postmenopausal women who use estrogen with progestin

NURSING ACTIONS: Rule out estrogen-dependent breast cancer prior to starting therapy.

CLIENT EDUCATION: Examine breasts regularly. Obtain yearly breast exams by a provider, and periodic mammograms.

Altered coagulation

- Estrogen either suppresses blood coagulation or promotes it; the effect depends on genetic influences. Monitor for embolic event (MI, pulmonary embolism, DVT, stroke).
- Increased risk of myocardial infarction and coronary heart disease (clients who are older than 60 years of age).

ESTROGEN NURSING ACTIONS: Monitor for pain, swelling, warmth, or erythema of lower legs.

CLIENT EDUCATION
- Avoid all nicotine products.
- Reduce risk of cardiovascular disease.

CONTRAINDICATIONS/PRECAUTIONS

- **Warnings**
  - Pregnancy: Conjugated equine estrogens contraindicated.
  - Lactation: Conjugated equine estrogens contraindicated; can alter the quality and quantity of breast milk.
- Contraindicated for clients who have the following. Qs
  - Client or family history of heart disease
  - Atypical vaginal bleeding that is undiagnosed
  - Breast or estrogen-dependent cancer
- Estrogens are not indicated for prepubertal children.

INTERACTIONS

Estrogens can reduce the effectiveness of warfarin.
NURSING ACTIONS
- If used concurrently, monitor international normalized ratio (INR) and prothrombin time (PT).
- Warfarin doses might need to be adjusted.

Concurrent use of phenytoin can decrease the effectiveness of estrogens.
NURSING ACTIONS: Monitor for decreased estrogen effects. An alternative form of contraception might be indicated.

Concurrent use of corticosteroids can increase effects of the corticosteroid.
NURSING ACTIONS: Monitor for increased corticosteroid effects.

Smoking increases risk for thrombophlebitis.
CLIENT EDUCATION
- Avoid smoking. Use alternative treatment if smoking persists.
- Decreases effects of anticoagulants, oral hypoglycemics, or thyroid medications when used concurrently.

NURSING ACTIONS: Monitor for decreased effects, and adjust dosages as needed. Monitor glucose and thyroid levels.

NURSING ADMINISTRATION

- Apply estrogen patches to the skin of the trunk. Avoid the breasts and waistline.
- Discontinue prior to knee or hip surgery or any surgical procedures that can cause extensive immobilization.

CLIENT EDUCATION
- Take medication at the same time each day, such as at bedtime.
- Report menstrual changes (dysmenorrhea, amenorrhea, breakthrough bleeding), or breast changes.
- Notify the provider of any swelling or redness in legs, shortness of breath, or chest pain.
- Ensure regular self- and clinical breast examination.

NURSING EVALUATION OF MEDICATION EFFECTIVENESS

Depending on therapeutic intent, effectiveness is evidenced by the following.
- Avoidance of conception
- Relief of severe postmenopausal manifestations (hot flashes, mood changes)
- Reduction in dysfunctional uterine bleeding
- Decrease in spread of prostate cancer

Progesterones (Progestin)

SELECT PROTOTYPE MEDICATION: Medroxyprogesterone

OTHER MEDICATIONS
- Norethindrone
- Megestrol acetate

ROUTES OF ADMINISTRATION: Oral, IM, subcutaneous, transdermal, and intravaginal

PURPOSE

EXPECTED PHARMACOLOGICAL ACTION: Bind with progesterone receptors in the cell nucleus. Often prescribed in combination with estrogen.

THERAPEUTIC USES
- Contraception, alone or with estrogens
- Counter adverse effects of estrogen in menopausal hormone therapy
- Dysfunctional uterine bleeding due to hormonal imbalance
- Amenorrhea (initiates menses)
- Endometriosis (counter adverse effects of proliferation related estrogen)
- Advanced cancer of the endometrium, breast, and kidney (provides palliation)
- Facilitation of in vitro fertilization (support early pregnancy)
- Prevention of preterm birth

COMPLICATIONS

Breast cancer

In postmenopausal clients when used in combination with estrogens

CLIENT EDUCATION: Encourage regular breast self-exams, mammograms and clinical breast exams as recommended

Thromboembolic events

MI, pulmonary embolism, thrombophlebitis, stroke

NURSING ACTIONS
- Discourage clients from smoking.
- Monitor for pain, swelling, warmth, or erythema of lower legs.

CLIENT EDUCATION: Notify the provider of chest pain or shortness of breath.

Breakthrough bleeding, amenorrhea, breast tenderness

CLIENT EDUCATION
- Obtain baseline clinical breast exam and Pap smear.
- Report abnormal vaginal bleeding.

Edema

NURSING ACTIONS: Monitor blood pressure, I&O, and weight gain.

Jaundice

NURSING ACTIONS: Monitor for indications of jaundice (yellowing of the skin and sclera of the eyes). Monitor liver enzymes.

Migraine headaches

NURSING ACTIONS: Notify the provider of severe headache.

CONTRAINDICATIONS/PRECAUTIONS

- **Warnings**
  - Pregnancy: Progesterones contraindicated.
  - Lactation: Progesterones contraindicated; enters breast milk.
  - Reproductive: Notify provider if pregnancy is planned or suspected.
- Contraindicated in clients who have the following. Qs
  - Undiagnosed vaginal bleeding
  - History of thromboembolic disease, cardiovascular, or cerebrovascular disease
  - History of breast or genital cancers
- Use cautiously in clients who have diabetes mellitus, seizures disorders, and migraine headaches.

INTERACTIONS

Use of carbamazepine, phenobarbital, phenytoin, and rifampin can decrease contraceptive effectiveness.
NURSING ACTIONS: Additional contraceptive measures might be needed with concurrent use of these medications.

Concurrent use with corticosteroids and anticoagulants can cause decreased bone density.
CLIENT EDUCATION: Increase calcium and vitamin D intake when taken together. Avoid concurrent use.

Smoking increases risk for thrombophlebitis.
CLIENT EDUCATION: Avoid smoking or stop using progestins if unable to stop.

NURSING ADMINISTRATION

Administer progestins through oral, IM, subcutaneous, intrauterine, intravaginal, or transdermal routes. Vaginal inserts are administered using an applicator from the manufacturer.

CLIENT EDUCATION: Anticipate withdrawal bleeding 3 to 7 days after stopping the medication. Qpcc

NURSING EVALUATION OF MEDICATION EFFECTIVENESS

Depending on therapeutic intent, effectiveness is evidenced by the following.
- Restoration of hormonal balance with control of uterine bleeding
- Restoration of menses
- Decrease in endometrial hyperplasia in postmenopausal clients receiving concurrent estrogen
- Control of the spread of endometrial cancer

Hormonal contraceptives

- Estrogen–progestin combinations contain estrogen and progestin and are referred to as combination oral contraceptives (OCs). OCs that contain progestin only are often referred to as minipills.
- Combination oral contraceptives are classified as monophasic, biphasic, triphasic, or quadriphasic. With monophasic OCs, the dosage of estrogen to progestin remains the same throughout the cycle. With the other classifications, the estrogen/progestin changes to duplicate a typical menstrual cycle.

SELECT PROTOTYPE MEDICATIONS
- Combination oral contraceptives with estrogen plus a progestin
  - Ethinyl estradiol and norethindrone
  - Ethinyl estradiol and drospirenone
- Progestin-only oral contraceptives: Norethindrone

OTHER MEDICATIONS
- Transdermal patch: Ethinyl estradiol and norelgestromin
- Vaginal contraceptive ring: Ethinyl estradiol and etonogestrel
- Parenteral: Depot medroxyprogesterone acetate available for IM use and for subcutaneous use
- Etonogestrel implants
- Hormonal IUD

PURPOSE

EXPECTED PHARMACOLOGICAL ACTION: Oral contraceptives stop conception by preventing ovulation. They also thicken the cervical mucus and alter the endometrial lining to reduce the chance of fertilization.

THERAPEUTIC USES
- Prevention of pregnancy
- Premenstrual dysphoric disorder (PDD)
- Acne
- Fibrocystic breast
- Leiomyomas (manage discomfort and bleeding)
- Reducing menstrual blood loss, which can help with iron deficiency anemia
- Reducing menstrual cramping, which can help with dysmenorrhea
- Protection against endometrial and ovarian cancers

COMPLICATIONS

Thromboembolic events

- MI, pulmonary embolism, thrombophlebitis, stroke
- Unlikely with progestin-only OCs

CLIENT EDUCATION
- Avoid smoking.
- Report warmth, edema, tenderness, or pain in lower legs, chest pain, shortness of breath, severe headache.

Hypertension

CLIENT EDUCATION: Monitor for and report high blood pressure and vision changes.

Breakthrough or irregular uterine bleeding

CLIENT EDUCATION
- Record duration and frequency of breakthrough bleeding.
- Evaluate for possible pregnancy if two or more menstrual periods are missed.
- If taking OCs, take pill every day at approximately the same time, and for any missed pills, follow provider instructions for catching up and use a back-up contraceptive method for pregnancy prevention.

Breast cancer

NURSING ACTIONS: Oral contraceptives can increase growth of a pre-existing breast cancer. Do not administer to clients who have breast cancer.

Hyperglycemia

NURSING ACTIONS: Monitor glucose in clients who have diabetes mellitus. Adjust antihyperglycemics as needed.

Hyperkalemia

With combination OC that contains drospirenone

NURSING ACTIONS: Do not use combination OC with drospirenone in clients at risk for hyperkalemia (renal or adrenal insufficiency).

CONTRAINDICATIONS/PRECAUTIONS

- **Warnings**
  - Pregnancy: Hormonal contraceptives contraindicated.
  - Lactation: Combination oral contraceptives contraindicated. Progestin only (mini pills) is safe.
  - Reproductive: Notify provider if pregnancy is planned or suspected.
- Contraindicated for clients who ⓆS
  - Are smokers and older than 35 years of age.
  - Have a history of thrombophlebitis and cardiovascular events.
  - Have suspected or known breast cancer.
  - Have liver conditions
  - Are experiencing abnormal vaginal bleeding.
- Use cautiously in clients who have hypertension, diabetes mellitus, gallbladder disease, uterine leiomyoma, seizures, and migraine headaches.

INTERACTIONS

Oral contraceptive effectiveness decreases with use of carbamazepine, phenobarbital, ritonavir, rifampin, St. John's wort. Some sources suggest that antibiotics can decrease the effectiveness of oral contraceptives.
NURSING ACTIONS: For clients using hormonal contraceptives to prevent pregnancy, suggest using a secondary method of birth control while taking these medications or antibiotic therapy.

Oral contraceptives decrease the effects of warfarin and oral hypoglycemics.
NURSING ACTIONS: Monitor INR, PT, and glucose levels, and provider may need to adjust dosages accordingly. Monitor for breakthrough bleeding or spotting.

Oral contraceptives can increase the effects of theophylline, imipramine, tricyclic antidepressants, chlordiazepoxide, diazepam.
NURSING ACTIONS: Monitor for indications of toxicity. Provider may need to decrease dosage.

NURSING ADMINISTRATION

- Nurses or others administering the medication who are of childbearing age should avoid directly handling hormonal medications to avoid potential effects on the reproductive system.
- Rule out client pregnancy prior to start of therapy. Ⓠpcc
- Most combination OCs are given in a cyclic pattern, usually in a 28-day regimen. Extended-cycle OCs are taken for longer than the typical 28-day cycle. Eighty-four days is common, but some preparations are taken continuously.

  > For example, for extended-cycle OC taken for 84 days, the client has withdrawal bleeding four times per year. Some extended-cycle OC are taken continuously, and the client does not have withdrawal bleeding.

- Administer IM or subcutaneous contraception when it can be assumed the client is not pregnant (the sixth postpartum week if exclusively breastfeeding, within the first 5 postpartum days if not exclusively breastfeeding, or within the first 5 days of menstruation). Inform the client the injection is repeated every 3 months.

CLIENT EDUCATION

- Quit smoking.
- Report abdominal pain, chest pain, headache (severe), eye problems, and severe leg pain, swelling or redness in legs, or shortness of breath.
- Take pills at the same time each day.
- Take medication for 21 days followed by 7 days of no medication (or inert pill). For the traditional 28-day cycle OCs, begin the sequence on the first day or first Sunday after the onset of menses.
  - If one or more pills are missed in the first week, take one pill as soon as possible and continue on with the pack. Use an additional form of contraception for 7 days.
  - If one or two pills are missed in the second or third week, take one as soon as possible and continue on with the active pills in the pack but skip the placebos and go straight to the new pack once all of the active pills have been taken.
  - If three or more pills are missed during the second or third week, follow the same instructions for missing two pills. Use an additional form of contraception for 7 days.
- For transdermal patches, apply to the lower abdomen, upper arm or torso, or the buttock. Place a new patch on clean, dry skin weekly for 3 weeks, then omit the patch for the fourth week to allow menstruation.
- For the vaginal ring, insert the ring and leave in place for 3 weeks, removing the fourth week to allow for menstruation. If the ring falls out early, rinse the ring and replace it as soon as possible. If the ring is out more than 3 hr, use backup contraception for the next 7 days to prevent pregnancy.
- Contraceptive implants are inserted under the dermis of the skin in the inner upper arm and must be replaced every 3 years.
- Intrauterine devices (IUDs) are placed within 7 days of menses and can be replaced regardless of the timing of menstruation. IUDs are replaced between 3 and 10 years, depending on the type.

NURSING EVALUATION OF MEDICATION EFFECTIVENESS

Depending on therapeutic intent, effectiveness is confirmed by no evidence of conception.

Emergency oral contraceptive

SELECT PROTOTYPE MEDICATION: Progestin with levonorgestrel

OTHER MEDICATIONS: Levonorgestrel, ulipristal, estrogen/progestin

ROUTE OF ADMINISTRATION: PO (over-the-counter medication, self-administration)

PURPOSE

EXPECTED PHARMACOLOGICAL ACTION: Inhibits ovulation and the transport of sperm if taken within at least 72 hr following unprotected sexual intercourse

THERAPEUTIC USES
- Prevention of fertilization of sperm and ovum
- Cessation/delay of ovulation

COMPLICATIONS

Menorrhagia

A common adverse effect.

NURSING ACTIONS: Monitor bleeding

CLIENT EDUCATION
- Be aware of possible medication effects.
- Discuss these effects with the provider. If effects are undesirable, medication might need to be stopped to prevent permanent changes.

Nausea

Common adverse effect of mediation

NURSING ACTIONS: A provider will recommend an over-the-counter antiemetic to be taken 1 hr prior to each dose to counteract the adverse effects of nausea that can occur with high doses of estrogen and progestin

CONTRAINDICATIONS/PRECAUTIONS

- **Warnings**
  - Pregnancy: Contraindicated
- Method is contraindicated if a client is pregnant or has undiagnosed abnormal vaginal bleeding.

CLIENT EDUCATION
- Be evaluated for pregnancy if menstruation does not begin within 21 days.
- Monitor adverse effects of abdominal pain, headache, nausea, menorrhagia, and dizziness.
- Consider counseling about contraception and modification of sexual behaviors that are risky.
- This method is not taken on a regular basis.
- Anyone, regardless of age, is allowed to purchase emergency oral contraceptive at a pharmacy.
- Directions are easy to understand.
- Does not terminate an established pregnancy.
- Does not protect against STIs.

NURSING EVALUATION OF MEDICATION EFFECTIVENESS

- Depending on therapeutic intent, effectiveness is evidenced by the following:
- Absence of fertilization (absence of pregnancy)

Therapeutic/Medical termination of Pregnancy

SELECT PROTOTYPE MEDICATION: mifepristone also known as (RU 486)

OTHER MEDICATIONS
- Misoprostol
- Methotrexate

ROUTE OF ADMINISTRATION: PO

PURPOSE

EXPECTED PHARMACOLOGICAL ACTION: Binds to progesterone receptors and prevents the action of progesterone (maintaining pregnancy)

THERAPEUTIC USES
- Prevention of pregnancy (if taken within 5 days of unprotected intercourse) – not current FDA approved as an emergency contraceptive
- Medical induction of termination of pregnancy (can be given up to 70 days after last menstrual period)

COMPLICATIONS

Incomplete termination of pregnancy

CLIENT EDUCATION: May require surgical intervention.

Prolonged excessive bleeding

CLIENT EDUCATION: Notify provider if saturating pads every hour.

CONTRAINDICATIONS/PRECAUTIONS

- Ectopic pregnancy
- IUD
- Hemorrhagic conditions (anticoagulant use)
- Long-term corticosteroid use

NURSING ACTIONS: Be aware of state laws regarding elective and therapeutic termination of pregnancy, in some states these are not allowed or restricted.

CLIENT EDUCATION
- Follow up with provider within 2 weeks following administration (exam, ultrasound).
- May require surgical intervention if medication was not effective.
- Monitor adverse effects of abdominal cramping, bleeding, headache, fever, chills, and dizziness.
- Consider counseling about contraception and modification of sexual behaviors that are risky.

NURSING EVALUATION OF MEDICATION EFFECTIVENESS

Depending on therapeutic intent, effectiveness is evidenced by the following:
- Absence of fertilization
- Absence of current pregnancy

Androgens

SELECT PROTOTYPE MEDICATION: Testosterone

OTHER MEDICATIONS: Methyltestosterone

ROUTE OF ADMINISTRATION: PO, IM, Sub-cut (implantable pellets), transdermal, topical, intranasal, buccal

PURPOSE

EXPECTED PHARMACOLOGICAL ACTION: The hormone-receptor complex acts on cellular DNA to promote specific mRNA molecules and production of proteins, resulting in the following:
- Development of sex traits in males and the production and maturation of sperm
- Increase in skeletal muscle
- Increase in synthesis of erythropoietin

THERAPEUTIC USES
- Hypogonadism in males
- Delayed puberty in males
- Androgen replacement in testicular failure or menopause
- Anemia not responsive to traditional therapy
- Postmenopausal breast cancer
- Muscle wasting in male clients who have AIDS
- Unlabeled use: Gender affirming therapy

COMPLICATIONS

Androgenic (virilization) effects

- For clients who are assigned female at birth, these medications can cause irregularity or cessation of menses, hirsutism, weight gain, acne, lowering of voice, growth of clitoris, vaginitis, and baldness.
- For clients who are assigned male at birth, these medications can cause acne, priapism, increased facial and body hair, and penile enlargement.

CLIENT EDUCATION
- Be aware of possible medication effects.
- Discuss these effects with the provider. If effects are undesirable medication might need to be stopped to prevent permanent changes.

Epiphyseal closure

Premature closure of epiphysis in boys can reduce mature height.

NURSING ACTIONS: Monitor epiphysis with serial X-rays.

Cholestatic hepatitis, jaundice

NURSING ACTIONS
- Monitor for indications of jaundice (yellowing of the skin and sclera of the eyes).
- Monitor liver enzymes.

Hypercholesterolemia

These medications can decrease high-density lipoproteins (HDL) and increase LDL.

CLIENT EDUCATION
- Monitor cholesterol levels.
- Adjust diet to reduce cholesterol levels.

Increase in growth of prostate cancer

NURSING ACTIONS
- Do not give to clients who have prostate cancer.
- Monitor for prostate cancer.

Polycythemia

NURSING ACTIONS: Monitor hemoglobin and hematocrit.

Edema from salt and water retention

NURSING ACTIONS: Medication can be discontinued.

CLIENT EDUCATION: Monitor for weight gain and swelling of extremities, and report these to the provider.

Potential for misuse

NURSING ACTIONS: Recognize that androgens are controlled medications. Identify high-risk groups and provide information about potential misuse and health risks.

Hypercalcemia

NURSING ACTIONS: Monitor electrolytes and for manifestations of hypercalcemia, (lethargy, nausea, vomiting, and constipation).

Hypoglycemia in clients who have diabetes mellitus

NURSING ACTIONS: Monitor glucose and adjust antidiabetic medications.

CONTRAINDICATIONS/PRECAUTIONS

- **Warnings**
  - Pregnancy: Androgens contraindicated.
  - Lactation: Androgens contraindicated.
  - Reproductive: Notify provider if pregnancy is planned or suspected.
- Contraindicated in older adult clients and males who have prostate or breast cancer, severe cardiac, renal, or liver disease. Ⓒ
- Use cautiously in clients who have heart failure, hypercalcemia, or hypertension.

INTERACTIONS

Androgens can alter effects of oral anticoagulants.
NURSING ACTIONS: Monitor PT and INR.

Androgens can alter effects of insulins and antidiabetic agents.
NURSING ACTIONS: Monitor glucose level and adjust dosages.

Concurrent use of androgens and hepatotoxic medications can increase risk for hepatotoxicity.
NURSING ACTIONS: Monitor liver enzymes. Assess for jaundice.

NURSING ADMINISTRATION

- Instruct clients using gel formulations to wash their hands after every application due to the possibility of skin-to-skin transfer to others. Cover application with clothing after gel has dried and wash off before skin to skin contact with another person.
- Inject IM formulations into a large muscle and rotate injection sites. Ⓠpcc
- Obtain daily weights.

CLIENT EDUCATION
- Use a barrier method of birth control.
- Reduce cholesterol in the diet.

NURSING EVALUATION OF MEDICATION EFFECTIVENESS

Depending on therapeutic intent, effectiveness is evidenced by the following:
- Puberty is induced in males.
- Increased blood testosterone levels.
- There is a decrease in the progression of breast cancer in females. Medication produces expected results with minimal adverse effects.

5-Alpha reductase inhibitors

SELECT PROTOTYPE MEDICATIONS: Finasteride

OTHER MEDICATIONS: Dutasteride

ROUTE OF ADMINISTRATION: Oral

PURPOSE

EXPECTED PHARMACOLOGICAL ACTION: Decreases usable testosterone by inhibiting the converting enzyme, causing a reduction of the prostate size and increased hair growth

THERAPEUTIC USES
- Benign prostatic hyperplasia (BPH)
- Alopecia (androgenetic)

COMPLICATIONS

Decreased libido, ejaculate volume

CLIENT EDUCATION: Notify the provider if adverse effects occur.

Gynecomastia

CLIENT EDUCATION: Notify the provider if adverse effects occur.

CONTRAINDICATIONS/PRECAUTIONS

- **Warnings**
  - Pregnancy: Finasteride contraindicated in females.
  - Lactation: Finasteride contraindicated in females.
  - Reproductive
    - Notify provider of changes in breast tissue.
    - Can cause erectile dysfunction, decreased libido, decreased ejaculate.
    - Females should avoid exposure to semen.
- Contraindicated in clients who have medication hypersensitivity.
- Use with caution in clients who have liver disease.

INTERACTIONS

None significant

NURSING ADMINISTRATION

Pregnant clients should not handle crushed or broken medication. Qs

CLIENT EDUCATION
- Therapeutic effects can take 6 months or longer.
- Do not donate blood unless medication has been discontinued for at least 1 month.

NURSING EVALUATION OF MEDICATION EFFECTIVENESS

Depending on therapeutic intent, effectiveness is evidenced by the following:.
- Prostate size is decreased, and the client can urinate effectively.
- Prostate-specific antigen (PSA) levels have decreased from baseline.
- Client has increased hair growth.

Alpha₁ adrenergic antagonists

SELECT PROTOTYPE MEDICATION
Selective alpha₁ receptor antagonist: Tamsulosin

OTHER MEDICATIONS
- Selective alpha₁ receptor antagonist: Silodosin
- Nonselective alpha₁ receptor antagonists
- Alfuzosin
- Terazosin
- Doxazosin

ROUTE OF ADMINISTRATION: Oral

PURPOSE

EXPECTED PHARMACOLOGICAL ACTION
- Decrease mechanical obstruction of the urethra by relaxing smooth muscles of the bladder neck and prostate.
- Nonselective agents also cause vasodilation and can lower blood pressure. These agents are used for clients who have BPH and hypertension.

THERAPEUTIC USES
- BPH, thus increasing urinary flow
- Off-label use for females for treatment of urinary hesitancy or urinary retention

COMPLICATIONS

Hypotension, dizziness, nasal congestion, sleepiness, faintness

More likely with nonselective antagonists

NURSING ACTIONS: Monitor blood pressure.

CLIENT EDUCATION
- Rise slowly from sitting or lying position.
- Do not drive or operate machinery when starting therapy or with change in dose until response is known.

Problems with ejaculation

Failure, decreased volume with silodosin and tamsulosin

CLIENT EDUCATION: Be aware of possible adverse effects.

Floppy iris syndrome following cataract surgery

NURSING ACTIONS: Hold the medication before cataract surgery.

CONTRAINDICATIONS/PRECAUTIONS

- **Warnings**
  - Pregnancy
    - Terazosin and doxazosin safety not established.
    - Tamsulosin only used for treatment of BPH.
  - Lactation: Terazosin and doxazosin safety not established.
  - Reproductive: Clients of childbearing age should not handle these medications.
- Contraindicated in clients who have medication sensitivity. Qs
- Alfuzosin is contraindicated in females and in clients who have severe liver failure.
- Silodosin is contraindicated in clients who have renal failure or liver failure.
- Doxazosin should be used cautiously in clients who have liver impairment.
- Tamsulosin should be used cautiously in clients who have hepatic or renal impairment.

INTERACTIONS

Cimetidine can decrease clearance of tamsulosin.
NURSING ACTIONS: Use concurrently with caution.

Antihypertensives, PDE5 inhibitors, or nitroglycerin used concurrently with nonselective agents can cause severe hypotension.
NURSING ACTIONS
- Use with caution.
- Monitor blood pressure.

Erythromycin or HIV protease inhibitors (ritonavir) will increase levels of alfuzosin and silodosin when used concurrently.
NURSING ACTIONS: Avoid concurrent use.

NURSING ADMINISTRATION

Monitor blood pressure, especially at the start of therapy and with changes of dose. Qpcc

CLIENT EDUCATION: Take medication daily as prescribed:
- Tamsulosin: 30 min after a meal at the same time each day
- Silodosin: With the same meal each day
- Alfuzosin: Right after the same meal each day
- Terazosin: At bedtime
- Doxazosin: At the same time each day

NURSING EVALUATION OF MEDICATION EFFECTIVENESS

Depending on therapeutic intent, effectiveness is evidenced by improved urinary flow with minimal adverse effects.

Phosphodiesterase type 5 inhibitors (PDE5 inhibitors)

SELECT PROTOTYPE MEDICATIONS: Sildenafil

OTHER MEDICATIONS
- Tadalafil
- Vardenafil
- Avanafil

PURPOSE

EXPECTED PHARMACOLOGICAL ACTION: Augments the effects of nitric oxide released during sexual stimulation, resulting in enhanced blood flow to the corpus cavernosum and penile erection

THERAPEUTIC USES
- Erectile dysfunction
- BPH: Decrease severity of urinary symptoms (frequency, urgency, straining)

COMPLICATIONS

MI, sudden death

NURSING ACTIONS: Monitor risk factors and history regarding cardiovascular health.

Priapism

CLIENT EDUCATION: If erection lasts more than 4 hr (seek immediate medical attention because may lead to irreversible damage)

Sudden hearing loss

CLIENT EDUCATION: Discontinue medication if hearing is affected.

CONTRAINDICATIONS/PRECAUTIONS

- **Warnings**
  - Pregnancy: Sildenafil contraindicated.
  - Lactation: Use sildenafil with caution.
  - Reproductive: Does not protect against STIs.
- Contraindicated in clients taking any medications in the nitrate family (nitroglycerin).
- Use cautiously in clients who have cardiovascular disease, including QT prolongation. Qs

INTERACTIONS

Organic nitrates, such as nitroglycerin and isosorbide dinitrate, can lead to fatal hypotension.
NURSING ACTIONS: Do not use with organic nitrates or alpha blockers.

Ketoconazole, erythromycin, cimetidine, ritonavir, and grapefruit juice inhibit metabolism of sildenafil, thereby increasing plasma levels of medication.
NURSING ACTIONS: Use these medications cautiously in clients taking PDE5 inhibitors.

NURSING ADMINISTRATION

- If using sildenafil to treat pulmonary artery hypertension, administer three times daily at least 4 hr apart. Clients should take a missed dose as soon as remembered, unless it is almost time for the next dose.
- Instruct clients taking these medications for erectile dysfunction not to exceed one dose in 24 hr. Qpcc

CLIENT EDUCATION

- Take sildenafil at least 1 hr before sexual activity, depending on dosage. May use only once per day.
- Tadalafil is approved to be taken daily or prior to sexual activity.
- Take vardenafil 1 hr prior to sexual activity. It can last for up to 36 hr.
- Avanafil is effective 15 minutes after administration and lasts about 2 hr.

NURSING EVALUATION OF MEDICATION EFFECTIVENESS

Depending on therapeutic intent, effectiveness is evidenced by erection sufficient for sexual intercourse.

Active Learning Scenario

A nurse in a provider's office is instructing a client who has a new prescription for finasteride to treat benign prostatic hyperplasia. Use the ATI Active Learning Template: Medication to complete this item.

EXPECTED PHARMACOLOGICAL ACTION

COMPLICATIONS: Identify two adverse effects.

Application Exercises

1. A nurse is reviewing the health care record of a client who is asking about conjugated equine estrogens. The nurse should inform the client this medication is contraindicated in which of the following conditions?

   A. Atrophic vaginitis

   B. Dysfunctional uterine bleeding

   C. Osteoporosis

   D. Thrombophlebitis

2. A nurse is teaching about the mechanism of action of combination oral contraceptives with a group of clients. The nurse should tell the clients that which of the following actions occur with the use of combination oral contraceptives? (Select all that apply.)

   A. Thickening the cervical mucus

   B. Inducing maturation of ovarian follicle

   C. Increasing development of the corpus luteum

   D. Altering the endometrial lining

   E. Inhibiting ovulation

3. A nurse is providing teaching to a female client who is taking testosterone to treat advanced breast cancer. The nurse should tell the client that which of the following are adverse effects of this medication? (Select all that apply.)

   A. Deepening voice

   B. Weight gain

   C. Low blood pressure

   D. Dry mouth

   E. Facial hair

4. A nurse is reinforcing teaching to a client who will start alfuzosin for treatment of benign prostatic hyperplasia. The nurse should instruct the client that which of the following is an adverse effect of this medication?

   A. Bradycardia

   B. Edema

   C. Hypotension

   D. Tremor

5. A nurse is caring for a client who has angina and asks about obtaining a prescription for sildenafil to treat erectile dysfunction. Which of the following medications should the nurse recognize as contraindicated with sildenafil?

Application Exercises Key

1. A. Atrophic vaginitis occurs when there is estrogen deficiency. This medication is used to treated atrophic vaginitis.
   B. Dysfunctional uterine bleeding can occur when there is estrogen deficiency. This medication is used to treat dysfunctional uterine bleeding.
   C. Females are at risk for osteoporosis after the onset of menopause. Estrogen is used to slow the progression of osteoporosis.
   D. **CORRECT:** Estrogen increases the risk of thrombolytic events. Estrogen use is contraindicated for a client who has a history of thrombophlebitis.

   Ⓝ *NCLEX® Connection: Pharmacological and Parenteral Therapies, Adverse Effects/Contraindications/Adverse Effects/Interactions*

2. A. **CORRECT:** Oral contraceptives cause thickening of the cervical mucus, which slows sperm passage.
   D. **CORRECT:** Oral contraceptives alter the lining of the endometrium, which inhibits implantation of the fertilized egg and they prevent pregnancy by inhibiting ovulation.
   E. **CORRECT:** Inducing maturation of ovarian follicles and increasing the development of the corpus luteum are not actions of oral contraceptives.

   Ⓝ *NCLEX® Connection: Pharmacological and Parenteral Therapies, Medication Administration*

3. A, B, E. **CORRECT:** When reviewing adverse effects of testosterone, the nurse should include adverse effects such as virilization, the development of adult male characteristics because they can be an adverse effect of testosterone which includes deepening of the voice, edema, weight gain, high blood pressure, nasal congestion, and the development of facial hair.

   Ⓝ *NCLEX® Connection: Pharmacological and Parenteral Therapies, Adverse Effects/Contraindications/Adverse Effects/Interactions*

4. A. Alfuzosin can cause tachycardia.
   B. Edema and tremors are not adverse effects of this medication.
   C. **CORRECT:** Alfuzosin relaxes muscle tone in veins and cardiac output decreases, which leads to hypotension. Clients taking this medication are advised to rise slowly from a sitting or lying position.
   D. Alfuzosin can cause dizziness. Tremors are not an adverse effect of this medication.

   Ⓝ *NCLEX® Connection: Pharmacological and Parenteral Therapies, Adverse Effects/Contraindications/Adverse Effects/Interactions*

5. Isosorbide is an organic nitrate that manages pain from angina. Concurrent use of it is contraindicated because fatal hypotension can occur. The client should avoid taking a nitrate medication for 24 hr after taking isosorbide.

   Ⓝ *NCLEX® Connection: Pharmacological and Parenteral Therapies, Adverse Effects/Contraindications/Adverse Effects/Interactions*

Active Learning Scenario Key

Using the ATI Active Learning Template: Medication

EXPECTED PHARMACOLOGICAL ACTION: Finasteride slows the production of testosterone, which reduces the size of the prostate and subsequently promotes urinary elimination.

COMPLICATIONS
- Decreased libido
- Decreased ejaculate volume
- Gynecomastia
- Orthostatic hypotension

Ⓝ *NCLEX® Connection: Pharmacological and Parenteral Therapies, Medication Administration*

UNIT 7   MEDICATIONS AFFECTING THE
REPRODUCTIVE SYSTEM

CHAPTER 30 *Medications Affecting Labor and Delivery*

Understanding medications affecting labor and delivery is imperative to promote positive maternal and fetal outcomes. These include medications used to induce or augment labor, and medication used in the management of preterm labor and provide comfort.

Uterine stimulants: Oxytocics

SELECT PROTOTYPE MEDICATION: Oxytocin

OTHER MEDICATIONS
- Dinoprostone
- Methylergonovine maleate
- Misoprostol
- Carboprost tromethamine
- Tranexamic acid

PURPOSE

EXPECTED PHARMACOLOGICAL ACTION: Uterine stimulants increase the strength, frequency, and length of uterine contractions.

THERAPEUTIC USES

Oxytocin
- Induction of labor (postterm pregnancy, premature rupture of membranes, preeclampsia)
- Enhancement of labor (dysfunctional labor)
- Delivery of placenta (postpartum, miscarriage)
- Management of postpartum hemorrhage
- Stress testing

Dinoprostone is a prostaglandin used to promote cervical ripening and to stimulate uterine contractions.

Misoprostol is an alternative to dinoprostone. It has an off-label use for cervical ripening which can result in uterine simulation.

Methylergonovine maleate contracts the uterus and is used for emergency intervention for serious postpartum hemorrhage.

Carboprost tromethamine is a prostaglandin F_2-alpha that is used to manage postpartum hemorrhage by causing strong uterine contractions.

Tranexamic acid is an antifibrinolytic used to improve blood clotting as an emergency intervention for serious postpartum hemorrhage.

COMPLICATIONS

OXYTOCIN

Uterine rupture, uterine tachysystole, placental abruption, water intoxication

NURSING ACTIONS
- Pre-assess risk factors (multiple deliveries).
- Monitor the length, strength, and duration of contractions.
- Assess fetal status.
- Monitor vital signs.
- Monitor I&O.
- Monitor for water intoxication with large doses (rare at dosages used for labor induction). Findings include hyponatremia, hypochloremia, listlessness, confusion, headache.
- For uterine tachysystole, follow institution protocol for interventions depending on FHR stability.

DINOPROSTONE

Uterine tachysystole, gastrointestinal reactions, cervical or uterine lacerations

NURSING ACTIONS
- Monitor the length, strength, and duration of contractions.
- Assess fetal status.
- Monitor vital signs.
- Monitor for gastrointestinal reactions (vomiting and diarrhea), cervical or uterine lacerations, fever.

MISOPROSTOL

Uterine tachysystole, non-reassuring fetal heart rate

NURSING ACTIONS
- Monitor the length, strength, and duration of contractions.
- Assess fetal status.
- Monitor vital signs.

METHYLERGONOVINE MALEATE

Hypertensive crisis

NURSING ACTIONS
- Monitor vital signs.
- Monitor for manifestations of hypertensive crisis (headache, nausea, vomiting, increased blood pressure).
- Monitor for uterine tone and vaginal bleeding.
- Provide emergency interventions.

CARBOPROST TROMETHAMINE

GI effects (nausea, vomiting, diarrhea)

NURSING ACTIONS
- Monitor and educate client about common adverse effects.
- May need to administer an antiemetic or antidiarrheal medication

TRANEXAMIC ACID

Venous/arterial thrombosis

NURSING ACTIONS
- Monitor arterial thrombosis (retina) by assessing the client for changes with vision.
- Monitor for vaginal bleeding.

CONTRAINDICATIONS/PRECAUTIONS

OXYTOCIN

Maternal factors: Sepsis, an unripe cervix, active genital herpes, history of multiple births, scheduled cesarean section, history of uterine surgery Qs

Fetal factors: Immature lungs, cephalopelvic disproportion, fetal malpresentation, prolapsed umbilical cord, fetal distress, placental abnormalities, threatened spontaneous abortion

DINOPROSTONE

Prior history of cesarean birth or uterine surgery, fetal distress, vaginal bleeding

NURSING ACTIONS
- Avoid use with maternal history of multiparity, hypotension, hypertension, diabetes mellitus, and asthma.
- Use with caution for clients who have active heart, lung, or kidney/liver disease.

MISOPROSTOL

Cesarean birth, previous uterine surgery

NURSING ACTIONS: Use with caution in clients who have kidney failure.

METHYLERGONOVINE MALEATE

Hypertension, preeclampsia, asthma and cardiac disease

NURSING ACTIONS
- Use with caution with maternal history of severe kidney or hepatic disease, and sepsis.
- Use only after delivery, and not during labor.
- Contraindicated for clients who are breastfeeding (may resume breastfeeding 12 following last dose)

CARBOPROST TROMETHAMINE

History of hypertension or respiratory problems

NURSING ACTIONS
- Can cause constriction of bronchi (Monitor for respiratory problems.)
- Monitor vital signs.

TRANEXAMIC ACID

History of thrombosis

NURSING ACTIONS
- Monitor for thrombosis.
- Contraindicated for client who take oral contraceptives

INTERACTIONS

OXYTOCIN

Severe hypertension can occur if oxytocin follows the administration of vasopressors.

NURSING ACTIONS: Monitor vital signs, uterine activity, and fetal status.

DINOPROSTONE

Other oxytocics increase effects.

NURSING ACTIONS
- Avoid concurrent use.
- Monitor vital signs, uterine activity, and fetal status.

MISOPROSTOL

Increased risk for diarrhea when administered concurrently with aluminum- or magnesium-containing antacids.

NURSING ACTIONS: Avoid concurrent use.

METHYLERGONOVINE

Vasopressors and consumption of grapefruit juice (ergots increase effects), tobacco use (smoking can cause vasoconstriction)

NURSING ACTIONS
- Avoid concurrent use.
- Monitor vital signs.

NURSING ADMINISTRATION

OXYTOCIN

- Use an infusion pump to administer IV oxytocin. Gradually increase the flow rate per prescribed low-dose or high-dose parameters. The starting rates will vary from 0.5 to 6 milliunits/min every 15 to 40 min. ⓠEBP
  - Monitor blood pressure, respiratory rate, and pulse every 30 to 60 min and with every dosage change.
  - Carefully monitor uterine contractions (frequency and duration) every 15 min and with every dosage change during the first stage of labor and every 5 min the second stage of labor. Generally, the goal is contractions that last 45 to 60 seconds or less every 2 to 3 min.
- Monitor for uterine tachysystole (more than five contractions in 10 min, contractions occurring within 1 min of each other, or a series of single contractions lasting greater than 1 min).
- Continuously monitor the fetal heart rate and rhythm. Report findings of fetal distress.

DINOPROSTONE OR MISOPROSTOL

- Place the client in a supine position with a lateral tilt.
- Have the client remain in position 30 to 40 min after administering misoprostol.
- Allow dinoprostone gel to warm to room temperature before insertion (do not use external warming.)
- Have the client remain in position for 2 hr following administration of a dinoprostone vaginal insert.

METHYLERGONOVINE MALEATE

- Administer IM after passage of placenta (IV administration is reserved for emergencies).
- Can be administered orally every 6 to 8 hr for one week to promote uterine involution
- Monitor uterine activity and response.

CARBOPROST TROMETHAMINE

- Administer IM.
- Can repeat every 15 to 90 minutes for a max dose of 2 mg (about 8 doses)
- Monitor and educate client about common GI adverse effects (nausea, vomiting, diarrhea).
- May administer antiemetic or antidiarrheal to manage adverse effects
- Monitor for medication induced fever or other underlying cause.

TRANEXAMIC ACID

- Recommended to administer to clients who experience postpartum hemorrhage within 3 hr of birth
- Educate client about common adverse effects: headache, back pain, fatigue, nasal/sinus problems.

NURSING EVALUATION OF MEDICATION EFFECTIVENESS

Depending on therapeutic intent, effectiveness can be evidenced by the following.

- Effective contractions (lasting less than 45 to 60 seconds and occurring every 2 to 3 min)
- Increase in uterine tone and no evidence of postpartum hemorrhage

Tocolytic medications

SELECT PROTOTYPE MEDICATION

- Terbutaline
- Hydroxyprogesterone caproate

OTHER MEDICATIONS

- Nifedipine
- Magnesium sulfate
- Indomethacin

PURPOSE

THERAPEUTIC USES

Terbutaline (beta$_2$-adrenergic agonist) that selectively activates beta$_2$-adrenergic receptors, resulting in uterine smooth muscle relaxation. Subcutaneous terbutaline can be used for up to 48 hr to delay but not to prevent preterm labor.

Hydroxyprogesterone caproate is a progestin hormone and the only FDA-approved medication to decrease the risk of recurrent preterm labor. Its mechanism of action is unknown. It is only for use in pregnancy with a single fetus and history of at least one preterm birth.

Nifedipine is a calcium channel blocker that is used to temporarily suppress preterm labor for at least 48 hours.

Magnesium sulfate is a central nervous system depressant and relaxes smooth muscles. Its primary use is to prevent seizures in clients who have preeclampsia. It has significant adverse maternal effects and increases fetal mortality. Although magnesium sulfate is not recommended for management of preterm labor, it can be prescribed to decrease the risk of cerebral palsy.

Indomethacin is a cyclooxygenase inhibitor that is used to suppress labor by inhibiting the synthesis of prostaglandins. Reserved for use for clients who are having early preterm labor

COMPLICATIONS

TERBUTALINE

Multiple effects

Maternal
- Tachycardia, palpitations, chest pain, hypotension, hypokalemia, hyperglycemia, pulmonary edema
- Intolerable: Blood pressure less than 90/60 mm Hg, heart rate greater than 120/min, chest pain, pulmonary edema, cardiac arrhythmias

Fetal: Tachycardia

NURSING ACTIONS
- Monitor vital signs, blood glucose, and potassium levels.
- Notify the provider for intolerable adverse effects.
- Monitor fetal heart rate and frequency of contractions.

HYDROXYPROGESTERONE CAPROATE

Injection-site reactions, glucose intolerance, fluid retention, depression: Can promote glucose intolerance, clinical depression, and fluid retention

NURSING ACTIONS
- Monitor for common adverse effects at the injection site: pain, swelling, itching, and appearance of hives.
- Monitor clients who have diabetes, mellitus, history of depression, conditions which could cause fluid retention (i.e., preeclampsia, cardiac or kidney dysfunction) with caution.

NIFEDIPINE

Hypotension, headache, dizziness, nausea, maternal tachycardia

NURSING ACTIONS
- Monitor for manifestations of adverse effects.
- Monitor intake and output.

MAGNESIUM SULFATE

Maternal
- Hypocalcemia, hot flashes, dyspnea, transient hypotension
- Intolerable: Respirations less than 12/min, pulmonary edema, altered level of consciousness, severe hypotension, urine output less than 25 mL/hr, blood magnesium level 10mEq/L or greater

Fetal: Nonreactive NST, reduced fetal heart rate (FHR) variability

NURSING ACTIONS
- Monitor deep tendon reflexes.
- Obtain vital signs.
- Monitor blood magnesium level.
- Limit IV fluids to 125 mL/hr.
- Have calcium gluconate available.
- Discontinue infusion with any intolerable adverse effects.

INDOMETHACIN

Partial closure of ductus arteriosus (high doses), interstitial nephritis, gastric irritation

NURSING ACTIONS: Monitor for manifestations of adverse effects (nausea).

CONTRAINDICATIONS/PRECAUTIONS

TERBUTALINE

Hypersensitivity

NURSING ACTIONS: Use caution with heart disease, chronic/active hepatic disease, kidney disease.

HYDROXYPROGESTERONE CAPROATE

Uncontrolled hypertension, liver disease, history of thrombosis, breast cancer

NIFEDIPINE

Hypersensitivity, AV heart blocks

NURSING ACTIONS: Use caution with hypotension (systolic BP less than 90 mm Hg), hepatic or kidney disease, unstable angina, or acute MI. Avoid concurrent use with magnesium sulfate or terbutaline.

MAGNESIUM SULFATE

Hypersensitivity, abdominal pain, heart block

NURSING ACTIONS: Avoid concurrent use with nifedipine.

INDOMETHACIN

Hypersensitivity, active GI bleeding, ulcer disease, hypertension

NURSING ACTIONS: Use with caution for clients who have a history of kidney or liver conditions.

INTERACTIONS

TERBUTALINE

Increase effect: MAOIs, green tea, caffeine (tea, soda-cola)

Decrease effect: Beta blockers

NURSING ACTIONS
- Monitor for hypertensive crisis.
- Avoid using with beta blockers.

NIFEDIPINE

Increase effect: Level of digoxin, ketoconazole, erythromycin, beta blockers, antihypertensives, ginkgo biloba, ginseng, grapefruit juice

Decrease effect: phenytoin phenobarbital carbamazepine

Increase toxicity: Cimetidine, St. John's wort, melatonin

NURSING ACTIONS
- Avoid using with grapefruit juice, ginkgo biloba, ginseng, melatonin, and St. John's wort.
- Risk of skeletal muscle blockade when used with magnesium sulfate
- Avoid concurrent use.

MAGNESIUM SULFATE

Increase effect: Calcium channel blockers, neuromuscular blockers

Decrease effect: Digoxin

NURSING ACTIONS
- Monitor blood pressure.
- Monitor for toxicity (thirst, confusion, decreased or absent reflexes).

INDOMETHACIN

Increase effect: NSAIDs (increase GI effects), insulin and antihyperglycemic agents (can cause hypoglycemia)

Decrease effect: aspirin, diuretics, antihypertensives

NURSING ADMINISTRATION

Monitor FHR, uterine contractions, pulse, blood pressure, respirations, lung sounds, and daily weights.

TERBUTALINE

- Administer subcutaneously. Monitor injection site for infection.
- Assess maternal heart rate before and after administering terbutaline.
  - Withhold terbutaline and contact the provider for reports of chest pain, maternal heart rate greater than 120/min, or presence of cardiac arrhythmias.
- Limit client fluid intake to 2,500 to 3,000 mL/day.
- Notify the provider if contractions persist or increase in frequency or duration.

MAGNESIUM SULFATE

- Monitor for magnesium sulfate toxicity and discontinue for any of the following adverse effects: loss of deep tendon reflexes, urinary output less than 25 to 30 mL/hr or 100 mL/4 hr, respirations less than 12/min, pulmonary edema, severe hypotension, or chest pain. Calcium gluconate should be available to administer IV as an antidote for magnesium sulfate toxicity.
- Administer magnesium sulfate IV when possible as a loading dose followed by a maintenance infusion for up to 48 hr (not to exceed 125 mL/hr total). Monitor magnesium levels during therapy.

HYDROXYPROGESTERONE CAPROATE

Administer IM. Monitor for fluid retention during therapy.

NIFEDIPINE

Administer PO every 3 to 6 hr until contractions to decrease frequency of contraction, then long-acting nifedipine every 6 to 8 hr.

INDOMETHACIN

- Administer indomethacin PO or rectally. Client may take with food to decrease GI effects.
- Monitor blood glucose of clients who have diabetes mellitus and gestational diabetes.

NURSING EVALUATION OF MEDICATION EFFECTIVENESS

Depending on therapeutic intent, effectiveness can be evidenced by cessation of preterm labor (20 to 36 weeks).

Glucocorticoid medications

SELECT PROTOTYPE MEDICATIONS
- Betamethasone
- Dexamethasone

PURPOSE

EXPECTED PHARMACOLOGICAL ACTION: Releases enzymes that produce and release lung surfactant to stimulate lung maturity in a fetus

THERAPEUTIC USES: Reduce neonatal respiratory distress syndrome, intraventricular hemorrhage, necrotizing enterocolitis, and death
- The therapeutic action is to enhance fetal lung maturity and surfactant production in fetuses between 24- and 34-weeks of gestation.
- Betamethasone is a glucocorticoid that requires 24 hours to be effective.

COMPLICATIONS

Fetal decreased breathing and body movements

Transient

NURSING ACTIONS: Maintain continuous fetal monitoring.

NURSING ADMINISTRATION

- Administer deep IM to clients who are between 24 to 34 weeks of gestation, at least 24 hr before delivery but no more than 7 days before.
  - Administer betamethasone IM in two injections at least 24 hr apart.
  - Administer dexamethasone IM for four doses 12 hr apart.
- Administer deep IM using the ventral gluteal or vastus lateralis muscle.
- Monitor for maternal hyperglycemia.
- Monitor lung sounds of newborn.

NURSING EVALUATION OF MEDICATION EFFECTIVENESS

Depending on therapeutic intent, effectiveness can be evidenced by fetal lung maturity at birth.

Opioid analgesics

SELECT PROTOTYPE MEDICATION: Fentanyl

OTHER MEDICATIONS
- Butorphanol
- Nalbuphine

PURPOSE

EXPECTED PHARMACOLOGICAL ACTION
- These medications adhere to opioid receptors in the central nervous system to decrease the perception of pain without the loss of consciousness.
- Fentanyl is an opioid agonist.
- Butorphanol and nalbuphine are opioid agonist–antagonist analgesics.

THERAPEUTIC USES: Provide partial, temporary pain relief, particularly during early, active labor.

COMPLICATIONS

Respiratory depression

Risk increases with increased dosage of fentanyl but not with nalbuphine and butorphanol increases.

Dry mouth

NURSING ACTIONS: Provide ice chips.

Nausea and vomiting

More likely with fentanyl

NURSING ACTIONS: Administer antiemetic as prescribed.

Neonatal depression

NURSING ACTIONS: Have naloxone available at birth.

Tachycardia, hypotension, decreased FHR variability

NURSING ACTIONS: Monitor vital signs and FHR per facility protocol.

Sedation

NURSING ACTIONS: Provide safety.

CONTRAINDICATIONS/PRECAUTIONS

- Avoid nalbuphine and butorphanol for clients who have a history of opioid dependence to prevent abstinence syndrome in the mother and newborn.
- Delivery within 1 to 4 hr of administration

NURSING ADMINISTRATION

- Prior to administering analgesic or anesthetic pain relief, verify that labor is well established by performing a vaginal exam showing cervical dilation to be at least 4 cm with the fetus engaged. Q EBP
- Naloxone is administered to reverse the effects of opioids for the client (respiratory depression, pruritus) or for severe respiratory depression in the newborn. Qs
- Administer antiemetics as prescribed.
- Monitor vital signs and uterine contraction pattern. Provide continuous FHR monitoring.
- The client can be given opioid analgesics IM or IV, but the IV route is recommended during labor because of its quicker action.
- If the opioid is given too soon, it can delay the progression of labor. If given too late (within 1 to 4 hr of birth), it can depress neonatal respirations.

CLIENT EDUCATION
- The medication will cause drowsiness.
- Request assistance with ambulation.

NURSING EVALUATION OF MEDICATION EFFECTIVENESS

Depending on therapeutic intent, effectiveness can be evidenced by decreased pain during labor.

Application Exercises

1. A nurse is caring for a client who has a new prescription for oxytocin to stimulate uterine contractions. Which of the following actions should the nurse take? (Select all that apply.)

   A. Use an infusion pump for medication administration.

   B. Obtain vital signs frequently and with every dosage change.

   C. Stop infusion if uterine contractions occur every 4 min and last 45 seconds.

   D. Increase medication infusion rate rapidly.

   E. Monitor fetal heart rate continuously.

2. A nurse is caring for a client who is in labor and is receiving oxytocin. The nurse should monitor the client for what 4 complications of oxytocin?

3. A nurse is teaching a client about terbutaline. Which of the following statements by the client indicates understanding of the teaching?

   A. "This medication will stop my contractions."

   B. "This medication will prevent vaginal bleeding."

   C. "This medication will promote blood flow to my baby."

   D. "This medication will increase my prostaglandin production."

4. A nurse is caring for a client who has preeclampsia and is receiving magnesium sulfate IV continuous infusion. Which of the following findings should the nurse report to the provider?

   A. 2+ deep tendon reflexes

   B. 2+ pedal edema

   C. 24 mL/hr urinary output

   D. Respirations 12/min

5. A nurse is reviewing a new prescription for terbutaline with a client who has a history of preterm labor. Which of the following client statements indicates understanding of the teaching?

   A. "I can increase my activity now that I've started on this medication."

   B. "I will increase my daily fluid intake to 3 quarts."

   C. "I will report increasing intensity of contractions to my doctor."

   D. "I am glad this will prevent preterm labor."

Active Learning Scenario

A nurse is reviewing a new prescription for methylergonovine for a client who is postpartum. What information should the nurse include in this review? Use the ATI Active Learning Template: Medication to complete this item.

THERAPEUTIC USES

COMPLICATIONS: Describe one adverse effect.

CONTRAINDICATIONS/PRECAUTIONS: Describe one contraindication.

NURSING INTERVENTIONS: Describe at least three.

Active Learning Scenario Key

Using the ATI Active Learning Template: Medication

THERAPEUTIC USES: Prevents postpartum hemorrhage

COMPLICATIONS: Hypertensive crisis

CONTRAINDICATIONS/PRECAUTIONS: Hypertension, preeclampsia, cardiac disease: Use with caution with maternal history of severe renal or hepatic disease, and sepsis.

NURSING INTERVENTIONS
- Monitor vital signs for increase in blood pressure.
- Monitor for manifestations of hypertensive crisis (headache, nausea, vomiting, and increased blood pressure).
- Monitor for uterine tone and vaginal bleeding.
- Provide emergency interventions.

Ⓝ *NCLEX® Connection: Pharmacological and Parenteral Therapies, Medication Administration*

Application Exercises Key

1. A. **CORRECT:** Oxytocin must be administered by an infusion pump to ensure precise dosage.
   B. **CORRECT:** Vital signs are monitored to assess for hypertension, an adverse effect of oxytocin.
   C. If contractions are occurring every 4 min and lasting 45 seconds, the nurse should continue the infusion or gradually increase the infusion rate of oxytocin, because the therapeutic effect has not been achieved.
   D. Oxytocin rate is increased gradually to prevent hypertonic uterine contractions.
   E. **CORRECT:** Continuous FHR monitoring is required to assess for fetal distress.

Ⓝ *NCLEX® Connection: Pharmacological and Parenteral Therapies, Medication Administration*

2. Uterine rupture is a potential complication of oxytocin administration because the medication increases the force of uterine contractions. Uterine tachysystole is a potential complication of oxytocin administration because the medication increases the frequency of uterine contractions. Placental abruption is a potential complication of oxytocin administration. Hyponatremia is a potential complication of oxytocin administration because the medication can cause water intoxication.

Ⓝ *NCLEX® Connection: Pharmacological and Parenteral Therapies, Parenteral/Intravenous Therapies*

3. A. **CORRECT:** The nurse understands that the clients understands the teaching about terbutaline when the client states, "This medication will stop my contractions." Terbutaline blocks beta2-adrenergic receptors, which causes uterine smooth muscle relaxation. It does not prevent bleeding, promote placental blood flow, or increase the production of prostaglandin production.

Ⓝ *NCLEX® Connection: Pharmacological and Parenteral Therapies, Expected Actions/Outcomes*

4. A. This is an expected finding and does not need to be reported to the provider.
   B. This is an expected finding and does not need to be reported to the provider.
   C. **CORRECT:** Urine output less than 25 to 30 mL/hr is associated with magnesium sulfate toxicity and should be reported to the provider.
   D. A respiratory rate of 12/min is an expected finding and does not need to be reported to the provider.

Ⓝ *NCLEX® Connection: Pharmacological and Parenteral Therapies, Expected Actions/Outcomes*

5. A. The action of terbutaline is to relax uterine smooth muscle. Clients taking this medication are instructed to limit activity, which stimulates smooth muscle, to delay preterm labor.
   B. Fluid intake should be limited to 2,400 mL/day.
   C. **CORRECT:** The nurse determines the client understands the teaching regarding terbutaline when they state, "I will report increasing intensity of contractions to my provider."
   D. Terbutaline delays preterm labor; it does not prevent it.

Ⓝ *NCLEX® Connection: Pharmacological and Parenteral Therapies, Medication Administration*

When reviewing the following chapters, keep in mind the relevant topics and tasks of the NCLEX outline, in particular:

Client Needs: Pharmacological and Parenteral Therapies

ADVERSE EFFECTS/CONTRAINDICATIONS/SIDE EFFECTS/INTERACTIONS

Monitor for anticipated interactions among the client's prescribed medications and fluids.

Provide information to the client on common side effects/adverse effects/potential interactions of medications, and inform the client of when to notify the primary health care provider.

EXPECTED ACTIONS/OUTCOMES

Evaluate the client's use of medications over time.

Use clinical decision making/critical thinking when addressing expected effects/outcomes of medications.

MEDICATION ADMINISTRATION

Administer and document medications given by common routes.

Prepare and administer medications, using rights of medication administration.

Educate client about medications.

UNIT 8   MEDICATIONS FOR JOINT AND BONE CONDITIONS

CHAPTER 31   *Connective Tissue Disorders*

Rheumatoid arthritis (RA) is a chronic, progressive disorder with autoimmune and inflammatory components. Pharmacological management relieves manifestations and can slow disease progression. Categories of medications in this section include disease-modifying antirheumatic medications (DMARDs), glucocorticoids, and nonsteroidal anti-inflammatory drugs (NSAIDs), which can be used individually or in combination to manage RA.

Gout (aka gouty arthritis) is a painful type of arthritis that is caused by elevated levels of uric acid, which can accumulate and cause localized inflammation in synovial areas. Gout can result in severe joint pain caused by crystallization of sodium urate in the synovial space. Antigout medications act either by reducing inflammation or decreasing blood uric acid levels. Categories of medications in this section include anti-inflammatory agents, NSAIDs, glucocorticoids, and agents for hyperuricemia.

Systemic lupus erythematous (SLE) is an autoimmune condition that can cause damage to joints, skin, blood vessels, CNS, and organs. Medications for treating lupus include anti-inflammatory medications, NSAIDs, corticosteroids, antimalarials, immunomodulators, and monoclonal antibodies. Topical cortisone can reduce inflammation of the typical skin rash of SLE.

Fibromyalgia is a syndrome characterized by muscle pain and fatigue. There are three FDA-approved medications for treating this syndrome: pregabalin, duloxetine, and milnacipran. Other medications used to treat fibromyalgia syndrome (but not FDA-approved for this use) include amitriptyline, cyclobenzaprine, tramadol, NSAIDs, and opioids. In addition, medications that facilitate sleep (zolpidem) and treat restless leg syndrome (gabapentin) are sometimes prescribed for manifestations of this condition.

Disease-modifying antirheumatic drugs

DMARDS I: Major nonbiologic DMARDs
- Immunomodulator medications: methotrexate, leflunomide
- Antimalarial agent: hydroxychloroquine
- Anti–inflammatory medication: sulfasalazine

DMARDS II: Major biologic DMARDs
- Tumor necrosis factor (TNF) antagonists
  - Etanercept
  - Infliximab
  - Adalimumab
  - Certolizumab pegol
  - Golimumab
- B-lymphocyte–depleting agent: Rituximab
- T-cell activation inhibitor: Abatacept

DMARDS III: Minor nonbiologic and nonbiologic DMARDs
- Gold salts: Auranofin
- Penicillamine
- Immunosuppressant medications (Reserved for severe RA that has not responded to safer DMARD medications)
  - Azathioprine
  - Cyclosporine

GLUCOCORTICOIDS
- Prednisone
- Prednisolone

NSAIDS
- Aspirin (salicylate)
- Ibuprofen
- Diclofenac
- Indomethacin
- Meloxicam
- Naproxen sodium
- Oxaprozin
- Celecoxib (second–generation NSAID [COX-2 inhibitor])

PURPOSE

EXPECTED PHARMACOLOGICAL ACTION
- DMARDs slow joint degeneration and progression of rheumatoid arthritis.
- Glucocorticoids provide relief of inflammation and pain. Glucocorticoids can also delay disease progression.
- NSAIDs provide rapid relief of inflammation and pain but do not slow disease progression.

THERAPEUTIC USES
- Analgesia for pain, swelling, and joint stiffness
- Maintenance of joint function
- Slow/delay the worsening of the disease (DMARDs, glucocorticoids)
- Short-term therapy for temporary relief (with NSAIDs, glucocorticoids) until long-acting DMARDs take effect
- Prevention of organ rejection in clients who have transplants (kidney, liver, and heart transplants [glucocorticoids, immunosuppressants])
- Management of inflammatory bowel disease (glucocorticoids, immunosuppressants, DMARDs)

COMPLICATIONS

Cytotoxic agent/immunomodulator: methotrexate

Increased risk of infection
CLIENT EDUCATION: Notify the provider immediately for manifestations of infection (fever or sore throat).

Hepatic fibrosis and toxicity
- NURSING ACTIONS
  - Monitor liver function tests and kidney function tests.
  - Dosing with folic acid is recommended to reduce GI and hepatic toxicity.
- CLIENT EDUCATION: Observe for anorexia, abdominal fullness, and jaundice, and notify the provider if findings occur.

Bone marrow suppression
NURSING ACTIONS: Obtain baseline CBC, including platelet counts. Repeat every 3 to 6 months.

Ulcerative stomatitis/other GI ulcerations
- Early finding with toxicity
- NURSING ACTIONS
  - Inspect mouth, gums, and throat daily for ulcerations, bleeding, or color changes.
  - Stop the medication if findings occur.
  - Monitor CBC, platelet counts.
- CLIENT EDUCATION: Use soft toothbrush when performing oral care.

Fetal death/congenital abnormalities
- NURSING ACTIONS: Avoid use during pregnancy.
- CLIENT EDUCATION: Use adequate contraception if taking this medication.

Gold salts: auranofin

Toxicity (severe pruritus, rashes, stomatitis)
NURSING ACTIONS: Notify the provider if these manifestations occur.

Renal toxicity (proteinuria)
NURSING ACTIONS: Monitor I&O, BUN, creatinine, and urinalysis.

Blood dyscrasias
- Thrombocytopenia, leukopenia, agranulocytosis, aplastic anemia
- NURSING ACTIONS: Monitor CBC, WBC, and platelet counts periodically.
- CLIENT EDUCATION: Observe for bruising and gum bleeding and notify the provider if these occur.

Hepatitis
NURSING ACTIONS: Monitor liver function tests.

GI discomfort (nausea, vomiting, abdominal pain)
NURSING ACTIONS: Observe for manifestations and notify the provider if they occur.

Sulfasalazine

Safe to administer during pregnancy and lactation.

GI discomfort
- Nausea, vomiting, diarrhea, abdominal pain
- NURSING ACTIONS: Use an enteric-coated preparation and divide dosage daily.

Hepatic dysfunction
NURSING ACTIONS: Monitor liver function tests.

Bone marrow suppression
NURSING ACTIONS: Monitor CBC, including platelet counts.

Dermatologic reaction (rash)
NURSING ACTIONS: Do not administer to clients who have a sulfa allergy.

Antimalarial agent: hydroxychloroquine

Retinal damage (blindness)
- NURSING ACTIONS: Stop the medication and notify the provider if any visual disturbances are noted.
- CLIENT EDUCATION: Have baseline eye examination and follow-up eye exams every 6 months with an ophthalmologist.

Tumor necrosis factor (TNF) antagonists: etanercept, infliximab

Subcutaneous injection–site irritation
- Redness, swelling, pain, itching
- NURSING ACTIONS: Monitor the injection site and stop the medication if manifestations of irritation occur.

IV infusion reactions (infliximab)
- Flu-like findings, hypotension, possible anaphylaxis
- NURSING ACTIONS
  - Stop infusion and notify provider immediately for severe reaction.
  - Continue to monitor for reaction 2 hr after IV infusion.

Risk of infection, including invasive fungal infections and other opportunistic pathogens

- Invasive fungal infections (histoplasmosis, TB, reactivation of hepatitis B)
- NURSING ACTIONS: Test for hepatitis B and TB.
- CLIENT EDUCATION: Monitor for infection (fever, sore throat, inflammation) and notify the provider if findings occur. Medication should be discontinued.

Severe skin reactions

- Including Stevens-Johnson syndrome
- CLIENT EDUCATION: Monitor for adverse skin reactions and notify the provider if findings occur. Medication should be discontinued.

Heart failure

NURSING ACTIONS: Monitor for development or worsening of heart failure (distended neck veins, crackles in lungs, dyspnea). Medication should be discontinued.

Blood dyscrasias

- NURSING ACTIONS: Monitor for manifestations of a blood disorder (bleeding, bruising, persistent fever) and seek immediate medical attention. Medication should be discontinued.
- CLIENT EDUCATION: If manifestations of a blood disorder (persistent fever, bruising, bleeding, pallor) develop, seek immediate medical attention.

Penicillamine

Bone marrow suppression

NURSING ACTIONS: Obtain baseline CBC including platelet counts and repeat every 3 to 6 months.

Toxicity (severe pruritus, rashes)

NURSING ACTIONS

- Stop the medication.
- Notify the provider if findings occur.

Cyclosporine

Risk of infection

- Flu-like findings, painful urination (nephrotoxicity)
- CLIENT EDUCATION: Notify the provider immediately if findings occur.

Hepatotoxicity (jaundice)

NURSING ACTIONS: Monitor liver function and adjust dosage.

Nephrotoxicity

NURSING ACTIONS

- Monitor BUN and creatinine throughout treatment.
- Monitor I&O.

Hirsutism

NURSING ACTIONS: This effect is reversible with discontinuation of the medication.

Gingival hyperplasia

CLIENT EDUCATION: Perform good dental hygiene and regular dental check-ups.

Glucocorticoids: prednisone

Risk of infection (fever and/or sore throat)

CLIENT EDUCATION: Notify the provider immediately if findings occur.

Osteoporosis

- NURSING ACTIONS: Observe clients for manifestations of vertebral compression fractures, and for indications of fractures in other bones. Monitor bone density studies
- CLIENT EDUCATION: Take calcium supplements, vitamin D, and/or bisphosphonate (etidronate).

Adrenal suppression

- Nausea, vomiting, hypotension, and confusion can occur if glucocorticoids are stopped abruptly.
- NURSING ACTIONS
  - Administer IV fluids (0.9% sodium chloride and hydrocortisone). Advise clients not to discontinue the medication suddenly.
  - Increase in glucocorticoid dosage can be needed during times of stress (e.g., surgery, acute illness).
- CLIENT EDUCATION
  - Observe for manifestations, and notify the provider if manifestations occur.
  - Carry Medic Alert identification to ensure proper dosing during emergency.

Fluid retention

NURSING ACTIONS: Monitor for manifestations of fluid excess (crackles, weight gain, and edema).

GI discomfort/gastric ulceration

- NURSING ACTIONS
  - H2-receptor antagonists can be used prophylactically.
  - To provide early detection of ulcer formation, stools should be periodically checked for occult blood.
- CLIENT EDUCATION
  - Observe for findings and to notify the provider if findings occur.
  - Report findings of GI bleeding (coffee-ground emesis or black, tarry stools).

Hyperglycemia

NURSING ACTIONS: Monitor blood glucose level.

Hypokalemia

- NURSING ACTIONS
  - Monitor blood potassium levels.
  - Administer potassium supplements.
- CLIENT EDUCATION: Eat potassium-rich foods.

CONTRAINDICATIONS/PRECAUTIONS

Methotrexate
- **Warnings**
  - Pregnancy
    - Methotrexate: Contraindicated due to fetal death and congenital abnormalities.
    - Cyclosporine: Do not administer unless the benefits to the client outweigh the risk to the fetus.
    - Sulfasalazine: Use with caution due to the potential of neural tube defects.
  - Lactation
    - Methotrexate: Contraindicated.
    - Cyclosporine: Do not administer unless the benefits to the client outweigh the risk to the fetus.
    - Sulfasalazine: Safety not established.
  - Reproductive
    - Methotrexate: Teratogenic properties; contraception should be employed by males during therapy and for at least 3 months following treatment and for one ovulatory cycle for females. Fertility can be impaired in all sexes.
    - Sulfasalazine: Can cause male infertility
- Methotrexate is contraindicated in clients who have liver failure, alcohol use disorder, or blood dyscrasias.
- Use with caution in clients who have liver or kidney dysfunction, cancer and suppressed bone marrow function, peptic ulcer disease, ulcerative colitis, impaired nutritional status, or infections.
- Use cautiously with children, or clients who are breastfeeding.

Etanercept is contraindicated in clients who have malignancies, active infection, hematologic disorder, or during lactation. Use caution in clients who have heart failure, CNS demyelinating disorders (multiple sclerosis), blood dyscrasias, pre-existing liver dysfunction.

Cyclosporine is contraindicated in pregnancy, recent vaccination with live virus vaccines, and recent contact with or active infection of chickenpox or herpes zoster.

Glucocorticoids
- Glucocorticoids are contraindicated in systemic fungal infections and live virus vaccines.
- Warn clients against abrupt discontinuation of glucocorticoids. Dosage of glucocorticoids is always adjusted and withdrawn gradually.

INTERACTIONS

Methotrexate

- Salicylates, other NSAIDs, sulfonamides, penicillin, and tetracyclines can cause methotrexate toxicity. Monitor for toxic effects.
- Folic acid is often prescribed with methotrexate to prevent hepatic and GI toxicity.

Etanercept

- Concurrent use of etanercept with a live vaccine increases the risk of getting or transmitting infection. Avoid live virus vaccines.
- Concurrent use with immunosuppressants increases the client's chance of serious infection. Use precautions against illness if taking immunosuppressants.

Cyclosporine

- Concurrent use of phenytoin, phenobarbital, rifampin, carbamazepine, and trimethoprim-sulfamethoxazole decreases cyclosporine level, which can lead to organ rejection. Monitor cyclosporine levels and adjust dosage accordingly.
- Concurrent use of ketoconazole, erythromycin, and amphotericin B can increase cyclosporine level, leading to toxicity. Monitor cyclosporine dosage, and adjust accordingly to prevent toxicity.
- Amphotericin B, aminoglycoside, and NSAIDs are nephrotoxic. Concurrent use with cyclosporine increases the risk for kidney dysfunction. Monitor BUN, creatinine, and I&O.
- Consumption of grapefruit juice increases cyclosporine levels by 50% to 200%, which poses an increased risk of toxicity. Advise clients to avoid drinking grapefruit juice.

Glucocorticoids

- Diuretics that promote potassium loss increase the risk of hypokalemia. Monitor potassium level, and administer supplements as needed.
- Because of the risk for hypokalemia, concurrent use of glucocorticoids with digoxin increases the risk of digoxin-induced dysrhythmias. Monitor for digoxin-induced dysrhythmias and toxicity. Monitor potassium levels.
- NSAIDs increase the risk of GI ulceration. Advise clients to avoid use of NSAIDs. If GI distress occurs, instruct clients to notify the provider.
- Glucocorticoids promote hyperglycemia, thereby counteracting the effects of insulin and oral hypoglycemics. The dose of hypoglycemic medications might need to be increased.

NURSING ADMINISTRATION

- Advise clients that effects of DMARDs are delayed and can take 3 to 6 weeks, with full therapeutic effect taking several months. Q PCC
- Administer adalimumab subcutaneously every 2 weeks.
- Administer etanercept by subcutaneous injection once per week. Ensure solution is clear without particles present.
- Glucocorticoids can be used as oral agents or as intra-articular injections. Short-term therapy can be used to control exacerbations of findings and also can be used while waiting for the effects of DMARDs to develop.

Cyclosporine

- Administer the initial IV dose of cyclosporine over 2 to 6 hr.
- Monitor for hypersensitivity reactions. Stay with clients for 30 min after administration of cyclosporine.
- Mix oral cyclosporine with milk or orange juice right before ingestion to increase palatability.
- Instruct clients regarding the importance of lifelong therapy if used to prevent organ rejection.

NURSING EVALUATION OF MEDICATION EFFECTIVENESS

Depending on the therapeutic intent, effectiveness can be evidenced by the following.
- Improvement of findings of rheumatoid arthritis (reduced swelling of joints, absence of joint stiffness, ability to maintain joint function, absence of pain)
- Decrease in systemic complications (weight loss and fatigue)

Antigout medication

ANTI-INFLAMMATORY AGENTS

SELECT PROTOTYPE MEDICATION: Colchicine
Once considered drug of choice for acute gout, colchicine is now usually reserved for clients who do not respond to or cannot tolerate safer agents.

OTHER MEDICATIONS
- NSAIDs
  - Indomethacin
  - Naproxen
  - Diclofenac
- Glucocorticoids: Prednisone

PURPOSE

EXPECTED PHARMACOLOGICAL ACTION
- Colchicine is only effective for inflammation caused by gout.
- These medications decrease inflammation.

THERAPEUTIC USES
- Abort an acute gout attack in response to precursor findings.
- Treatment of acute attacks.
- Prednisone is used for clients who have acute gout who are unable to take or unresponsive to NSAIDs. This medication is not for clients who have hyperglycemia.

ROUTE OF ADMINISTRATION: Colchicine: Oral

AGENTS FOR HYPERURICEMIA

For clients who have chronic gout or frequent gout attacks

SELECT PROTOTYPE MEDICATION: Allopurinol

OTHER MEDICATIONS: Febuxostat, probenecid, pegloticase, and rasburicase

PURPOSE

EXPECTED PHARMACOLOGICAL ACTION: Allopurinol and febuxostat inhibit uric acid production. Probenecid inhibits uric acid reabsorption by renal tubules.

THERAPEUTIC USES: Hyperuricemia due to chronic gout or secondary to cancer chemotherapy

ROUTE OF ADMINISTRATION
- Allopurinol (oral, IV)
- Febuxostat, probenecid (oral)
- Pegloticase, rasburicase (IV)

COMPLICATIONS

Colchicine

Most characteristic side effects result from injury to rapidly proliferating cells

Mild GI distress, which can progress to GI toxicity
- Abdominal pain, diarrhea, nausea, vomiting
- CLIENT EDUCATION
  - Take oral medications with food.
  - Take antidiarrheal agents as prescribed.
  - If severe GI distress occurs, stop colchicine and notify provider.

Thrombocytopenia, suppressed bone marrow
CLIENT EDUCATION: Notify the provider of bleeding, bruising or sore throat.

Rhabdomyolysis
- Sudden onset of muscle pain, tenderness
- More likely with long-term, low-dose therapy, or for clients taking statins for high cholesterol and those who have impaired kidneys or liver.
- CLIENT EDUCATION: Notify provider for new onset of these findings.

Probenecid

Renal calculi and renal injury
- Occur from deposition of urate in the kidney
- Should not be initiated at the beginning of an acute gout attack (may exacerbate acute episodes)
- CLIENT EDUCATION
  - Drink 2.5 to 3 L fluid daily to decrease risk by alkalinizing the urine during the first few days of treatment.
  - Do not take concurrently with aspirin or other salicylates.

Gastrointestinal effects
NURSING ACTIONS: Take medication with food to decrease GI effects.

Hypersensitivity reactions (e.g., rash)
CLIENT EDUCATION: Report any rash to provider.

Allopurinol

Hypersensitivity syndrome, fever, rash, and kidney and liver damage
NURSING ACTIONS: If administering IV, stop infusion. Severe reaction can require hemodialysis or glucocorticoids.

Kidney injury
NURSING ACTIONS: Alkalinize the urine and encourage intake of 2 to 3 L of fluids/day. Monitor I&O, BUN, and creatinine.

Hepatitis
NURSING ACTIONS: Monitor liver enzymes.

GI distress (nausea and vomiting)
NURSING ACTIONS: Administer with food.

Increase in gout attacks
- During the first months of treatment
- CLIENT EDUCATION: Report increased gout attacks to provider. Colchicine or an NSAID can be prescribed along with allopurinol to prevent this.

CONTRAINDICATIONS/PRECAUTIONS

Colchicine

- Pregnancy Risk Category C.
- Contraindicated for clients who have severe renal, cardiac, hepatic, or gastrointestinal dysfunction.
- Use cautiously in older adults and clients who are debilitated or have blood disorders or mild to moderate hepatic dysfunction. Ⓖ

Probenecid

- Pregnancy Risk Category C.
- Can precipitate acute gout. Do not give within 2 to 3 weeks of an acute attack.

Allopurinol

- Pregnancy Risk Category C.
- This medication is contraindicated in clients who have medication hypersensitivity or idiopathic hemochromatosis.

INTERACTIONS

Colchicine

Grapefruit or grapefruit juice can increase adverse effects. Advise clients to avoid eating grapefruit or drinking grapefruit juice when taking colchicine.

Probenecid

- Salicylates can lessen the effectiveness of probenecid and can precipitate gout.
- Salicylates (aspirin) interfere with probenecid's therapeutic effect.

Allopurinol

Allopurinol slows the metabolism of warfarin within the liver, which places clients at risk for bleeding.
- Instruct clients to observe for manifestations of bleeding (bruising, petechiae, hematuria).
- Monitor prothrombin time and INR levels and adjust warfarin dosages accordingly.

NURSING ADMINISTRATION

- When clients are taking medications for gout, monitor uric acid levels, CBC, urinalysis, and liver and kidney function tests.
- Allopurinol IV should be well diluted and administered as an infusion over 30 to 60 min.
- Allopurinol and probenecid: If a rash develops, advise clients to stop the medication and report the occurrence to the provider.

CLIENT EDUCATION
- Take oral gout medication with food or after meals to minimize GI distress.
- Implement actions to prevent gout attacks (avoiding alcohol and foods high in purine [red meat, other foods that seem to precipitate attacks], ensuring an adequate intake of water, exercise regularly, and maintaining a healthy BMI). ⓆPcc

NURSING EVALUATION OF MEDICATION EFFECTIVENESS

Depending on the therapeutic intent, effectiveness can be evidenced by the following.
- Improvement of pain caused by a gout attack (decrease in joint swelling, redness, uric acid levels)
- Decrease in number of gout attacks
- Decrease in uric acid levels

Medication for systemic lupus erythematosus

MONOCLONAL ANTIBODY MEDICATION: Belimumab

PURPOSE

EXPECTED PHARMACOLOGICAL ACTION: Disrupts activation of B–lymphocytes through interference with BLyS, a protein needed for B-cell activation and survival

THERAPEUTIC USES: SLE

COMPLICATIONS

GI effects (nausea, vomiting, diarrhea)
CLIENT EDUCATION: Utilize natural GI remedies (e.g., ginger tea or hard candy). If severe GI distress occurs, notify provider.

Headache, depressed mood
NURSING ACTIONS: If suicidal thoughts are present, notify the provider.

Insomnia
CLIENT EDUCATION: Utilize strategies to promote adequate sleep. (Make sure bedroom is quiet, dark, and relaxing. Avoid large meals before bedtime.)

Infusion reaction
- Erythema, edema, pruritus around IV site.
- Anaphylaxis can occur, manifesting as angioedema, hypotension, and dyspnea.
- NURSING ACTIONS
  - Infuse slowly over an hour. If anaphylaxis occurs, discontinue infusion and begin emergency treatment.
  - Premedication might be prescribed to minimize hypersensitivity reactions.

Increased risk of infection
CLIENT EDUCATION: Avoid being around sick people, do not receive live virus vaccines within 30 days of medication, and notify provider if fever, painful urination, or bloody diarrhea is present.

CONTRAINDICATIONS/PRECAUTIONS

- Pregnancy Risk Category C. Avoid breastfeeding.
- Not for clients who have severe renal impairment or SLE affecting CNS.
- Use caution in older adult clients, and clients who have depression, cardiac disorders, or infections. ©

INTERACTIONS

Cyclophosphamide or immune suppressants increase risk for infection.
CLIENT EDUCATION: Avoid being around sick people, no live virus vaccines within 30 days of medication, and notify provider if fever, painful urination, or bloody diarrhea is present.

NURSING ADMINISTRATION

- Reconstitute with sterile water, and dilute only with 0.9% saline solution. Q EBP
- Refrigerate solution no longer than 8 hr after reconstitution. Allow solution to stand at room temperature for 10 to 15 min before using.
- Administered by IV infusion, and given slowly, over about 1 hr. Monitor closely for infusion reactions and hypersensitivity.
- Discard unused solution.
- No administration of live virus vaccines within 30 days.

NURSING EVALUATION OF MEDICATION EFFECTIVENESS

Decrease in manifestations of SLE

Medications for fibromyalgia

SEROTONIN–NOREPINEPHRINE REUPTAKE INHIBITORS (SNRI)
- Duloxetine
- Milnacipran

GAMMA-AMINOBUTYRIC ACID ANALOGUE (GABA): Pregabalin

PURPOSE

Serotonin–norepinephrine reuptake inhibitors (SNRIs)

EXPECTED PHARMACOLOGICAL ACTION: Restores balance of neurotransmitters, serotonin, and norepinephrine

THERAPEUTIC USES
- Fibromyalgia (duloxetine and milnacipran)
- Depression (duloxetine)
- Diabetic peripheral neuropathy (duloxetine)

GABA (pregabalin)

EXPECTED PHARMACOLOGICAL ACTION: It is thought that pregabalin binds to alpha–2–delta in CNS tissue.

THERAPEUTIC USES: Fibromyalgia, seizures, neuropathic pain

COMPLICATIONS

Serotonin–norepinephrine reuptake inhibitors

Drowsiness, dizziness, blurred vision
CLIENT EDUCATION
- Do not drive or operate heavy machinery while taking this medication.
- Change positions slowly.
- Employ fall prevention strategies (e.g., sensible shoes, removing home hazards).

Nausea, anorexia, weight loss
NURSING ACTIONS: Monitor weight and food intake.

Headache, insomnia, anxiety
NURSING ACTIONS: Monitor for these findings.

Hypertension, tachycardia
NURSING ACTIONS: Monitor vital signs, and report changes.

Withdrawal syndrome
- Results in headache, nausea, visual disturbances, anxiety, dizziness, and tremors
- CLIENT EDUCATION: Withdraw from medication gradually.

Sexual dysfunction
- No orgasm, decreased libido, impotence, menstrual changes
- CLIENT EDUCATION: Report sexual dysfunction to the provider.

GABA

Drowsiness, fatigue, dizziness, blurred vision, lightheadedness
CLIENT EDUCATION: Do not drive or operate heavy machinery while taking this medication; change positions slowly; and employ fall prevention strategies (e.g., sensible shoes, removing home hazards).

Increased appetite, weight gain, constipation, abdominal pain
CLIENT EDUCATION
- Utilize ways to prevent weight gain (eating a balanced diet, eliminating high-fat, high-sugar foods from the diet).
- Develop an exercise plan.

Hypersensitivity reactions (angioedema)
CLIENT EDUCATION: Stop taking the medication and notify the provider or call 911 immediately for rash, hives, dyspnea, or swelling of the face or tongue.

Rhabdomyolysis
- Acute onset of severe muscle weakness and tenderness with elevation of blood creatinine kinase
- CLIENT EDUCATION: Notify the provider for manifestations. Medication will need to be discontinued if rhabdomyolysis occurs.

Erectile dysfunction and anorgasmia
CLIENT EDUCATION: Report manifestations of sexual dysfunction.

CONTRAINDICATIONS/PRECAUTIONS

Serotonin-norepinephrine reuptake inhibitors

- Pregnancy Risk Category C
- Contraindicated in clients who have hepatic or renal impairment or those taking MAOI within 14 days
- Caution in clients who have cardiac problems, hypertension, tachycardia, diabetes, gastrointestinal disorders, and glaucoma

GABA

- Pregnancy Risk Category C.
- Dose might need to be adjusted in older adult clients and clients who have renal impairment. Ⓖ
- Use with caution in clients who have cardiac problems, hypertension, diabetes, renal impairment, mental illness, angioedema, and thrombocytopenia.

INTERACTIONS

Serotonin-norepinephrine reuptake inhibitors

Antidepressants
NURSING ACTIONS
- SSRIs increase risk for serotonin syndrome.
- Notify provider if suicidal thoughts are present.

Anticoagulants, warfarin, and NSAIDs, which increase the risk of bleeding (e.g., GI bleed)
NURSING ACTIONS: Notify provider for manifestations of internal bleeding (e.g., blood in stools).

Diuretics increase risk of low blood sodium levels.
NURSING ACTIONS: Monitor blood sodium levels.

GABA

- **ACE inhibitors** increase risk of angioedema. Advise cool compresses and notify provider.
- **Benzodiazepines** increase drowsiness. Do not drive or operate heavy machinery.
- **Thiazolidinedione** (antidiabetic agent) increases risk of weight gain and peripheral edema. Advise healthy, well-balanced diet and regular activity to help counteract weight gain and elevating extremities for peripheral edema.
- **Alcohol** increases drowsiness and dizziness. Advise clients not to consume alcohol while taking this medication.

NURSING ADMINISTRATION

Serotonin-norepinephrine reuptake inhibitors

- Administered orally without regard to food.
- Swallow capsule whole.
- Taper withdrawal dosage gradually over 2 weeks.

GABA

- Administered orally with or without food.
- Notify provider if suicidal thoughts are present. Ⓠs
- Taper withdrawal gradually over at least 1 week.

NURSING EVALUATION OF MEDICATION EFFECTIVENESS

Decrease in manifestations of fibromyalgia

Application Exercises

1. A nurse is caring for a client who has a new prescription for adalimumab for rheumatoid arthritis. Based on the route of administration of adalimumab, which of the following should the nurse plan to monitor?

   A. The vein for thrombophlebitis during IV administration

   B. The subcutaneous site for redness following injection

   C. The oral mucosa for ulceration after oral administration

   D. The skin for irritation following removal of transdermal patch

2. A nurse is evaluating teaching for a client who has rheumatoid arthritis and a new prescription for methotrexate. Which of the following statements by the client indicates understanding of the teaching?

   A. "I will be sure to return to the clinic at least once a year to have my blood drawn."

   B. "I can receive live-virus vaccines."

   C. "I'll let the doctor know if I develop sores in my mouth."

   D. "I should stop taking oral contraceptives."

3. A nurse is providing teaching for a client who has gout and a new prescription for allopurinol. For which of the following adverse effects should the client be taught to monitor? (Select all that apply.)

   A. Stomatitis

   B. Insomnia

   C. Nausea

   D. Rash

   E. Increased gout pain

4. A nurse is preparing to administer belimumab for a client who has systemic lupus erythematosus. Which of the following actions should the nurse plan to take?

   A. Warm the medication to room temperature over 1 hr before administering.

   B. Administer the medication by IV bolus over 5 min.

   C. Dilute the medication in 5% dextrose and water solution.

   D. Monitor the client for hypersensitivity reactions.

5. A nurse is caring for a client who has a new diagnosis of fibromyalgia. Which of the following medications should the nurse expect to administer to this client?

   A. Colchicine

   B. Hydroxychloroquine

   C. Auranofin

   D. Duloxetine

Active Learning Scenario

A nurse is teaching a client who has rheumatoid arthritis (RA) about a new prescription for etanercept. What should the nurse teach the client about this medication? Use the ATI Active Learning Template: Medication to complete this item.

THERAPEUTIC USES: Describe the therapeutic use for etanercept in this client.

COMPLICATIONS: Describe at least three adverse effects the client should monitor for.

NURSING INTERVENTIONS: Describe one for each of the adverse effects above.

MEDICATION ADMINISTRATION: Describe at least three important factors.

Using the ATI Active Learning Template: Medication

THERAPEUTIC USES: Etanercept is a biologic DMARD classified as a tumor necrosis factor antagonist. It suppresses manifestations of moderate to severe RA and slows the progression of the disorder.

COMPLICATIONS
- Severe infections, including tuberculosis or reactivation of hepatitis B
- Heart failure
- Severe skin reactions, such as Stevens-Johnson syndrome
- Hematologic disorders

NURSING INTERVENTIONS
- Instruct clients to monitor for infection, and to report sore throat and other manifestations.
- Discuss reasons for TB testing and possible hepatitis B testing.
- Clients should notify the provider for edema, shortness of breath, and other manifestations of heart failure.
- Report skin rash to provider.
- Report easy bruising, bleeding, or unusual fatigue to provider.

MEDICATION ADMINISTRATION
- Teach clients to administer by subcutaneous injection twice weekly.
- Discard solutions that are discolored or that contain particulate matter.
- Monitor for injection-site reactions, and report them to provider.
- Rotate injection sites.
- Avoid skin areas that are bruised or reddened when injecting.

Ⓝ *NCLEX® Connection: Pharmacological and Parenteral Therapies, Medication Administration*

1. A. Adalimumab is not administered IV. Assessing for thrombophlebitis during administration is not necessary.
   B. **CORRECT:** Adalimumab is administered subcutaneously, and injection-site redness and swelling are common. It is appropriate to assess the site for redness following injection.
   C. Adalimumab is not administered orally. Assessing oral mucosa for ulceration following administration is not necessary.
   D. Adalimumab is not administered transdermally. Inspecting the skin for irritation is not necessary.

Ⓝ *NCLEX® Connection: Pharmacological and Parenteral Therapies, Medication Administration*

2. A. CBC including platelet count, and liver and kidney function tests will be monitored at baseline and frequently during treatment with methotrexate to check for adverse effects.
   B. Methotrexate causes bone marrow suppression. The client should be instructed not to receive vaccinations without first consulting their provider.
   C. **CORRECT:** Ulcerations in the mouth, tongue, or throat are often the first manifestations of methotrexate toxicity and should be reported to the provider immediately.
   D. Methotrexate is a Pregnancy Category X medication and can cause severe fetal damage. The client should have a pregnancy test before starting the medication and should use a reliable form of birth control during methotrexate therapy. Oral contraceptives are not contraindicated with methotrexate therapy.

Ⓝ *NCLEX® Connection: Pharmacological and Parenteral Therapies, Medication Administration*

3. A. Stomatitis occurs with medications that increase the risk of infection (many of the DMARDs used to treat rheumatoid arthritis). Allopurinol does not increase a client's risk for infection.
   B. Insomnia is not an adverse effect caused by allopurinol.
   C. **CORRECT:** Nausea and vomiting are adverse effects that can be caused by allopurinol.
   D. **CORRECT:** Rash and other hypersensitivity reactions can be caused by allopurinol. The client should be taught to contact the provider for any manifestation of hypersensitivity so that the medication can be discontinued.
   E. **CORRECT:** An increase in gout attacks can occur during the first few months in a client who is taking allopurinol.

Ⓝ *NCLEX® Connection: Pharmacological and Parenteral Therapies, Adverse Effects/Contraindications/Side Effects/Interactions*

4. A. The solution of belimumab should be carefully refrigerated and allowed to sit at room temperature for only 10 to 15 min after being taken from the refrigerator.
   B. Belimumab is administered by intermittent IV infusion over 1 hr.
   C. Belimumab should be diluted only in 0.9% saline solution.
   D. **CORRECT:** Belimumab can cause severe infusion reactions and can cause anaphylaxis. Carefully monitor the client during infusion of this medication and be prepared to slow or stop the medication if a reaction occurs.

Ⓝ *NCLEX® Connection: Pharmacological and Parenteral Therapies, Adverse Effects/Contraindications/Side Effects/Interactions*

5. A. Colchicine is an anti-inflammatory medication used to treat gout.
   B. Hydroxychloroquine is an anti-malarial medication used as a DMARD along with methotrexate to treat rheumatoid arthritis.
   C. Auranofin is a gold salt used to relief joint pain and stiffness in clients who have rheumatoid arthritis.
   D. **CORRECT:** Duloxetine is a serotonin-norepinephrine reuptake inhibitor used to treat fibromyalgia. Other uses for this medication include treating depression and diabetic peripheral neuropathy.

Ⓝ *NCLEX® Connection: Pharmacological and Parenteral Therapies, Medication Administration*

CHAPTER 32 *Bone Disorders*

Calcium and vitamin D are necessary for the proper functioning of the heart, bones, nerves, muscles, and for blood coagulation. They can be given as supplements when dietary intake is insufficient. Other medications are also used for prevention and treatment of osteoporosis and prevention of fractures.

Medication classifications include calcium supplements, selective estrogen receptor modulators (also known as estrogen agonists/antagonists), bisphosphonates, and calcitonin.

Calcium supplements

SELECT PROTOTYPE MEDICATION: Calcium citrate

OTHER MEDICATIONS
- Calcium carbonate
- Calcium acetate
- For IV administration
  - Calcium chloride
  - Calcium gluconate

PURPOSE

EXPECTED PHARMACOLOGICAL ACTION: Maintenance of musculoskeletal, neurologic, and cardiovascular function

THERAPEUTIC USES
- Oral calcium supplements are used for clients who have hypocalcemia or deficiencies of parathyroid hormone, vitamin D, or dietary calcium.
- Oral dietary supplements are used for adolescents, older adults, and clients who are postmenopausal, pregnant, or breastfeeding. ⓖ
- IV medications are used for clients who have critically low levels of calcium.
- Oral vitamin D supplements can assist with the absorption of dietary calcium.
- Calcium and vitamin D supplements used in conjunction with calcitonin or a bisphosphonate can reduce the risk of osteoporosis.

COMPLICATIONS

Hypercalcemia

Calcium level greater than 10.5 mg/dL

FINDINGS: Initially, tachycardia and elevated blood pressure eventually leading to bradycardia and hypotension. Other findings include muscle weakness, hypotonia, constipation, nausea, vomiting, abdominal pain, lethargy, and confusion.

NURSING ACTIONS
- Monitor blood calcium levels to maintain between 9 and 10.5 mg/dL.
- Infuse 0.9% sodium chloride IV.
- Medications used to reverse hypercalcemia include IV furosemide, and calcium chelators (plicamycin).
- Medications used to prevent hypercalcemia include bisphosphonates (alendronate and oral inorganic phosphates).

CLIENT EDUCATION: Monitor for manifestations and report them to the provider.

CONTRAINDICATIONS/PRECAUTIONS

- Calcium supplements are contraindicated in clients who have hypercalcemia, renal calculi, hypophosphatemia, digoxin toxicity, and ventricular fibrillation. Ⓠs
- Use cautiously in clients who have kidney disease or a decrease in GI function.

INTERACTIONS

Glucocorticoids

Concurrent use of glucocorticoids reduces absorption of calcium.
NURSING ACTIONS: Give at least 1 hr apart.

Tetracyclines and thyroid hormone

Concurrent use of calcium decreases absorption of tetracyclines and thyroid hormone.
NURSING ACTIONS: Ensure 1 hr between administration of tetracyclines and calcium and at least 4 hr between the administration of thyroid hormone and calcium.

Thiazide diuretics

Concurrent administration of thiazide diuretics increases risk of hypercalcemia.
NURSING ACTIONS
- Assess for hypercalcemia.
- Avoid concurrent use.

Foods

Spinach, rhubarb, beets, bran, and whole grains can decrease calcium absorption.

NURSING ACTIONS
- Do not administer calcium with foods that decrease absorption.
- Instruct clients to avoid consuming these foods at the same time as taking calcium.

Phosphates, carbonates, sulfates, and tartrates

IV calcium precipitates with phosphates, carbonates, sulfates, and tartrates.

NURSING ACTIONS: Do not mix parenteral calcium with compounds that cause precipitation.

Digoxin

Concurrent use of digoxin and parenteral calcium can lead to severe bradycardia.

NURSING ACTIONS: IV injection of calcium must be given slowly with careful monitoring of client cardiac status. Qs

NURSING ADMINISTRATION

- Chewable tablets provide more consistent bioavailability.
- Recommended doses of oral calcium vary widely depending on the specific calcium preparation. Instruct the client to follow the prescription.
- Prior to administration, warm IV infusions of calcium to body temperature.
- Administer IV bolus doses at 0.5 to 2 mL/min.
- Monitor IV injection site carefully to prevent extravasation.

CLIENT EDUCATION
- Take a calcium supplement at least 1 hr apart from glucocorticoids and tetracyclines and at least 4 hr apart from thyroid hormone.
- Take oral calcium with 8 oz of water.

NURSING EVALUATION OF MEDICATION EFFECTIVENESS

Depending on therapeutic intent, effectiveness is evidenced by blood calcium level within expected reference range: 9 to 10.5 mg/dL.

Selective estrogen receptor modulator (agonist/antagonist)

SELECT PROTOTYPE MEDICATION: Raloxifene

PURPOSE

EXPECTED PHARMACOLOGICAL ACTION

- Works as endogenous estrogen in bone, lipid metabolism, and blood coagulation
- Decreases bone resorption, which slows bone loss and preserves bone mineral density
- Works as an antagonist to estrogen on breast and endometrial tissue
- Can decrease plasma levels of cholesterol

THERAPEUTIC USES

- Prevent and treat postmenopausal osteoporosis to prevent spinal fractures in female clients.
- Protect against breast cancer.

COMPLICATIONS

Increased risk for pulmonary embolism and deep-vein thrombosis (DVT)

NURSING ACTIONS
- Medication should be stopped prior to scheduled immobilization (surgery or extended bedrest). Medication can be resumed when the client is fully mobile.
- Monitor for manifestations of DVT (red, swollen extremity).
- Discourage long periods of sitting and inactivity (e.g., when traveling long distances).

Hot flashes

CLIENT EDUCATION: The medication can exacerbate hot flashes.

CONTRAINDICATIONS/PRECAUTIONS

- Raloxifene is Pregnancy Risk Category X.
- This medication is contraindicated in clients who have a history of or risk for venous thrombosis.
- The medication should be stopped 72 hrs prior to periods of prolonged immobility (surgery or travel). Qs

INTERACTIONS

Concurrent use with estrogen hormone therapy is discouraged.

NURSING ADMINISTRATION

- Take medication with or without food once per day.
- Monitor bone density. Clients should undergo a bone density scan every 12 to 18 months.
- Monitor blood calcium. Expected reference range is 9 to 10.5 mg/dL.
- Monitor liver function tests. Raloxifene levels can increase in clients who have hepatic impairment.

CLIENT EDUCATION

- For maximum benefit of the medication, consume adequate amounts of calcium (from dairy products) and vitamin D (from egg yolks). Inadequate amounts of dietary calcium and vitamin D cause release of parathyroid hormone, which stimulates calcium release from the bone.
- Perform weight-bearing exercises daily (walking 30 to 40 min each day).
- Minimize periods of restricted activity (e.g., when traveling).

NURSING EVALUATION OF MEDICATION EFFECTIVENESS

Depending on therapeutic intent, effectiveness is evidenced by the following.
- Increase in bone density
- No fractures

Bisphosphonates

SELECT PROTOTYPE MEDICATION: Alendronate

OTHER MEDICATIONS

- Ibandronate
- Risedronate
- For IV infusion: Zoledronic

PURPOSE

EXPECTED PHARMACOLOGICAL ACTION

Bisphosphonates decrease the number and action of osteoclasts and inhibit bone resorption.

THERAPEUTIC USES

- Prophylaxis and treatment of postmenopausal osteoporosis
- For male clients who have osteoporosis
- Prophylaxis and treatment of osteoporosis produced by long-term glucocorticoid use
- For clients who have Paget's disease of the bone
- Hypercalcemia due to malignancy

COMPLICATIONS

Esophagitis, esophageal ulceration (oral formulations)

NURSING ACTIONS
- Instruct the client to sit upright or ambulate for 30 min after taking this medication orally. Q EBP
- Clients taking ibandronate must remain upright and not ingest food or other medications for 1 hr after taking the medication orally.
- Instruct the client to take tablets with at least 240 mL (8 oz) water and liquid formulation with at least 60 mL (2 oz).
- Discontinue the medication and contact the provider for difficulty swallowing or new heartburn.

GI disturbances (all bisphosphonates)

Abdominal pain, nausea, diarrhea, constipation

NURSING ACTIONS: Notify provider for GI problems that prevent adequate intake.

Musculoskeletal pain

CLIENT EDUCATION
- Take a mild analgesic.
- Notify the provider if pain persists. Alternate medication can be prescribed.

Visual disturbances (caused by ocular inflammation)

Blurred vision and eye pain

CLIENT EDUCATION: Watch for manifestations and report them to the provider. Medication should be discontinued.

Bisphosphonate-related osteonecrosis of the jaw

With IV infusion

NURSING ACTIONS: See dentist prior to beginning treatment. Avoid dental work during administration of medication.

Kidney toxicity with IV infusion

NURSING ACTIONS: Monitor kidney function and hydration status.

Atypical femoral fractures

NURSING ACTIONS: Monitor the need for continued treatment after 5 years (risk increases with duration of treatment).

CONTRAINDICATIONS/PRECAUTIONS

- Most bisphosphonates are Pregnancy Risk Category D. Ibandronate and etidronate are Pregnancy Risk Category C.
  - Zoledronate has been associated with an increase in stillbirths and a decreased survivability of neonates.
- These medications are contraindicated for clients who have dysphagia, esophageal stricture, esophageal disorders, serious kidney impairment, and hypocalcemia. This medication should not be administered to clients who cannot sit upright or stand for at least 30 min after medication administration.
- Use cautiously for clients who are lactating and in clients who have upper GI disorders, infection, and liver impairment.
- Older adults are at slight risk for femoral fractures, which can occur without trauma while taking bisphosphonates. ⊙

INTERACTIONS

Alendronate absorption decreases when taken with calcium, iron, magnesium supplements, antacids, orange juice, and caffeine.
- NURSING ACTIONS: Wait at least 2 hr after administration to administer antacids or supplements.
- CLIENT EDUCATION: Take the medication in the morning on an empty stomach with at least 240 mL (8 oz) water.

NURSING ADMINISTRATION

- Bisphosphonates are available in varying forms and in varying schedules of administration.
- Monitor bone density. Clients should have a bone density scan every 12 to 18 months.
- Monitor blood calcium. Expected reference range is 9 to 10.5 mg/dL.

CLIENT EDUCATION Qpcc
- Take the medication first thing in the morning after getting out of bed.
- Wait at least 2 hours after administration before taking calcium products, mineral supplements, or antacids.
- Take oral medication on an empty stomach, drinking at least 240 mL (8 oz) water with tablets and at least 60 mL (2 oz) water with liquid formulation.
- Sit or ambulate for 30 min after taking the medication.
- Avoid all calcium-containing foods and liquids or any medications within 2 hr of taking alendronate.
- Avoid chewing or sucking on the tablet.
- Perform weight-bearing exercises daily (walking 30 to 40 min each day).
- Notify the provider of difficulty swallowing, painful swallowing, or new or worsening heartburn.
- If a dose is skipped, wait until the next day 30 min before eating breakfast to take the dose. Do not take two tablets on the same day.
- For maximum benefit of the medication, consume adequate amounts of calcium and vitamin D.

NURSING EVALUATION OF MEDICATION EFFECTIVENESS

Depending on therapeutic intent, effectiveness is evidenced by the following.
- Increase in bone density
- No fractures

Calcitonin

SELECT PROTOTYPE MEDICATION: Calcitonin-salmon

PURPOSE

EXPECTED PHARMACOLOGICAL ACTION

- Decreases bone resorption by inhibiting the activity of osteoclasts in osteoporosis
- Increases renal calcium excretion by inhibiting tubular resorption

THERAPEUTIC USES

Treats (but does not prevent) postmenopausal osteoporosis, moderate to severe Paget's disease, hypercalcemia caused by hyperparathyroidism, and cancer

COMPLICATIONS

Nausea

CLIENT EDUCATION: Nausea is usually self-limiting.

Nasal dryness and irritation with intranasal route

NURSING ACTIONS: Inspect nasal mucosa periodically for ulceration.

CLIENT EDUCATION: Alternate nostrils daily.

CONTRAINDICATIONS/PRECAUTIONS

- This medication is Pregnancy Risk Category C.
- The medication is contraindicated in clients who have hypersensitivity to the medication or fish protein. Perform an allergy skin test prior to administration if the client is at risk.
- Use cautiously with children, clients who are lactating, and clients who have kidney disease.
- Intranasal spray is only approved for treatment of postmenopausal osteoporosis.

INTERACTIONS

Concurrent use with lithium can decrease blood lithium levels.
NURSING ACTIONS: Monitor lithium levels closely.

NURSING ADMINISTRATION

- Calcitonin-salmon is administered IM, subcutaneously, or intranasally. The intranasal route is reserved for clients who have postmenopausal osteoporosis. Qᴘᴄᴄ
- Keep the container in an upright position.
- Check for Chvostek's or Trousseau's signs to monitor for hypocalcemia.
- Monitor bone density scans periodically.

CLIENT EDUCATION

- Consume a diet high in calcium and vitamin D.
- Rotate subcutaneous injection sites to prevent inflammation.
- Administer intranasal formulation in a different nostril each day.

NURSING EVALUATION OF MEDICATION EFFECTIVENESS

Depending on therapeutic intent, effectiveness is evidenced by the following.
- Increase in bone density
- Blood calcium level within the expected reference range of 9 to 10.5 mg/dL

Active Learning Scenario

A nurse in a provider's office is teaching a client who is postmenopausal and at high risk for osteoporosis about a new prescription for alendronate. What should the nurse teach the client about this medication? Use the ATI Active Learning Template: Medication to complete this item.

THERAPEUTIC USES: Identify the therapeutic use for alendronate.

COMPLICATIONS: List two adverse effects of this medication.

NURSING INTERVENTIONS

- Describe two diagnostic tests to monitor.
- Describe two nursing actions.

Application Exercises

1. A nurse is providing teaching to a client who is taking raloxifene to prevent postmenopausal osteoporosis. The nurse should advise the client that which of the following are adverse effects of this medication? (Select all that apply.)

   A. Hot flashes

   B. Lump in breast

   C. Swelling or redness in calf

   D. Shortness of breath

   E. Difficulty swallowing

2. A nurse is teaching a client who has osteoporosis and a new prescription for alendronate. Which of the following instructions should the nurse provide? (Select all that apply.)

   A. Take medication in the morning before eating.

   B. Chew tablets to increase bioavailability.

   C. Drink 8 oz of water with each tablet.

   D. Take medication with an antacid if heartburn occurs.

   E. Avoid lying down after taking this medication.

3. A nurse is caring for a client who has a new prescription for calcitonin-salmon for osteoporosis. Which of the following tests should the nurse tell the client to expect before beginning this medication?

   A. Skin test for allergy to the medication

   B. ECG to rule out cardiac dysrhythmias

   C. Mantoux test to rule out exposure to tuberculosis

   D. Liver function tests to assess risk for medication toxicity

4. A nurse is providing instruction to a client who has a new prescription for calcitonin-salmon for postmenopausal osteoporosis. Which of the following instructions should the nurse include in the teaching?

   A. Swallow tablets on an empty stomach with plenty of water.

   B. Watch for skin rash and redness when applying calcitonin-salmon topically.

   C. Mix the liquid medication with juice and take it after meals.

   D. Alternate nostrils each time calcitonin-salmon is inhaled.

5. A nurse is caring for a client whose blood calcium is 8.8 mg/dL. Which of the following medications should the nurse anticipate administering to this client? (Select all that apply.)

   A. Calcitonin-salmon

   B. Calcium carbonate

   C. Zoledronic acid

   D. Ibandronate

   E. Vitamin D

Active Learning Scenario Key

Using the ATI Active Learning Template: Medication

THERAPEUTIC USES: In this client who is at high risk for osteoporosis, the purpose of alendronate is to prevent osteoporosis from occurring by decreasing resorption of bone. The medication also is used to treat existing osteoporosis and Paget's disease.

COMPLICATIONS: Alendronate can cause esophagitis and esophageal ulceration; other GI effects (nausea, diarrhea, and constipation); muscle pain; and visual disturbances. Rarely, it can cause atraumatic femoral fracture.

NURSING INTERVENTIONS

Diagnostic tests: Blood calcium, bone density scans

Nursing interventions
- Assess the client's ability to follow administration directions (must be able to sit upright or stand for at least 30 min after taking alendronate).
- Teach the client to take this medication first thing in the morning with at least 240 mL (8 oz) water and wait 30 min before eating or drinking anything else or taking any other medications or supplements.
- Teach the client other ways to help prevent osteoporosis, such as performing weight-bearing exercises daily and obtaining adequate amounts of calcium and vitamin D.

Ⓝ *NCLEX® Connection: Pharmacological and Parenteral Therapies, Medication Administration*

Application Exercises Key

1. A. **CORRECT:** Raloxifene can cause hot flashes or increase existing hot flashes.
   B. Raloxifene does not cause breast lumps. It is used therapeutically to protect against breast and endometrial cancer.
   C. **CORRECT:** Raloxifene increases the risk for thrombophlebitis, which can cause swelling or redness in the calf or other extremity.
   D. **CORRECT:** Raloxifene increases the risk for pulmonary embolism, which can cause shortness of breath.
   E. Difficulty swallowing due to esophagitis is an adverse effect of bisphosphonates, such as alendronate, but is not an adverse effect of taking raloxifene.

Ⓝ *NCLEX® Connection: Pharmacological and Parenteral Therapies, Adverse Effects/Contraindications/Side Effects/Interactions*

2. A. **CORRECT:** Take alendronate first thing in the morning before eating to increase absorption.
   B. Chewing alendronate tablets can cause esophageal ulcers. Swallow the tablets whole.
   C. **CORRECT:** Clients should drink at least 240 mL (8 oz) water with alendronate tablets.
   D. Do not take alendronate within 2 hr of an antacid.
   E. **CORRECT:** Clients should sit upright or stand for at least 30 min after taking alendronate.

Ⓝ *NCLEX® Connection: Pharmacological and Parenteral Therapies, Medication Administration*

3. A. **CORRECT:** Anaphylaxis can occur if the client is allergic to calcitonin-salmon. A skin test to determine allergy might be done before starting this medication. The nurse also should ask the client about previous allergies to fish.
   B. An ECG to rule out cardiac dysrhythmias is not necessary before beginning calcitonin-salmon. This medication does not affect heart rhythm.
   C. A Mantoux test to rule out exposure to tuberculosis is not necessary before beginning calcitonin-salmon. This medication does not affect resistance to TB.
   D. Liver function tests are not necessary before beginning calcitonin-salmon. This medication is metabolized in the kidneys and does not affect the liver.

Ⓝ *NCLEX® Connection: Pharmacological and Parenteral Therapies, Expected Actions/Outcomes*

4. A. Clients should drink at least 240 mL (8 oz) water with alendronate tablets and take it on an empty stomach to promote absorption and prevent esophagitis.
   B. Calcitonin-salmon is not supplied as a topical preparation.
   C. Clients should drink at least 60 mL (2 oz) water with alendronate liquid solution.
   D. **CORRECT:** Calcitonin-salmon can be administered IM or subcutaneously, but is commonly administered intranasally for postmenopausal osteoporosis. The client should alternate nostrils daily.

Ⓝ *NCLEX® Connection: Pharmacological and Parenteral Therapies, Medication Administration*

5. A. Calcitonin-salmon increases excretion of calcium and should not be given to a client who has a blood calcium of 8.8 mg/dL.
   B. **CORRECT:** The client's blood calcium level is below the expected reference range. Calcium carbonate is an oral form of calcium used to increase blood calcium to the expected reference range.
   C. Zoledronic acid is an IV bisphosphonate used to treat osteoporosis. This medication can decrease blood calcium levels by inhibiting bone resorption of calcium, and should not be given to a client who has a blood calcium of 8.8 mg/dL.
   D. Ibandronate is a bisphosphonate used to treat osteoporosis. This medication can decrease blood calcium levels by inhibiting bone reabsorption of calcium. It should not be given to a client who has a blood calcium of 8.8 mg/dL.
   E. **CORRECT:** Vitamin D is often prescribed to ensure calcium absorption.

Ⓝ *NCLEX® Connection: Pharmacological and Parenteral Therapies, Expected Actions/Outcomes*

When reviewing the following chapters, keep in mind the relevant topics and tasks of the NCLEX outline, in particular:

Pharmacological and Parenteral Therapies

MEDICATION ADMINISTRATION

Evaluate appropriateness and accuracy of medication order for client.

Educate client about medications.

Administer and document medications given by parenteral routes.

PARENTERAL/INTRAVENOUS THERAPIES: Monitor the use of an infusion pump.

PHARMACOLOGICAL PAIN MANAGEMENT

Administer medications for pain management.

Assess client's need for administration of a PRN pain medication.

Evaluate and document the client's use and response to pain medications.

ADVERSE EFFECTS/CONTRAINDICATIONS/SIDE EFFECTS/INTERACTIONS

Assess the client for actual or potential side effects and adverse effects of medications.

Identify a contraindication to the administration of a medication to the client.

Monitor for anticipated interactions among the client's prescribed medications and fluids.

Provide information to the client on common side effects/adverse effects/potential interactions of medications, and inform the client of when to notify the primary health care provider.

EXPECTED ACTIONS/OUTCOMES: Evaluate client's response to medication.

CHAPTER 33 # Non-Opioid Analgesics

Non-opioid analgesics can have anti-inflammatory, antipyretic, and analgesic actions. These medications include nonsteroidal anti-inflammatory drugs (NSAIDs) and acetaminophen.

Nonsteroidal anti-inflammatory drugs

SELECT PROTOTYPE MEDICATIONS

First-generation NSAIDs (COX-1 and COX-2 inhibitors)
- Aspirin
- Ibuprofen
- Naproxen
- Indomethacin
- Diclofenac
- Ketorolac
- Meloxicam
- Piroxicam
- Ketoprofen

Second-generation NSAIDs (selective COX-2 inhibitor):
Celecoxib

PURPOSE

EXPECTED PHARMACOLOGICAL ACTION

Inhibition of cyclooxygenase: Inhibition of COX-1 can result in decreased platelet aggregation and kidney damage while inhibition of COX-2 results in decreased inflammation, fever, and pain and does not decrease platelet aggregation.

THERAPEUTIC USES
- Inflammation suppression
- Analgesia for mild to moderate pain (with osteoarthritis and rheumatoid arthritis)
- Fever reduction
- Dysmenorrhea
- Inhibition of platelet aggregation, which protects against ischemic stroke and myocardial infarction (aspirin)
- Celecoxib suppresses inflammation, relieves pain, decreases fever, and can protect against colorectal cancer.

COMPLICATIONS

Gastrointestinal discomfort

Dyspepsia, abdominal pain, heartburn, nausea

NURSING ACTIONS
- Damage to gastric mucosa can lead to gastrointestinal (GI) bleeding and perforation, especially with long-term use.
- Risk is increased in older adults, clients who smoke or have alcohol use disorder, and those who have a history of peptic ulcers or previous inability to tolerate NSAIDs.
- Observe for indications of GI bleeding (passage of black or dark-colored stools, severe abdominal pain, nausea, vomiting).
- Administer a proton pump inhibitor (omeprazole) or an H2 receptor antagonist (cimetidine) to decrease the risk of ulcer formation.
- Use prophylaxis agents (misoprostol).

CLIENT EDUCATION
- Take medication with food or with an 8 oz glass of water or milk.
- Avoid alcohol.

Impaired kidney function

Decreased urine output, weight gain from fluid retention, increased BUN, and creatinine levels

NURSING ACTIONS
- Use cautiously with older adults and clients who have heart failure.
- Monitor I&O and kidney function (BUN, creatinine).

Increased risk of heart attack and stroke

With non-aspirin NSAIDs

NURSING ACTIONS: Use the smallest effective dose for clients who have cardiovascular disease.

Salicylism (can occur with aspirin)

MANIFESTATIONS: Tinnitus, sweating, headache, dizziness, and respiratory alkalosis

CLIENT EDUCATION: Notify the provider and stop taking aspirin if manifestations occur.

Reye syndrome (rare but serious complication)

This occurs when aspirin is used for fever reduction in children and adolescents who have a viral illness (chickenpox or influenza).

CLIENT EDUCATION: Avoid giving aspirin when a child or adolescent has a viral illness (chickenpox or influenza). Qs

Aspirin toxicity

Progresses from the mild findings in salicylism to sweating, high fever, acidosis, dehydration, electrolyte imbalances, coma, and respiratory depression

NURSING ACTIONS
- Aspirin toxicity should be managed as a medical emergency in the hospital.
- Activated charcoal can be given to decrease absorption.
- Hemodialysis can be indicated.
- Cool the client with tepid water.
- Correct dehydration and electrolyte imbalance with IV fluids.
- Reverse acidosis and promote salicylate excretion with bicarbonate.
- Perform gastric lavage.

CONTRAINDICATIONS/PRECAUTIONS

FIRST-GENERATION NSAIDS

- Pregnancy (Pregnancy Risk Category D)
- Peptic ulcer disease
- Bleeding disorders (hemophilia and vitamin K deficiency)
- Hypersensitivity to aspirin and other NSAIDs
- Aspirin is contraindicated in children and adolescents who have a viral illness (chickenpox, influenza).

NURSING ACTIONS: Use NSAIDs cautiously in the following.
- Older adult clients ©
- Clients who smoke cigarettes
- Clients who have *Helicobacter pylori* infection, hypovolemia, asthma, chronic urticaria, bleeding disorders
- Clients taking ACE inhibitors and ARBs

Ketorolac is contraindicated in clients who have advanced kidney disease. Use should be no longer than 5 days because of the risk for gastrointestinal, cardiovascular, and renal complications. Qs

SECOND-GENERATION NSAIDS

- Celecoxib, an NSAID COX-2 inhibitor, is a last-choice medication for chronic pain due to the increased risk of myocardial infarction (MI) and stroke due to secondary suppression of vasodilation.
- Celecoxib is contraindicated in clients who have an allergy to sulfonamides.

INTERACTIONS

Anticoagulants (heparin and warfarin) increase the risk of bleeding.
NURSING ACTIONS: Monitor PTT, PT, and INR.

CLIENT EDUCATION: Remain aware of the potential risk of bleeding when an NSAID is combined with an anticoagulant. Report indications of bleeding.

Glucocorticoids increase the risk of gastric bleeding.
CLIENT EDUCATION: Take antiulcer prophylaxis (misoprostol) to decrease the risk for gastric ulcer.

Alcohol increases the risk of bleeding and gastric ulceration.
CLIENT EDUCATION: Avoid consuming alcoholic beverages to decrease the risk of GI bleeding.

Ibuprofen decreases the antiplatelet effects of low-dose aspirin used to prevent MI.
CLIENT EDUCATION: Do not take ibuprofen concurrently with aspirin.

Ketorolac and concurrent use of other NSAIDs increase the risk of known adverse effects.
NURSING ACTIONS: Ketorolac should not be used concurrently with other NSAIDs.

Celecoxib can decrease the diuresis of furosemide and the antihypertensive effects of ACE inhibitors.
Clients prescribed ACE inhibitors and ARBs should avoid taking NSAIDS as the combination increases the risk for acute renal failure.

Over-the-counter medications
- Supplements (feverfew, garlic, ginger) can increase the risk for bleeding in clients who are taking NSAIDs.
- The supplement ginkgo biloba can suppress coagulation and is used with caution in clients who are taking NSAIDs.

CLIENT EDUCATION: Tell the provider about any over-the-counter medications, vitamins, or herbal supplements before taking them.

NURSING ADMINISTRATION

- Ketorolac can be used for short-term treatment of moderate to severe pain (that's associated with postoperative recovery).
  - Concurrent use with opioids allows for lower dosages of opioids and thus minimizes adverse effects (constipation and respiratory depression).
  - Ketorolac is usually first administered parenterally and then switched to oral doses. Use should not be longer than 5 days because of the risk for gastrointestinal, cardiovascular, and renal complications.
- Administer IV ibuprofen as an infusion over 30 min. The client should be hydrated before infusion to prevent kidney damage.

CLIENT EDUCATION
- Stop aspirin 1 week before an elective surgery or expected date of childbirth. Q EBP
- Take NSAIDs with food, milk, or an 8 oz glass of water to reduce gastric discomfort.
- Do not chew or crush enteric-coated or sustained-release aspirin tablets.

NURSING EVALUATION OF MEDICATION EFFECTIVENESS

Depending on therapeutic intent, effectiveness can be evidenced by the following.

- Reduction in inflammation
- Reduction of fever
- Relief from mild to moderate pain
- Relief from dysmenorrhea

Acetaminophen

PURPOSE

EXPECTED PHARMACOLOGICAL ACTION: Slows the production of prostaglandins in the central nervous system

THERAPEUTIC USES

- Analgesic (relief of pain) effect
- Antipyretic (reduction of fever) effects
- Preferred to NSAIDs for children suspected of having a viral infection (e.g., chicken pox, influenza)

COMPLICATIONS

Adverse effects are rare at therapeutic dosages.

Acute toxicity

- Results in liver damage with early manifestations of nausea, vomiting, diarrhea, sweating, and abdominal discomfort progressing to hepatic failure, coma, and death
- Overt indications of hepatic injury appear 48 to 72 hr after ingestion.

NURSING ACTIONS
- Ensure the client's daily acetaminophen total intake does not exceed recommended limits (4 g/day for most clients, 3 g/day for undernourished clients, and 2 g/day for clients who consume more than three servings of alcohol daily).
- Administer the antidote, acetylcysteine, via duodenal tube to prevent emesis and subsequent aspiration.

CLIENT EDUCATION: Take acetaminophen as prescribed and do not exceed recommended daily dosages. Parents should carefully follow the provider's advice regarding administration to children.

CONTRAINDICATIONS/PRECAUTIONS

- Pregnancy Risk Category B for oral, rectal use, and C for IV use
- Avoid in clients who have hypersensitivity to a component, severe liver impairment or disease, kidney impairment, chronic alcohol use disorder, or malnutrition.
- Use IV form cautiously for clients who are breastfeeding.

INTERACTIONS

Alcohol increases the risk of liver damage.
CLIENT EDUCATION: Remain aware of the potential risk of liver damage with consumption of alcohol.

Acetaminophen slows the metabolism of warfarin, leading to increased levels of warfarin. This places clients at risk for bleeding.
NURSING ACTIONS: Monitor prothrombin time and INR levels and adjust dosages of warfarin accordingly.

CLIENT EDUCATION: Observe for indications of bleeding (bruising, petechiae, hematuria).

NURSING ADMINISTRATION

- Teach clients to read medication labels carefully to determine the amount of medication contained in each dose and to only take one product containing acetaminophen at a time.
- Administer orally with a full glass of water, with or without food.

CLIENT EDUCATION: If pain or fever persists for more than 3 days, contact the provider. Adults should not take acetaminophen for more than 10 days or children for more than 5 days without provider approval.

NURSING EVALUATION OF MEDICATION EFFECTIVENESS

Depending on therapeutic intent, effectiveness can be evidenced by the following.

- Relief of pain
- Reduction of fever

Active Learning Scenario

A nurse at a provider's office is providing teaching to a client who has osteoarthritis and is starting long-term therapy with NSAIDs. What should the nurse include in the teaching? Use the ATI Active Learning Template: Medication to complete this item.

THERAPEUTIC USES

COMPLICATIONS: Describe two adverse effects.

NURSING INTERVENTIONS: Describe three nursing actions, including two laboratory values the nurse should monitor.

Application Exercises

1. A nurse is assessing a client who has salicylism. Which of the following findings should the nurse expect? (Select all that apply.)
   - A. Dizziness
   - B. Diarrhea
   - C. Jaundice
   - D. Tinnitus
   - E. Headache

2. A nurse in an emergency department is performing an admission assessment for a client who has severe aspirin toxicity. Which of the following findings should the nurse expect? (Select all that apply.)
   - A. Body temperature 35° C (95° F)
   - B. Dehydration
   - C. Lung crackles
   - D. Cool, dry skin
   - E. Respiratory depression

3. A nurse is taking a history for a client who reports taking aspirin about four times daily for a sprained wrist. Which of the following prescribed medications taken by the client is contraindicated with aspirin?
   - A. Digoxin
   - B. Metformin
   - C. Warfarin
   - D. Nitroglycerin

4. A nurse is teaching a client about a new prescription for celecoxib. Which of the following information should the nurse include in the teaching?
   - A. Increases the risk for a myocardial infarction
   - B. Decreases the risk of stroke
   - C. Inhibits COX-1
   - D. Increases platelet aggregation

5. A nurse is admitting a client to the hospital following acetaminophen toxicity. Which of the following medications should the nurse expect to administer to this client?
   - A. Acetylcysteine
   - B. Pegfilgrastim
   - C. Misoprostol
   - D. Naltrexone

Application Exercises Key

1. A. **CORRECT:** The client who has salicylism can have dizziness, which is an expected finding.
   B. The client who takes aspirin is not expected to develop diarrhea. However, monitor the color of the client's stools to determine if the client has a gastric bleed from taking aspirin.
   C. The client who takes aspirin will metabolize the medication through the liver. Jaundice is not an expected finding in salicylism.
   D. **CORRECT:** The client who has salicylism can have tinnitus, which is an expected finding.
   E. **CORRECT:** The client who has salicylism can have a headache, which is an expected finding.

   Ⓝ *NCLEX® Connection: Pharmacological and Parenteral Therapies, Expected Actions/Outcomes*

2. A. Expect hyperthermia as a manifestation of severe aspirin toxicity.
   B. **CORRECT:** Expect dehydration as a manifestation of severe aspirin toxicity.
   C. Lung crackles are not an expected finding.
   D. Expect diaphoresis as a manifestation of severe aspirin toxicity. Cool, dry skin is not an expected finding.
   E. **CORRECT:** Respiratory depression due to increasing respiratory acidosis is an expected late manifestation of severe aspirin toxicity.

   Ⓝ *NCLEX® Connection: Pharmacological and Parenteral Therapies, Adverse Effects/Contraindications/Side Effects/Interactions*

3. A. Digoxin does not interact with aspirin and therefore is not contraindicated.
   B. Metformin does not interact with aspirin and therefore is not contraindicated.
   C. **CORRECT:** The effect of warfarin and other anticoagulants is increased by aspirin, which inhibits platelet aggregation. This client would have an increased risk for bleeding. Use of aspirin generally is contraindicated for clients who take warfarin.
   D. Nitroglycerin does not interact with aspirin and therefore is not contraindicated.

   Ⓝ *NCLEX® Connection: Pharmacological and Parenteral Therapies, Adverse Effects/Contraindications/Side Effects/Interactions*

4. A. **CORRECT:** The client who takes celecoxib has an increased risk for a myocardial infarction secondary to suppressing vasodilation.
   B. The client who takes celecoxib has an increased risk for stroke secondary to suppressing vasodilation.
   C. Celecoxib inhibits COX-2, which suppresses inflammation, relieves pain, decreases fever, and protects against colorectal cancer.
   D. Celecoxib does not have an effect on platelet aggregation. However, the medication suppresses vasodilation.

   Ⓝ *NCLEX® Connection: Pharmacological and Parenteral Therapies, Dosage Calculations*

5. A. **CORRECT:** Administer acetylcysteine, which is the antidote for acetaminophen toxicity.
   B. To increase the body's production of neutrophils, administer pegfilgrastim.
   C. To prevent the formation of gastric ulcers, administer misoprostol, which is a prostaglandin hormone.
   D. To prevent alcohol craving, administer naltrexone, which is an opioid antagonist.

   Ⓝ *NCLEX® Connection: Pharmacological and Parenteral Therapies, Expected Actions/Outcomes*

Active Learning Scenario Key

Using the ATI Active Learning Template: Medication

THERAPEUTIC USES: NSAIDs will treat mild to moderate joint pain and stiffness, and decrease inflammation in the client who has osteoarthritis.

COMPLICATIONS
- Gastrointestinal effects can occur, including anorexia, abdominal pain, nausea, vomiting, and heartburn.
- GI bleeding can occur because NSAIDs affect platelet function.
- Nephrotoxicity can occur.
- NSAIDs can cause CNS effects (dizziness, headache, blurred vision, and tinnitus).
- Allergy can occur, including cross allergy with other NSAIDs (aspirin).

NURSING INTERVENTIONS
- Monitor Hgb/Hct and kidney function tests.
- Assess the client for previous allergy to NSAIDs.
- Assess the GI system, and ask about any history of GI bleed or peptic ulcer disease.
- Advise the client to take the medication with food, milk, or an 8 oz glass of water to prevent GI distress.
- Advise the client to tell provider about any over-the-counter medications, vitamins, or herbal supplements before taking them.

Ⓝ *NCLEX® Connection: Pharmacological and Parenteral Therapies, Medication Administration*

CHAPTER 34

Opioid Agonists and Antagonists

Opioid analgesics are medications used to treat moderate to severe pain. Most opioid analgesics reduce pain by attaching to a receptor in the central nervous system, altering perception and response to pain.

Opioids are classified as agonists, agonist-antagonists, and antagonists. An agonist attaches to a receptor and produces a response (analgesia, euphoria, sedation, respiratory depression, and other effects). An agonist-antagonist causes an analgesic response when administered alone and prevents an analgesic response when administered with a pure agonist. An antagonist does not produce analgesia or any other effects of opioids. Its main use is to reverse respiratory and CNS depression caused by overdose of opioids.

The desired outcome is to reduce pain and increase activity with few adverse effects. Opioid agonists are in Schedule II under the Controlled Substances Act.

Opioid agonists

SELECT PROTOTYPE MEDICATION: Morphine

OTHER MEDICATIONS
- Fentanyl
- Meperidine
- Methadone
- Codeine
- Oxycodone
- Hydromorphone

ROUTE OF ADMINISTRATION
- Morphine: Oral, subcutaneous, IM, IV, epidural, intrathecal Qpcc
- Fentanyl: IV, IM, transmucosal, transdermal
- Meperidine: Oral, subcutaneous, IM, IV
- Codeine: Oral, subcutaneous, IM, IV
- Methadone: Oral, subcutaneous, IM
- Oxycodone: Oral, rectal
- Hydromorphone: Oral, subcutaneous, IM, IV

PURPOSE

EXPECTED PHARMACOLOGICAL ACTION: Opioid agonists and other morphine-like medications (fentanyl), act on the mu receptors and, to a lesser degree, on kappa receptors. Activation of mu receptors produces analgesia, respiratory depression, euphoria, and sedation, whereas kappa receptor activation produces analgesia, sedation, and decreased GI motility. Activation of mu receptors can also be linked to physical dependence.

THERAPEUTIC USES
- Relief of moderate to severe pain (postoperative, myocardial infarction, following childbirth, cancer)
- Sedation
- Reduction of bowel motility relief of diarrhea
- Cough suppression (codeine)

COMPLICATIONS

Respiratory depression

NURSING ACTIONS
- Monitor vital signs.
- Stop opioids if the client's respiratory rate is less than 12/min, and notify the provider.
- Have naloxone and resuscitation equipment available.
- Avoid use of opioids with CNS depressant medications (barbiturates, benzodiazepines, consumption of alcohol).

Constipation

NURSING ACTIONS
- Teach the client to increase fluid/fiber intake and physical activity.
- Administer a stimulant laxative (bisacodyl) to counteract decreased bowel motility or a stool softener (docusate sodium) to prevent constipation.
- For clients who have end-stage disorders (cancer or AIDS), administer an opioid antagonist (methylnaltrexone) designed to treat severe constipation in opioid-dependent clients.

Orthostatic hypotension

NURSING ACTIONS
- Advise clients to sit or lie down if lightheadedness or dizziness occurs.
- Due to the dilation effect to the peripheral arterioles and veins, avoid sudden changes in position by slowly moving clients from a lying to a sitting or standing position.
- Provide assistance with ambulation as needed.

Urinary retention

NURSING ACTIONS
- Monitor I&O.
- Assess the bladder for distention by palpating the lower abdominal area every 4 to 6 hr because opioid medication can suppress awareness that the bladder is full.

CLIENT EDUCATION
- Void every 4 hr.
- Medications with anticholinergic properties (tricyclic antidepressants, antihistamines) can increase manifestations.

Cough suppression

NURSING ACTIONS: Auscultate the lungs for crackles and instruct clients to increase intake of fluid to liquefy secretions.

CLIENT EDUCATION: Cough at regular intervals to prevent accumulation of secretions in the airway.

Sedation

CLIENT EDUCATION: Avoid hazardous activities (driving or operating heavy machinery).

Biliary colic

NURSING ACTIONS: Avoid giving morphine to clients who have a history of biliary colic. Use meperidine as an alternative.

Nausea/vomiting

NURSING ACTIONS: Administer an antiemetic.

Opioid toxicity triad

Coma, respiratory depression, and pinpoint pupils

NURSING ACTIONS
- Monitor vital signs.
- Provide mechanical ventilation.
- Administer naloxone, an opioid antagonist that reverses respiratory depression and other manifestations of toxicity.

CONTRAINDICATIONS/PRECAUTIONS

- **Warnings**
  - Pregnancy: Use opioids with caution; avoid chronic use.
  - Lactation: Use opioids with caution; avoid chronic use (can cause withdrawal in the newborn and respiratory depression).
  - Reproductive: Notify provider if pregnancy is planned or suspected.
- Morphine is contraindicated after biliary tract surgery. Qs
- Morphine is contraindicated for premature infants during and after delivery because of respiratory depressant effects.
- Meperidine is contraindicated for clients who have kidney failure because of the accumulation of normeperidine, which can result in seizures and neurotoxicity.

- Use cautiously with the following.
  - Clients who have asthma, emphysema, or head injuries; infants; and older adult clients (risk of respiratory depression) Ⓖ
  - Clients who are extremely obese (greater risk for prolonged adverse effects because of the accumulation of medication that is metabolized at a slower rate)
  - Clients who have inflammatory bowel disease (risk of megacolon or paralytic ileus)
  - Clients who have an enlarged prostate (risk of acute urinary retention)
  - Clients who have hepatic or renal disease

INTERACTIONS

CNS depressants (barbiturates, phenobarbital, benzodiazepines, alcohol) have additive CNS depression action.
CLIENT EDUCATION
- Avoid the use of these medications in conjunction with opioid agonists.
- Avoid consumption of alcohol.

Anticholinergic agents (atropine or scopolamine), antihistamines (diphenhydramine), and tricyclic antidepressants (amitriptyline) have additive anticholinergic effects (constipation, urinary retention).
CLIENT EDUCATION: Increase fluids and dietary fiber to prevent constipation.

Meperidine can interact with monoamine oxidase inhibitors (MAOIs) and cause hyperpyrexic coma, characterized by excitation, delirium, seizures, and respiratory depression.
NURSING ACTIONS: Avoid the use of meperidine with MAOIs to prevent occurrence of this syndrome.

Antihypertensives have additive hypotensive effects.
CLIENT EDUCATION: Refrain from using opioids with antihypertensive agents.

Additional medications (amphetamines, clonidine, and dextromethorphan) can increase opioid-induced analgesia.
CLIENT EDUCATION: Avoid taking other medications that have a CNS effect with opioid medication.

NURSING ADMINISTRATION

- Assess pain level on a regular basis. Document the client's response. QEBP
- Take baseline vital signs. If the respiratory rate is less than 12/min, notify the provider and withhold the medication.
- Follow controlled substance procedures.
- Double-check opioid doses with another nurse prior to administration.
- Administer IV opioids slowly over 4 to 5 min. Have naloxone and resuscitation equipment available.
- Warn clients not to increase dosage without consulting the provider.

- For clients who have cancer, administer opioids on a fixed schedule around the clock. Administer supplemental doses as needed.
- Advise clients who have physical dependence not to discontinue opioids abruptly. Opioids should be withdrawn slowly, and the dosage should be tapered over a period of 3 days.
- Closely monitor patient-controlled analgesia (PCA) pump settings (dose, lockout interval, 4-hr limit). Reassure clients regarding safety measures that safeguard against self-administration of excessive doses. Encourage clients to use PCA prophylactically prior to activities likely to augment pain levels.
- When switching clients from PCA to oral doses of opioids, make sure the client receives adequate PCA dosing until the onset of oral medication takes place.
- The first administration of a transdermal fentanyl patch will take several hours (up to 24 hours) to achieve the desired therapeutic effect. Administer short-acting opioids as needed prior to onset of therapeutic effects and for breakthrough pain.

NURSING EVALUATION OF MEDICATION EFFECTIVENESS

Depending on the therapeutic intent, effectiveness can be evidenced by the following.
- Relief of moderate to severe pain (postoperative pain, cancer pain, myocardial pain)
- Cough suppression
- Resolution of diarrhea

Agonist-antagonist opioids

SELECT PROTOTYPE MEDICATION: Butorphanol

OTHER MEDICATION
- Nalbuphine
- Buprenorphine
- Pentazocine

ROUTE OF ADMINISTRATION
- Butorphanol: IV, IM, intranasal
- Nalbuphine: IV, IM, subcutaneous
- Buprenorphine: IV, IM, sublingual, transdermal
- Pentazocine: PO, IV, IM, subcutaneous

PURPOSE

EXPECTED PHARMACOLOGICAL ACTION
- These medications act as antagonists on mu receptors and agonists on kappa receptors, except for buprenorphine, whose agonist/antagonist activity is on opposite receptors.
- Compared to pure opioid agonists, agonist-antagonists have the following.
  - Low potential for abuse, causing little euphoria. In fact, high doses can cause adverse effects (anxiety, restlessness, mental confusion).
  - Less respiratory depression
  - Less analgesic effect

THERAPEUTIC USES
- Relief of mild to moderate pain
- Treatment of opioid dependence (buprenorphine)
- Adjunct to balanced anesthesia
- Relief of labor pain

COMPLICATIONS

Abstinence syndrome

Cramping, hypertension, vomiting, fever, and anxiety

NURSING ACTIONS
- This syndrome can be precipitated when these medications are given to clients who are physically dependent on opioid agonists.
- Advise clients to stop opioid agonists (morphine) before using agonist-antagonist medications (pentazocine).
- Avoid giving to clients if undisclosed opioid use is suspected.

Sedation, respiratory depression

NURSING ACTIONS
- Have naloxone and resuscitation equipment available.
- Monitor for respiratory depression.

Dizziness

CLIENT EDUCATION: Use caution in standing up and avoid driving or using heavy machinery.

Headache

NURSING ACTIONS
- Monitor for headache.
- Assess level of consciousness.

CONTRAINDICATIONS/PRECAUTIONS

Use cautiously in clients who have a history of myocardial infarction, kidney or liver disease, respiratory depression, or head injury and clients who are physically dependent on opioids. Qs

INTERACTIONS

CNS depressants and alcohol can cause additive effects.
NURSING ACTIONS
- Use together cautiously.
- Monitor respirations.

Opioid agonists can antagonize and reduce analgesic effects of the opioid.
NURSING ACTIONS: Do not use concurrently.

NURSING ADMINISTRATION

- Obtain baseline vital signs. If the respiratory rate is less than 12/min, withhold the medication and notify the provider. ○EBP
- Have naloxone and resuscitation equipment available.
- Assess clients for opioid dependence prior to administration. Agonist-antagonists can trigger withdrawal manifestations.

CLIENT EDUCATION
- Do not increase dosage without consulting the provider.
- Use caution when getting out of bed or standing. Do not operate heavy machinery or drive until CNS effects are known.

NURSING EVALUATION OF MEDICATION EFFECTIVENESS

Monitor for improvement of manifestations (relief of pain).

Opioid antagonists

SELECT PROTOTYPE MEDICATION: Naloxone

OTHER MEDICATIONS
- Naltrexone
- Methylnaltrexone
- Alvimopan
- Naloxegol
- Naldemedine

ROUTE OF ADMINISTRATION
- Naloxone: IV, IM, subcutaneous
- Naltrexone: Oral, IM
- Methylnaltrexone: Subcutaneous
- Alvimopan: Oral
- Naloxegol: Oral
- Naldemedine: Oral

PURPOSE

EXPECTED PHARMACOLOGICAL ACTION: Opioid antagonists interfere with the action of opioids by competing for opioid receptors. Opioid antagonists have no effect in the absence of opioids.

THERAPEUTIC USES
- Treatment of opioid abuse by preventing euphoria (naltrexone)
- Reversal of effects of opioids (respiratory depression [naloxone])
- Reversal of respiratory depression in an infant (naloxone)
- Reversal of severe opioid-caused constipation in clients who have late-stage cancer or other disorders (methylnaltrexone, alvimopan)
- Reversal of post-operative opioid effects (respiratory depression, ileus)

COMPLICATIONS

Tachycardia and tachypnea

NURSING ACTIONS
- Monitor heart rhythm (risk of ventricular tachycardia) and respiratory function.
- Have resuscitative equipment, including oxygen, on standby during administration.

Abstinence syndrome

Cramping, hypertension, vomiting, and reversal of analgesia

NURSING ACTIONS: These manifestations can occur when given to clients physically dependent on opioid agonists.

CONTRAINDICATIONS/PRECAUTIONS

- **Warnings**
  - Pregnancy
    - Naloxone: Contraindicated; can cause withdrawal syndrome in a client who has opioid dependence
    - Naltrexone: Use with caution.
  - Lactation
    - Naloxone: Safety not established
    - Naltrexone: Use with caution.
- Naloxone and naltrexone are contraindicated in clients who have opioid dependency.
- Naltrexone is contraindicated for clients who have acute hepatitis or liver failure and during lactation.

NURSING ADMINISTRATION

- Naloxone has rapid first-pass inactivation and should be administered IV, IM, or subcutaneously. Do not administer orally.
- Observe withdrawal manifestations or abrupt onset of pain. Be prepared to address the need for analgesia if given for postoperative opioid-related respiratory depression. ○EBP
- Titrate naloxone dosage to achieve reversal of respiratory depression without full reversal of pain management effects.
- Rapid infusion of naloxone can cause hypertension, tachycardia, nausea, and vomiting.
- Half-life of opioid analgesic can exceed the half-life of naloxone (60 to 90 min). Repeated dosing is required until the crisis has passed.
- Monitor respirations for up to 2 hr after use to assess for recurrence of respiratory depression and the need for repeat dosage of naloxone.
- Alvimopan is only administered for a 7-day period due to increased risk for myocardial infarction in prolonged administration.

NURSING EVALUATION OF MEDICATION EFFECTIVENESS

- Reversal of respiratory depression
  - Respirations are regular.
  - Client is without shortness of breath.
  - Respiratory rate is 12 to 20/min in adults and 30 to 60/min in newborns.
- Reduced euphoria in alcohol dependency and decreased craving for alcohol in alcohol dependency (naltrexone)
- Severe opioid–induced constipation (methylnaltrexone, naloxegol) and opioid–induced ileus (alvimopan) are relieved.

Active Learning Scenario

A nurse is providing discharge teaching for a client who is postoperative and has a new prescription for an opioid medication for incisional pain. What should the nurse include in the teaching? Use the ATI Active Learning Template: Medication to complete this item.

THERAPEUTIC USES: Describe for oxycodone.

COMPLICATIONS: List three adverse effects for oxycodone.

NURSING INTERVENTIONS: List three.

Application Exercises

1. A nurse is preparing to administer morphine to a client who has acute pain. For which of the following manifestations should the nurse monitor as an adverse effect of this medication?

   A. Urinary retention

   B. Tachypnea

   C. Hypertension

   D. Irritating cough

2. A nurse is planning to administer morphine IV to a client who is postoperative. Which of the following actions should the nurse take?

   A. Monitor for seizures and confusion with repeated doses.

   B. Protect the client's skin from the severe diarrhea that occurs with morphine.

   C. Withhold this medication if respiratory rate is less than 12/min.

   D. Give morphine intermittent via IV bolus over 30 seconds or less.

3. A nurse is reviewing the medication administration record for a client who is receiving transdermal fentanyl for severe pain. The nurse should identify that which of the following medications can cause an adverse effect when administered concurrently with fentanyl?

   A. Ampicillin

   B. Diazepam

   C. Furosemide

   D. Prednisone

4. A nurse is preparing to administer butorphanol to a client who has a history of substance use disorder. The nurse should consider which of the following information prior to administration regarding butorphanol?

   A. Butorphanol has a greater risk for abuse than morphine.

   B. Butorphanol causes a higher incidence of respiratory depression than morphine.

   C. Butorphanol cannot be reversed with an opioid antagonist.

   D. Butorphanol can cause abstinence syndrome in opioid-dependent clients.

5. A nurse is caring for a client who has end-stage cancer and is receiving morphine. The client's family member asks why the provider prescribed methylnaltrexone. Which of the following responses should the nurse make?

   A. "The medication will increase respirations."

   B. "The medication will prevent dependence on the morphine."

   C. "The medication will relieve constipation."

   D. "The medication works with the morphine to increase pain relief."

Active Learning Scenario Key

Using the ATI Active Learning Template: Medication

THERAPEUTIC USES: Opioid medication is indicated for relief of moderate to severe pain.

COMPLICATIONS

- Sedation
- Nausea/vomiting
- Constipation
- Orthostatic hypotension
- Urinary retention

NURSING INTERVENTIONS

- Instruct the client not to drive or perform other hazardous activities while using this medication.
- Notify the provider for severe nausea or vomiting.
- Prevent constipation by increasing intake of liquids and foods with fiber. Consider use of a stool softener or laxatives if necessary.
- Move the client slowly from lying or sitting to standing to minimize effects of orthostatic hypotension.
- Instruct the client to void every 4 hr. Contact the provider for manifestations of dysuria.

Ⓝ *NCLEX® Connection: Pharmacological and Parenteral Therapies, Medication Administration*

Application Exercises Key

1. A. **CORRECT:** Monitor for urinary retention because morphine can suppress awareness that the bladder is full.
   B. Monitor for respiratory depression because the activation of mu receptors has an effect on respirations.
   C. Monitor for hypotension because opioid medications can lower blood pressure by dilating peripheral arterioles and veins.
   D. Administer an opioid medication to suppress a cough because opioid receptors affect the medulla.

   Ⓝ *NCLEX® Connection: Pharmacological and Parenteral Therapies, Adverse Effects/Contraindications/Side Effects/Interactions*

2. A. When administering repeated doses of meperidine, a toxic metabolite can build up and cause severe CNS effects (agitation, confusion, and seizures).
   B. Plan to monitor for constipation because morphine affects the mu opioid receptors in the GI tract.
   C. **CORRECT:** Withhold all opioids if the respiratory rate is 12/min or less, and notify the provider.
   D. Administer morphine IV bolus slowly over 3 to 5 min to determine the client's response, and monitor the respiratory rate and blood pressure.

   Ⓝ *NCLEX® Connection: Pharmacological and Parenteral Therapies, Medication Administration*

3. A. Ampicillin, an antibiotic, does not interact with fentanyl and should not cause an adverse effect.
   B. **CORRECT:** Diazepam, a benzodiazepine, is a CNS depressant, which can interact by causing the client to become severely sedated when administered concurrently with an opioid agonist or agonist/antagonist.
   C. Furosemide, a loop diuretic, does not interact with fentanyl and should not cause an adverse effect.
   D. Prednisone, a glucocorticoid, does not interact with fentanyl and should not cause an adverse effect.

   Ⓝ *NCLEX® Connection: Pharmacological and Parenteral Therapies, Adverse Effects/Contraindications/Side Effects/Interactions*

4. A. Butorphanol has less risk for misuse than morphine.
   B. Butorphanol is less likely to cause respiratory depression than morphine.
   C. Manifestations of butorphanol toxicity can be reversed with an opioid antagonist if necessary.
   D. **CORRECT:** Opioid agonist/antagonist medications (butorphanol) can cause abstinence syndrome in opioid-dependent clients. Manifestations include abdominal pain, fever, and anxiety.

   Ⓝ *NCLEX® Connection: Pharmacological and Parenteral Therapies, Expected Actions/Outcomes*

5. A. Methylnaltrexone does not decrease analgesia or increase a depressed respiratory rate.
   B. Methylnaltrexone does not prevent dependence on opioids, such as morphine.
   C. **CORRECT:** Methylnaltrexone is an opioid antagonist used for treating severe constipation that is unrelieved by laxatives in clients who are opioid-dependent. The medication blocks the mu opioid receptors in the GI tract.
   D. Methylnaltrexone is not an adjunct to opioids for pain relief.

   Ⓝ *NCLEX® Connection: Pharmacological and Parenteral Therapies, Medication Administration*

UNIT 9   MEDICATIONS FOR PAIN AND INFLAMMATION

CHAPTER 35 *Adjuvant Medications for Pain*

Adjuvant medications for pain are used with a primary pain medication, usually an opioid agonist, to increase pain relief while reducing the dosage of the opioid agonist. Reduced dosage of the opioid results in reduced adverse reactions (respiratory depression, sedation, and constipation). Targeting pain stimulus using different types of medications often provides improved pain reduction.

Although adjuvants can relieve pain, all of them were developed to treat other conditions. Categories of medications include tricyclic antidepressants, anticonvulsants, CNS stimulants, antihistamines, glucocorticoids, bisphosphonates, and nonsteroidal anti-inflammatory drugs (NSAIDs). The use of these medications to assist in the alleviation of pain can be an off-label use.

SELECT PROTOTYPE MEDICATIONS

- **Tricyclic antidepressants:** Amitriptyline (oral)
- **Anticonvulsants:** Carbamazepine, gabapentin (oral)
- **CNS stimulants:** Methylphenidate (oral, transdermal)
- **Antihistamines:** Hydroxyzine (oral, IM)
- **Glucocorticoids:** Dexamethasone (oral, IV, IM)
- **Bisphosphonates:** Etidronate (oral)
- **NSAIDs:** Ibuprofen (oral, IV)

OTHER MEDICATIONS

- **Tricyclic antidepressants:** Imipramine, amitriptyline (oral)
- **Anticonvulsants:** Phenytoin (oral, IV)
- **CNS stimulants:** Dextroamphetamine (oral)
- **Glucocorticoids:** Prednisone (oral)
- **Bisphosphonates:** Pamidronate (IV)
- **NSAIDs:** Ketorolac (oral, IM, IV, intranasal)

PURPOSE

EXPECTED PHARMACOLOGICAL ACTION: Adjuvant medications for pain enhance the effects of opioids. ⓠEBP

THERAPEUTIC USES: These medications are used in combination with opioids and cannot be used as a substitute for opioids.

- **Tricyclic antidepressants** are used to treat depression, fibromyalgia syndrome, and neuropathic pain (cramping; aching; burning; darting; and sharp, stabbing pain).
- **Anticonvulsants** are used to relieve neuropathic pain and neuralgia.
- **CNS stimulants** augment analgesia and decrease sedation.
- **Antihistamines** decrease anxiety, prevent insomnia, and relieve nausea and vomiting.
- **Glucocorticoids** improve appetite and decrease pain from intracranial pressure, spinal cord compression, and rheumatoid arthritis.
- **Bisphosphonates** manage hypercalcemia and bone pain.
- **NSAIDs** are used to treat inflammation and fever and relieve mild to moderate pain and dysmenorrhea.

COMPLICATIONS

Tricyclic antidepressants: amitriptyline

Orthostatic hypotension
NURSING ACTIONS
- Provide assistance with ambulation as needed.
- Monitor blood pressure while the client is lying, sitting, and standing.
- Withhold the medication and notify the provider for low blood pressure or increased heart rate.
- Dose at bedtime, because this can take advantage of sedative effects and minimize hypotension during the day.

CLIENT EDUCATION: Sit or lie down if lightheadedness or dizziness occurs and change positions slowly.

Sedation
CLIENT EDUCATION: Avoid hazardous activities (driving or operating heavy machinery).

Anticholinergic effects: Dry mouth, urinary retention, constipation, and blurred vision
NURSING ACTIONS
- Administer a stimulant laxative (bisacodyl) to counteract decreased bowel motility, and a stool softener (docusate sodium) to prevent constipation.
- If blurred vision is present, instruct clients to avoid hazardous activities, wear dark glasses for intolerance to light, and report blurred vision to the provider.
- Monitor I&O, and assess the bladder for distention by palpating the lower abdomen area every 4 to 6 hr.

CLIENT EDUCATION

- Void just prior to taking medication and then every 4 hr. Report urinary retention to the provider.
- Increase fluid intake, sip fluids throughout the day, chew sugarless gum or suck on sugarless hard candy, and use an alcohol-free mouthwash.
- Increase daily fiber intake.
- Increase physical activity by engaging in a regular exercise routine.

Anticonvulsants: carbamazepine, gabapentin

NURSING ACTIONS: The effectiveness of oral contraceptives can be reduced by concurrent therapy with carbamazepine.

CLIENT EDUCATION: Use a second form of contraception if pregnancy is not desired.

Bone marrow suppression
NURSING ACTIONS

- The risk of myelosuppression is greater with carbamazepine.
- Periodically monitor complete blood count, including platelets.

CLIENT EDUCATION: Observe for indications of bone marrow suppression (easy bruising) and bleeding, fever, or sore throat, and notify the provider if they occur.

Gastrointestinal distress: Nausea, vomiting, diarrhea, and constipation
CLIENT EDUCATION

- Take the medication with food.
- If constipation occurs, increase physical activity and daily fluid and fiber intake; administer a stimulant laxative (bisacodyl) and a stool softener (docusate sodium).

Drowsiness
CLIENT EDUCATION: Avoid activities that require alertness.

Rash
NURSING ACTIONS: Withhold the medication and notify the provider.

CNS stimulants: methylphenidate

Weight loss
NURSING ACTIONS

- Monitor the client's weight.
- Encourage good nutrition.

Insomnia
CLIENT EDUCATION

- Take the last dose of the day no later than 4 p.m.
- Decrease caffeine consumption.

Antihistamines: hydroxyzine

Sedation
NURSING ACTIONS: Reduce dosage in older adult clients. Ⓖ

CLIENT EDUCATION: Avoid hazardous activities (driving or operating heavy machinery).

Dry mouth
CLIENT EDUCATION: Increase fluid intake, sip fluids throughout the day, and chew sugarless gum or suck on hard sugarless candy.

Glucocorticoids: dexamethasone

CLIENT EDUCATION: Avoid social interactions where there is potential for being exposed to infectious materials.

Adrenal insufficiency: Hypotension, dehydration, infection, weakness, lethargy, vomiting, diarrhea associated with prolonged use
CLIENT EDUCATION: Observe for indications and notify the provider if they occur.

Osteoporosis
CLIENT EDUCATION: The risk of osteoporosis can be reduced by giving calcium supplements and vitamin D along with calcitonin or a bisphosphonate (etidronate).

Fluid and electrolyte disturbances: Hypokalemia and sodium and water retention
NURSING ACTIONS

- Monitor potassium levels and administer potassium supplements as needed.
- Restrict sodium intake.

CLIENT EDUCATION

- Increase intake of potassium-rich foods (potatoes, bananas, citrus fruits).
- Report fluid retention or edema to the provider.

Glucose intolerance
NURSING ACTIONS: Monitor blood glucose levels.

Peptic ulcer disease
NURSING ACTIONS: Regularly check stools for occult blood.

CLIENT EDUCATION

- Take the medication with meals.
- Report black, tarry stools.
- Utilize an antiulcer medication.

Bisphosphonates: etidronate, pamidronate

Transient flu-like manifestations (pamidronate)
NURSING ACTIONS: Monitor for fever.

CLIENT EDUCATION: Notify the provider if manifestations occur.

Abdominal cramps, nausea, diarrhea, esophagitis (etidronate)
CLIENT EDUCATION

- Administer this medication with a full glass of water and sit or stand upright for 30 to 60 min after taking. Ⓠs
- For maximum absorption, wait 2 hr before ingesting food, antacids, or vitamins.

Venous irritation at injection site (pamidronate)
NURSING ACTIONS: Monitor the injection site and infuse with sufficient IV fluids.

Hypocalcemia
NURSING ACTIONS: Monitor calcium, magnesium, potassium, and phosphate levels. Instruct clients to report numbness/tingling around the mouth, spasms, or seizures to provider.

CLIENT EDUCATION: Take supplemental calcium and vitamin D.

NSAIDs: ibuprofen

Bone marrow suppression
NURSING ACTIONS: Periodically monitor CBC, including platelets.

CLIENT EDUCATION: Observe for indications of easy bruising and bleeding, fever, or sore throat, and notify the provider if they occur.

Gastrointestinal distress: Abdominal pain, ulceration, nausea, vomiting, and diarrhea or constipation
NURSING ACTIONS: Monitor for GI bleeding (coffee-ground emesis; bloody or black tarry stools; abdominal pain).

CLIENT EDUCATION: Take with food, milk, or antacid.

MI or stroke
NURSING ACTIONS: Monitor cardiac and neurologic status, especially in older adult clients and those who have a history of cardiac disease or risk factors for MI or stroke. Ⓖ

CONTRAINDICATIONS/PRECAUTIONS

Tricyclic antidepressants: amitriptyline

- These medications should only be used in pregnancy if maternal benefits outweigh risk to fetus, and can cause sedation to infant during lactation.
- These medications are contraindicated in clients recovering from an MI and within 14 days of taking a MAOI.
- Use caution with clients who have a seizure disorder, urinary retention, prostatic hyperplasia, angle-closure glaucoma, hyperthyroidism, hypotension, and liver or kidney disease.

Anticonvulsants: carbamazepine, gabapentin

- These medications are contraindicated in clients who have bone marrow suppression and within 14 days of taking a MAOI.
- Avoid use in pregnancy.
- Gabapentin: Safety in pregnancy not established; discontinue medication with lactation and bottle feeding.
- Carbamazepine: Should only be used in pregnancy if maternal benefits outweigh risk to fetus with additional vitamin K recommended during last week of gestation; discontinue drug during lactation and bottle feeding.

CNS stimulants: methylphenidate

- **Warnings**: Pregnancy: Use only if the benefit to the client outweighs the risks to the fetus.
- Clients should not take methylphenidate within 14 days of taking a MAOI.
- Use caution with clients who have hypertension. Methylphenidate can result in hypertensive crisis.
- Use caution with clients who have agitation or tics.
- Use caution with clients who have a history of substance use disorder.

Antihistamines: hydroxyzine

- Clients who have acute asthma should not take hydroxyzine.
- Clients who are in the first trimester of pregnancy or breastfeeding should not take hydroxyzine.
- Use caution with older adults and those in the second or third trimester of pregnancy.

Glucocorticoids: dexamethasone

- Safety in pregnancy is not established, so avoid chronic use during lactation.
- Dexamethasone is contraindicated in clients who have fungal infection, seizure disorders, ulcerative colitis, or coagulopathy.
- Use caution with clients who have hypertension, hypothyroidism, glucose intolerance, diabetes mellitus, osteoporosis, or liver disease.

Bisphosphonate: etidronate

- Safety in pregnancy is not established. Discontinue the medication prior to becoming pregnant. Discontinue medication with lactation and bottle feeding.
- Etidronate is contraindicated in clients who have achalasia, esophageal structure, or osteomalacia.
- Use caution with clients who have kidney disease.

NSAIDs: ibuprofen

- Avoid after 30 weeks of gestation, use cautiously with lactation.
- Ibuprofen is contraindicated in clients who have a history of bronchospasms with aspirin or other NSAIDs and those who have severe kidney/hepatic disease.
- Use caution with clients who have bleeding, GI, or cardiac disorders.
- Use caution with older adult clients. Ⓖ

INTERACTIONS

Tricyclic antidepressants: amitriptyline

Barbiturates, CNS depressants, antihistamines, over-the-counter (OTC) sleep aids, and alcohol can cause additive CNS depression.
NURSING ACTIONS: Do not use together.

Anticonvulsants: carbamazepine, gabapentin

Carbamazepine causes a decrease in the effectiveness of oral contraceptives and warfarin.
NURSING ACTIONS: Monitor for therapeutic effects of warfarin with PT and INR. Dosage might need to be adjusted.

CLIENT EDUCATION: Discuss possible contraceptive changes with the provider.

Carbamazepine can result in CNS toxicity with lithium and a fatal reaction with MAOIs.
NURSING ACTIONS: Concurrent use should be avoided.

Grapefruit juice inhibits metabolism, and thus increases carbamazepine levels.
CLIENT EDUCATION: Advise clients to avoid intake of grapefruit juice.

Phenytoin and phenobarbital decrease the effects of carbamazepine.
NURSING ACTIONS: Concurrent use is not recommended.

CNS depression occurs with gabapentin and all other CNS depressants (alcohol, sedatives, and antihistamines).
CLIENT EDUCATION: Do not use together.

CNS stimulants: methylphenidate

Alkalizing medications can cause increase in reabsorption.
NURSING ACTIONS: Monitor for increase in amphetamine effects.

Acidifying medications can increase excretion of amphetamine.
NURSING ACTIONS: Monitor for decrease in amphetamine effects.

Insulin and oral antidiabetic medications can decrease glucose level.
NURSING ACTIONS: Monitor glucose level.

Methylphenidate decreases the effect of antihypertensives.
NURSING ACTIONS: Monitor blood pressure. Check more frequently in clients who have cardiac disease.

MAOIs can cause severe hypertension.
NURSING ACTIONS: Avoid concurrent use.

Caffeine can increase stimulant effect.
CLIENT EDUCATION: Avoid caffeine.

OTC medications with sympathomimetic action can lead to increased CNS stimulation.
CLIENT EDUCATION: Avoid use of OTC medications.

Antihistamines: hydroxyzine

Barbiturates, CNS depressants, and alcohol can cause additive CNS depression.
NURSING ACTIONS: Do not use together.

Glucocorticoids: dexamethasone

Glucocorticoids promote hyperglycemia, thereby counteracting the effects of insulin and oral hypoglycemics.
NURSING ACTIONS: The dose of hypoglycemic medications might need to be increased.

Concurrent use of salicylates and NSAIDs with glucocorticoids can increase the risk for GI bleed.
NURSING ACTIONS
- Monitor for GI bleed.
- Use together cautiously.

Because of the risk for hypokalemia, there is an increased risk of dysrhythmias caused by digoxin when taken with glucocorticoids.
NURSING ACTIONS
- Monitor blood potassium levels and cardiac rhythm.
- Encourage clients to eat potassium-rich foods.
- Administer potassium supplements.

Diuretics that promote potassium loss increase the risk for hypokalemia.
NURSING ACTIONS
- Monitor blood potassium level.
- Administer potassium supplements.

CLIENT EDUCATION: Eat potassium-rich foods.

Glucocorticoids decrease the antibody response to vaccines and increase the risk of infection from live virus vaccines.
NURSING ACTIONS: Clients should not receive immunizations while on glucocorticoid therapy.

Bisphosphonates: etidronate, pamidronate

Decreased absorption with calcium or iron supplements and high calcium foods
CLIENT EDUCATION: Take etidronate on an empty stomach 2 hr before meals, with an 8 oz glass of water.

NSAIDs: ibuprofen

NSAIDs can reduce effectiveness of antihypertensives, furosemide, thiazide diuretics, and oral antidiabetic medications.
NURSING ACTIONS: Monitor for medication effectiveness.

Aspirin, corticosteroids, alcohol, and tobacco can increase GI effects.
CLIENT EDUCATION: Do not use together.

NSAIDs can increase levels of oral anticoagulants and lithium.
NURSING ACTIONS: Monitor medication levels.

There is an increased risk of bleeding with the use of other NSAIDs, thrombolytics, antiplatelets, anticoagulants, and salicylates.
NURSING ACTIONS
- Clients who take medications together should use caution.
- Monitor for bleeding.

NURSING ADMINISTRATION

- The client's self-report is the key element in the assessment of pain. Q_{PCC}
- Clients should receive a pain management plan.
- Older adult clients need careful monitoring because they are at risk for increased adverse effects and adverse medication interactions with pain medications.
- Because some medications used as adjuvants are an off-label use, it is important to explain to clients the medications are being given to reduce pain, and not for the original purpose.

CLIENT EDUCATION

- If client has cancer, the client should voice fears and concerns about cancer, cancer pain, and pain treatment.
- Pain medications should be given on a fixed schedule around the clock, and not as-needed. Q_{EBP}
- Physical dependence is not considered addiction.

NURSING EVALUATION OF MEDICATION EFFECTIVENESS

Depending on the therapeutic intent, effectiveness can be evidenced by the following.
- Relief of depression, seizures, dysrhythmias, and other manifestations that aggravate the client's pain level
- Decreased opioid adverse effects
- Relief of neuropathic pain
- Decreased cancer bone pain
- Relief of neuralgia

Active Learning Scenario

A nurse in an acute care facility is teaching a client who has metastatic cancer and is receiving morphine and carbamazepine for pain. What information should the nurse provide about the use of these medications? Use the ATI Active Learning Template: Medication to complete this item.

THERAPEUTIC USES: Describe the therapeutic use for carbamazepine in this client.

COMPLICATIONS: Describe two adverse effects the client should monitor for.

INTERACTIONS: Describe two interactions with carbamazepine.

NURSING INTERVENTIONS: Describe two.

Active Learning Scenario Key

Using the ATI Active Learning Template: Medication

THERAPEUTIC USES: Carbamazepine relieves neuropathic (nerve) pain, which can be described as sharp, burning, or aching.

COMPLICATIONS: Adverse effects of carbamazepine include GI manifestations (abdominal pain, nausea, and vomiting). It also can cause bone marrow suppression, affecting all blood cell types.

INTERACTIONS

- The medication can cause hypertensive crisis if taken within 14 days of an MAOI antidepressant.
- Toxicity can result if the client drinks grapefruit juice while taking carbamazepine.

NURSING INTERVENTIONS

- Monitor CBC, including platelet counts.
- Assess for abnormal bleeding, bruising, or infection.
- Monitor for GI manifestations, and advise the client to take the medication with food.

Ⓝ *NCLEX® Connection: Pharmacological and Parenteral Therapies, Medication Administration*

Application Exercises

1. A nurse is caring for a client who has cancer and is taking morphine and carbamazepine for pain. Which of the following effects should the nurse monitor for when giving the medications together? (Select all that apply.)

   A. Need for reduced dosage of the opioid

   B. Reduced adverse effects of the opioid

   C. Increased analgesic effects

   D. Enhanced CNS stimulation

   E. Increased opioid tolerance

2. A nurse is planning care for a client who has brain cancer and is experiencing headaches. For which of the following adjuvant medications should the nurse expect the provider to prescribe?

   A. Dexamethasone

   B. Methylphenidate

   C. Hydroxyzine

   D. Amitriptyline

3. A nurse is preparing to administer pamidronate to a client who has bone pain related to cancer. Which of the following precautions should the nurse take when administering pamidronate?

   A. Inspect the skin for redness and irritation when changing the intradermal patch.

   B. Assess the IV site for thrombophlebitis frequently during administration.

   C. Instruct the client to sit upright or stand for 30 min following oral administration.

   D. Watch for manifestations of anaphylaxis for 20 min after IM administration.

4. A nurse is administering amitriptyline to a client who is experiencing cancer pain. For which of the following adverse effects should the nurse monitor?

   A. Decreased appetite

   B. Explosive diarrhea

   C. Decreased pulse rate

   D. Orthostatic hypotension

5. A nurse is planning care for a client who has cancer and is taking a glucocorticoid as an adjuvant medication for pain control. The nurse should include monitoring for which of the following in the plan of care? (Select all that apply.)

   A. Urinary retention

   B. Blood glucose

   C. Blood potassium level

   D. Gastric bleeding

   E. Respiratory depression

Application Exercises Key

1. A. **CORRECT:** Dosage of the opioid can be reduced when adjuvant medications are added for pain.
   B. **CORRECT:** Adverse effects of the opioid can be reduced when adjuvant medications are added for pain.
   C. **CORRECT:** Analgesic effects are increased when adjuvant medications are added for pain.
   D. CNS stimulation is not enhanced when morphine and carbamazepine are used together for pain relief.
   E. Opioid tolerance can be decreased when an adjuvant medication is added for pain.

   Ⓝ *NCLEX® Connection: Pharmacological and Parenteral Therapies, Pharmacological Pain Management*

2. A. **CORRECT:** Dexamethasone, a glucocorticoid, decreases inflammation and swelling. It is used to reduce cerebral edema and relieve pressure from the tumor.
   B. The use of methylphenidate as an adjuvant is to elevate mood and increase pain relief.
   C. The use of hydroxyzine as an adjuvant is to decrease anxiety and help the client sleep.
   D. The use of amitriptyline as an adjuvant is to relieve neuropathic pain and elevate mood.

   Ⓝ *NCLEX® Connection: Pharmacological and Parenteral Therapies, Pharmacological Pain Management*

3. A. This medication is not administered by the intradermal route.
   B. **CORRECT:** Pamidronate is administered by IV infusion. This medication is irritating to veins, and assess for thrombophlebitis during administration.
   C. This medication is not administered orally.
   D. This medication is not administered by the IM route.

   Ⓝ *NCLEX® Connection: Pharmacological and Parenteral Therapies, Pharmacological Pain Management*

4. A. Amitriptyline can cause increased appetite and weight gain.
   B. Amitriptyline can cause constipation.
   C. Amitriptyline can cause increased pulse rate.
   D. **CORRECT:** Amitriptyline can cause orthostatic hypotension. Assess for this effect and instruct the client to move slowly from lying down or sitting after taking this medication.

   Ⓝ *NCLEX® Connection: Pharmacological and Parenteral Therapies, Adverse Effects/Contraindications/Side Effects/Interactions*

5. A. Monitoring for urinary retention is not necessary because glucocorticoids do not cause this effect.
   B. **CORRECT:** Monitoring blood glucose is important because glucocorticoids raise the glucose level, especially in clients who have diabetes mellitus.
   C. **CORRECT:** Monitoring blood potassium level is important because glucocorticoids can cause hypokalemia.
   D. **CORRECT:** Monitoring for gastric bleeding is important because glucocorticoids irritate the gastric mucosa and put the client at risk for a peptic ulcer.
   E. Monitoring for respiratory depression is not necessary because glucocorticoids do not depress respirations.

   Ⓝ *NCLEX® Connection: Pharmacological and Parenteral Therapies, Pharmacological Pain Management*

UNIT 9   MEDICATIONS FOR PAIN AND INFLAMMATION

CHAPTER 36 *Miscellaneous Pain Medications*

Pain is subjective and can be indicative of current or impending tissue injury. Pain can result from the release of chemical mediators, inflammation, or pressure.

Migraine headaches can be caused by the inflammation and vasodilation of cerebral blood vessels. Medications for migraine headaches can be used to stop a migraine (abortive) or prevent one from occurring (prophylactic). First-line treatment for migraine headaches includes nonspecific analgesics (aspirin-like medications) and migraine-specific medications (serotonin receptor agonists [also known as triptans]). Ergot alkaloid medications are second-line treatment for migraines, and prophylactic medications include beta blockers, anticonvulsants, tricyclic antidepressants, and estrogens.

Local anesthetics block motor and sensory neurons to a specific area. They can be given topically; injected directly into an area; or given regionally, epidurally, or into the subarachnoid (spinal) space.

Migraine medications

SELECT PROTOTYPE MEDICATIONS

Aspirin-like medications: Acetaminophen, NSAIDs (aspirin, naproxen)

Serotonin receptor agonists (triptans): Sumatriptan (oral, subcutaneous, inhalation, transdermal)

Ergot alkaloids
- Ergotamine (oral, sublingual, rectal)
- Dihydroergotamine (IV, IM, subcutaneous, intranasal)

Beta blockers: Propranolol (oral), metoprolol (oral)

Anticonvulsants: Divalproex (oral), topiramate

Tricyclic antidepressants: Amitriptyline (oral)

Estrogens: Estrogen (gel, patches)

OTHER MEDICATIONS

Triptans: Almotriptan, frovatriptan, naratriptan, zolmitriptan

Ergot alkaloids: Ergotamine and caffeine

Combination OTC analgesics: Acetaminophen, aspirin, caffeine

Other combinations: Isometheptene, dichloralphenazone/acetaminophen
- Isometheptene relieves headaches through vasoconstriction of arterioles.
- Dichloralphenazone has sedative properties.
- Acetaminophen is a mild analgesic.

PURPOSE

EXPECTED PHARMACOLOGICAL ACTION: Migraine medications prevent inflammation and dilation of the intracranial blood vessels, thereby relieving migraine pain.

THERAPEUTIC USES
- Some medications are used as abortive therapy to stop a migraine after it begins or after prodromal manifestations start. These include nonsteroidal anti-inflammatory drugs (NSAIDs) and combination anti-inflammatory medications, triptans, and ergot alkaloids.
- Other medications are used as prophylactic therapy to help prevent a migraine headache. Preventive agents include beta blockers, anticonvulsants, amitriptyline, and estrogens.

COMPLICATIONS

Aspirin-like drugs: NSAIDs, acetaminophen combination

Bone marrow suppression
NURSING ACTIONS: Periodically monitor CBC, including platelets.

CLIENT EDUCATION: Observe for indications of easy bruising and bleeding, fever, or sore throat, and notify the provider if they occur.

Gastrointestinal (GI) distress: Abdominal pain, ulceration, nausea, vomiting, and diarrhea or constipation
NURSING ACTIONS: Monitor for GI bleeding (coffee-ground emesis; bloody or black tarry stools; abdominal pain).

CLIENT EDUCATION: Take with food, milk, or antacid.

Myocardial infarction (MI) or stroke
NURSING ACTIONS
- Monitor cardiac status, especially in older adult clients and clients who have a history of cardiac disease.
- All NSAIDs except aspirin increase the risk of thrombotic events.

Serotonin receptor agonists (triptans): sumatriptan

Chest pressure (heavy arms or chest tightness)
CLIENT EDUCATION
- Medications have increased risk for these manifestations; however, the manifestations are self-limiting and not dangerous.
- Notify the provider for continuous or severe chest pain.

Coronary artery vasospasm/angina
NURSING ACTIONS: Do not administer to a client who has or is at risk for coronary artery disease (CAD).

Dizziness or vertigo
CLIENT EDUCATION: Avoid driving or operating heavy machinery until medication effects are known.

Ergot alkaloids: ergotamine and dihydroergotamine

Gastrointestinal discomfort: Nausea and vomiting
NURSING ACTIONS: Administer an antiemetic (metoclopramide).

Acute or chronic toxicity (ergotism): Muscle pain, paresthesia in fingers and toes; peripheral ischemia (can result in gangrene)
NURSING ACTIONS: Stop medication and immediately notify the provider if manifestations occur.

Physical dependence
NURSING ACTIONS
- Medication should not be taken daily on a long-term basis.
- Notify the provider if manifestations occur.

CLIENT EDUCATION
- Do not exceed the prescribed dose or exceed the recommended duration of treatment.
- Medications can cause manifestations of withdrawal (headache, nausea, vomiting, restlessness).

Beta blockers: propranolol

Extreme tiredness, fatigue, depression, asthma exacerbation
CLIENT EDUCATION: Observe for manifestations and notify the provider if they occur.

Bradycardia, hypotension
NURSING ACTIONS
- Monitor heart rate and blood pressure.
- Notify the provider of significant change.

CLIENT EDUCATION: Take apical pulse prior to dosing.

Anticonvulsants: divalproex

GI distress: Nausea, vomiting, diarrhea, dyspepsia, indigestion
NURSING ACTIONS: Report manifestations to the provider.

Hepatitis
NURSING ACTIONS
- Monitor liver enzymes.
- Notify the provider of lethargy or fever.

Pancreatitis
CLIENT EDUCATION: Report abdominal pain, nausea, vomiting, and anorexia. Medication should be discontinued. Other adverse effects include fatigue, weight gain, tremor, bone loss, and reversible hair loss.

Tricyclic antidepressants: amitriptyline

Anticholinergic effects: Dry mouth, constipation, urinary retention, blurred vision, tachycardia, hypotension
NURSING ACTIONS
- Increase daily fiber intake.
- Increase physical activity by engaging in regular exercise.
- Monitor vital signs.
- Administer stimulant laxatives (bisacodyl) to counteract reduced bowel motility, or stool softeners (docusate sodium) to prevent constipation.

CLIENT EDUCATION
- Increase fluid intake, sip fluids throughout the day, chew sugarless gum or suck on sugarless hard candy, and use an alcohol-free mouthwash.
- Void just before taking medication and then every 4 hr. Report urinary retention to the provider.
- Report blurred vision.

Drowsiness or dizziness
CLIENT EDUCATION: Avoid driving or operating heavy machinery until medication effects are known.

CONTRAINDICATIONS/PRECAUTIONS

Ergotamine

- **Warnings**
  - Pregnancy: Avoid taking this medication (risk of fetal harm or abortion).
  - Lactation: Avoid while taking this medication.
  - Reproductive: Recommend the use of contraceptive measures to avoid pregnancy while taking this medication.
- Contraindicated in clients who have renal and/or liver dysfunction, sepsis, hypertension, history of myocardial infarction, and CAD

Triptans

- **Warnings**
  - Pregnancy: Use only if maternal benefit outweighs fetal risk.
  - Lactation: Use only if maternal benefit outweighs fetal risk.
  - Reproductive: Recommend the use of contraceptive measures to avoid pregnancy while taking this medication.
- Contraindicated in clients who have liver failure, ischemic heart disease, a history of myocardial infarction, uncontrolled hypertension, and other heart diseases

Propranolol

- **Warnings**
  - Pregnancy: Crosses the placenta and can cause fetal/neonatal bradycardia, hypotension, hypoglycemia, or respiratory depression
  - Lactation: Appears in breast milk; use formula while taking this medication.
- Contraindicated in clients who have greater than first-degree heart block, bradycardia, bronchial asthma, cardiogenic shock, or heart failure
- Use with caution in clients taking other antihypertensives or who have liver or renal impairment, diabetes mellitus, or Wolff-Parkinson-White syndrome.

Divalproex

- **Warnings**
  - Pregnancy: Can cause fetal harm and other major congenital malformations. Contraindicated for migraine prophylaxis only
  - Lactation: Passes into breast milk. Consider using formula while taking this medication.
- Contraindicated in clients who have liver or pancreatic disease

Amitriptyline

- **Warnings**
  - Pregnancy: Use only if maternal benefit outweighs fetal risk.
  - Lactation: Can cause sedation in infant
- Contraindicated in clients who have recent MI or within 14 days of a MAOI
- Use with caution in clients who have seizure history, urinary retention, prostatic hyperplasia, angle-closure glaucoma, hyperthyroidism, and liver or kidney disease.

Aspirin-like drugs

- **Warnings**
  - Pregnancy: Aspirin should be avoided during pregnancy, especially in the third trimester.
  - Lactation: Safety not established
- Contraindicated in clients who have severe renal/hepatic disease
- Use caution with clients who have bleeding, GI or cardiac disorders, and with older adult clients.

Acetaminophen

- **Warnings**
  - Pregnancy: IV use in pregnancy only if clearly needed
  - Lactation: IV use with caution during lactation
- Should not be used alone, but only in combination with other medications

INTERACTIONS

Aspirin-like medications: NSAIDs, acetaminophen combination

NSAIDs can reduce the effectiveness of antihypertensives, furosemide, thiazide diuretics, and oral antidiabetic medications.
NURSING ACTIONS: Monitor for medication effectiveness.

Corticosteroids, alcohol, and tobacco can increase GI effects.
Client Education: Do not use these together.

NSAIDs can increase levels of oral anticoagulants and lithium.
NURSING ACTIONS: Monitor medication levels.

There is an increased risk of bleeding with the use of other NSAIDs, thrombolytics, antiplatelets, anticoagulants, and salicylates.
NURSING ACTIONS
- Clients who take medications together should use caution.
- Monitor for bleeding.

Serotonin receptor agonists (triptans): sumatriptan

Concurrent use of MAOIs can lead to MAOI toxicity.
NURSING ACTIONS: Do not give triptans within 2 weeks of stopping MAOIs.

Concurrent use with ergotamine or another triptan can cause a vasospastic reaction.
NURSING ACTIONS: Avoid concurrent use of these medications.

Selective serotonin reuptake inhibitors (SSRIs) taken with triptans can cause serotonin syndrome (confusion, agitation, hyperthermia, diaphoresis, possible death).
NURSING ACTIONS: Do not use medications together.

Ergotamine and dihydroergotamine

Concurrent use with triptans can cause a vasospastic reaction.
NURSING ACTIONS: Triptans should be taken at least 24 hr apart from an ergotamine medication.

Some HIV protease inhibitors, antifungal medications, macrolide antibiotics, and grapefruit juice can increase ergotamine levels, causing increased vasospasm.
NURSING ACTIONS: Do not use together.

Beta blockers: propranolol

Verapamil and diltiazem have additive cardiosuppression effects.
NURSING ACTIONS: If medications are used together, monitor ECG, heart rate, and blood pressure.

Diuretics and antihypertensive medications have additive hypotensive effects.
NURSING ACTIONS: Monitor blood pressure. Hold and notify the provider if systolic blood pressure is less than 90 mm Hg.

Propranolol can mask the hypoglycemic effect of insulin and prevent the breakdown of fat in response to hypoglycemia.
NURSING ACTIONS
- Use with caution.
- Monitor blood glucose.

Anticonvulsants: divalproex

NSAIDs, erythromycin, and salicylates can cause divalproex toxicity.
NURSING ACTIONS: Monitor medication levels.

Benzodiazepines, opioids, antihistamines, and alcohol can cause CNS depression.
NURSING ACTIONS: Do not use together.

Divalproex can increase levels of phenobarbital and phenytoin.
NURSING ACTIONS: Monitor medication levels.

Increase the effects of warfarin.
NURSING ACTIONS
- Monitor for therapeutic effects of warfarin with PT and INR. Dosage can need to be adjusted.
- Monitor for bleeding.

Tricyclic antidepressants: amitriptyline

Barbiturates, CNS depressants, antihistamines, over-the-counter sleep aids, and alcohol can cause additive CNS depression.
NURSING ACTIONS: Do not use together.

Cimetidine can increase amitriptyline levels.
NURSING ACTIONS: Monitor medication effects.

MAOIs can increase CNS excitation or cause seizures.
NURSING ACTIONS: Do not give amitriptyline within 2 weeks of stopping MAOIs.

NURSING ADMINISTRATION

- Antiemetics, preferably metoclopramide, are useful as adjunct medications in migraine treatment.
- Use caution in case of orthostatic hypotension (amitriptyline, propranolol).

CLIENT EDUCATION

- Abortive medications should not be used more than 2 days a week.
- If having migraines, avoid trigger factors that cause stress and fatigue (consumption of alcohol and tyramine-containing foods [wine, aged cheese]).
- Lying down in a dark, quiet place can help ease manifestations. Qᴘᴄᴄ
- Check apical pulse before dosage (propranolol).
- Dosage can be taken with food to reduce GI distress (divalproex) and increase absorption (propranolol).
- Protect skin and eyes from sun (amitriptyline) and avoid driving or operating heavy machinery until medication effects are known (amitriptyline, sumatriptan).

NURSING EVALUATION OF MEDICATION EFFECTIVENESS

Effectiveness can be evidenced by the following.
- Reduction in intensity and frequency of migraine attacks
- Prophylaxis against migraine attacks
- Termination of migraine headaches
- Reduction in size and frequency of medication doses used

Local anesthetics

SELECT PROTOTYPE MEDICATIONS

Amide type: Lidocaine

OTHER MEDICATIONS

Ester type: Tetracaine, procaine, chloroprocaine

Amide type: EMLA (eutectic mixture of 2.5% lidocaine/2.5% prilocaine)

PURPOSE

EXPECTED PHARMACOLOGICAL ACTION

These medications decrease pain by blocking conduction of pain impulses in a circumscribed area. Loss of consciousness does not occur.

THERAPEUTIC USES

PARENTERAL ADMINISTRATION
- Pain management for dental procedures, minor surgical procedures, labor and birth, and diagnostic procedures
- Regional anesthesia (spinal, epidural)

TOPICAL ADMINISTRATION
- Skin and mucous membrane disorders
- Control laryngeal and esophageal reflexes prior to endoscopic procedures
- Minor procedures (IV insertion, injection [pediatric], wart removal)

COMPLICATIONS

CNS excitation

Seizures, followed by respiratory depression, leading to unconsciousness

NURSING ACTIONS
- Monitor for indications of seizure activity, sedation, and change in mental status (decrease in level of consciousness).
- Monitor vital signs and respiratory status.
- Have equipment ready for resuscitation.
- Administer benzodiazepines (midazolam or diazepam) to treat seizures.

Hypotension, cardiosuppression

Evidenced by bradycardia, heart block, reduced contractile force, and cardiac arrest (common in spinal anesthesia due to sympathetic block)

NURSING ACTIONS
- Monitor vital signs and ECG.
- If manifestations occur, administer treatment as prescribed.

Allergic reactions

More likely with ester-type agents (procaine). Reactions ranging from allergic dermatitis to anaphylaxis.

NURSING ACTIONS
- Clients who are allergic to one ester-type agent are likely allergic to all other ester-type agents.
- Amide-type anesthetic agents are less likely to cause allergic reactions, and therefore are used for injection; they have largely replaced ester-type agents.
- Observe for manifestations of allergy to anesthetics (allergic dermatitis or anaphylaxis).
- Treat with antihistamines or agency protocol.

Labor and birth

- Labor can be prolonged due to a decrease in uterine contractility.
- Local anesthetics can cross the placenta and result in fetal bradycardia and CNS depression.

NURSING ACTIONS
- Use cautiously in clients who are in labor.
- Monitor uterine activity for effectiveness.
- Monitor fetal heart rate for bradycardia and decreased variability.

Spinal headache

NURSING ACTIONS: Monitor for indications of severe headache.

CLIENT EDUCATION: Remain flat in bed for 12 hr post procedure.

Urinary retention

Can occur with spinal anesthesia

NURSING ACTIONS
- Monitor urinary output.
- Notify the provider if the client has not voided within 8 hr.

CONTRAINDICATIONS/PRECAUTIONS

- **Warnings**
  - Pregnancy: Use only if maternal benefit outweighs fetal risk.
  - Lactation: Use only if maternal benefit outweighs fetal risk.
- Supraventricular dysrhythmias and/or heart block.
- Use cautiously in clients who have liver and kidney dysfunction, heart failure, and myasthenia gravis.

- Epinephrine added to the local anesthetic is contraindicated for use in fingers, nose, and other body parts with end arteries. Gangrene can result due to vasoconstriction.
- Advise clients to use caution against self-inflicted injury until the anesthetic effect wears off.
- Avoid topical benzocaine in children under the age of two.
- Allergic reactions are more likely with ester-type anesthetics.

INTERACTIONS

Antihypertensive medications have additive hypotensive effects with parenteral administration of local anesthetics.
NURSING ACTIONS: Monitor heart rate and blood pressure.

NURSING ADMINISTRATION

Maintain clients in a comfortable position during recovery.

Injection of local anesthetic
- Vasoconstrictors (epinephrine) often are used in combination with local anesthetics to prevent the spread of the local anesthetic.
  - Keeping the anesthetic contained prolongs the anesthesia and decreases the chance of systemic toxicity.
  - Epinephrine added to the local anesthetic is contraindicated for use in fingers, nose, and other body parts with end arteries.
  - Gangrene can result due to vasoconstriction.
- Prepare injection site for local anesthetic by cleansing and shaving if indicated.
- Monitor vital signs and level of consciousness.
- Maintain IV access for administration of emergency medications if necessary.
- Have equipment ready for resuscitation.
- For regional block, protect the area of numbness from injury.

Spinal or epidural nerve blocks
- Monitor during insertion for hypotension, anaphylaxis, seizure, and dura puncture. Q EBP
- Monitor for respiratory depression and sedation.
- Monitor insertion site for hematoma and indications of an infection.
- Assess level of sensory block. Evaluate leg strength prior to ambulating.
- Prepare IV fluids to administer to compensate for the sympathetic blocking effects of regional anesthetics.
- Have client lie supine for 12 hr following spinal anesthesia to minimize headache.
- Notify provider if the client is unable to void after 8 hr.

Topical cream (EMLA)
- Apply to intact skin 1 hr before routine procedures or superficial puncture and 2 hr before more extensive procedures or deep puncture.
- Apply to the smallest surface area needed to minimize systemic absorption. Avoid wrapping or heating the area.

- Prior to the procedure, remove the dressing and clean the skin with aseptic solution.
- Keep the client NPO following oral administration until normal pharyngeal sensation returns (approximately 1 hr). Monitor the client's first oral intake.
- EMLA can be applied at home prior to coming to a health care facility for a procedure.
- Monitor vital signs and level of consciousness to monitor for systemic absorption.

CLIENT EDUCATION
- Avoid hazardous activities when recovering from anesthesia.
- Notify the provider for indications of infection (fever, swelling, and redness; increase in pain or severe headache; sudden weakness to lower extremities; or decrease in bowel or bladder control). Qs
- Notify the provider for indications of systemic infusion (a metallic taste, ringing in ears, perioral numbness, and seizures).
- Sanitize hands before and after administration of topical anesthetic.

NURSING EVALUATION OF MEDICATION EFFECTIVENESS

Depending on the therapeutic intent, effectiveness can be evidenced by the following.
- Client undergoes procedure without experiencing pain.
- Pain is relieved.

Active Learning Scenario

A nurse is teaching a client who has frequent migraine headaches about a new prescription for sumatriptan. What should the nurse teach the client about this medication? Use the ATI Active Learning Template: Medication to complete this item.

THERAPEUTIC USES: Describe the therapeutic use for sumatriptan in this client.

COMPLICATIONS: Describe two adverse effects the client should monitor for.

INTERACTIONS: Describe two interactions the nurse should teach the client about.

NURSING INTERVENTIONS: Describe two for this client.

Application Exercises

1. A nurse is providing teaching to a client who is experiencing migraine headaches. Which of the following instructions should the nurse provide? (Select all that apply.)
   A. Take ergotamine as a prophylaxis to prevent a migraine headache.
   B. Identify and avoid trigger factors.
   C. Lie down in a dark, quiet room at the onset of a migraine.
   D. Avoid foods that contain tyramine.
   E. Avoid exercise that can increase heart rate.

2. A nurse is reviewing the health history of a client who has migraine headaches and is to begin prophylaxis therapy with propranolol. Which of the following findings in the client history should the nurse report to the provider?
   A. The client had a prior myocardial infarction.
   B. The client takes warfarin for atrial fibrillation.
   C. The client takes an SSRI for depression.
   D. An ECG indicates a first-degree heart block.

3. A nurse is providing teaching to a client who has migraine headaches and a new prescription for ergotamine. For which of the following manifestations indicating a possible adverse reaction should the nurse instruct the client to stop taking the medication and notify the provider?
   A. Nausea
   B. Visual disturbances
   C. Numbness and tingling in fingers
   D. Muscle tremors

4. A nurse is planning care for a client who is to receive tetracaine prior to a bronchoscopy. Which of the following actions should the nurse include in the plan of care?
   A. Monitor client for seizure activity.
   B. Monitor the insertion site for a hematoma.
   C. Palpate the bladder to detect urinary retention.
   D. Maintain the client on bed rest for 12 hr following the procedure.

5. A nurse is caring for a client who is receiving a local anesthetic of lidocaine during the repair of a skin laceration. For which of the following manifestations should the nurse monitor as an adverse reaction to the anesthetic?
   A. Drowsiness
   B. Tachycardia
   C. Hypertension
   D. Fever

Application Exercises Key

1. A. Ergotamine is used at the onset of a migraine to abort headache manifestations. It should not be used regularly because it can cause physical dependence and toxicity.
   B. **CORRECT:** Identifying and avoiding trigger factors is an important action that can help to prevent some migraines.
   C. **CORRECT:** Lying down in a dark, quiet room at the onset of a migraine can prevent the onset of more severe manifestations.
   D. **CORRECT:** Foods that contain tyramine can be a trigger for some migraines and should be avoided.
   E. Exercise should be encouraged between migraines because it can relieve stress, which can trigger headaches.

   Ⓝ *NCLEX® Connection: Pharmacological and Parenteral Therapies, Medication Administration*

2. A. A prior MI is not a contraindication to taking propranolol.
   B. Concurrent use of warfarin is not a contraindication to taking propranolol.
   C. Concurrent use of an SSRI is not a contraindication to taking propranolol. Taking sumatriptan with SSRIs can lead to serotonin syndrome. The medications should not be used together.
   D. **CORRECT:** Propranolol is contraindicated in clients who have a first-degree heart block. Report this finding to the provider.

   Ⓝ *NCLEX® Connection: Pharmacological and Parenteral Therapies, Medication Administration*

3. C. **CORRECT:** When taking actions and teaching a client about taking ergotamine, the nurse should instruct the client to monitor and report any numbness and tingling in the fingers or toes which can be a manifestation of ergotamine toxicity.

   Ⓝ *NCLEX® Connection: Pharmacological and Parenteral Therapies, Adverse Effects/Contraindications/Side Effects/Interactions*

4. A. **CORRECT:** The nurse should plan to generate solutions to include actions in the plan of care to address the safety of a client who received tetracaine. The nurse should plan to monitor the client for seizure activity and have resuscitative equipment available.

   Ⓝ *NCLEX® Connection: Pharmacological and Parenteral Therapies, Adverse Effects/Contraindications/Side Effects/Interactions*

5. A. **CORRECT:** The nurse should plan to generate solutions to monitor the client for potential adverse effects of receiving a local anesthetic injection. The nurse should monitor the client for drowsiness which can indicate a depressive adverse effect and lead to coma or even death if not treated.

   Ⓝ *NCLEX® Connection: Pharmacological and Parenteral Therapies, Adverse Effects/Contraindications/Side Effects/Interactions*

Active Learning Scenario Key

Using the ATI Active Learning Template: Medication

THERAPEUTIC USES: Sumatriptan is used to abort a migraine headache and associated manifestations (nausea and vomiting) after it begins by causing cranial artery vasoconstriction.

COMPLICATIONS: The nurse should monitor for chest and arm heaviness/pressure, angina caused by coronary vasospasm, dizziness, and vertigo.

INTERACTIONS: Toxicity can result if sumatriptan is given concurrently or within 2 weeks of an MAOI antidepressant. Sumatriptan should not be given concurrently with other triptan medications or within 24 hr of ergotamine or dihydroergotamine.

NURSING INTERVENTIONS
- Teach clients to take sumatriptan at the first finding of migraine manifestations.
- Teach client how to administer sumatriptan if it is prescribed intranasally or by subcutaneous injection.
- Monitor cardiovascular risk factors and vital signs while taking this medication.
- Advise clients to notify the provider immediately for onset of angina pain. Teach clients to distinguish transient chest or arm heaviness caused by sumatriptan from angina pain.

Ⓝ *NCLEX® Connection: Pharmacological and Parenteral Therapies, Medication Administration*

When reviewing the following chapters, keep in mind the relevant topics and tasks of the NCLEX outline, in particular:

Pharmacological and Parenteral Therapies

ADVERSE EFFECTS/CONTRAINDICATIONS/SIDE EFFECTS/ INTERACTIONS

Identify actual and potential incompatibilities of prescribed client medications.

Provide information to the client on common side effects/adverse effects/ potential interactions of medications, and inform the client of when to notify the primary health care provider.

Assess the client for actual or potential side effects and adverse effects of medications.

DOSAGE CALCULATIONS: Use clinical decision–making/critical thinking when calculating dosages.

MEDICATION ADMINISTRATION:

Mix medications from two vials when necessary.

Educate client about medications.

Prepare and administer medications, using rights of medication administration.

Review pertinent data prior to medication administration.

EXPECTED ACTIONS/OUTCOMES: Evaluate client's response to medication.

CHAPTER 37 *Diabetes Mellitus*

Diabetes mellitus is a chronic illness that results from an absolute or relative deficiency of insulin, often combined with a cellular resistance to insulin's actions. Various insulins are available to manage diabetes. These medications differ in their onset, peak, and duration.

Oral antidiabetic medications work in various ways to increase available insulin or modify carbohydrate metabolism. Newer injectable medications are used to supplement insulin or oral agents to manage glucose control.

Insulin

SELECT PROTOTYPE MEDICATIONS

Rapid-acting: Lispro insulin
- Onset: 15 to 30 min
- Peak: 0.5 to 3 hr
- Duration: 3 to 5 hr

Short-acting: Regular insulin
- Onset: 0.5 to 1 hr
- Peak: 1 to 5 hr
- Duration: 6 to 10 hr

Intermediate-acting: NPH insulin
- Onset: 1 to 2 hr
- Peak: 4 to 14 hr
- Duration: 14 to 24 hr

Long-acting: Insulin glargine U-100
- Onset: 1 to 4 hr
- Peak: None
- Duration: 24 hr

OTHER MEDICATIONS

Rapid-acting
- Insulin aspart
- Insulin glulisine
- Inhaled human insulin

Short-acting: Regular insulin (U-500, U-100 strength)

Long-acting: Insulin detemir is dose-dependent. The greater units/kg the client receives, the longer the duration of the insulin; up to 24 hr with higher doses.

Ultra-long (longer duration) insulin: U-300 insulin glargine, insulin degludec; duration of more than 24 hr.

PREMIXED INSULINS

70% NPH and 30% regular: Mixture of intermediate- and short-acting insulin

75% insulin lispro protamine and 25% insulin lispro: Mixture of intermediate- and rapid-acting insulin

PURPOSE

EXPECTED PHARMACOLOGICAL ACTION

- Promotes cellular uptake of glucose (decreases glucose levels)
- Converts glucose into glycogen and promotes energy storage
- Moves potassium into cells (along with glucose)

THERAPEUTIC USES

- Insulin is used for glycemic control of diabetes mellitus (type 1, type 2, gestational) to prevent complications.
- Clients who have type 2 diabetes mellitus can require insulin when:
  - Oral antidiabetic medications, diet, and exercise are unable to control blood glucose levels.
  - Severe renal or liver disease is present.
  - Painful neuropathy is present.
  - Undergoing surgery or diagnostic tests.
  - Experiencing severe stress (infection and trauma).
  - Undergoing emergency treatment of diabetes ketoacidosis (DKA) and hyperosmolar hyperglycemic nonketotic syndrome.
  - Requiring treatment of hyperkalemia.

COMPLICATIONS

Hypoglycemia

- Hypoglycemia occurs when blood glucose is less than 70 mg/dL.
- Hypoglycemia can result from the following.
  - Toxic dose of insulin
  - Too little food
  - Vomiting and diarrhea
  - Alcohol intake
  - Strenuous exercise
  - Childbirth

NURSING ACTIONS

- Monitor clients for hypoglycemia. If abrupt onset, client will experience sympathetic nervous system (SNS) effects (tachycardia, palpitations, diaphoresis, shakiness). If gradual onset, client will experience parasympathetic (PNS) manifestations (headache, tremors, weakness, lethargy, disorientation).
- Administer glucose. For conscious clients, administer a snack of 15 g carbohydrate (4 oz orange juice, 2 oz grape juice, 8 oz milk, glucose tablets per manufacturer's suggestion to equal 15 g).
- If the client is not fully conscious, do not risk aspiration. Administer glucose parenterally (IV glucose) or subcutaneous/IM glucagon.

CLIENT EDUCATION: Wear a medical alert bracelet and always have a snack with glucose handy.

Hypokalemia

Insulin can decrease blood potassium levels. Clients who take large doses of insulin are at risk.

NURSING ACTIONS: Monitor clients taking large doses a significant amount of insulin across multiple doses for indications of hypokalemia (muscle cramping and cardiac dysrhythmias).

Lipohypertrophy

CLIENT EDUCATION: Systematically rotate injection sites and allow 1 inch between injection sites.

CONTRAINDICATIONS/PRECAUTIONS

Warnings
- Pregnancy: Use with caution; the requirements for insulin can be increased.
- Lactation: Use with caution; can inhibit milk production.
- Reproductive: Notify the provider if pregnancy is planned or suspected.

INTERACTIONS

Sulfonylureas, meglitinides, beta blockers, and alcohol have additive hypoglycemic effects with concurrent use.
NURSING ACTIONS: Monitor blood glucose levels for hypoglycemia (less than 70 mg/dL) and adjust insulin or oral antidiabetic dosages accordingly.

Concurrent use of thiazide diuretics and glucocorticoids can raise blood glucose levels and thereby counteract the effects of insulin.
NURSING ACTIONS: Monitor blood glucose levels for hyperglycemia and adjust insulin doses accordingly. Higher insulin doses can be indicated.

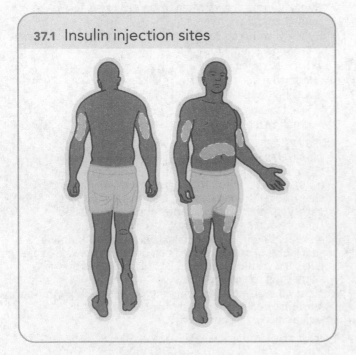

37.1 Insulin injection sites

Beta blockers can mask SNS response to hypoglycemia (tachycardia, tremors), making it difficult for clients to identify hypoglycemia. Beta blockers also impair the body's natural ability to breakdown glycogen stores to raise blood glucose levels.
CLIENT EDUCATION
- Monitoring glucose levels is important when taking this medication, and do not rely on SNS manifestations as an alert to developing hypoglycemia.
- Maintain a regular eating schedule to ensure adequate glucose during times of hypoglycemic action.

NURSING ADMINISTRATION

- Adjust the insulin dosage to meet insulin needs.
  - The dosage can need to be increased in response to increase in caloric intake, infection, stress, growth spurts, and in the second and third trimesters of pregnancy. Qpcc
  - The dosage can need to be decreased in response to level of exercise or first trimester of pregnancy.
- Ensure adequate glucose is available at the time of onset of insulin and during all peak times.
- When mixing short-acting insulin with longer-acting insulin, draw the short-acting insulin up into the syringe first, then the longer-acting insulin. This prevents the possibility of accidentally injecting some of the longer-acting insulin into the shorter-acting insulin vial. (This can pose a risk for unexpected insulin effects with subsequent uses of the vial.)
- For insulin suspensions, gently rotate the vial between the palms to disperse the particles throughout the vial prior to withdrawing insulin.
- NPH and premixed insulins should appear cloudy. Do not administer other insulins if they are cloudy or any insulins that are discolored or if a precipitate is present.
- Insulin glargine and insulin detemir are both clear in color, not administered IV, and should not be mixed in a syringe with any other insulin.
- Administer lispro, aspart, glulisine, and regular insulin by subcutaneous injection, continuous subcutaneous infusion, and IV route.
- Administer NPH by subcutaneous route.
- Instruct clients to administer subcutaneous insulin in the appropriate site and in one general area to have consistent rates of absorption. Absorption rates from subcutaneous tissue increase from thigh to upper arm to abdomen.
- Use only insulin-specific syringes that correspond to the concentration of insulin being administered. Administer U-100 insulin with a U-100 syringe; administer U-500 insulin with a U-500 syringe.
- Select an appropriate needle length to ensure insulin is injected into subcutaneous tissue vs. intradermal (too short) or intramuscular (too long).
- Encourage clients to enhance diabetes medication therapy with a proper diet and consistent activity.

- Ensure proper storage of insulin.
  - Unopened vials of a single type of insulin can be stored in the refrigerator until their expiration date. ◯EBP
  - Vials of premixed insulins can be stored for up to 3 months under refrigeration.
  - Insulins premixed in syringes can be kept for 1 to 2 weeks under refrigeration. Keep the syringes in a vertical position, with the needles pointing up. Prior to administration, the insulin should be resuspended by gently moving the syringe.
  - Store the vial that is in use at room temperature, avoiding proximity to sunlight and intense heat. Discard after 1 month.
- Inhaled human insulin is available as dry powder, packed in cartridges for use in an inhaler. Cartridges are available in 4, 8, or 12 units. Ensure the correct dose is administered; multiple cartridges might be required to administer the full prescribed dose (i.e. use two-12 unit cartridges to administer a 12 unit dose).
- IV administration of insulin can be required for clients that require rapid glucose reduction who are being monitored in an inpatient facility.
  - Regular insulin is the most common type of insulin administered. The typical concentration is 100 units/100 mL of 0.9% sodium chloride solution (1 unit/mL).
  - Insulin aspart, insulin glulisine, and insulin lispro are the only other insulins appropriate for IV administration.

> **!** Safety alert: When insulin is administered via IV infusion, allow 50 mL of solution to flow through the IV tubing and waste. Insulin binds to the tubing, so this ensures the fluid the client receives will have the appropriate concentration of insulin.

Oral antidiabetics

Sulfonylureas

SELECT PROTOTYPE MEDICATIONS
- **First generation:** Chlorpropamide
- **Second generation:** Glipizide

OTHER MEDICATIONS
- **First generation:** Tolazamide
- **Second generation:** Glyburide, glimepiride

Meglitinides (glinides; non-sulfonylurea insulin secretagogues)

SELECT PROTOTYPE MEDICATION: Repaglinide

OTHER MEDICATION: Nateglinide

Biguanides

SELECT PROTOTYPE MEDICATION: Metformin

Thiazolidinediones (glitazones)

SELECT PROTOTYPE MEDICATION: Pioglitazone

OTHER MEDICATION: Rosiglitazone

Alpha-glucosidase inhibitors

SELECT PROTOTYPE MEDICATION: Acarbose

OTHER MEDICATIONS: Miglitol

Dipeptidyl peptidase-4 (DPP-4) inhibitors (gliptins)

SELECT PROTOTYPE MEDICATION: Sitagliptin

OTHER MEDICATIONS: Saxagliptin, linagliptin, alogliptin

Sodium-glucose co-transporter 2 (SGLT-2) inhibitors

SELECT PROTOTYPE MEDICATION: Canagliflozin

OTHER MEDICATIONS: Dapagliflozin, empagliflozin

Glucagon-like Peptide 1 (GLP-1)

SELECT PROTOTYPE MEDICATION: Semaglutide

PURPOSE

EXPECTED PHARMACOLOGICAL ACTION

Sulfonylureas: Insulin release from the pancreas; can increase tissue sensitivity to insulin over time

Meglitinides (glinides): Insulin release from the pancreas

Biguanides
- Reduces the production of glucose within the liver through suppression of gluconeogenesis
- Increases glucose uptake and use in fat and skeletal muscles
- Decreases glucose absorption in the gastrointestinal tract
- First choice medication for most clients who have type 2 diabetes

Thiazolidinediones (glitazones)
- Increases cellular response to insulin by decreasing insulin resistance
- Increases glucose uptake and decreased glucose production

Alpha-glucosidase inhibitors
- Slows carbohydrate absorption and digestion
- Miglitol was particularly effective for clients of Latino or African heritage in clinical trials

DPP-4 inhibitors (gliptins)
- Augments naturally occurring incretin hormones, which promote release of insulin and decrease secretion of glucagon
- Lowers fasting and postprandial blood glucose levels

SGLT-2 inhibitors
- Indicated for the management of type 2 diabetes
- Limits the rise of glucose postprandial
- Excretes glucose through the urine by preventing its reabsorption in the kidney
- Promotes weight loss

Glucagon-like Peptide 1 (GLP-1): Reduces the incretin hormone GLP-1 the body uses

THERAPEUTIC USES

- Antidiabetic agents control blood glucose levels in clients who have type 2 diabetes mellitus and are used in conjunction with diet and exercise lifestyle changes.
- Metformin is also used to treat polycystic ovary syndrome (PCOS) (off-label use).

COMPLICATIONS

Glipizide and repaglinide

Hypoglycemia
NURSING ACTIONS
- Monitor for manifestations of hypoglycemia.
- Ensure the client knows how to treat hypoglycemia orally, or that glucagon is available.

CLIENT EDUCATION: Notify the provider if there is a recurrent problem.

Weight gain
CLIENT EDUCATION: Adhere to a proper diet and increase physical activity.

Metformin

Gastrointestinal effects: Anorexia, nausea, and diarrhea, which frequently result in weight loss of 3 to 4 kg (6.6 to 8.8 lb)
NURSING ACTIONS
- Effects usually subside with use.
- Monitor for severity of these effects.
- Discontinue the medication if necessary.

Vitamin B$_{12}$ and folic acid deficiency: Caused by altered absorption
NURSING ACTIONS: Provide supplements as needed.

Lactic acidosis: Hyperventilation, myalgia, sluggishness, somnolence: 50% mortality rate
NURSING ACTIONS
- Severe lactic acidosis can be treated with hemodialysis.
- Clients with renal insufficiency should not use metformin (can rapidly accumulate to toxic levels).

CLIENT EDUCATION: Withhold medication if these findings occur and inform the provider immediately.

Pioglitazone

Fluid retention
NURSING ACTIONS: Monitor for edema, weight gain, and/or indications of heart failure.

Elevations in low density lipoproteins (LDL) cholesterol
NURSING ACTIONS: Monitor cholesterol levels.

Hepatotoxicity
NURSING ACTIONS: Perform baseline and periodic liver function tests.

CLIENT EDUCATION: Report any hepatotoxicity manifestations (jaundice or dark urine).

Ovulation in females who had been anovulatory (perimenopausal)
CLIENT EDUCATION: There is an increased risk for pregnancy; discuss contraceptive options if desired.

Acarbose

Gastrointestinal effects: Abdominal distention and cramping, hyperactive bowel sounds, diarrhea, excessive gas

NURSING ACTIONS
- Monitor impact of these effects on the client.
- Discontinue the medication if necessary.

Anemia due to the decrease of iron absorption

NURSING ACTIONS
- Monitor hemoglobin and iron levels.
- Discontinue the medication if necessary.

Hepatotoxicity with long-term use

NURSING ACTIONS
- Check baseline liver function and perform periodic liver function tests.
- Discontinue the medication if elevations occur.
- Liver function will return to normal after the medication is discontinued.

Impaired breakdown of sucrose

NURSING ACTIONS: Use glucose to treat hypoglycemia.

Sitagliptin

Generally well tolerated; can cause headache, nausea, joint pain, hypersensitivity reaction pancreatitis (rare)

CLIENT EDUCATION: This medication can cause manifestations of pancreatitis; notify the provider if they occur.

Canagliflozin

Cystitis, candidiasis, and polyuria in males and females
NURSING ACTIONS: Monitor for manifestations of infection.

Dizziness and risk for hypotension: In older adults with concurrent use of diuretics
NURSING ACTIONS: Use caution if medications are given together.

CLIENT EDUCATION: Rise slowly from a seated position and report episodes of dizziness to the provider.

Semaglutide

Nausea, loss of appetite, pancreatitis
NURSING ACTIONS: Monitor for nausea, weight loss

CLIENT EDUCATION: Advise client to notify provider for manifestations of pancreatitis (nausea, vomiting, abdominal pain radiating to back)

CONTRAINDICATIONS/PRECAUTIONS

- **Warnings**
  - Pregnancy
    - Sulfonylureas, meglitinides, biguanides, alpha-glucosidase inhibitors: Safety not established.
    - Thiazolidinediones: Contraindicated.
    - DPP-4 inhibitors: Use only if needed.
    - SGLT-2 inhibitors: Use only if the benefit to the client outweighs the risks to the fetus.
  - Lactation
    - Sulfonylureas, meglitinides, biguanides, DPP-4 inhibitors: Safety not established.
    - Thiazolidinediones, SGLT-2 inhibitors: Contraindicated.
  - Reproductive
    - Insulin is recommended during pregnancy for glycemic control.
    - Oral antidiabetics can decrease the effectiveness of oral contraceptives.
    - Clients should notify the provider if pregnancy is planned or suspected.
- Use cautiously in clients who have renal failure, hepatic dysfunction, or heart failure due to the risk of medication accumulation and resulting hypoglycemia. Severity of disease can indicate contraindication.
- All oral diabetic medications are contraindicated in the treatment of DKA.
- **Metformin** is contraindicated for clients who have severe infection, shock, kidney impairment, and any hypoxic condition. The medication should not be used by clients who have alcohol use disorder. The safety of metformin during pregnancy and lactation is unknown.
- **Acarbose** is contraindicated for clients who have gastrointestinal disorders (inflammatory disease, ulceration, or obstruction).
- **Pioglitazone** is contraindicated for clients who have severe heart failure, history of bladder cancer, and active hepatic disease. Use cautiously in clients who have mild heart failure and in older adults. Ⓖ
- **Canagliflozin** is contraindicated for clients who have renal failure and are undergoing dialysis.
- **Semaglutide** is contraindicated for clients who have type 1 diabetes mellitus.

INTERACTIONS

Glipizide

Use of alcohol can result in disulfiram-like reaction (intense nausea and vomiting, flushing, palpitations).
CLIENT EDUCATION: This medication increases this risk and should avoid alcohol.

NSAIDs, sulfonamide antibiotics, and cimetidine have additive hypoglycemic effect.
NURSING ACTIONS: Dosage adjustment of the oral antidiabetic medication might be indicated.

CLIENT EDUCATION: Closely monitor glucose levels when these other agents are used concurrently.

Beta blockers can mask SNS response to hypoglycemia (tachycardia, tremors, palpitations, diaphoresis), making it difficult for clients to identify hypoglycemia.
CLIENT EDUCATION
- Monitoring glucose levels is important, and do not rely on SNS manifestations as an alert to developing hypoglycemia.
- Maintain a regular eating schedule to ensure adequate glucose during times of hypoglycemic action.

Beta blockers decrease effectiveness by inhibiting insulin release.
CLIENT EDUCATION: Closely monitor glucose levels.

Repaglinide

Concurrent use of gemfibrozil results in inhibition of repaglinide metabolism, leading to an increased risk for hypoglycemia.
NURSING ACTIONS
- Avoid concurrent use of repaglinide or pioglitazone and gemfibrozil.
- Closely monitor for manifestations of hypoglycemia.

Pioglitazone

Use with insulin can lead to fluid retention.
NURSING ACTIONS: Avoid concurrent use.

Increased levels with ketoconazole and CYP2C8 inhibitors (gemfibrozil).
NURSING ACTIONS: Monitor glucose levels. Dosage of pioglitazone might need to be reduced.

Decreased levels with rifampin and cimetidine.
NURSING ACTIONS: Monitor glucose levels. Dosage of pioglitazone might need to be increased.

Metformin

Alcohol or cimetidine can increase the risk of lactic acidosis with concurrent use.
CLIENT EDUCATION: This medication increases these risks and avoid consuming alcohol. If a histamine$_2$ receptor blocker is required, take something other than cimetidine.

Concurrent use of iodine-containing contrast media can result in acute kidney failure.
CLIENT EDUCATION: If taking metformin, discontinue medication 24 to 48 hr prior to procedure. Medication can be continued 48 hr after test if lab results indicate normal kidney function.

Acarbose

Concurrent use of acarbose with sulfonylureas or insulin increases the risk for hypoglycemia.
NURSING ACTIONS: Monitor carefully for hypoglycemia.

Sitagliptin

Concurrent use of insulin, glyburide, glipizide or glimepiride increases the risk of hypoglycemia.
NURSING ACTIONS: Monitor for hypoglycemia. Dose reduction of insulin or sulfonylurea medication might be required.

Canagliflozin

Decreased effect if used concurrently with rifampin, phenytoin, or phenobarbital
NURSING ACTIONS: Monitor glucose levels, as dosage might need to be increased.

Increases the effect of thiazide and loop diuretics
NURSING ACTIONS: Monitor for dehydration and hypotension. Use caution if medications are used together.

Semaglutide

Concurrent use with agents that increase insulin secretion (sulfonylureas, insulin) can increase the risk of hypoglycemia
NURSING ACTIONS: Monitor glucose levels, as dosage might of agents increasing insulin secretion may need to be decreased.

NURSING ADMINISTRATION

- Consider referring clients to a registered dietitian or diabetic nurse educator. Qтс
- Administer medications orally and at appropriate times.
  - **Glipizide:** Best taken 30 min before breakfast. Withhold dose if client will not be able to eat.
  - **Repaglinide:** Instruct clients to take the medication within 30 min of mealtime, three times per day.
  - **Metformin:** Instruct clients to take immediate release tablets two times per day with breakfast and dinner and to take sustained-release tablets once daily with dinner.
  - **Pioglitazone:** Instruct clients to take once a day, with or without food.
  - **Acarbose:** Instruct clients to take with the first bite of food, three times per day. If a dose is missed, take the dose at the next meal but do not take two doses.
  - **Sitagliptin:** Instruct clients to take once a day with or without food.
  - **Canagliflozin:** Instruct clients to take once a day, before breakfast.

CLIENT EDUCATION
- Exercise consistently and follow appropriate dietary guidelines.
- Maintain a log of glucose levels and note patterns that affect glucose levels (increased dietary intake, infection).
- Formulations can combine two medications.
- If also taking insulin, monitor for manifestations of hypoglycemia.

Non-insulin injectable antidiabetics

Amylin mimetics

SELECT PROTOTYPE MEDICATION: Pramlintide

Incretin mimetics

SELECT PROTOTYPE MEDICATION: Exenatide

OTHER MEDICATIONS
- Liraglutide
- Albiglutide
- Lixisenatide
- Dulaglutide
- Semaglutide

PURPOSE

EXPECTED PHARMACOLOGICAL ACTION

Amylin mimetics: Pramlintide mimics the actions of the naturally occurring peptide hormone amylin to decrease gastric emptying time and inhibit secretion of glucagon, which reduces postprandial glucose levels. It also satiates, which helps decrease caloric intake.

Incretin mimetics: Mimics the effects of naturally occurring glucagon-like peptide-1 one type of incretin hormone. It promotes release of insulin, decreases secretion of glucagon, and slows gastric emptying. Fasting and postprandial blood glucose levels are lowered. Incretin mimetics decrease appetite which can lead to weight loss.

THERAPEUTIC USES

Amylin mimetics

- Supplemental glucose control for clients who have type 1 or type 2 diabetes mellitus, who have had ineffective glucose control with insulin therapy.
- Used in conjunction with insulin therapy

Incretin mimetics

- Supplemental glucose control for clients who have type 2 diabetes
- Can be used in conjunction with an oral antidiabetic medication, usually metformin or a sulfonylurea

COMPLICATIONS

Amylin mimetics

Nausea
CLIENT EDUCATION: Report manifestations to the provider. Dose can be decreased.

Reaction at injection sites: Generally self-limiting.

Incretin mimetics

GI effects (nausea, vomiting, diarrhea)
CLIENT EDUCATION: Notify the provider if manifestations are intolerable.

Pancreatitis (severe and intolerable abdominal pain)
CLIENT EDUCATION: Withhold medication and notify the provider.

CONTRAINDICATIONS/PRECAUTIONS

Warnings
- Pregnancy
  - Pramlintide: Safety not established.
  - Exenatide: Safety unknown, risk for possible birth defects.
- Lactation
  - Pramlintide: Safety not established.
  - Exenatide: Unknown.
- Reproductive: Take exenatide within 1 hr of oral contraceptives

Amylin mimetics

- This medication is contraindicated for clients who have kidney failure or are receiving dialysis.
- Use cautiously in clients who have thyroid disease, osteoporosis, or alcohol use disorder.

Incretin mimetics

- Contraindicated for clients who have kidney failure, ulcerative colitis, Crohn's disease, or a history of pancreatitis.
- Use cautiously in older adult clients and clients who have renal impairment or thyroid disease. Ⓖ

INTERACTIONS

Amylin mimetics

Concurrent use of insulin severely increases the risk for hypoglycemia.
NURSING ACTIONS: The provider should decrease the client's premeal rapid- or short-acting insulin dose by 50% when pramlintide therapy is initiated. Avoid use in clients unable to self-monitor blood glucose levels.

Concurrent use of pramlintide with medications that slow gastric emptying (opioids) or medications that delay food absorption (acarbose) can further slow gastric emptying time.
NURSING ACTIONS: Avoid concurrent use.
Oral medication absorption is delayed.

NURSING CONSIDERATIONS: Administer oral medications 1 hr before or 2 hr after injection of pramlintide.

Incretin mimetics

Oral medication absorption is delayed, especially oral contraceptives, antibiotics, and acetaminophen.
NURSING ACTIONS: Administer oral medications 1 hr before injection of exenatide.

Concurrent use of sulfonylurea increases risk of hypoglycemia.
CLIENT EDUCATION: A lower dose of sulfonylurea can be required. Monitor blood glucose levels.

NURSING ADMINISTRATION

Amylin mimetics

- Administer subcutaneously prior to meals, using the thigh or abdomen. Ensure the injection is at least 5 cm (2 in) from the injection site for any insulin given at that time. Ⓠ EBP
- Administer oral medications 1 hr before or 2 hr after pramlintide injections, to prevent delayed absorption of the oral medication.

CLIENT EDUCATION
- Keep unopened vials in the refrigerator and do not allow to freeze. Opened vials can be kept cool or at room temperature but should be discarded after 28 days. Keep vials out of direct sunlight.
- Do not mix medication with insulin in the same syringe.

Incretin mimetics

- This medication is supplied in prefilled injector pens.
- Administer subcutaneously in the thigh, abdomen, or upper arm. Ⓠ EBP
- Give exenatide injection within 60 min before the morning and evening meal. Never administer after a meal. Exenatide is also available in a longer-acting formula that can be administered once weekly.
- Other incretin mimetics have varied dosing requirements for frequency and regard to meals. Verify the dosing information for the specific medication prior to administration.

CLIENT EDUCATION: Keep the injection pen in the refrigerator and discard after 30 days.

NURSING EVALUATION OF MEDICATION EFFECTIVENESS

Incretin mimetics

Depending on therapeutic intent, effectiveness can be evidenced by the following.
- Preprandial glucose levels 90 to 130 mg/dL and postprandial levels less than 180 mg/dL
- HbA1c less than 7%

Hyperglycemic agent

SELECT PROTOTYPE MEDICATION: Glucagon

PURPOSE

EXPECTED PHARMACOLOGICAL ACTION: Increases blood glucose levels by increasing the breakdown of glycogen into glucose

THERAPEUTIC USES

- Emergency management of hypoglycemic reactions (insulin toxicity) in clients who are unable to take oral glucose or if IV glucose is not an option
- Decrease in gastrointestinal motility in clients undergoing radiological procedures of the stomach and intestines

COMPLICATIONS

GI distress (nausea, vomiting)

NURSING ACTIONS: Turn clients onto the left side following administration to reduce the risk of aspiration if emesis occurs.

CONTRAINDICATIONS/PRECAUTIONS

- **Warnings**
  - Pregnancy: Glucagon safe only if indicated.
  - Lactation: Glucagon safety not established.
- Glucagon might not be effective for hypoglycemia resulting from inadequate glycogen stores (starvation).
- Use cautiously in clients who have cardiovascular disease.

NURSING ADMINISTRATION

- Administer glucagon subcutaneously, IM, or IV immediately following reconstitution parameters. ⓆEBP
- Provide oral glucose as soon as the client regains full consciousness and is able to swallow.

CLIENT EDUCATION: Maintain access to a source of glucose and glucagon kit at all times and replace glucagon immediately when it reaches the expiration date.

NURSING EVALUATION OF MEDICATION EFFECTIVENESS

Depending on therapeutic intent, effectiveness can be evidenced by elevation in blood glucose level to greater than 70 mg/dL

37.2 Case study

Scenario introduction

Lisa is a nurse at an urgent care center caring for Ms. Smith, a 65-year-old Caucasian female. She was brought to the clinic by her daughter who is visiting from out of town.

Ms. Smith's social history is as follows:

- Lives alone in a one-bedroom low-income apartment complex
- Does not have a landline or a cellular phone
- BMI of 38, appropriately dressed for the weather
- Does not have medical insurance, has not been to a provider's office in 3 years
- Works part time at a bakery and states that she is often able to bring home merchandise at the end of the day that did not sell. She travels to and from work using public transportation
- Quit school due to pregnancy, stated she gained a great deal of weight during pregnancy
- Widowed and has one adult child who lives three hours away

Scene 1

Nurse Lisa: "Hello, Ms. Smith. My name is Lisa, and I will be caring for you. Can you tell me what brings you here to the urgent care center today?"

Ms. Smith: "My daughter insisted I come in because I haven't been feeling well for about a month now. I am thirsty all the time, my vision is blurry, and I am so tired even after sleeping all night. I have gained about 10 pounds over the past two months, and I really don't know what could be wrong with me."

Nurse Lisa: "Okay, thank you for providing this information. Mrs. Smith, do you have a family history of diabetes?"

Ms. Smith: "Yes, I think my mother may have had it. But I'm not sure."

Scene 2

Nurse Lisa: "Ms. Smith, I would like to check your blood sugar if that is okay with you. Have you eaten anything today?"

Ms. Smith: "No, I've not eaten any food today."

Nurse Lisa: "Ms. Smith, your blood glucose reading is 358. This is elevated and could indicate diabetes mellitus. I will inform your provider, who will be by to see you soon."

Scene 3

Nurse Lisa: "Since your provider has discussed your new diagnosis of type 2 diabetes mellitus with you, the laboratory technician will be in shortly to draw some additional blood for further testing. In the meantime, I would like to review some information about diabetes mellitus and your provider prescriptions."

Ms. Smith: "Okay, sure."

Nurse Lisa: "Your provider would like for you to monitor your blood sugar at home at least twice each day. You have a prescription for 500 mg of metformin to be taken twice a day by mouth. You will need to follow up with a primary care provider in approximately 3 weeks. Here is a list of our local providers. If you're unable to see a primary provider, you can make an appointment at the community health center. I am providing you with several pamphlets about diabetes as well as information about metformin."

Scenario conclusion

Ms. Smith looks briefly at the information Nurse Lisa provides and becomes tearful. She tells her that she does not know how she can possibly cope with this news. Nurse Lisa reviews the social determinants of health (SDOH) for Ms. Smith to gain a better understanding of her situation.

Case study exercise

1. Nurse Lisa reviews the client's social history. Which of the following social determinants of health (SDOH) may be impacting Ms. Smith's feelings of inability to cope? (Select all that apply.)

   A. Economic stability

   B. Education

   C. Health and health care

   D. Neighborhood and built environment

   E. Social and community context

   F. Food security/insecurity

Application Exercises

1. A nurse is teaching clients about the use of insulin to treat type 1 diabetes mellitus. For which of the following types of insulin should the nurse tell the clients to expect a peak effect 1 to 5 hr after administration?

   A. Insulin glargine

   B. NPH insulin

   C. Regular insulin

   D. Insulin lispro

2. A nurse is providing teaching for a client who has a new prescription for metformin. Which of the following findings should the nurse instruct the client to report as an adverse effect of metformin?

   A. Somnolence

   B. Constipation

   C. Fluid retention

   D. Weight gain

3. A nurse is caring for a client who has been taking acarbose for type 2 diabetes mellitus. Which of the following laboratory tests should the nurse plan to monitor?

   A. WBC

   B. Amylase

   C. Platelet count

   D. Liver function tests

4. A nurse is providing teaching to a client who has type 2 diabetes mellitus and is starting repaglinide. Which of the following statements by the client indicates understanding of the administration of this medication?

   A. "I'll take this medication after I eat."

   B. "I'll take this medicine 30 minutes before I eat."

   C. "I'll take this medicine just before I go to bed."

   D. "I'll take this medication at least 1 hour before I eat."

5. A nurse is providing teaching to a client who has a prescription for pramlintide for type 1 diabetes mellitus. Which of the following should the nurse include in the teaching? (Select all that apply.)

   A. "Take oral medications 30 min before injection."

   B. "Use upper arms as preferred injection sites."

   C. "Mix pramlintide with the breakfast dose of insulin."

   D. "Inject pramlintide just before a meal."

   E. "Allow the medication to warm to room temperature."

Active Learning Scenario

A nurse is teaching a client who has type 2 diabetes mellitus and is taking exenatide along with an oral antidiabetic agent. What should the nurse teach the client about this medication? Use the ATI Active Learning Template: Medication to complete this item.

THERAPEUTIC USES: Identify the therapeutic use for exenatide in this client.

COMPLICATIONS: Identify two adverse effects the client should watch for.

NURSING INTERVENTIONS: Describe two laboratory tests the nurse should monitor.

CLIENT EDUCATION: Describe teaching points to give a client taking exenatide.

Application Exercises Key

1. C. **CORRECT:** When taking actions, the nurse should instruct the client that regular insulin has a peak effect around 1 to 5 hr following administration. Insulin glargine has no set peak. NPH insulin has a peak of 4-14 hours. Insulin lispro has a peak of 0.5 hr. to 3 hr.

   Ⓝ *NCLEX® Connection: Pharmacological and Parenteral Therapies, Medication Administration*

2. A. **CORRECT:** When taking actions, the nurse should instruct the client that somnolence can indicate lactic acidosis, which is manifested by extreme drowsiness, hyperventilation, and muscle pain. It is a rare but very serious adverse effect caused by metformin and should be reported to the provider.

   Ⓝ *NCLEX® Connection: Pharmacological and Parenteral Therapies, Adverse Effects/Contraindications/Side Effects/Interactions*

3. D. **CORRECT:** The nurse should plan to generate solutions to address potential adverse effects of a client's medications. Acarbose can cause liver toxicity when taken long-term. The nurse should monitor the client's liver function while taking this medication.

   Ⓝ *NCLEX® Connection: Pharmacological and Parenteral Therapies, Expected Actions/Outcomes*

4. B. **CORRECT:** When taking actions, the nurse should instruct the client that repaglinide causes a rapid, short-lived release of insulin. The client should take this medication within 30 min before each meal so that insulin is available when food is digested. N

   Ⓝ *NCLEX® Connection: Pharmacological and Parenteral Therapies, Medication Administration*

5. D, E. **CORRECT:** When taking actions, the nurse should instruct the client that pramlintide can cause hypoglycemia, especially when the client also takes insulin, so it is important to eat a meal after injecting this medication.

   The nurse should also inform the client that the medication should be allowed to warm to room temperature prior to administration.

   Ⓝ *NCLEX® Connection: Pharmacological and Parenteral Therapies, Medication Administration*

Case Study Exercises Key

1. A, B, C, F. **CORRECT:** Type 2 diabetes is more common among those who have poor SDOH. Cost-related nonadherence (CRN) among clients who have diabetes is prevalent and the negative health consequences can be significant. Health care costs for clients who have diabetes are 3 times higher than for those without diabetes. The nurse should analyze the cues from the client's history and determine that Ms. Smith's economic stability (only works at a part time job) impacts her ability to pay for her prescription.

   Health and health care impacts Ms. Smith's access to healthcare (uses public transportation), her lack of a primary care provider, and health literacy can be a factor in her understanding the pamphlets and medication information.

   Ms. Smith is also impacted by food insecurity due to a minimal income and her admission of taking home baked goods to supplement her food intake.

Active Learning Scenario Key

Using the ATI Active Learning Template: Medication

THERAPEUTIC USES: Exenatide is prescribed along with an oral antidiabetic medication (metformin or a sulfonylurea medication) for clients who have type 2 diabetes mellitus to improve diabetes control. Exenatide improves insulin secretion by the pancreas, decreases secretion of glucagon, and slows gastric emptying.

COMPLICATIONS
- GI effects (nausea and vomiting)
- Pancreatitis manifested by acute abdominal pain and possibly severe vomiting
- Hypoglycemia, especially when taken concurrently with a sulfonylurea medication (glipizide)

NURSING INTERVENTIONS: Monitor daily blood glucose testing by the client, periodic HbA1c tests, and periodic kidney function testing. Exenatide should be used cautiously in clients who have any renal impairment.

CLIENT EDUCATION
- Inject exenatide subcutaneously.
- Take exenatide within 60 min before the morning and evening meal but not following the meal.
- Withhold exenatide and notify the provider for severe abdominal pain.
- Recognize and treat hypoglycemia.
- Exenatide should not be given within 1 hr of oral medications, particularly antibiotics, acetaminophen, or contraceptives due to its ability to slow gastric emptying.

Ⓝ *NCLEX® Connection: Pharmacological and Parenteral Therapies, Medication Administration*

UNIT 10   MEDICATIONS AFFECTING THE
ENDOCRINE SYSTEM

CHAPTER 38 *Endocrine Disorders*

The endocrine system is made up of glands that secrete hormones, which act on specific receptor sites. Hormones target receptor sites to regulate response to stress, growth, metabolism, and homeostasis.

An endocrine disorder usually involves the oversecretion or undersecretion of hormones, or an altered response by the target area or receptor.

Medications used to treat disorders of the thyroid, anterior and posterior pituitary, and adrenal glands are discussed in this chapter.

Thyroid hormone

SELECT PROTOTYPE MEDICATION: Levothyroxine

OTHER MEDICATIONS
- Liothyronine
- Liotrix
- Thyroid USP

PURPOSE

EXPECTED PHARMACOLOGICAL ACTION: Thyroid hormone preparations are a synthetic form of thyroxine (T_4), a form of liothyronine (T_3), or a combination of T_3 and T_4, that increase metabolic rate, protein synthesis, cardiac output, renal perfusion, oxygen use, body temperature, blood volume, and growth processes.

THERAPEUTIC USES
- Thyroid hormone replacement is used for treatment of hypothyroidism (all ages, all forms).
- Thyroid hormones are used for the emergency treatment of myxedema coma (IV route), a severe deficiency of thyroid hormone. They are also used to manage cretinism and simple goiter.
- Maintenance of thyroid hormone levels after surgery or radiation of the thyroid.

ROUTE OF ADMINISTRATION: Oral, IV (myxedema coma)

COMPLICATIONS

Overmedication

Overmedication can result in manifestations of thyrotoxicosis (anxiety, tachycardia, chest pain, nervousness, tremors, palpitations, abdominal cramping, heat intolerance, fever, diaphoresis, weight loss).

CLIENT EDUCATION: Report manifestations of overmedication to the provider.

Chronic overtreatment

Chronic overtreatment can cause atrial fibrillation and an increased risk of fractures from accelerated bone loss, especially in older adults.

NURSING ACTIONS: TSH levels should be monitored at least once a year.

CONTRAINDICATIONS/PRECAUTIONS

- Warnings
  - Pregnancy: Levothyroxine is safe.
  - Lactation: Use levothyroxine with caution.
- Use is contraindicated for clients who have thyrotoxicosis and adrenal insufficiency.
- Because of cardiac stimulant effects, use is contraindicated following a MI. Use cautiously in clients who have cardiovascular problems (hypertension, angina pectoris, ischemic heart disease).
- Use cautiously in older adults, who may require lower dosages. ©
- Use cautiously in clients who have diabetes.
- Thyroid hormone replacement is not for use in the treatment of obesity.

INTERACTIONS

Increases cardiac responsiveness to catecholamines (epinephrine, dopamine, dobutamine) thereby increasing the risk of dysrhythmias.
NURSING ACTIONS: Use catecholamines cautiously with clients who take levothyroxine.

Can increase requirements for insulin and digoxin.

Binding agents, antiulcer medications, calcium and iron supplements, magnesium salts, and food reduce levothyroxine absorption with concurrent use.
- Binding agents include cholestyramine and colestipol. Antiulcer medications include sucralfate, cimetidine, lansoprazole, and antacids.
- NURSING ACTIONS: Allow at least 4 hr between medication administration.

Many antiseizure and antidepressant medications, including carbamazepine, phenytoin, phenobarbital, and sertraline, can increase levothyroxine metabolism.
NURSING ACTIONS: Monitor for therapeutic effects of levothyroxine. Dosages of levothyroxine might need to be increased.

Levothyroxine can increase the anticoagulant effects of warfarin by breaking down vitamin K.

NURSING ACTIONS

- Monitor prothrombin time (PT) and international normalized ratio (INR).
- Decreased dosages of warfarin may be needed.

CLIENT EDUCATION: Report bleeding (bruising, petechiae).

NURSING ADMINISTRATION

- Obtain baseline vital signs, weight, and height, and monitor periodically throughout treatment.
- Monitor and report manifestations of cardiac excitability (angina, chest pain, palpitations, dysrhythmias). Check apical pulse.
- Daily therapy begins with a low dose that increases gradually over several weeks. Full effect of medication can take 6 to 8 weeks.
- Monitor T_4 and TSH levels.
- Medication is generally dosed in micrograms.
- Prepare and administer IV doses cautiously. Medication requires reconstituting and verification of the final concentration should be obtained prior to administering medication. Qs

CLIENT EDUCATION

- Take the medication daily on an empty stomach 30 to 60 min before breakfast.
- Lifelong replacement is important even after improvement. Do not discontinue the medication without checking with the provider.
- Check with the provider before switching to another brand of levothyroxine because different brands might have varied effects, and dosage adjustments can be necessary. Qtc

NURSING EVALUATION OF MEDICATION EFFECTIVENESS

Depending on therapeutic intent, evidence of effectiveness can include the following.

- Decreased TSH levels. Evaluation of TSH should not be done until 6 to 8 weeks following the start of treatment.
- T_4 levels within expected reference range
- Absence of hypothyroidism manifestations (depression, weight gain, bradycardia, anorexia, cold intolerance, dry skin, menorrhagia)

Thionamides

SELECT PROTOTYPE MEDICATION: Methimazole

OTHER MEDICATION: Propylthiouracil (PTU)

PURPOSE

EXPECTED PHARMACOLOGICAL ACTION

- Blocks the synthesis of thyroid hormones
- Prevents the oxidation of iodide
- Blocks conversion of T_4 into T_3 (PKU)

THERAPEUTIC USES

- Treatment of Graves' disease
- Produces a euthyroid state prior to thyroid removal surgery
- As an adjunct to irradiation of the thyroid gland
- In the emergency treatment of thyrotoxicosis
- Methimazole is considered first-line therapy

ROUTE OF ADMINISTRATION: Oral

COMPLICATIONS

Hypothyroidism

Overmedication can result in manifestations of hypothyroidism (drowsiness, depression, weight gain, edema, bradycardia, anorexia, cold intolerance, dry skin, menorrhagia).

NURSING ACTIONS: Reduced dosages and/or temporary administration of thyroid supplements can be needed.

CLIENT EDUCATION: Report manifestations of overmedication to the provider.

Agranulocytosis

NURSING ACTIONS

- Monitor for early manifestations of agranulocytosis (sore throat, fever), and instruct clients to report them promptly to provider.
- Monitor blood counts at baseline and periodically.
- If agranulocytosis occurs, stop treatment, and monitor the client for reversal of agranulocytosis.
- Filgrastim can be indicated to treat agranulocytosis.

Liver injury, hepatitis (propylthiouracil)

NURSING ACTIONS: Monitor for jaundice, dark urine, light-colored stools, and elevated liver function tests during treatment.

CONTRAINDICATIONS/PRECAUTIONS

- **Warnings**: Pregnancy/Lactation:
  ○ Methimazole: Caution in clients who are pregnant; use only if the benefit to the client outweighs the risks to the fetus. Can use during the second and third trimester.
- Propylthiouracil does not cross the placenta and can be used during the first trimester; use only if the benefit to the client outweighs the risks to the fetus.
- Methimazole, propylthiouracil: Present in breastmilk; however, can be prescribed at low dose.
- Use cautiously in clients who have bone marrow depression and/or immunosuppression, and in clients at risk for liver failure.

INTERACTIONS

Concurrent use of antithyroid medications and anticoagulants can increase anticoagulation.
NURSING ACTIONS: Monitor PT, INR, and activated partial thromboplastin time (aPTT), and adjust dosages of anticoagulants accordingly.

Concurrent use of antithyroid medications and digoxin can increase glycoside level.
NURSING ACTIONS: Monitor digoxin level and reduce digoxin dose as needed.

NURSING ADMINISTRATION

- Methimazole and propylthiouracil do not destroy the thyroid hormone that is present, but rather prevent continued synthesis of TH.
- Monitor vital signs, weight, and I&O at baseline and periodically.
- Monitor thyroid levels before, during and after therapy. Monitor for manifestations of hyperthyroidism (indicating inadequate medication).
- Clients who have hyperthyroidism may be given a beta-adrenergic antagonist (propranolol) to decrease tremors and tachycardia.
- Monitor for manifestations of hypothyroidism (indicating overmedication), including drowsiness, depression, weight gain, edema, bradycardia, anorexia, cold intolerance, and dry skin.
- Monitor CBC for leukopenia or thrombocytopenia.
- Health care workers of childbearing age should handle methimazole with caution. Qs

CLIENT EDUCATION

- Report fever, chills, headache, malaise, and weakness.
- Therapeutic effects can take 1 to 2 weeks to be evident, while full benefit can take 3 to 12 weeks. Qpcc
- Take medication at consistent times each day and with meals to maintain a consistent therapeutic level and decrease gastric distress.
- Do not discontinue the medication abruptly (risk of thyroid crisis due to stress response).
- Do not take any OTC medications or herbals without consent of provider.
- May cause drowsiness, use caution with driving or other activities that require alertness.
- Check weight 2 to 3 times per week.
- Products that contain iodine may not always be a contraindication in clients who have a shellfish allergy. Further assessment may be needed.

NURSING EVALUATION OF MEDICATION EFFECTIVENESS

Depending on therapeutic intent, evidence of effectiveness can include the following.
- Weight gain
- Vital signs within expected reference range
- Decreased T_4 levels
- Absence of manifestations of hyperthyroidism (anxiety, tachycardia, palpitations, increased appetite, abdominal cramping, heat intolerance, fever, diaphoresis, weight loss, menstrual irregularities)

Radiopharmaceuticals

SELECT PROTOTYPE MEDICATION: Radioactive iodine (I–131)

PURPOSE

EXPECTED PHARMACOLOGICAL ACTION: Radioactive iodine is absorbed by the thyroid and destroys some of the thyroid hormone–producing cells.

THERAPEUTIC USES
- At high doses:
  - Hyperthyroidism
  - Thyroid cancer
  - Clients who have not responded to other antithyroid treatments
- At low doses: Thyroid function studies (Visualization of the degree of iodine uptake by the thyroid gland is helpful in the diagnosis of thyroid disorders.)

ROUTE OF ADMINISTRATION: Oral

COMPLICATIONS

Radiation sickness

NURSING ACTIONS
- Monitor for manifestations of radiation sickness (hematemesis, epistaxis, intense nausea, vomiting).
- Stop treatment and notify the provider.

Bone marrow depression

Leukemia may be induced.

NURSING ACTIONS: Monitor for leukemia, anemia, leukopenia, and thrombocytopenia.

Hypothyroidism

Intolerance to cold, edema, bradycardia, weight gain, depression

CLIENT EDUCATION: Instruct clients to report manifestations of hypothyroidism to the provider.

CONTRAINDICATIONS/PRECAUTIONS

- **Warnings**
  - Pregnancy: Radioactive iodine contraindicated.
  - Lactation: Radioactive iodine contraindicated.
- Young children are considered inappropriate candidates. Qs

INTERACTIONS

Concurrent use of other antithyroid medications reduces uptake of radioactive iodine. Also known as Lugol's solution.
NURSING ACTIONS: Discontinue use of other antithyroid medications for a week prior to therapy.

NURSING ADMINISTRATION

Clients and secretions will be radioactive until the iodide decays.

CLIENT EDUCATION
- Maintain a distance of 6 feet from others.
- Do not prepare food for others or share utensils. Qpcc
- Avoid close contact with a young children or clients who are pregnant (limit exposure to about 1 hr daily).
- Increase fluid intake, usually 2 to 3 L/day.
- Dispose of body wastes as instructed (saliva, stool, emesis, bronchial secretions).

Iodine products

SELECT PROTOTYPE MEDICATION: Strong iodine solution: nonradioactive iodine (also known as Lugol's Solution)

OTHER MEDICATIONS
- Sodium iodide
- Potassium iodide

PURPOSE

EXPECTED PHARMACOLOGICAL ACTION: Nonradioactive iodine creates high levels of iodide that will reduce iodine uptake (by the thyroid gland), inhibit thyroid hormone production, and block the release of thyroid hormones into the bloodstream.

THERAPEUTIC USES
- Nonradioactive iodine is used for the development of euthyroid state and reduction of thyroid gland size prior to thyroid removal surgery.
- Nonradioactive iodine is used for the emergency treatment of thyrotoxicosis.

ROUTE OF ADMINISTRATION: Oral

COMPLICATIONS

Iodism

- Due to corrosive property (metallic taste, stomatitis, sore teeth and gums, frontal headache, skin rash).
- Iodism (early toxicity) can progress to toxicity (severe GI distress and swelling of the glottis).

NURSING ACTIONS: Prepare to administer sodium thiosulfate (to reverse effects of iodine). Assist with gastric lavage as needed.

CLIENT EDUCATION: Notify provider for any manifestations of toxicity.

CONTRAINDICATIONS/PRECAUTIONS

Warnings
- Pregnancy: Strong iodine solution safety unknown.
- Lactation: Strong iodine solution safety unknown.

INTERACTIONS

Concurrent intake of foods high in iodine (iodized salt, seafood containing iodine) increases risk for iodism.
NURSING ACTIONS: Monitor for iodism (brassy taste in mouth, burning sensation in mouth, sore teeth).

CLIENT EDUCATION: Avoid foods high in iodine.

Concurrent use of potassium-sparing diuretics, potassium supplements, and ACE inhibitors increases the risk of hyperkalemia.
NURSING ACTIONS: Do not use medications together.

NURSING ADMINISTRATION

- Nonradioactive iodine can be used in conjunction with other therapy because effects are not usually complete or permanent. Qpcc
- Obtain baseline vital signs, weight, and I&O, and monitor periodically.

CLIENT EDUCATION
- Dilute strong iodine solution with juice to improve taste.
- Take at the same time each day to maintain therapeutic levels.
- Increase fluid intake, unless contraindicated.
- Do not take any OTC medications that contain iodine.
- Do not discontinue medication abruptly.

NURSING EVALUATION OF MEDICATION EFFECTIVENESS

Depending on therapeutic intent, effectiveness can be evidenced by the following.

- Weight gain
- Vital signs within expected reference range
- Decreased circulating levels of T_3 and T_4
- Reduction in size of thyroid gland
- Client will be able to get adequate sleep, achieve and maintain appropriate weight, maintain blood pressure and heart rate within expected reference range, and be free of complications of hyperthyroidism.

Anterior pituitary hormones/ growth hormones

SELECT PROTOTYPE MEDICATION: Somatropin

PURPOSE

EXPECTED PHARMACOLOGICAL ACTION: Anterior pituitary hormones/growth hormones stimulate overall growth and the production of protein and decrease the use of glucose.

THERAPEUTIC USES

- Anterior pituitary hormones/growth hormones are used to treat growth hormone deficiencies (pediatric and adult growth hormone deficiencies, Turner's syndrome, Prader-Willi syndrome, chronic renal insufficiency, cachexia, and short bowel syndrome).
- AIDS wasting syndrome
- Pediatric growth failure associated with chronic renal insufficiency, cachexia, and short bowel syndrome.

ROUTES OF ADMINISTRATION: IM or subcutaneous (preferred route)

COMPLICATIONS

Hyperglycemia

NURSING ACTIONS

- Observe for manifestations of hyperglycemia (polyphagia, polydipsia, polyuria).
- Monitor glucose levels when used in clients who have diabetes. Insulin doses may need to be adjusted.

Inactivation

Neutralizing antibodies: over the course of treatment, clients may develop neutralizing antibodies that bind with growth hormones and render it inactive.

NURSING ACTIONS: Must use mecasermin for further treatment.

CONTRAINDICATIONS/PRECAUTIONS

- **Warnings**
  - Pregnancy: Somatropin safety not established.
  - Lactation: Safety not established.
- Use is contraindicated in clients who are severely obese or have severe respiratory impairment (sleep apnea) because of higher risk of fatality.
- Use cautiously in clients who have diabetes because of the risk of hyperglycemia.
- Use cautiously in clients who have hypothyroidism, as thyroid function can be suppressed. Evaluate thyroid function prior to administering and periodically.
- Treatment should be stopped prior to epiphyseal closure.

INTERACTIONS

Concurrent use of glucocorticoids can counteract growth-promoting effects.
NURSING ACTIONS: Avoid concurrent use of glucocorticoids and growth hormones if possible. When giving concurrently, glucocorticoid dosage should be adjusted cautiously to prevent this effect.

NURSING ADMINISTRATION

- Obtain baseline height and weight.
- Monitor growth patterns during medication administration, usually monthly. Qᴾᶜᶜ
- Reconstitute medication per directions. Mix gently, and do not shake prior to administration. Do not administer if medication contains particulates or is discolored.
- Rotate injection sites. Abdomen (subcutaneous) and thighs (subcutaneous, IM) are preferred.

NURSING EVALUATION OF MEDICATION EFFECTIVENESS

Depending on therapeutic intent, effectiveness can be evidenced by the client increasing height and weight.

Antidiuretic hormone

SELECT PROTOTYPE MEDICATION: Vasopressin

OTHER MEDICATION: Desmopressin

PURPOSE

EXPECTED PHARMACOLOGICAL ACTION

- Antidiuretic hormone (ADH), produced by the hypothalamus and stored in the posterior pituitary, promotes reabsorption of water within the kidney through vasoconstriction.
- Both medications simulate natural ADH effects, with vasopressin being more potent than desmopressin.

THERAPEUTIC USES

- These hormones are used to treat diabetes insipidus (DI). Desmopressin is the agent of choice for DI.
- Antidiuretic hormone (vasopressin) is sometimes used during CPR to temporarily decrease blood flow to the periphery and increase flow to the brain and heart.
- Desmopressin can be used for nocturnal enuresis (decreases the production of urine) and hemophilia (promote release of certain clotting factors).

ROUTE OF ADMINISTRATION

- Desmopressin: Oral, intranasal, subcutaneous, IV
- Vasopressin: Subcutaneous, IM, IV

COMPLICATIONS

Water intoxication (retention of too much water)

NURSING ACTIONS

- Monitor for and report manifestations of overhydration (sleepiness, pounding headache).
- In general, clients should reduce fluid intake during therapy.
- Clients should use the smallest effective dosage of desmopressin.

Myocardial ischemia

From excessive vasoconstriction (vasopressin) of coronary arteries. Manifestations include angina pectoris, coronary insufficiency, and MI.

NURSING ACTIONS: Monitor ECG and blood pressure.

CLIENT EDUCATION: Notify the provider of chest pain, tightness, or diaphoresis.

CONTRAINDICATIONS/PRECAUTIONS

- **Warnings**
  - Pregnancy
    - Vasopressin: Use with caution.
    - Desmopressin: Safety not established.
  - Lactation
    - Vasopressin: Use with caution.
    - Desmopressin: Safety not established.
- Use of vasopressin is contraindicated in clients who have coronary artery disease (risk for angina, MI), decreased peripheral circulation (risk for gangrene), or chronic nephritis. Qs
- Use caution in clients who have renal impairment, as risk of water intoxication is increased.

INTERACTIONS

Carbamazepine and tricyclic antidepressants can increase the antidiuretic action.
NURSING ACTIONS: Use cautiously together.

Concurrent use of alcohol, heparin, lithium, or phenytoin can decrease antidiuretic effects.
NURSING ACTIONS: Establish baseline I&O and weight (monitor frequently).

NURSING ADMINISTRATION

- Desmopressin might be preferred due to ease of administration and less severe adverse effects.
- Monitor vital signs, central venous pressure, I&O, specific gravity, and laboratory studies (potassium, sodium, BUN, creatinine, specific gravity, osmolality).
- Monitor blood pressure, daily weight, and heart rate.
- Monitor for headache, drowsiness, confusion, or other manifestations of water intoxication.
- Desmopressin starts with a bedtime dosing. I&O is monitored. When nocturia is controlled, doses are given PO twice daily.
- If toxicity is suspected, notify the provider, who might restrict water intake and discontinue therapy.

NURSING EVALUATION OF MEDICATION EFFECTIVENESS

Depending on therapeutic intent, evidence of effectiveness can include the following.

- Reduction in the large volumes of urine output associated with diabetes insipidus to normal levels of urine output (1.5 to 2 L/24 hr)
- Cardiac arrest survival

Adrenal hormone replacement

SELECT PROTOTYPE MEDICATION: Hydrocortisone

OTHER MEDICATIONS
- Glucocorticoids
  - Prednisone
  - Dexamethasone
- Mineralocorticoid: Fludrocortisone

PURPOSE

EXPECTED PHARMACOLOGICAL ACTION: Mimic effect of natural steroid hormones

THERAPEUTIC USES
- Acute and chronic replacement therapy for adrenocortical insufficiency (Addison's disease, adrenal crisis).
- Nonendocrine disorders include cancer, inflammation, and allergic reactions.

ROUTE OF ADMINISTRATION: Oral, IV, IM

COMPLICATIONS

Glucocorticoids: hydrocortisone

Glucose intolerance: Glucocorticoids can increase plasma glucose levels, causing hyperglycemia and glycosuria

Fluid and electrolyte disturbance: Can cause sodium and water retention and potassium loss. Can lead to hypertension, edema, and serious dysrhythmias

Osteoporosis

CLIENT EDUCATION: Take calcium supplements, vitamin D, and/or bisphosphonate, and to get regular exercise.

Adrenal suppression

NURSING ACTIONS: Increase dose with stress. Do not stop the medication suddenly. Taper dose to discontinue.

CLIENT EDUCATION: Observe for manifestations (fatigue, muscle weakness, weight loss, nausea, vomiting, confusion, hypotension), and notify the provider if they occur.

Peptic ulcer, GI discomfort

CLIENT EDUCATION: Observe for manifestations (coffee-ground emesis, bloody or tarry stools, abdominal pain), and notify the provider if they occur.

Infection

NURSING ACTIONS

- Can cause immunosuppression and mask the manifestations of infection.
- Monitor for any manifestations of infection (fever).

CLIENT EDUCATION: Avoid contact with people who have a communicable disease.

Cushing's syndrome

NURSING ACTIONS: Risks are associated with long-term use of glucocorticoids and excessive doses.

CLIENT EDUCATION: Observe for manifestations (muscle weakness, moon face, buffalo hump, cutaneous striations), and notify the provider if they occur.

Mineralocorticoid: fludrocortisone

Retention of sodium and water: This can lead to hypertension, edema, heart failure and hypokalemia.

NURSING ACTIONS

- Monitor weight, blood pressure, and blood potassium. Monitor breath sounds and urine output.
- Educate clients on manifestations of sodium and water retention (weight gain, peripheral edema) and hypokalemia (muscle weakness, irregular pulse), and to notify provider if they occur.

CONTRAINDICATIONS/PRECAUTIONS

- **Warnings**
  - Pregnancy: Glucocorticoids safety not established.
  - Lactation: Glucocorticoids contraindicated.
  - Reproductive: Glucocorticoids can decrease the effectiveness of oral contraceptives.
- Use is contraindicated in clients who have an active infection not controlled by antibiotics.
- Use with caution in clients who have had a recent MI, gastric ulcer, hypertension, kidney disorder, osteoporosis, diabetes mellitus, cirrhosis, hypothyroidism, myasthenia gravis, glaucoma, or seizure disorder.

INTERACTIONS

Oral antidiabetics

Clients who have diabetes mellitus may require increased doses of glucose-lowering drug.
NURSING ACTIONS: Monitor blood glucose levels.

Glucocorticoids: hydrocortisone

NSAIDs, acetaminophen, or alcohol use can cause increased gastric distress or bleed.
NURSING ACTIONS: Use together with caution. Concurrent use with potassium depleting agents can cause hypokalemia (loop and thiazide diuretics).

NURSING ACTIONS: Monitor blood potassium and ECG.

Concurrent use with vaccines and toxoids can reduce the antibody response.
NURSING ACTIONS: Do not use together.

Mineralocorticoid: fludrocortisone

Barbiturates and phenytoin can reduce effects of fludrocortisone.
NURSING ACTIONS: Monitor for reduced medication effects.

Antidiabetic effects of insulin and sulfonylureas decrease with concurrent use of fludrocortisone.
NURSING ACTIONS: Closely monitor blood glucose levels in clients who have diabetes mellitus.

NURSING ADMINISTRATION

- Monitor weight, blood pressure, and electrolytes.
- Monitor glucose levels in clients who have diabetes mellitus or prediabetes.
- Give with food to reduce gastric distress.
- Do not stop the medication suddenly. Taper dosage if discontinuing.

CLIENT EDUCATION

- Observe for manifestations of peptic ulcer (coffee-ground emesis, bloody or tarry stools, abdominal pain) and notify the provider if they occur.
- Notify the provider of manifestations of acute adrenal insufficiency (fever, muscle and joint pain, weakness, fatigue).
- Dosages need to be increased during times of stress (infection, surgery, trauma).
- Replacement therapy for Addison's disease must continue for life.
- Carry an extra supply of glucocorticoids for emergencies and wear medical identification at all times.

NURSING EVALUATION OF MEDICATION EFFECTIVENESS

Depending on therapeutic intent, evidence of effectiveness can include relief of effects of adrenocortical deficiency (weakness, hypoglycemia, hyperkalemia, and fatigue) with minimal adverse effects.

Hyperpituitarism medications

SELECT PROTOTYPE MEDICATION: Octreotide

OTHER MEDICATIONS
- Lanreotide
- Pegvisomant

PURPOSE

EXPECTED PHARMACOLOGICAL ACTION: Suppresses growth hormone release. Used when surgery and radiation are ineffective or not optional.

THERAPEUTIC USES: Gigantism in children, acromegaly in adults.

ROUTE OF ADMINISTRATION
- Octreotide (IM, subcutaneous, IV)
- Lanreotide (subcutaneous)
- Pegvisomant (subcutaneous)

COMPLICATIONS

Octreotide

Gastrointestinal disturbances
- Cholesterol gallstones can develop within a year
- Nausea, cramps, diarrhea, flatulence, ileus

NURSING ACTIONS
- Give injections without food or at bedtime to minimize manifestations.
- Assess stools for quantity and consistency.

CLIENT EDUCATION: Manifestations usually subside in 1 to 2 weeks.

Hypo/hyperglycemia
NURSING ACTIONS: Monitor glucose levels regularly.

Lanreotide

Injection-site reactions

Gastrointestinal disturbances: Diarrhea, cholelithiasis
CLIENT EDUCATION: Notify the provider if manifestations occur.

Pegvisomant

Nausea, diarrhea
CLIENT EDUCATION: Notify the provider of manifestations.

Liver injury

NURSING ACTIONS: Monitor liver function studies.

Chest pain
CLIENT EDUCATION: Notify the provider of manifestations promptly.

Flu-like manifestations
CLIENT EDUCATION: Notify the provider of manifestations of infection.

CONTRAINDICATIONS/PRECAUTIONS

Octreotide

- **Warnings**
  - Pregnancy: Safety not established.
  - Lactation: Safety not established.
- Use cautiously in clients who have diabetes, hypothyroidism, renal disease, gallbladder disease, and in older adult clients.

INTERACTIONS

Octreotide

Conduction delays can occur if used with antidysrhythmics.
NURSING ACTIONS: Monitor cardiac status.

Octreotide can alter requirements for insulin.
NURSING ACTIONS: Monitor blood glucose levels

Lanreotide: Bradycardia can occur with concurrent use of medications that affect heart rate.
NURSING ACTIONS: Monitor cardiac status.

Pegvisomant: Concurrent use with opioids can reduce the effect of pegvisomant.
NURSING ACTIONS: Dosage can need to be increased.

NURSING ADMINISTRATION

- Teach clients proper technique for subcutaneous injection. Qs
- Minimize injection site pain by rotating sites. The abdomen, hip, and thigh are the preferred sites.
- IM injection of octreotide should be to a large muscle (do not use deltoid muscle). Teach clients to minimize injection site pain by administering slowly, after the medication reaches room temperature.

NURSING EVALUATION OF MEDICATION EFFECTIVENESS

Depending on therapeutic intent, evidence of effectiveness can include the suppression of excess growth hormone for the management of acromegaly when surgery or radiation has failed.

Application Exercises

1. A nurse is caring for an older adult client who has hypothyroidism and a new prescription for levothyroxine. Which of the following dosage schedules should the nurse expect for this client?

   A. The client will start at a high dosage, and the amount will be tapered as needed.

   B. The client will remain on the initial dosage during the course of treatment.

   C. The client's dosage will be adjusted daily based on blood levels.

   D. The client will start on a low dosage, which can be gradually increased.

2. A nurse is caring for a client who is taking propylthiouracil. For which of the following findings should the nurse monitor the client as a potential adverse effect of this medication?

   A. Cold intolerance

   B. Tachycardia

   C. Insomnia

   D. Weight loss

3. A nurse is teaching a client who has Graves' disease and a new prescription for propranolol. Which of the following client statements indicates effective teaching?

   A. "Propranolol helps increase blood flow to my thyroid gland."

   B. "Propranolol is used to prevent excess glucose in my blood."

   C. "Propranolol will decrease my tremors and fast heartbeat."

   D. "Propranolol promotes a decrease of thyroid hormone in my body."

4. A nurse is caring for a client who is taking for somatropin to stimulate growth. The nurse should plan to monitor the client for which of the following as an adverse effect of this medication?

   A. Tachycardia

   B. Hyperthyroidism

   C. Sweating

   D. Hyperglycemia

5. A nurse is reviewing the medical record of a client who takes desmopressin for diabetes insipidus. Which of the following findings is an adverse effect of desmopressin?

   A. Hypovolemia

   B. Hypercalcemia

   C. Agitation

   D. Headache

Active Learning Scenario

A nurse in a provider's office is providing instructions to a client who has a new prescription for levothyroxine to treat hypothyroidism. Use the *ATI Active Learning Template: Medication* to complete this item.

THERAPEUTIC USES: Describe the therapeutic use of levothyroxine in this client.

COMPLICATIONS: Identify two adverse effects of this medication.

NURSING INTERVENTIONS: Describe two laboratory tests the nurse should monitor.

CLIENT EDUCATION: Describe teaching points for a client taking levothyroxine.

Active Learning Scenario Key

Using the ATI Active Learning Template: Medication

THERAPEUTIC USES: Levothyroxine replaces T_4 and is used as thyroid hormone replacement therapy. Replacement of T_4 also raises T_3 levels, because some T_4 is converted into T_3.

COMPLICATIONS: Adverse effects are essentially the same as manifestations of hyperthyroidism: cardiac manifestations (hypertension and angina pectoris); insomnia; anxiety; weight loss; heat intolerance; increased body temperature; tremors; and menstrual irregularities.

NURSING INTERVENTIONS: Monitor thyroid function tests: T_3, T_4, and TSH.

CLIENT EDUCATION
- Take levothyroxine on an empty stomach, usually 1 hr before breakfast.
- Thyroid replacement therapy is usually required for life.
- Monitor for adverse effects that indicate that the dosage needs to be adjusted.

Ⓝ *NCLEX® Connection: Pharmacological and Parenteral Therapies, Medication Administration*

Application Exercises Key

1. A. Starting a new medication at a high dosage can cause harm.
   B. The client's dosage will change periodically throughout treatment.
   C. The client's dosage will be based on blood levels, but daily monitoring is not required.
   D. **CORRECT:** Expect that levothyroxine will be started at a low dosage and gradually increased over several weeks. This is especially important in older adult clients to prevent toxicity.

   Ⓝ *NCLEX® Connection: Pharmacological and Parenteral Therapies, Expected Actions/Outcomes*

2. A. **CORRECT:** When analyzing cues, the nurse should identify that intolerance to cold, a manifestation of hypothyroidism, can be an adverse effect of propylthiouracil.
   B. Bradycardia is an adverse effect of propylthiouracil. Monitor for bradycardia.
   C. Drowsiness, rather than insomnia, is an adverse effect of propylthiouracil.
   D. Weight gain, rather than weight loss, is an adverse effect of propylthiouracil.

   Ⓝ *NCLEX® Connection: Pharmacological and Parenteral Therapies, Adverse Effects/Contramanifestations/Adverse Effects/Interactions*

3. A. Propranolol lowers blood pressure, but does not increase blood flow to the thyroid gland.
   B. Propranolol does not help prevent hyperglycemia.
   C. **CORRECT:** Propranolol is a beta-adrenergic antagonist that decreases heart rate and controls tremors.
   D. Propranolol does not promote a decrease of thyroid hormone.

   Ⓝ *NCLEX® Connection: Pharmacological and Parenteral Therapies, Medication Administration*

4. D. **CORRECT:** The nurse should plan to generate solutions to address the potential adverse effects of somatropin by monitoring the client for manifestations of hyperglycemia (polyphagia, polydipsia, polyuria) which can be a potential adverse effect of this medication.

   Ⓝ *NCLEX® Connection: Pharmacological and Parenteral Therapies, Adverse Effects/Contramanifestations/Adverse Effects/Interactions*

5. A. Edema and hypervolemia, rather than hypovolemia, are adverse effects of desmopressin.
   B. Calcium imbalance is not an adverse effect of desmopressin.
   C. Sleepiness, rather than agitation, is an adverse effect of desmopressin, which can indicate water intoxication.
   D. **CORRECT:** Headache during desmopressin therapy is an indication of water intoxication.

   Ⓝ *NCLEX® Connection: Pharmacological and Parenteral Therapies, Adverse Effects/Contramanifestations/Adverse Effects/Interactions*

When reviewing the following chapters, keep in mind the relevant topics and tasks of the NCLEX outline, in particular:

Pharmacological and Parenteral Therapies

ADVERSE EFFECTS/CONTRAINDICATIONS/SIDE EFFECTS/INTERACTIONS

Identify a contraindication to the administration of a medication to the client.

Provide information to the client on common side effects/adverse effects/potential interactions of medications, and inform the client of when to notify the primary health care provider.

EXPECTED ACTIONS/OUTCOMES: Obtain information on a client's prescribed medications.

MEDICATION ADMINISTRATION

Administer and document medications given by parenteral routes.

Educate client about medications.

UNIT 11   MEDICATIONS AFFECTING THE IMMUNE SYSTEM

CHAPTER 39 *Immunizations*

Administration of a vaccine causes the immune system to produce antibodies that target a specific microbe. Vaccines are made from killed viruses or live, attenuated (weakened) viruses.

IMMUNITY

Active immunity develops when the immune system produces antibodies in response to the entry of antigens into the body. Active immunity develops over several days to weeks and is long lasting.

- **Active-artificial immunity** develops when a vaccine is administered, and the body produces antibodies in response to exposure to a killed or attenuated virus.
- **Active-natural immunity** develops when an antigen enters the body naturally, without human assistance, stimulating the immune system to produce antibodies to the antigen.

Passive immunity is temporary and develops when antibodies are created by another human or animal and then transferred to the client. Because the client does not independently develop antibodies, passive immunity is temporary.

- **Passive-natural immunity** develops when antibodies are passed from a client to their fetus through the placenta, or parent to newborn/infant via colostrum and breast milk.
- **Passive-artificial immunity** develops after antibodies in the form of immune globulins are administered to an individual who requires immediate protection against a disease after exposure has occurred (following a bite from a poisonous snake or an animal who has rabies). After several weeks or months, the individual is no longer protected.

RECOMMENDED CHILDHOOD IMMUNIZATIONS

See the CDC's website for updates. Q EBP

Diphtheria and tetanus toxoids and acellular pertussis vaccine (DTaP): Administer doses at 2, 4, 6, 15 to 18 months, and 4 to 6 years.

Tetanus and diphtheria toxoids and pertussis vaccine (Tdap): Administer one dose at 11 to 12 years.

Tetanus and diphtheria (Td) booster: Administer one dose every 10 years following Tdap.

Haemophilus influenzae type B (Hib): Administer 4-dose series at 2, 4, 6 and 12 to 15 months. Administer 3-dose series at 2,4, and 12 to 15 months. If PedvaxHIB or Comvax is used for the first two doses, the 6- month dose can be omitted.

39.1 Case study

Scenario introduction

Molly is a nurse caring for Chloe and her primary caregivers Annie and David at the pediatric clinic.

Scene 1

Molly: "Now that Chloe is 2 months old, she is scheduled to receive several of her immunizations today. They will include the second dose of the hepatitis B (Hep B), and the 1st dose of each of the following: Rotavirus (RV); diphtheria, tetanus, and acellular pertussis (DTaP); haemophilus influenzae type b (Hib); pneumococcal conjugate (PCV13); and inactivated poliovirus (IPV)."

Annie: "I know it is important to have Chloe vaccinated, I just hate to see her get so many shots in one day."

Molly: "Some of the vaccines can be combined so there are only 2 injections containing the vaccine medications, and some are given orally."

Scene 2

Molly: "I can't believe that Chloe is 5 years old now and starting kindergarten next month."

David: "Yes, that is why we are here today. We want her to have the necessary immunizations prior to starting school."

Molly: "Sounds great. Here is a list of the immunizations Chloe will receive today."

Scene 3

Molly: "Yes, this is Molly. We can certainly schedule Chloe for her seasonal influenza vaccine. Also, now that she is 11 years old, have you considered having Chloe receive the human papillomavirus (HPV) vaccination? ...... No problem, I can send you some information for you to review and we can discuss any questions or concerns you may have."

Rotavirus (RV) oral vaccine

- Two formulations are available. The infant may receive either formulation. The first dose of either form should not be initiated for infants 14 weeks, 6 days or older.
  - RV-5 vaccine should be administered as a three-dose series at ages 2, 4, and 6 months.
  - RV-1 vaccine should be administered as two-dose series at 2 and 4 months.
- Maximum age for the final dose of RV vaccine is 8 months, 0 days.

Inactivated poliovirus vaccine (IPV): Administer subcutaneous doses at 2, 4, and 6 to 18 months, and 4 to 6 years.

Measles, mumps, and rubella vaccine (MMR): Administer doses at 12 to 15 months and 4 to 6 years.

Varicella vaccine: Administer one dose at 12 to 15 months and 4 to 6 years or two doses administered a minimum of 4 weeks apart if administered after age 13 years (catch-up schedule).

Pneumococcal conjugate vaccine (PCV13): Administer doses at 2, 4, 6, and 12 to 15 months. Pneumovax 23 is ineffective for children under age 2.

Hepatitis A: Administer the first dose between 12 and 23 months. Administer the second dose at least 6 months after the first.

Hepatitis B: Administer within 12 to 24 hr after birth with additional doses at age 1 to 2 months and 6 to 18 months. The third dose should not be given prior to 24 weeks of age.

Seasonal influenza vaccine

- Annually, beginning at age 6 months, administer inactivated influenza vaccine (IIV).
- Starting at age 2 years the live-attenuated influenza vaccine (LAIV) nasal spray can be used. LAIV is contraindicated for children age 2 to 17 years who are receiving aspirin-containing products, children age 2 to 4 years who have asthma or have had wheezing during the past year, or anyone who has taken an antiviral medication in the 48 hr prior to vaccine administration. Children who are six months through 8 years and are receiving an initial influenza vaccine or never received a previous dose, should obtain 2 doses.
- Administration recommendations can change yearly because the vaccine is created with different influenza strains each year. The vaccine is typically available beginning in early fall.

COVID-19 vaccine

- Refer to CDC guidelines for various age groups.
- Not recommended for children less than 6 months of age.
- Current Recommendations are as follows: two-dose mRNA vaccine (recommend doses given 4 to 8 weeks apart); three-dose mRNA vaccine (recommend dose 1 to 2 to be administered 3 to 8 weeks apart; dose 2 to 3 to be administered at least 8 weeks to 5 months apart).
- Age 6 months to 5 years: 2-dose mRNA vaccine (at least 4 to 8 weeks apart); 3-dose mRNA vaccine (dose 1 to 2 at least 3 to 8 weeks apart; dose 2 to 3 at least 8 weeks apart.)
- Age 5 to 11 and 12 to 17 years: appropriate dose given intramuscularly in the deltoid. Two-dose mRNA vaccine (recommend doses given 4 to 8 weeks apart); three-dose mRNA vaccine (recommend dose 1 and 2 to be administered 3 to 8 weeks apart; dose 2 to 3 to be administered at least to 5 months apart).

Meningococcal vaccine (MenACWY, MenB)

- MenACWY2: doses are recommended for children (1 dose at 11 to 12 years of age, second dose (booster) at 16 years of age
- MenB is recommended for those who are at increased risk for meningococcal disease (2 doses between 16 to 23 years of age at least 1 to 6 months apart

Human papillomavirus (HPV)

- There are different types of HPV. Types 6 and 11 can cause genital warts. Types 16, 18, 31, 33, 45, 52 and 58 can cause cancer of the anus, vagina, vulva, and cervix.
- While there are 3 different HPV vaccines available, only the 9-valent formulation is available in the United States and is FDA approved for use through age 45.
- 9-valent human papillomavirus (9vHPV) prevents HPV 6, 11, 16, 18, plus HPV 31,33,45, 52, and 58 noninfectious virus-like particles (VLP).
- The immunization is recommended initially for adolescents between 11 to 12 years but can be given as early as 9 years.

- Recommend a 2-to 3-dose series depending on age of initial dose. Do not restart if vaccine schedule was interrupted.
  - 9 to 14 years of age for initial dose: 2 dose series at (0, 6 to 12 months)
  - Greater than 15 years of age for initial dose: 3 dose series (0, 1 to 2 months, 6 months)

RECOMMENDED ADULT IMMUNIZATIONS

- For adults age 19 and older.
- See the CDC's website for updates.

Td/Tdap: Administer one dose of Tdap instead of Td, and then give Td booster every 10 years. Give one dose of Tdap to clients who are pregnant (with each pregnancy) between 27 and 36 weeks gestation.

MMR: Follow recommendations for administering one or two doses to clients between the ages of 19 and 49 who lack documentation of immunization or prior infection, or laboratory proof of immunity.

- People born before 1957 are considered immune to measles and mumps.
- A client who is pregnant should not receive the MMR vaccine.
- Anaphylactic-like reaction to gelatin or neomycin is also a contradiction for not administering the MMR vaccine.

Varicella vaccine: Administer two doses to adults who do not have evidence of immunity. Administer a second dose to adults who had only one previous dose and lack evidence of immunity, or one dose depending on the type of zoster vaccine. Varicella vaccine is contraindicated for pregnant clients, individuals with certain cancers, and hypersensitivity to neomycin and gelatin. Additionally, the vaccine is not recommended for clients who have HIV, congenital immune deficiencies, or those taking immunosuppressive drugs.

Pneumococcal polysaccharide vaccine (PPSV23) and pneumococcal conjugate vaccine (PCV15 and PCV20): Follow recommendations for administration to adults who are immunocompromised, have certain chronic diseases, smoke cigarettes, or live in a long-term care facility or received previous doses of PCV13 and or PPSV23. PCV13 is no longer recommended. For adults 65 years and older who have not been immunized with PCV or vaccination history is unknown, administer PCV15 or PCV20 (if the client received PCV15, then they should receive a dose of PPSV23 within 12 months). Ⓖ

Hepatitis A: Administer single-antigen vaccines as two doses spaced 6 to 12 months, or 6 to 18 months apart to high-risk individuals.

Hepatitis B: Administer three doses to high-risk individuals who lack completion of the series. There must be at least 1 month between doses one and two, and at least 2 months between doses two and three. A minimum of 4 months are required between doses one and three.

Influenza vaccine

- One dose annually is recommended for all adults.
- Inactivated influenza vaccine (IIV) is approved for individuals 6 months of age or older, including those who are pregnant.
- Recombinant influenza vaccine (RIV) is approved for adults 18 years of age and older.
- Live attenuated influenza vaccine (LAIV) is a nasal spray and is approved for individuals between aged 2 to 49 years who are healthy and not pregnant.

COVID-19

- Recommendations are as follows. (Refer to CDC website for current updates.)
  - mRNA vaccine: administered intramuscularly, dose 1 to 2 given 3 to 8 weeks apart, dose 2 to 3 given at least 5 months apart, dose 3 to 4 can be given at least 4 months (clients who are greater than 50 years of age). This can vary depending on manufacturer recommendations.
  - Viral vector vaccine: administered intramuscularly, dose 1 to 2 administered at least 8 weeks apart, dose 2 to 3 at least 4 months apart for client who are greater than 50 years of age (the second dose can be with a mRNA vaccine).

Meningococcal vaccines (MenACWY, Men B)

- **MenACWY:** Administer to clients greater than 16 years of age at high risk (history sickle cell disease, history of HIV, travel outside the US frequently to hyperendemic areas or live in high-risk areas, military, college student (living in dorms. Two doses recommended if not vaccinated previously. Adults who are at high risk should receive reimmunization every 5 years.
- **MenB:** for clients who are 16 to 23 years of age; receive 2 dose series if at high risk (history of sickle cell disease, military, college student). May reimmunize every 2 to 3 years if remain at high risk.

Human papilloma vaccine (HPV): Vaccine is not recommended for client who are greater than 26 years of age. Can be administered to clients 27 to 45 years of age after shared decision making with provider. (Refer to children schedule for more information)

Zoster vaccine: Recommended as two doses of recombinant vaccine to all adults age 50 years and older. Second doses should be administered 2 to 6 months after the first

PURPOSE

EXPECTED PHARMACOLOGICAL ACTION

Vaccines cause the immune system to produce antibodies that provide active artificial immunity. Immunizations can take months to have an effect but confer long-lasting protection against infectious diseases.

THERAPEUTIC USES

- Eradication of infectious diseases (polio, smallpox)
- Prevention of childhood and adult infectious diseases (measles, diphtheria, mumps, rubella, tetanus, H. influenzae) and their complications

COMPLICATIONS, CONTRAINDICATIONS, AND PRECAUTIONS

- Anaphylactic reaction to a vaccine is a contraindication for further doses of that vaccine. Qs
- Anaphylactic reaction to any component of a vaccine is a contraindication to use of subsequent vaccines containing that substance.
- Do not administer live virus vaccines (varicella or MMR), to a client who is severely immunocompromised. Severe febrile illness is a precaution for all immunizations.
- Precautions to immunizations require the provider to analyze data and weigh the risks that come with immunizing or not immunizing. Qpcc
- Moderate or severe illnesses with or without fever are precautions to receiving immunizations.
- The common cold and other minor illnesses are not a contraindication or precaution for receiving immunizations.

DTaP

ADVERSE EFFECTS

- **Mild**
  - Redness, swelling, and tenderness at the injection site
  - Low fever
  - Behavioral changes (drowsiness, irritability, anorexia)
- **Moderate**
  - Inconsolable crying for 3 hr or more
  - Fever 40.6° C (105° F) or greater
  - Seizures (with or without fever)
  - Shock-like state
- **Severe:** Acute encephalopathy (rare)

CONTRAINDICATIONS: Occurrence of encephalopathy within 7 days following prior dose of the vaccine

PRECAUTIONS

- Occurrence of Guillain-Barré syndrome within 6 weeks of prior dose of tetanus toxoid
- Progressive neurologic disorders; uncontrolled seizures
- Fever 40.6° C (105° F) or greater within 48 hr of prior dose
- Shock-like state within 48 hr of prior dose
- Seizures within 3 days of prior dose
- Inconsolable crying for 3 hr or more within 48 hr of prior dose

Haemophilus influenzae type B

ADVERSE EFFECTS

- Redness, swelling, warmth, and tenderness at the injection site
- Fever greater than 37.8° C (101° F), vomiting, diarrhea, and crying

CONTRAINDICATION: Age less than 6 weeks

COVID-19

ADVERSE EFFECTS

- Pain, redness and swelling at the injection site
- Fatigue, headache, muscle pain, chills, fever, nausea
- Severe allergic reaction (rare)

CONTRAINDICATIONS

- Severe allergic reaction (anaphylaxis) following a previous dose to a component of the COVID-19 vaccine
- Known diagnosed allergy to a component of the COVID-19 vaccine

PRECAUTIONS

- Moderate or severe acute illness
- History of an immediate allergic reaction to any non-COVID-19 vaccine or injectable therapy

Rotavirus

ADVERSE EFFECTS

- Irritability
- Mild, temporary diarrhea or vomiting
- Intussusception

CONTRAINDICATIONS

- History of intussusception
- Severe combined immunodeficiency (SCID), which is a rare disorder that is inherited

PRECAUTIONS

- Chronic gastrointestinal disease
- Spina bifida
- Bladder exstrophy
- Immunocompromised (other than SCID)

Inactivated poliovirus vaccine

ADVERSE EFFECTS: Tenderness at the injection site

CONTRAINDICATION: Anaphylactic reaction to neomycin, streptomycin, or polymyxin B

PRECAUTION: Pregnancy

Measles, mumps, and rubella

ADVERSE EFFECTS

- **Mild:** Local reactions (rash; fever; swollen glands in cheeks or neck)
- **Moderate**
  - Joint pain and stiffness lasting for days to weeks
  - Febrile seizure
  - Low platelet count
- **Severe**
  - Transient thrombocytopenia
  - Deafness
  - Long-term seizures
  - Brain damage

CONTRAINDICATION: Pregnancy

PRECAUTIONS

- History of thrombocytopenia or thrombocytopenic purpura
- Anaphylactic reaction to eggs, gelatin, or neomycin
- Transfusion with blood product containing antibodies within the prior 3 to 11 months
- Simultaneous tuberculin skin testing

Varicella

ADVERSE EFFECTS

- **Mild**
  - Tenderness and swelling at injection site
  - Fever
  - Rash (mild) for up to 1 month after immunization
- **Moderate:** Seizures
- **Severe**
  - Pneumonia
  - Low blood count (extremely rare)
  - Severe brain reactions (extremely rare)

CONTRAINDICATIONS

- Pregnancy
- Anaphylactic reaction to gelatin or neomycin

PRECAUTIONS

- Transfusion with blood product containing antibodies within the prior 3 to 11 months
- Treatment with antiviral medication within 24 hr prior to immunization (avoid taking antivirals for 14 days following immunization)
- Extended use (2 weeks or longer) of corticosteroids or other medications that affect the immune system
- Cancer

Pneumococcal conjugate vaccine (PCV15 or 20)

ADVERSE EFFECTS

- Swelling, redness and tenderness at site of injection
- Fever
- Irritability
- Drowsiness
- Anorexia

CONTRAINDICATION: Anaphylactic reaction to any vaccine containing diphtheria toxoid

Pneumococcal polysaccharide vaccine (PPSV23)

ADVERSE EFFECTS

- Redness and tenderness at site of injection
- Fever
- Myalgia

CONTRAINDICATION: Age less than 2 years

PRECAUTION: Pregnancy

Hepatitis A

ADVERSE EFFECTS

- Tenderness at the injection site
- Headache
- Anorexia
- Malaise

CONTRAINDICATION: Previous hypersensitivity after previous dose or components of vaccine (neomycin, yeast)

PRECAUTION: Pregnancy

Hepatitis B

ADVERSE EFFECTS
- Tenderness at the injection site
- Temperature of 37.7° C (99.9° F) or greater

CONTRAINDICATION: Anaphylactic allergy to yeast

PRECAUTION: Infant weight less than 2 kg (4 lb, 6.5 oz)

Inactivated influenza vaccine

ADVERSE EFFECTS
- Swelling, redness and tenderness at the injection site
- Hoarseness
- Fever
- Malaise
- Headache
- Cough
- Aches
- Increased risk for Guillain–Barré syndrome
- Increased risk of seizures in children receiving PCV13 or DTaP simultaneously

PRECAUTIONS: Occurrence of Guillain–Barré syndrome within 6 weeks of prior influenza vaccine

Live, attenuated influenza vaccine

ADVERSE EFFECTS
- Vomiting, diarrhea
- Cough
- Fever
- Headache
- Myalgia
- Nasal congestion/runny nose

CONTRAINDICATIONS
- Age less than 2 years
- Age 50 years or older
- Pregnancy

PRECAUTIONS
- Occurrence of Guillain–Barré syndrome within 6 weeks of prior influenza vaccine
- Treatment with antiviral medication within 48 hr prior to immunization (avoid taking antivirals for 14 days following immunization)
- Some chronic conditions

> The Advisory Committee on Immunization Practices recommends the option of the live-attenuated influenza vaccine to clients regardless of the severity of egg allergy. Clients who have a history of an egg allergy, other than a hive-only reaction, should receive the immunization where a provider is present and emergency equipment is available. (At the time of publication, these recommendations were awaiting approval by the CDC. Please refer to the CDC's website for current approval status.)

Meningococcal MPSV4 and MCV4

ADVERSE EFFECTS
- Redness and tenderness at the injection site
- Fever

Human papilloma vaccine 9vHPV

ADVERSE EFFECTS
- Redness, swelling and tenderness at the injection site
- Mild to moderate fever
- Headache
- Fainting (shortly after receiving the vaccine)

CONTRAINDICATIONS
- Pregnancy
- Severe allergy to yeast

Zoster

ADVERSE EFFECTS
- Redness, edema, itching, and tenderness at the injection site
- Headache

CONTRAINDICATIONS
- Immunosuppression
- Pregnancy
- Treatment with medications that alter the immune system

INTERACTIONS
None significant

NURSING ADMINISTRATION

FOR INFANTS AND CHILDREN
- Obtain informed consent from the legal guardian prior to administration.
- Administer IM immunizations in the vastus lateralis or ventrogluteal muscle in infants and young children, and in the deltoid muscle for older children and adolescents.
- Administer subcutaneous injections in the outer aspect of the upper arm or anterolateral thigh.
- Use the appropriate size needle for route, site, age, and amount of medication. Adequate needle length reduces the incidence of swelling and tenderness at the injection site. Qpcc
- Use strategies to minimize discomfort (providing distraction, applying a topical anesthetic prior to injection, and giving infants a concentrated oral sucrose solution 2 min prior to, during, and 3 min after immunization administration).
- Do not allow the child to delay the procedure.
- Encourage caregivers to use comforting measures (cuddling and pacifiers) during procedure, and measures (application of cool compresses to injection site or gentle movement of the involved extremity) after the procedure.
- Provide praise afterward.
- Apply a colorful bandage if appropriate.
- Instruct parents to avoid administration of aspirin to children to treat fever or local reaction following administration of a live virus vaccine due to the risk of developing Reye syndrome.

FOR ADULTS
- Administer subcutaneous immunizations in the outer aspect of the upper arm or anterolateral thigh.
- Administer IM immunizations into the deltoid muscle.

FOR CLIENTS OF ALL AGES

- Have emergency medications and equipment on standby in case the client experiences an allergic response (anaphylaxis).
- Provide vaccine information sheets (VIS) and review the content with legal guardians or clients. Include the publication date of each VIS given in documentation.
- Instruct parents and clients to observe for complications and to notify the provider if adverse effects occur.
- Document the administration of the vaccine, including the date, route, and site of immunization; type, manufacturer, lot number, and expiration date of the vaccine; evidence of informed consent from the legal guardian, and name, address and title of the administering nurse. Qↄ
- Report any unusual or serious adverse effects to the Vaccine Adverse Event Reporting System (VAERS) by calling 800-822-7967, using the reporting form which can be printed from the FDA website (www.fda.gov) or the CDC website (www.cdc.gov).

NURSING EVALUATION OF MEDICATION EFFECTIVENESS

Depending on therapeutic intent, effectiveness can be evidenced by the following.

- Improvement of local reaction to immunization with absence of pain, fever, and swelling at the site of injection
- Development of immunity

Application Exercises

1. A nurse is teaching a group of new guardians about immunizations. The nurse should instruct the guardians that the series for which of the following vaccines is completed prior to the first birthday?

   A. Pneumococcal conjugate

   B. Meningococcal conjugate

   C. Varicella

   D. Rotavirus

2. Sort the following immunizations by route of administration: intramuscular (IM); subcutaneous or IM; or oral.

   A. DTaP

   B. Hep B

   C. Hib

   D. RV

   E. IPV

   F. PCV13

3. A nurse is preparing to administer immunizations to a 5-year-old child who will be entering kindergarten next month. Which of the following immunizations should the nurse plan to administer? (Select all that apply.)

   A. DTaP

   B. Hib

   C. RV

   D. Varicella (VAR)

   E. Measles, mumps, rubella (MMR)

   F. IPV

4. A nurse is caring for a group of clients who are not protected against varicella. The nurse should prepare to administer the varicella vaccine at this time to which of the following clients?

   A. 24-year-old client in the third trimester of pregnancy

   B. 12-year-old child who has a severe allergy to neomycin

   C. 2-month-old infant who has no health problems

   D. 32-year-old client who has essential hypertension

5. A nurse is caring for several clients who came to the clinic for a seasonal influenza immunization. The nurse should identify that which of the following clients is a candidate to receive the vaccine via nasal spray rather than an injection?

   A. 1-year-old who has no health problems

   B. 17-year-old who has a hypersensitivity to penicillin

   C. 25-year-old who is pregnant

   D. 52-year-old who takes a multivitamin supplement

6. A 12-month-old child just received the first measles, mumps, and rubella (MMR) vaccine. For which of the following findings should the nurse instruct the family to monitor for as adverse effects of the MMR vaccine?

   A. Rash

   B. Swollen glands

   C. Bruising

   D. Headache

   E. Inconsolable crying

7. A nurse is reviewing the medical record of an 11-year-old school-age child. Which of the following allergies would be a contraindication to receiving the HPV vaccination?

   A. Shellfish

   B. Eggs

   C. Yeast

   D. Gelatin

Application Exercises Key

1. D. **CORRECT:** When taking actions, the nurse should instruct the guardians that Rotavirus vaccine is administered only to infants less than 8 months, 0 days of age.

2. **INTRAMUSCULAR (IM):** A, B, C, F; **SUBCUTANEOUS OR IM:** E; **ORAL:** D

   The DTaP is administered IM in the mediolateral thigh. The Hep B is administered IM in the deltoid or anterolateral thigh. The Hib is administered IM in the mid-thigh or the outer aspect of the upper arm. RV is administered orally. IPV is administered subcutaneously in the anterolateral thigh. The PCV13 is administered IM in the deltoid or anterolateral thigh.

3. A, D, E, F. **CORRECT:** The DTaP, VAR, MMR, and IPV are all scheduled for administration to children ages 4 to 6 years of age. The final dose of Hib is administered at age 18 months and the final dose of RV is administered by age 6 months.

4. D. **CORRECT:** The nurse should analyze the cues from the client's medical history and determine that a 32-year-old client who has essential hypertension should be immunized. Essential hypertension is not a contraindication for this vaccine.

5. B. **CORRECT:** The nurse should analyze the cues from the client's medical history and determine that a 17-year-old can be immunized for influenza with the LAIV via nasal spray. A hypersensitivity to penicillin is not a contraindication for an influenza immunization.

6. A, B, C. **CORRECT:** When taking actions, the nurse should instruct the family to monitor for a rash and fever, and swollen glands which can develop in children 1 to 2 weeks following the MMR immunization. The nurse should also instruct the family to monitor for bruising due to a temporary low platelet count, which can cause bruising or bleeding.

7. C. **CORRECT:** The HPV vaccine should not be administered to clients who have an allergy to yeast or to those with a documented reaction to the first dose administered. It is also contraindicated in pregnancy and should not be administered to children younger than 9 years of age.

Active Learning Scenario

A nurse at a community health clinic is planning to administer the human papilloma virus (9vHPV) vaccine to an 11-year-old client. Use the *ATI Active Learning Template: Medication* to complete this item.

COMPLICATIONS: Identify two adverse effects the client should monitor for.

CLIENT EDUCATION: Describe two teaching points for a client who receives a first dose of the HPV vaccine.

Active Learning Scenario Key

Using the ATI Active Learning Template: Medication
COMPLICATIONS
- The 9vHPV vaccine can cause redness, tenderness, and swelling at the injection site.
- It has caused fainting in some clients shortly after the vaccine is administered.
- Headache and mild to moderate fever are also possible adverse effects the client should monitor for.

CLIENT EDUCATION
- Monitor for adverse effects; the common adverse effects are mild and temporary.
- The adolescent will require a second dose in 6 to 12 months since this one occurred before age 16. Initial administration after 16 years of age requires a three dose series.

- Ⓝ *NCLEX® Connection: Pharmacological and Parenteral Therapies, Medication Administration*

CHAPTER 40 *Chemotherapy Agents*

Chemotherapy is used to cure some cancers, augment the treatment of other cancers, and attempt to increase a client's survival rate and time. Depending on the agent, it can be given orally, parenterally, intravenous, intracavitary, or intrathecal. Specific training/certification is necessary for administration of some agents.

Combination chemotherapy uses more than one chemotherapy agent to treat the cancer. Medications used for combination chemotherapy should act on different phases of the cell cycle. Combination therapy is more effective than monotherapy and is used to reduce medication resistance, increase effectiveness, and, ideally, reduce toxic effects to healthy cells.

Personnel preparing and administering chemotherapeutic agents should follow safe handling procedures to prevent absorption through the skin.

If a chemotherapy spill occurs, follow institutional procedures. Generally, small spills can be handled by using supplies contained in a chemotherapy spill kit (goggles, mask, protective clothing, shoe covers, absorbent pads, detergent cleansers, and chemotherapy waste disposal bags). For large spills, contact the Occupational Safety and Health Administration. Qs

Cytotoxic chemotherapy agents

Cytotoxic chemotherapy agents are toxic to cancer cells.

- Cytotoxic chemotherapy agents kill fast-growing cancer cells as well as healthy cells, including skin, hair, intestinal mucosa, and hematopoietic cells. Many of the adverse effects of chemotherapeutic agents are related to the unintentional harm done to healthy rapidly proliferating cells (those found in the gastrointestinal [GI] tract, hair follicles, and bone marrow).
- Common adverse effects of cytotoxic chemotherapy agents include nausea, vomiting, myelosuppression, and alopecia. Many cytotoxic agents are vesicants that can cause severe damage if there is leakage into tissue. Extravasation of agents that are vesicants requires immediate attention to minimize tissue damage. Selection of the neutralizing solution is dependent on vesicant. Qs

PURPOSE

EXPECTED PHARMACOLOGICAL ACTION

Antimetabolites: Kill cancer cells by interrupting a specific phase of cell reproduction: known as S-phase specific

Antitumor antibiotics: Kill cancer cells by stopping the synthesis of RNA, DNA, or proteins

Antimitotics: Kill cancer cells by inhibiting mitosis and preventing cell division

Alkylating agents: Kill fast-growing cancer cells by altering DNA structure and preventing cell reproduction

Topoisomerase inhibitors: Kill cancer cells by interrupting DNA synthesis

Other: Kill cells by various mechanisms including interrupting DNA and RNA synthesis in leukemia cells

Antimetabolites

Folic acid analog

SELECT PROTOTYPE MEDICATION: Methotrexate (oral, IV, IM, intrathecal)

OTHER MEDICATIONS
- Pemetrexed (IV)
- Pralatrexate (IV)

Pyrimidine analog

SELECT PROTOTYPE MEDICATION: Cytarabine (IV, subcutaneous, intrathecal)

OTHER MEDICATIONS
- Fluorouracil (continuous IV)
- Floxuridine (infusion directly into the hepatic artery)
- Capecitabine (oral)
- Gemcitabine (IV)

Purine analogs

SELECT PROTOTYPE MEDICATION: Mercaptopurine (oral)
Interrupts the synthesis of DNA and RNA

OTHER MEDICATIONS
- Thioguanine (oral)
- Pentostatin (IV)
- Fludarabine (IV)
- Cladribine (IV)

PURPOSE

EXPECTED PHARMACOLOGICAL ACTION

Folic acid analog

Methotrexate
- Stops cell reproduction needed for the synthesis of DNA by inhibiting folic acid conversion
- S-phase specific

Pemetrexed
- Suppresses synthesis of DNA, RNA, and proteins
- S-phase specific

Pralatrexate
- Disrupts synthesis of DNA
- S-phase specific

Pyrimidine analog

Cytarabine
- Incorporates into DNA, then inhibits DNA and RNA synthesis of cancer cells which results in the death of rapid malignant cells
- S-phase specific

Fluorouracil, floxuridine
- Employed extensively to treat solid tumors
- Destroys cells mainly in the S-phase specificity
- Derivative of uracil

Capecitabine
- Active only against divided cells
- Has S-phase specificity

Gemcitabine
- Has S-phase specificity
- Inhibits DNA synthesis

Purine analogs

Mercaptopurine
- Interrupts the action of adenine and guanine present in DNA and RNA for the synthesis of the purine nucleotides needed to incorporate into the nucleic acid molecules.
- S-phase specific

Thioguanine
- Inhibits purine synthesis and DNA, and the interconversion of nucleotides
- S-phase specific

Pentostatin: Blocks DNA synthesis and promotes accumulation of a compound that is especially toxic to lymphocytes

Fludarabine: Inhibits DNA replication, impairs RNA function, and promotes apoptosis (destruction by a suppressive agent to eliminate cells)

THERAPEUTIC USES

Folic acid analog

Methotrexate: Choriocarcinoma, solid tumors (breast and lung), head and neck sarcomas, osteogenic sarcoma, acute lymphocytic leukemia, non-Hodgkin's lymphoma, T-cell lymphoma. Other uses include management of rheumatoid arthritis, psoriasis, and Crohn's disease.

Pemetrexed: Malignant pleural mesothelioma, non-small cell lung cancer

Pralatrexate: Peripheral T-cell lymphoma, non-Hodgkin's lymphoma

Pyrimidine analog

Cytarabine: Acute myelogenous leukemia, non-Hodgkin's lymphomas, and acute lymphocytic leukemia

Fluorouracil: Solid tumors: Colon, rectal, breast, stomach, and pancreatic cancer

Floxuridine: GI adenoma metastatic to the live

Capecitabine: Metastatic colorectal and breast cancer

Gemcitabine: Pancreatic, non-small cell lung cancer; advanced ovarian and breast cancer

Purine analogs

Mercaptopurine: Acute lymphocytic leukemia

Thioguanine: Acute nonlymphocytic leukemias

Pentostatin: Hairy cell leukemia

Fludarabine: Chronic lymphocytic leukemia, low-grade non-Hodgkin's lymphoma, follicular lymphoma, acute myelogenous leukemia

COMPLICATIONS

Bone marrow suppression
Low WBC count or neutropenia, bleeding caused by thrombocytopenia or low platelet count, and anemia or low RBCs

NURSING ACTIONS
- Monitor WBC, absolute neutrophil count, platelet count, Hgb, and Hct.
- Assess clients for bruising and bleeding gums.

CLIENT EDUCATION: Avoid crowds and contact with infectious individuals. Practice good hand hygiene.

GI discomfort (nausea and vomiting)
NURSING ACTIONS: Administer antiemetic (ondansetron in combination with dexamethasone, granisetron, or metoclopramide) before beginning chemotherapy.

Methotrexate

GI tract: Mucositis, gastric ulcers, perforation
NURSING ACTIONS
- Monitor for GI bleed (coffee-ground emesis or tarry black stools). Assess the mouth for sores.
- Provide frequent oral hygiene using soft toothbrushes and avoid alcohol mouthwashes.

Reproductive toxicity (congenital abnormalities)
CLIENT EDUCATION: Avoid becoming pregnant while taking these medications and for 6 months after.

Renal damage
Due to hyperuricemia or elevated levels of uric acid

NURSING ACTIONS
- Monitor kidney function, BUN, creatinine, and I&O.
- Encourage adequate fluid intake of 2 to 3 L/day.
- Administer allopurinol if uric acid level is elevated.
- Monitor urine pH, maintain a urine pH greater than 7.0

Cytarabine

Stomatitis, conjunctivitis.

Liver disease
NURSING ACTIONS
- Monitor liver enzymes.
- Monitor for jaundice.

Pulmonary edema
NURSING ACTIONS: Monitor breath sounds.

CLIENT EDUCATION: Notify the provider of shortness of breath.

Cytarabine syndrome
Can happen within 6 to 12 hr after administration. Findings include fever, myalgia, malaise, and conjunctivitis

NURSING ACTIONS: Administer corticosteroids.

Arachnoiditis
Indications include nausea, headache, and fever.

NURSING ACTIONS: Manifestations can be treated with dexamethasone.

CLIENT EDUCATION: Notify the provider of nausea, vomiting, headache, or fever.

Mercaptopurine

Liver toxicity
NURSING ACTIONS
- Monitor liver enzymes.
- Monitor for jaundice.

GI tract: Mucositis, gastric ulcers, perforation
NURSING ACTIONS
- Monitor for GI bleed (coffee-ground emesis or tarry black stools).
- Assess mouth for sores.
- Provide frequent oral hygiene using soft toothbrushes and avoiding alcohol mouthwashes.

Reproductive toxicity: Congenital abnormalities
CLIENT EDUCATION: Avoid becoming pregnant while taking these medications and for 6 months after.

CONTRAINDICATIONS/PRECAUTIONS

Methotrexate

- Contraindicated in renal or hepatic failure, blood dyscrasias, pregnancy or lactation.
- Use with caution in clients who have liver or kidney dysfunction, suppressed bone marrow, leukopenia, thrombocytopenia, anemia, or gastric ulcers, and in older adult clients.

Cytarabine

- Contraindicated include pregnancy or lactation.
- Use with caution in clients who have liver or renal disease.

Mercaptopurine

- Contraindicated in clients who are resistant to the medication.
- Contraindicated in clients who are pregnant or have liver disease.

INTERACTIONS

Methotrexate

Salicylates, other NSAIDs, sulfonamides, penicillin, and tetracyclines can cause methotrexate toxicity.
NURSING ACTIONS: Monitor for toxic effects.

Proton pump inhibitors
NURSING ACTIONS
- Avoid concurrent use.
- Monitor BUN and creatinine.

Cytarabine

Cytarabine can reduce the absorption of digoxin.
NURSING ACTIONS: Monitor digoxin level and ECG.

Live virus vaccines: Can decrease the antibody response and increase the risk for adverse reactions
NURSING ACTIONS: Avoid concurrent use.

Cytarabine can place the client at risk for bleeding if used with anticoagulants, salicylates, thrombolytics, NSAIDs, and platelet inhibitors.
NURSING ACTIONS: Monitor bleeding times and for manifestations of bleeding.

Mercaptopurine

Allopurinol can reduce breakdown of mercaptopurine.
NURSING ACTIONS: Reduce mercaptopurine dosage for clients taking allopurinol.

Mercaptopurine can either increase or decrease anticoagulant effect of warfarin.
NURSING ACTIONS: Monitor PT and INR.

NURSING ADMINISTRATION

- Reduce dosage in clients who have renal disease.
- Encourage 2 to 3 L of daily fluid intake from food and beverage sources. **Q**PCC
- Give with sodium bicarbonate capsules to alkalinize urine.
- Monitor for bleeding (bruising) and infection (fever, sore throat).
- Monitor CBC, BUN, creatinine, and liver enzymes.
- Monitor I&O. Monitor uric acid.
- Monitor for jaundice.
- Give an antiemetic for nausea and vomiting.
- Monitor for indications of gout (joint pain, increased uric acid levels).

CLIENT EDUCATION
- Prevent pregnancy during treatment. Can cause teratogenic effects to the fetus.
- Avoid use of alcohol during treatment.
- Consult provider before receiving vaccinations.
- Practice good oral hygiene and avoid mouthwash with alcohol.
- Monitor for dark urine and clay-colored stools.

For methotrexate

Administer with leucovorin rescue to reduce toxicity to healthy cells. Leucovorin is a folic acid derivative. It enters healthy cells and blocks methotrexate.

CLIENT EDUCATION
- Protect the skin from sunlight.
- Use birth control during and for 6 months after completing treatment .

For cytarabine

Monitor for indications of neurotoxicity, (nystagmus). Monitor for manifestations of chemical arachnoiditis (nausea, vomiting, headache, and fever). Coadministration of dexamethasone can reduce incidence and severity of reaction.

Antitumor (cytotoxic) antibiotics

Anthracyclines

SELECT PROTOTYPE MEDICATION: Doxorubicin (IV)

OTHER MEDICATIONS
- Liposomal doxorubicin (IV)
- Daunorubicin (conventional or liposomal; IV)
- Epirubicin (IV)
- Idarubicin (IV)
- Valrubicin (intravesical: directly into the bladder via urinary catheter)
- Mitoxantrone (IV)

Nonanthracyclines

SELECT PROTOTYPE MEDICATION: Dactinomycin (IV infusion)

OTHER MEDICATIONS
- Bleomycin (IM, IV, subcutaneous, intrapleural)
- Mitomycin (IV)

PURPOSE

EXPECTED PHARMACOLOGICAL ACTION

Anthracyclines

Doxorubicin, daunorubicin, epirubicin, idarubicin
- Binds to DNA, altering its structure; therefore, inhibits synthesis of DNA and RNA (intercalation).
- Cell cycle phase nonspecific
- Other mechanism-inhibition of topoisomerase II: prevents subsequent DNA repair.

Liposomal doxorubicin: Medication encapsulated within lipid vesicles (liposomes) to increase uptake to cancer cells and decrease uptake to healthy cells.

Valrubicin: Administered directly into the bladder by a urinary catheter and it stops cell growth by disrupting, not intercalating, with DNA.

Mitoxantrone
- Intercalates DNA and DNA strand breakage
- Cell-cycle phase nonspecific

Nonanthracyclines

Dactinomycin
- Binds to DNA, altering its structure, which inhibits RNA synthesis. DNA synthesis is not suppressed.
- Cell cycle phase nonspecific

Bleomycin: Binds to DNA

Mitomycin: Blockade of DNA synthesis

THERAPEUTIC USES

Anthracyclines

Doxorubicin: Includes solid tumors (lung, bone, stomach, and breast cancers); Hodgkin's and non-Hodgkin's lymphomas; sarcomas of soft tissue and bone; and carcinoma of ovaries, testes, and thyroid

Liposomal doxorubicin: AIDS-related Kaposi's sarcoma, metastatic ovarian and breast cancer, multiple myeloma

Daunorubicin: HIV-associated Kaposi's sarcoma, leukemia

Epirubicin: Breast cancer

Idarubicin: Acute myelogenous leukemia

Valrubicin: Bladder cancer

Mitoxantrone: Prostate cancer, acute nonlymphocytic leukemias

Nonanthracyclines

Dactinomycin: Includes Wilms' tumor, rhabdomyosarcoma, choriocarcinoma, Ewing's sarcoma, testicular cancer, and Kaposi's sarcoma

Bleomycin: Testicular carcinomas, lymphomas, squamous cell carcinomas, Hodgkin's disease

Mitomycin: Disseminated adenocarcinoma of the stomach and pancreas; carcinomas of the colon, rectum, esophagus, lung, breast, cervix, and bladder

COMPLICATIONS

Bone marrow suppression
Low WBC or neutropenia, bleeding caused by thrombocytopenia or low platelet count, and anemia or low RBCs

NURSING ACTIONS
- Monitor WBC, absolute neutrophil count, platelet count, Hgb, and Hct.
- Assess for bruising and bleeding gums.

CLIENT EDUCATION: Avoid crowds and contact with infectious individuals.

GI manifestations
Including nausea, vomiting, and stomatitis

NURSING ACTIONS
- Administer antiemetic (ondansetron in combination with dexamethasone, granisetron, or metoclopramide) before beginning chemotherapy.
- Provide gentle oral care. Rinse mouth with warmed saline solution.

Severe tissue damage
Due to extravasations of vesicants

NURSING ACTIONS
- Stop chemotherapeutic medications if extravasation occurs.
- Use central line for infusion.
- Only clinically trained personnel should give these medications IV.

Alopecia
CLIENT EDUCATION
- Hair loss can occur 7 to 10 days after the beginning of treatment and will last for a maximum of 2 months after the last administration of the chemotherapeutic agent.
- Select a hairpiece before the occurrence of hair loss.

Doxorubicin

Cardiac changes
Acute toxicity can cause dysrhythmias and ECG changes. Heart failure secondary to cardiomyopathy can occur months to years after treatment

NURSING ACTIONS
- Monitor ECG and echocardiogram.
- For acute changes, the client can be treated with dexrazoxane, but this medication can increase myelosuppression.
- If given early, ACE inhibitors may be able to prevent cardiac permanent damage.
- Dexrazoxane can protect the heart from toxicity but might reduce antitumor activity.

Red coloration to urine and sweat

CLIENT EDUCATION: This effect is not harmful.

Bleomycin

Pulmonary fibrosis and pneumonitis
NURSING ACTIONS: Monitor pulmonary function test

CONTRAINDICATIONS/PRECAUTIONS

Doxorubicin

- Contraindicated in clients who are pregnant or lactating, have severe myelosuppression and clients who have had a lifetime cumulative dose of 550 mg/m². Qs
- Use cautiously for clients who have liver impairment.

Dactinomycin

Contraindicated in clients who are pregnant or have acute infections.

INTERACTIONS

Doxorubicin

Calcium channel blockers can increase cardiotoxicity.
NURSING ACTIONS: Monitor ECG and heart function.

Phenobarbital can decrease metabolism of doxorubicin.
NURSING ACTIONS: Monitor for toxicities.

Paclitaxel can increase doxorubicin levels by decreasing clearance from the body.
NURSING ACTIONS: Monitor for toxicities.

Doxorubicin can increase effect of phenytoin levels.
NURSING ACTIONS: Monitor phenytoin level.

Live virus vaccines increase the risk for developing adverse reactions and decrease the antibody response
NURSING ACTIONS: Avoid concurrent use.

NURSING ADMINISTRATION

- Reduce dosage in liver disease.
- Monitor for bleeding (bruising) or infection (fever, sore throat).
- Monitor CBC and liver enzymes.
- Administer an antiemetic for nausea and vomiting.
- Stop chemotherapeutic medications if extravasation occurs.

CLIENT EDUCATION: Practice good oral hygiene and to avoid mouthwash with alcohol.

Doxorubicin

- Monitor ECG and cardiac function.
- IV vesicant; monitor IV site closely.

CLIENT EDUCATION
- Continue follow-up care after treatment is completed to monitor for delayed cardiac toxicity.
- Notify the provider if experiencing chest pain or shortness of breath.

Antimitotics

Vinca alkaloids

SELECT PROTOTYPE MEDICATION: Vincristine (conventional or liposomal; IV)

OTHER MEDICATIONS
- Vinblastine (IV)
- Vinorelbine (IV)

Taxanes

SELECT PROTOTYPE MEDICATION: Paclitaxel (IV)

OTHER MEDICATION: Docetaxel (IV)

PURPOSE

EXPECTED PHARMACOLOGICAL ACTION

Vinca alkaloids

Vincristine
- Useful in combination with other chemotherapy medications
- Stops cell division during mitosis
- Not bone marrow toxic
- M-phase specific

Vinblastine: Structural similar to vincristine. Toxic to peripheral nerves

Vinorelbine: Similar structure and actions to vincristine and vinblastine.

Taxanes

Paclitaxel
- Stop cell division during mitosis
- Inhibits cell division and produces apoptosis (programmed cell death)

Docetaxel: Similar structure and action of paclitaxel

THERAPEUTIC USE

Vinca alkaloids

Vincristine: Includes acute lymphocytic leukemia; Wilms' tumor; rhabdomyosarcoma; solid tumors, (bladder and breast cancers); Hodgkin's and non–Hodgkin's lymphomas; Kaposi's Sarcoma.

Vinblastine
- Kaposi's sarcoma, Hodgkin's and non–Hodgkin's lymphomas
- Carcinoma of the breast and testes

Vinorelbine: Non–small cell lung cancer

Taxanes

Paclitaxel: Includes ovarian, non–small cell lung tumors, and Kaposi's sarcoma; leukemias

Docetaxel: Metastatic breast cancer, metastatic non–small cell lung cancer, and prostate cancer

COMPLICATIONS

Vincristine

Nerve injury
- Injury to autonomic nerves (manifested by constipation, urinary hesitancy).
- Peripheral neuropathy (paresthesia, decreased reflexes, and sensory loss).

NURSING ACTIONS: Decreased dosage can be required.

CLIENT EDUCATION
- Report manifestations of decreased reflexes, weakness, paresthesia, and sensory loss.
- Use caution to prevent injury.

Severe tissue damage
Due to extravasations of vesicants

NURSING ACTIONS
- Stop chemotherapeutic medications if extravasation occurs.
- Only clinically trained personnel should administer these medications intravenously.
- Use a central line for infusion.

Alopecia
CLIENT EDUCATION
- Hair loss can occur 7 to 10 days after the beginning of treatment and will last for a maximum of 2 months after the last administration of the chemotherapeutic agent.
- Select a hairpiece before the occurrence of hair loss.

Paclitaxel

Bone marrow suppression
Low WBC count or neutropenia; bleeding caused by thrombocytopenia or low platelet count; anemia; or low RBCs

NURSING ACTIONS
- Monitor WBC, absolute neutrophil count, platelet count, Hgb, and Hct.
- Assess for bruising and bleeding gums.

CLIENT EDUCATION: Avoid crowds and contact with infectious individuals.

Bradycardia, heart block, MI, hypotension
NURSING ACTIONS
- Monitor for cardiac effects.
- Monitor ECG continuously during administration.

CLIENT EDUCATION: Report any chest pain or shortness of breath.

Alopecia
CLIENT EDUCATION
- Hair loss can occur 7 to 10 days after the beginning of treatment and will last for a maximum of 2 months after the last administration of the chemotherapeutic agent.
- Select a hairpiece before hair loss occurs.

Peripheral neuropathy: May need to decrease dosage.

Severe hypersensitivity reaction
- Monitor for hypotension, dyspnea, angioedema, urticaria.
- Manage with administering a glucocorticoid.

CONTRAINDICATIONS/PRECAUTIONS

Vincristine

- Contraindicated in pregnancy or lactation.
- Do not use with radiation therapy.
- Use with caution in clients who have liver disease or neuromuscular disease.

Paclitaxel

- Contraindicated in pregnancy
- Contraindicated in clients who have a neutrophil count less than 1,500/mm3. Use with caution in clients who have myelosuppression and liver impairment.

INTERACTIONS

Vincristine

Vincristine can reduce effects of digoxin.
NURSING ACTIONS: Monitor digoxin level and ECG.

Mitomycin can increase risk for bronchospasm.
NURSING ACTIONS: Monitor breath sounds.

Phenytoin can decrease vincristine effect.
NURSING ACTIONS: Monitor phenytoin level.

Live virus vaccines increase the risk for developing adverse reactions and decrease the antibody response.
NURSING ACTIONS: Avoid concurrent use.

Paclitaxel

Cisplatin or doxorubicin can increase myelosuppression.
NURSING ACTIONS: Use together with caution.

Cardiac medications that decrease heart rate (beta blockers, calcium channel blockers, and digoxin) can increase bradycardia.
NURSING ACTIONS: Monitor heart rate carefully.

Medications that increase risk for bleeding (NSAIDs and anticoagulants) can increase bleeding risk with paclitaxel.
NURSING ACTIONS: Monitor carefully for bleeding.

Live virus vaccines increase the risk for developing adverse reactions and decrease the antibody response.
NURSING ACTIONS: Avoid concurrent use.

NURSING ADMINISTRATION

- Assess for indications of neuropathy, including weakness, numbness, tingling, foot drop, ataxia, and paresthesia. Advise clients to use caution and report manifestations.
- Reduce dose for clients who have liver disease.
- Assess breath sounds for bronchospasm.
- Monitor for bleeding (bruising) or infection (fever, sore throat).
- Monitor CBC and liver enzymes.
- Give an antiemetic for nausea and vomiting.
- Stop chemotherapeutic medications if extravasation occurs.
- Monitor for cardiovascular effects, heart block, bradycardia, chest pain.

CLIENT EDUCATION
- Practice good oral hygiene.
- Prevent pregnancy during treatment

Alkylating agents

Nitrogen mustards

SELECT PROTOTYPE MEDICATION: Cyclophosphamide (oral, IV)

OTHER MEDICATIONS
- Mechlorethamine (IV, intracavitary, intrapleural)
- Bendamustine (IV)
- Chlorambucil (oral)
- Melphalan (oral or IV)

Nitrosoureas

SELECT PROTOTYPE MEDICATION: Carmustine (IV, topical implant to area where a brain tumor was removed)

OTHER MEDICATIONS
- Lomustine (oral)
- Streptozocin (IV)

Platinum compounds

SELECT PROTOTYPE MEDICATION: Cisplatin (IV)

OTHER MEDICATION: Carboplatin (IV)

PURPOSE

EXPECTED PHARMACOLOGICAL ACTION

Nitrogen mustards

Cyclophosphamide, mechlorethamine, bendamustine, chlorambucil
- Kills rapid growing cells by alkylation of DNA and RNA synthesis
- Cell cycle phase nonspecific. However, these medications are more toxic to dividing cells, especially those that divide rapidly.

Melphalan: Bifunctional agent that has two reactive sites to bind DNA

Nitrosoureas

Carmustine, lomustine
- Kills rapid growing cells by interrupting DNA and RNA synthesis
- Cell cycle phase nonspecific
- Crosses the blood–brain barrier. Therefore, is especially useful against primary and metastatic tumors of the brain.

Streptozocin: Selective uptake by the islet cells of the pancreas

Platinum compounds

Cisplatin
- Kills rapid growing cells by interrupting DNA and RNA synthesis
- Cell cycle phase nonspecific

Carboplatin: Cell kill resulting from cross-linking DNA

THERAPEUTIC USES

Nitrogen mustards

Effective against a broad spectrum of neoplastic diseases

Cyclophosphamide: Includes acute lymphomas; solid tumors (head, neck, ovary and breast cancers); Hodgkin's and non-Hodgkin's lymphomas; and multiple myeloma

Mechlorethamine: Bronchogenic carcinoma, Hodgkin's disease, leukemias, and mycosis fungoides

Bendamustine: Chronic lymphocytic leukemia, non–Hodgkin's lymphoma

Chlorambucil: Chronic lymphocytic leukemia, Hodgkin's disease, non-Hodgkin's lymphoma, multiple myeloma

Melphalan: Medication of choice for multiple myeloma, lymphoma, carcinoma of the ovary and breast.

Nitrosoureas

Carmustine: Includes brain tumors; Hodgkin's and non–Hodgkin's lymphomas; multiple myeloma; and adenocarcinoma of the stomach, colon, and rectum; malignant melanoma and hepatoma.

Lomustine: Brain cancer, Hodgkin's disease

Streptozocin: Metastatic islet cell tumors

Platinum compounds

Cisplatin: Includes bladder, testicular, and ovarian cancers

Carboplatin: Small cell cancer of the lung; squamous cell cancer of the head, neck; and endometrial cancer

COMPLICATIONS

Development of resistance to alkylating agents can occur due to decreased uptake of alkylating agents and increased production of enzymes that repair DNA.

Bone marrow suppression
Low WBC count or neutropenia, bleeding caused by thrombocytopenia or low platelet count, and anemia or low RBCs

NURSING ACTIONS
- Monitor WBC, absolute neutrophil count, platelet count, Hgb, and Hct.
- Assess for bruising and bleeding gums.

CLIENT EDUCATION: Avoid crowds and contact with infectious individuals.

GI discomfort (nausea and vomiting)
NURSING ACTIONS: Administer an antiemetic (ondansetron in combination with dexamethasone, granisetron, or metoclopramide) before beginning chemotherapy.

Cyclophosphamide

Acute hemorrhagic cystitis
NURSING ACTIONS
- Increase fluids to 3 L/day.
- Monitor for blood in urine.
- Mesna can be given if needed. Mesna is a uroprotectant agent that detoxifies metabolites to reduce hematuria.

Other effects: Can cause sterility or a decreased immune response.
NURSING ACTION: Instruct client about the possibility of these effects.

Alopecia
CLIENT EDUCATION
- Hair loss can occur 7 to 10 days after the beginning of treatment and will last for a maximum of 2 months after the last administration of the chemotherapeutic agent.
- Select a hairpiece before the occurrence of hair loss.

Carmustine

Severe nausea and vomiting

Pulmonary fibrosis
NURSING ACTIONS: Monitor lung function. The client can be treated with glucocorticoids.

Liver and kidney toxicity
NURSING ACTIONS: Monitor liver and kidney function.

Cisplatin

Severe nausea and vomiting
Nausea, vomiting can occur within 1 hr after administration and can continue for several days.

Renal toxicity
NURSING ACTIONS: Monitor kidney function. Increase fluids and give a diuretic if indicated.

Hearing loss
NURSING ACTIONS: Monitor for tinnitus and hearing loss.

CONTRAINDICATIONS/PRECAUTIONS

Cyclophosphamide
- Contraindicated in clients who are pregnant, lactating, and who have severe myelosuppression or severe infections. Qs
- Use with caution in clients who have kidney disorder, prostatic hypertrophy, liver disorders, leukopenia, or thrombocytopenia.

Carmustine: Contraindicated in clients who are pregnant or have severe myelosuppression or impaired pulmonary function.

Cisplatin: Contraindicated in clients who are pregnant, lactating, or have severe myelosuppression, kidney disorders, or hearing loss.

INTERACTIONS

Cyclophosphamide

Concurrent use of succinylcholine can cause increased neuromuscular blockage.
NURSING ACTIONS: Do not use together.

Carmustine

Concurrent use of cimetidine can increase bone marrow suppression.
NURSING ACTIONS: Do not use together.

Cisplatin

Concurrent use of aminoglycosides can increase risk for renal toxicity.
NURSING ACTIONS: Monitor kidney function.

Concurrent use of furosemide can increase hearing loss.
NURSING ACTIONS: Do not use together.

NURSING ADMINISTRATION

- Encourage adequate fluid intake of 2 to 3 L/day. Qᴘᴄᴄ
- Monitor for blood in urine. Mesna might be indicated.
- Reduce dose for clients who have liver disease.
- Monitor for bleeding (bruising) or infection (fever, sore throat).
- Monitor CBC, uric acid level, and liver enzymes.
- Give antiemetic for nausea and vomiting.
- Stop chemotherapeutic medications if extravasation occurs.
- Assess hearing prior to treatment with cisplatin.

CLIENT EDUCATION
- Practice good oral hygiene.
- Use birth control during treatment.

Topoisomerase inhibitors

Select prototype medication: Topotecan (IV)

PURPOSE

EXPECTED PHARMACOLOGICAL ACTION
- Interrupts DNA synthesis by making a cut in the DNA strand, thus altering its shape
- Cell cycle phase S–specific

THERAPEUTIC USES: Treats metastatic ovarian, cervical, colorectal, and small cell lung cancer.

COMPLICATIONS

Bone marrow suppression

- Low WBC count or neutropenia, bleeding caused by thrombocytopenia or low platelet count, and anemia or low RBCs
- Can occur 4 to 6 weeks after infusion

NURSING ACTIONS
- Monitor WBC, absolute neutrophil count, platelet count, Hgb, and Hct.
- Assess for bruising and bleeding gums.

CLIENT EDUCATION
- Continue precautions after treatment is completed.
- Avoid crowds and contact with infectious individuals.

GI discomfort (nausea, vomiting, abdominal pain, and diarrhea)

NURSING ACTIONS: Administer antiemetic (ondansetron in combination with dexamethasone, granisetron, or metoclopramide) before beginning chemotherapy.

Alopecia

CLIENT EDUCATION
- Hair loss can occur 7 to 10 days after the beginning of treatment and will last for a maximum of 2 months after the last administration of the chemotherapeutic agent.
- Select a hairpiece before the occurrence of hair loss.

CONTRAINDICATIONS/PRECAUTIONS

- Contraindicated in clients who are pregnant or lactating, or have severe myelosuppression with a neutrophil count less than 1,500/mm³ or hypersensitivity Qs
- Use caution for clients who have impaired renal function

INTERACTIONS

Cisplatin can increase myelosuppression.

NURSING ACTIONS: Use with caution.

Live virus vaccines increase the risk for developing adverse reactions and decrease the antibody response.

NURSING ACTIONS: Avoid concurrent use.

NURSING ADMINISTRATION

- Monitor for bleeding (bruising) or infection (fever, sore throat). Qpcc
- Monitor CBC.
- Give prophylactic antiemetics for nausea and vomiting.

CLIENT EDUCATION
- Perform good oral hygiene and avoid mouthwash with alcohol.
- Prevent pregnancy during treatment.
- Monitor for drowsiness for the first several days of therapy.

Other antineoplastic agents

- Asparaginase (IV, IM)
- Hydroxyurea (oral)
- Procarbazine (oral)

PURPOSE

EXPECTED PHARMACOLOGICAL ACTION

Asparaginase
- Kills cancer cells by interrupting protein synthesis in leukemia cells. Deprives the cell of asparagine.
- Cell cycle phase G1-specific

Hydroxyurea
- Kills cancer cells by interrupting DNA synthesis
- Cell cycle phase S-specific
- Can cross blood–brain barrier

Procarbazine
- Kills cancer cells by interrupting DNA, RNA, and protein synthesis by alkalizing.
- Cell cycle phase nonspecific
- Can cross blood–brain barrier

THERAPEUTIC USES

Asparaginase: Acute lymphocytic leukemia

Hydroxyurea: Includes chronic myelogenous leukemia, ovarian, sickle cell anemia, and squamous cell cancers.

Procarbazine: Includes brain tumors, and Hodgkin's and non–Hodgkin's lymphomas

COMPLICATIONS

Asparaginase, hydroxyurea, procarbazine

GI discomfort (nausea and vomiting)

NURSING ACTIONS: Administer antiemetic (ondansetron in combination with dexamethasone, granisetron, or metoclopramide) before beginning chemotherapy.

Asparaginase

Hypersensitivity reaction
Fatal anaphylaxis can occur.

NURSING ACTIONS
- Consider administering a test dose or premedicating to prevent hypersensitivity.
- Monitor for closely for wheezing or rash.
- Have epinephrine and resuscitation equipment readily available.

CNS effects
- From confusion to coma
- Temporary tremor can occur

NURSING ACTIONS: Monitor for CNS effects and evaluate frequently for changes.

Liver and pancreas toxicity
NURSING ACTIONS
- Monitor liver enzymes.
- Monitor for jaundice.
- Monitor pancreatic enzymes.

Renal toxicity
NURSING ACTIONS: Monitor kidney function. Increase fluids and administer a diuretic if indicated.

Hydroxyurea and procarbazine

Bone marrow suppression
- Low WBC count or neutropenia, bleeding caused by thrombocytopenia or low platelet count, and anemia or low RBCs
- Can occur 4 to 6 weeks after infusion

NURSING ACTIONS
- Monitor WBC, absolute neutrophil count, platelet count, hemoglobin, and hematocrit.
- Assess for bruising and bleeding gums.

CLIENT EDUCATION
- Avoid crowds and contact with infectious individuals.
- Continue precautions after treatment is completed.

Procarbazine

CNS depression, secondary leukemia, and sterility, especially in males.

Peripheral neuropathy manifestations
- Can include weakness and paresthesia
- CLIENT EDUCATION: Report manifestations. Use caution to prevent injury.

CONTRAINDICATIONS/PRECAUTIONS

Asparaginase

- Contraindicated in clients who are pregnant, or have a history of pancreatitis, thrombosis or hemorrhagic events following L–asparaginase therapy. Qs
- Use with caution in clients who have liver disease.

Hydroxyurea

- Contraindicated in clients who are pregnant or have severe myelosuppression or anemia.
- Use with caution in clients who have kidney disease.

Procarbazine

- Contraindicated in clients who are pregnant or have severe myelosuppression.
- Use with caution in clients who have liver or kidney disease.

INTERACTIONS

Asparaginase

Can decrease effects of methotrexate.
NURSING ACTIONS: Use with caution. Monitor for medication effect.

Prednisone and vincristine can increase the risk for asparaginase toxicity. Can cause hyperglycemia.
NURSING ACTIONS: Use with caution.

Increased risk for bleeding if used with anticoagulant, antiplatelet medication.
NURSING ACTIONS: Monitor blood coagulation panel.

Hydroxyurea

Cytotoxic medications and antivirals can increase risk for toxicity.
NURSING ACTIONS: Use with caution together.

Procarbazine

Can increase depressant effects of CNS depressants (opioids).
NURSING ACTIONS: Avoid concurrent use.

MAOI or tricyclic antidepressants, all sympathomimetic drugs, foods containing tyramine, and many OTC preparations (cough medicines) can cause hypertensive crisis.
NURSING ACTIONS: Discontinue medications in advance of procarbazine therapy. Advise client to avoid foods containing tyramine.

Alcohol can cause a disulfiram–type reaction.

Smoking increases the risk for secondary lung cancer.

Can reduce blood levels of digoxin when used concurrently.

NURSING ADMINISTRATION

Asparaginase

- Monitor for allergic reaction. Give a test dose. Have resuscitation equipment on hand. Qpcc
- Give an antiemetic for nausea and vomiting.
- Monitor glucose and liver function tests periodically during therapy.

CLIENT EDUCATION
- Prevent pregnancy during treatment.
- Practice good oral hygiene.

Hydroxyurea

- Monitor for bleeding (bruising) or infection (fever, sore throat). Withhold medication and notify the provider for a WBC less than 2,500/mm³ or a platelet count less than 100,000/mm³.
- Monitor CBC.
- Give an antiemetic for nausea and vomiting.

CLIENT EDUCATION
- Practice good oral hygiene.
- Prevent pregnancy during treatment.

Procarbazine

- Monitor for neurologic effects (confusion or paresthesia).
- Withhold the medication and notify the provider for a WBC less than 4,000/mm³ and a platelet count less than 100,000/mm³.

Noncytotoxic chemotherapy agents

Noncytotoxic chemotherapy medications are nontoxic to cells.

Hormonal agents are effective against tumors that are supported or suppressed by hormones.

- **Hormone agonists** cause an increase in a hormone that suppresses another hormone required for a tumor to grow. The use of androgenic hormones in a client who has estrogen-dependent cancer can suppress growth of this type of cancer. Conversely, the use of estrogenic hormones for a testosterone-dependent cancer can suppress growth of this type of cancer.
- **Hormone antagonists** block certain hormones and can be effective against tumors that require a particular hormone for support. The use of an antiestrogen hormone in a client who has estrogen-dependent cancer can suppress growth of this type of cancer. The same is true for ant testosterone hormones.

Biological response modulators act as immunostimulants to enhance the immune response and reduce proliferation of cancer cells.

Targeted antineoplastic agents are antibodies or small molecules that attach to specific target sites to stop cancer growth without injuring healthy tissue.

Hormonal agents: Prostate cancer medications

Gonadotropin-releasing hormone (GnRH) agonists

Select prototype medication: Leuprolide (subcutaneous, IM)

OTHER MEDICATIONS
- Triptorelin (subcutaneous, IM)
- Goserelin (subcutaneous, IM)
- Histrelin (subcutaneous, IM)

Androgen receptor blockers

Select prototype medication: Flutamide (oral)

OTHER MEDICATIONS
- Bicalutamide (oral)
- Nilutamide (oral)

Gonadotropin-releasing hormone antagonist

SELECT PROTOTYPE: Degarelix (SQ)

PURPOSE

EXPECTED PHARMACOLOGICAL ACTION

Gonadotropin-releasing hormone agonists: Prevents the release of luteinizing and follicle-stimulating hormones to prevent testosterone production by the testicles.

Androgen receptor blockers
- Blocks testosterone at receptor site.
- Used in conjunction with gonadotropin-releasing hormone agonists to block androgen receptors and suppress the growth of prostate cancer or in combination with surgical castration.

Gonadotropin-releasing hormone antagonists: Prevents the release of luteinizing and follicle-stimulating hormones to prevent testosterone production by the testicles.

THERAPEUTIC USES

Gonadotropin-releasing hormone agonists: Palliative therapy of advanced prostate cancer in clients who do not want surgical castration.

Androgen receptor blockers: Treatment of prostate cancer

Gonadotropin-releasing hormone antagonists: Use for clients who cannot use GnRH agonists and who do not want surgical castration.

COMPLICATIONS

Leuprolide

Hot flashes, decreased libido, erectile dysfunction, and gynecomastia
NURSING ACTIONS: Warn clients about adverse effects. Adverse reactions can be transient.

Decreased bone density
CLIENT EDUCATION
- Increase calcium and vitamin D intake.
- Increase bone mass with weight-bearing exercises.

Dysrhythmias, pulmonary edema
NURSING ACTIONS: Monitor for dysrhythmias and assess breath sounds.

Disease flare
NURSING ACTIONS: Manifestations of worsening of the prostate cancer after a dose of the medication. Use an androgen receptor blocker during the first weeks of leuprolide therapy to prevent leuprolide-induced tumor flare.

Flutamide

Hot flashes, decreased muscle and bone mass, decreased libido, and gynecomastia
NURSING ACTIONS: Warn clients about adverse effects.

Nausea, vomiting, diarrhea
NURSING ACTIONS: Monitor intake and output.

Liver toxicity
NURSING ACTIONS: Monitor liver enzymes.

Degarelix

Hot flashes, decreased muscle and bone mass, decreased libido, and gynecomastia
NURSING ACTIONS: Warn clients about adverse effects.

CONTRAINDICATIONS/PRECAUTIONS

Leuprolide: Contraindicated in clients who are pregnant or lactating, hypersensitive to gonadotropin-releasing agonists Qs

Flutamide: Contraindicated in clients who are pregnant or have severe liver disease.

Degarelix: Contraindicated in clients who are pregnant or have previous hypersensitivity.

INTERACTIONS

Leuprolide

Flutamide and megestrol increase antineoplastic action.

Flutamide

Concurrent use of flutamide and warfarin can increase anticoagulation.
NURSING ACTIONS: Monitor PT and INR.

Degarelix

Concurrent use with class IA or III antiarrhythmics increases the risk for dysrhythmia or QT prolongation.
NURSING ACTIONS: Monitor ECG periodically during treatment.

NURSING ADMINISTRATION

Leuprolide

- Perform bone density testing.
- Monitor for dysrhythmias and assess breath sounds.
- Monitor prostate-specific antigen (PSA) and testosterone levels, which should both decrease with treatment.

CLIENT EDUCATION
- Increase calcium and vitamin D intake. Minimize bone loss with weight-bearing exercises.
- Monitor for bone pain.
- Prostate manifestations can worsen at beginning of treatment (disease flare) and can be prevented by adding flutamide to treatment.

Flutamide

- Administered with a gonadotropin-releasing hormone agonist (such as leuprolide) or alone following surgical castration.
- Liver function should be assessed at baseline, and periodically thereafter.
- Warn clients of adverse effects of the medication (gynecomastia).

Degarelix

Administer two subcutaneous doses the first day, then a maintenance dose every 28 days.

CLIENT EDUCATION: Skin effects (swelling, itching, redness) at injection site usually resolve within 3 days.

Hormonal agents: Breast cancer medications

Estrogen receptor blockers

SELECT PROTOTYPE MEDICATION: Tamoxifen (oral)

OTHER MEDICATIONS
- Raloxifene (oral)
- Fulvestrant (IM)
- Toremifene (oral)

Aromatase inhibitors

SELECT PROTOTYPE MEDICATION: Anastrozole

OTHER MEDICATIONS
- Letrozole
- Exemestane (oral)

Monoclonal antibody

SELECT PROTOTYPE MEDICATION: Trastuzumab (IV)

PURPOSE

EXPECTED PHARMACOLOGICAL ACTION

Estrogen receptor blockers: Stops growth of breast cancer cells, which are estrogen-dependent cancers

Aromatase inhibitors: Stops growth of breast cancer cells by blocking estrogen production

Monoclonal antibody: Targets breast cancer cells, prevents cell growth, and causes cell death. Only effective against tumors that are HER2-positive.

THERAPEUTIC USES

Estrogen receptor blockers: Used to treat or prevent breast cancer

Aromatase inhibitors: Used to treat breast cancer in clients who are postmenopausal

Monoclonal antibody
- Used to treat metastatic breast cancer
- Can be used alone or in conjunction with paclitaxel

COMPLICATIONS

Tamoxifen

Endometrial cancer
NURSING ACTIONS: Monitor for abnormal bleeding.

CLIENT EDUCATION: Have a yearly gynecological exam and Pap smear.

Hypercalcemia (bone pain)
NURSING ACTIONS: Monitor calcium level.

Nausea and vomiting
NURSING ACTIONS
- Monitor fluid status.
- Administer fluids and antiemetics as prescribed.

Thromboembolic events (DVT, PE, stroke)
NURSING ACTIONS: Assess breath sounds.

CLIENT EDUCATION: Report chest pain edema of the leg or calf, or shortness of breath.

Hot flashes
NURSING ACTIONS: Warn clients about adverse effects.

Vaginal discharge or bleeding
NURSING ACTIONS: Monitor bleeding and discharge.

CLIENT EDUCATION: Have a yearly gynecological exam and Pap smear.

Anastrozole

Muscle and joint pain, headache
NURSING ACTIONS: Treat pain with a mild analgesic as prescribed.

Nausea
NURSING ACTIONS
- Monitor fluid status.
- Administer fluids and antiemetics as prescribed.

Vaginal bleeding
NURSING ACTIONS: Monitor bleeding and CBC.

Increased risk for osteoporosis
CLIENT EDUCATION: Take calcium and vitamin D supplements and perform weight-bearing exercises. Clients at high risk should take a bisphosphonate or denosumab.

Hot flashes
NURSING ACTIONS: Warn clients about adverse effects.

Trastuzumab

40% of clients experience a flu-like manifestations after first infusion (chills, fever, nausea, vomiting, weakness, pain, headache)

Cardiac toxicity, tachycardia, heart failure, pulmonary hypertension
NURSING ACTIONS
- Obtain baseline ECG and monitor.
- Monitor for dyspnea and edema.

CLIENT EDUCATION: Report chest pain or shortness of breath.

Hypersensitivity reaction
NURSING ACTIONS: Monitor closely during infusion. Have resuscitation equipment nearby.

Nausea and vomiting
NURSING ACTIONS: Monitor fluid status.

CONTRAINDICATIONS/PRECAUTIONS

Tamoxifen

Contraindicated in clients who are pregnant, taking warfarin, and in clients who have a history of blood clots or pulmonary embolism Qs

Anastrozole

- Contraindicated in clients who are pregnant, lactating, or before menopause and in severe liver disease.
- Use with caution in clients who have mild to moderate liver disease.

Trastuzumab

- Contraindicated in clients who are pregnant, lactating, or hypersensitive to the medication.
- Use with caution in clients who have heart disease or a pre-existing pulmonary condition.

INTERACTIONS

Tamoxifen

Tamoxifen can increase the anticoagulation action of warfarin.
NURSING ACTIONS
- Monitor PT and INR.
- Warfarin doses might need to be adjusted.

Some SSRI antidepressants (such as paroxetine) decrease effectiveness of tamoxifen.
NURSING ACTIONS: Avoid using together.

Anastrozole

Tamoxifen and estrogen-like medications can reduce anastrozole effects.
NURSING ACTIONS: Avoid using together.

Concurrent use of anastrozole and anthracyclines can increase the risk for cardiac effects.
NURSING ACTIONS: Monitor for cardiac effects.

NURSING ADMINISTRATION

- Monitor for dysrhythmias and assess breath sounds.
- Monitor CBC and calcium levels.
- Monitor fluid status.
- Monitor weights weekly and report weight gain.

CLIENT EDUCATION
- Increase calcium and vitamin D intake. Reduce bone loss with weight-bearing exercises.
- Prevent pregnancy during therapy.

Biologic response modifiers

SELECT PROTOTYPE MEDICATION: Interferon alfa-2b (subcutaneous, IM, IV)

OTHER MEDICATIONS
- Aldesleukin (IV infusion)
- Bacillus Calmette-Guerin (BCG) vaccine (intravesical into the bladder)

PURPOSE

EXPECTED PHARMACOLOGICAL ACTION: Increases immune response and decreases production of cancer cells.

THERAPEUTIC USES: Treat or prevent hairy cell leukemia, chronic myelogenous leukemia, malignant melanoma, follicular lymphoma, and AIDS-related Kaposi's sarcoma.

COMPLICATIONS

Flu-like manifestations
Fever, fatigue, headache, chills, myalgia

NURSING ACTIONS: Administer acetaminophen as prescribed. Flu-like manifestations tend to diminish with continued therapy.

Bone marrow suppression, alopecia, cardiotoxicity, thyroid dysfunction, and neurotoxicity (with prolonged therapy)
NURSING ACTIONS
- Monitor CBC, fatigue level, and indications of cardiotoxicity (dysrhythmias, palpitations, myocardial infarction, heart failure) and neurotoxicity (confusion, ataxia, inability to concentrate, paresthesia).
- Monitor for manifestations of infection.
- Monitor for bruising; bleeding; and blood in stools, urine, sputum, or emesis.

CLIENT EDUCATION: Report these manifestations to the provider.

Depression, anxiety, insomnia, altered mental states
NURSING ACTIONS: Monitor mood and mental status and assess for suicidal thoughts.

CONTRAINDICATIONS/PRECAUTIONS

- Contraindicated in clients who have hypersensitivity to the medication, suicidal thoughts, colitis, or pancreatitis
- Use caution in clients who are pregnant (can increase risk of spontaneous abortion), have severe liver, kidney, heart, or pulmonary disease; diabetes mellitus; or history of depression. Qs

INTERACTIONS

Concurrent use with theophylline can lead to theophylline toxicity.
NURSING ACTIONS: Monitor clients for indications of toxicity. Decreased theophylline dosage might be indicated.

Zidovudine can increase the risk of neutropenia or thrombocytopenia.
NURSING ACTIONS
- Monitor for neutropenia.
- Monitor for bleeding or easy bruising.

CLIENT EDUCATION: Avoid crowds and contact with infectious individuals.

Concurrent use with medications that are cardiotoxic or neurotoxic can increase cardiotoxicity or neurotoxicity.
NURSING ACTIONS: Monitor for cardiotoxicity or neurotoxicity.

Concurrent use with vaccines using a live virus can reduce antibody response.
NURSING ACTIONS: Avoid use together.

NURSING ADMINISTRATION

- Store the medication in the refrigerator and do not freeze. Administer at room temperature. Do not shake the vial.
- Monitor for flu manifestations. Premedicate with acetaminophen if prescribed.
- Monitor CBC, platelets, and electrolytes.
- Monitor fluid status.
- Monitor weight and nutritional status.

CLIENT EDUCATION: Practice good oral hygiene.

Targeted antineoplastic medications

Epidural growth factor receptor (EGFR)-tyrosine kinase inhibitors

SELECT PROTOTYPE MEDICATION: Cetuximab

OTHER MEDICATION
- Panitumumab (IV)
- Gefitinib (IV)
- Erlotinib (IV)
- Afatinib (IV)

BCR-ABL tyrosine kinase inhibitors

SELECT PROTOTYPE MEDICATION: Imatinib (oral)

CD20-directed antibodies

SELECT PROTOTYPE MEDICATION: Rituximab (IV)

Angiogenesis inhibitors

SELECT PROTOTYPE MEDICATION: Bevacizumab (IV)

PURPOSE

EXPECTED PHARMACOLOGICAL ACTION

EGFR-tyrosine kinase inhibitors: Antibody that stops cancer cell growth and increases apoptosis (cell death)

BCR-ABL tyrosine kinase inhibitors: Stops cancer growth by inhibiting intracellular enzymes

CD20-directed antibodies: Monoclonal antibody that binds to specific antigens on B-lymphocytes and then destroys cancer cells

Angiogenesis inhibitors: Suppresses formation of new blood vessels on solid tumors depriving them of the expanded blood supply they need for growth

THERAPEUTIC USES

EGFR-TYROSINE KINASE INHIBITORS: Treat EGFR-positive cancers (colorectal and solid tumors of the head and neck)

BCR-ABL TYROSINE KINASE INHIBITORS: Treat chronic myeloid leukemia

CD20-directed antibodies: Treat non-Hodgkin's lymphoma, B-cell chronic lymphocytic leukemia

Angiogenesis inhibitors: Treat colorectal and lung cancers

COMPLICATIONS

Cetuximab

Infusion reaction, rash, hypotension, wheezing
NURSING ACTIONS
- Monitor carefully for indications of a reaction.
- Premedicate if needed with diphenhydramine or corticosteroids.
- Stop treatment and administer antihistamines, epinephrine, glucocorticoids, bronchodilators, and oxygen as prescribed.

Pulmonary emboli
NURSING ACTIONS: Monitor breath sounds. Monitor SaO2.

Skin toxicity, rash
NURSING ACTIONS: Monitor for rash over 2 weeks of treatment. Treat with topical antibiotics if needed. Teach client to limit sun exposure, use a sunblock, and wear protective clothing.

Imatinib

GI discomfort (nausea and vomiting)
NURSING ACTIONS
- Administer antiemetic (ondansetron in combination with dexamethasone, granisetron, or metoclopramide) before beginning chemotherapy.
- Take with food.

Flu-like manifestations: Fever, fatigue, headache, chills, myalgia

NURSING ACTIONS: Administer acetaminophen as prescribed.

Edema
NURSING ACTIONS: Monitor for edema. Edema from fluid retention may lead to pleural effusion, pericardial effusion, pulmonary edema, or ascites.

Hypokalemia
NURSING ACTIONS: Monitor potassium level.

Neutropenia, anemia, thrombocytopenia
NURSING ACTIONS
- Monitor CBC.
- Assess for bruising and bleeding gums.

CLIENT EDUCATION: Avoid crowds and contact with infectious individuals.

Rituximab

Infusion reaction, rash, hypotension, wheezing
NURSING ACTIONS
- Monitor carefully for indications of a reaction.
- Premedicate if needed with diphenhydramine or corticosteroids.
- Stop treatment and administer epinephrine as prescribed.

Flu-like manifestations: Fever, fatigue, headache, chills, myalgia

NURSING ACTIONS: Administer acetaminophen as prescribed.

Tumor lysis syndrome due to rapid cell death: Can lead to kidney failure, hypocalcemia, hyperkalemia, and hyperuricemia

NURSING ACTIONS
- Monitor kidney function and administer dialysis if needed.
- Monitor fluids and electrolytes and correct abnormalities.

CLIENT EDUCATION: Report manifestation that begin 12 to 24 hr after the first medication infusion.

Bevacizumab

Thromboembolism
Including cerebrovascular accident, myocardial infarction, transient ischemic attacks (TIA)

NURSING ACTIONS: Monitor for thromboembolic disorders.

Alopecia
CLIENT EDUCATION
- Hair loss can occur 7 to 10 days after the beginning of treatment and will last for a maximum of 2 months after the last administration of the chemotherapeutic agent.
- Select a hairpiece before the occurrence of hair loss.

Hemorrhage
GI, vaginal, nasal, intracranial, or pulmonary

NURSING ACTIONS: Observe for signs of hemorrhage (intracranial, pulmonary, vaginal, nosebleeds).

Hypertension or hypotension
NURSING ACTIONS: Monitor blood pressure.

Gastric perforation
CLIENT EDUCATION: Notify the provider if they experience abdominal pain associated with vomiting and constipation.

CONTRAINDICATIONS/PRECAUTIONS

Cetuximab

Contraindicated in clients who are pregnant or lactating, or have hypersensitivity to the medication. Qs

Imatinib

- Contraindicated in clients who are pregnant or lactating, or have hypersensitivity to the medication.
- Use with caution in clients who have liver disease.

Rituximab

- Contraindicated in clients who are pregnant or lactating, or have hypersensitivity to the medication.
- Use with caution in clients who have liver or kidney failure.

Bevacizumab

- Contraindicated in clients who are pregnant or lactating, or have a low WBC, nephrotic syndrome, recent surgery or dental work, or hypertension.
- Use with caution in clients who have cardiac or renal disease history or hypersensitivity to the medication.

INTERACTIONS

Cetuximab

Sun exposure may increase skin toxicity.

CLIENT EDUCATION: Use sunscreen and avoid exposure.

Imatinib

Acetaminophen can increase chance of liver failure.
NURSING ACTIONS: Monitor liver enzymes.

Concurrent use with warfarin can increase anticoagulant effect.
NURSING ACTIONS
- Monitor for indications of bleeding.
- Monitor INR and PT and adjust warfarin dosage accordingly.

Clarithromycin, erythromycin, and ketoconazole can slow imatinib metabolism and cause toxicity by raising the levels of imatinib.
NURSING ACTIONS: Monitor for toxicity.

Carbamazepine and phenytoin can increase imatinib metabolism and reduce its levels.
NURSING ACTIONS: Monitor for effectiveness.

Rituximab

Calcium channel blockers and other antihypertensive medications increase chance of hypotension.
NURSING ACTIONS: Antihypertensives might be withheld up to 12 hr prior to rituximab infusions.

Bevacizumab

Bevacizumab can increase sunitinib level.
NURSING ACTIONS: Monitor medication levels.

NURSING ADMINISTRATION

- Monitor for infusion reaction and premedicate if prescribed.
- Monitor for infection.
- Monitor CBC, platelets, and electrolytes.
- Monitor fluid status.
- Assess for edema.

CLIENT EDUCATION
- Protect skin from the sun and assess for rash. Qpcc
- Notify the provider of shortness of breath.
- Practice good oral hygiene.
- Report adverse reactions (abdominal pain, skin lesions, headache, and episodes of bleeding).

Active Learning Scenario

A nurse is teaching a client who has prostate cancer and a new prescription for monthly injections of leuprolide IM. What should the nurse teach this client about leuprolide? Use the ATI Active Learning Template: Medication to complete this item.

THERAPEUTIC USES: Identify for leuprolide.

COMPLICATIONS: Identify two adverse effects.

NURSING INTERVENTIONS: Describe two diagnostic tests to monitor.

CLIENT EDUCATION: Include two teaching points.

Application Exercises

1. A nurse is caring for a client who has breast cancer. The client asks why the treatment plan contains a combination therapy of three different medications. Which of the following responses should the nurse make? (Select all that apply.)
   - A. "Combination chemotherapy decreases the risk of medication resistance."
   - B. "Combination chemotherapy attacks cancer cells at different stages of cell growth."
   - C. "Combination chemotherapy increases production of platelets."
   - D. "Combination chemotherapy stimulates the immune system."
   - E. "Combination chemotherapy reduces the risk of injury to healthy cells."

2. A nurse is teaching a client who is receiving methotrexate for non-Hodgkin lymphoma. Which of the following instructions should the nurse include?
   - A. "Drink 2 to 3 liters of fluid per day."
   - B. "Avoid grapefruit juice while taking this medication."
   - C. "Expect bruising while taking this medication."
   - D. "Weigh yourself two times per week."

3. A nurse is preparing to administer cyclophosphamide IV to a client who has Hodgkin's disease. What actions should the nurse take?

4. A nurse is teaching a group of nurses about chemotherapy agents. Match the chemotherapy agent with the corresponding action.

   A. Topoisomerase inhibitors   1. M-phase specific

   B. Antitumor antibiotics   2. S-phase specific

   C. Antimitotics   3. Cell cycle nonspecific

5. A nurse is teaching a client who has breast cancer about tamoxifen. What adverse effects of tamoxifen should the nurse discuss with the client?

6. A nurse is caring for a client who is being treated with interferon alfa-2b for malignant melanoma. The nurse should identify that which of the following findings are adverse effects of this medication? (Select all that apply.)
   - A. Tinnitus
   - B. Muscle aches
   - C. Peripheral neuropathy
   - D. Bone loss
   - E. Depression

Application Exercises Key

1. A. **CORRECT:** Medication resistance is decreased with combination therapy because the chance of developing resistance to several medications is less than to only one medication.
   B. **CORRECT:** Each medication kills cancer cells at a different stage of growth. A combination of medications can kill more cancer cells than only one medication.
   C. Chemotherapy agents are not blocked from entering healthy cells during combination therapy.
   D. Cancer chemotherapy with a combination of cytotoxic agents often causes infection rather than stimulating the immune system.
   E. **CORRECT:** Injury to normal body cells can be decreased by combination therapy because the medications used have different toxicities.

   Ⓝ *NCLEX® Connection: Pharmacological and Parenteral Therapies, Medication Administration*

2. A. **CORRECT:** When taking actions, the nurse should instruct the client to drink 2 to 3 L of fluids each day to promote excretion and reduce the risk of acute renal failure.

   Ⓝ *NCLEX® Connection: Pharmacological and Parenteral Therapies, Parenteral/Intravenous Therapies*

3. When taking actions, the nurse should encourage adequate fluid intake of 2 to 3 L/day. Monitor for blood in urine. Administer mesna, a uroprotectant agent that detoxifies metabolites, if indicated. Reduce dose for clients who have liver disease. Monitor the client for manifestations of bleeding, such as bruising, or infection, such as fever or sore throat. Monitor CBC, uric acid level, and liver enzymes. Administer antiemetic for nausea and vomiting. Stop chemotherapeutic medications if extravasation occurs.

   Ⓝ *NCLEX® Connection: Pharmacological and Parenteral Therapies, Intravenous Therapies*

4. A, 2; B, 3; C. 1

   When taking actions, the nurse should instruct that topoisomerase inhibitors are s-phase specific and kill cancer cells by interrupting DNA synthesis. Antitumor antibiotics kill cancer cells by altering DNA and are cell cycle nonspecific. Antimiotics kill cancer cells by blocking mitosis and are m-phase specific.

   Ⓝ *NCLEX® Connection: Pharmacological and Parenteral Therapies, Parenteral/Intravenous Therapies*

5. When taking actions, the nurse should instruct the client that adverse effects of tamoxifen can include endometrial cancer, hypercalcemia, nausea and vomiting, thromboembolic events, hot flashes, and vaginal discharge or bleeding. The nurse should instruct the client to monitor and report uterine bleeding, chest pain, edema of the leg or calf, or shortness of breath, and have a yearly gynecological exam and Pap smear. .

   Ⓝ *NCLEX® Connection: Pharmacological and Parenteral Therapies, Parenteral/Intravenous Therapies*

6. A. Tinnitus is not an adverse effect of interferon alfa-2b.
   B. **CORRECT:** Muscle aches and other flu-like manifestations are common adverse effects of interferon alfa-2b. Acetaminophen may be prescribed to relieve these manifestations.
   C. **CORRECT:** Peripheral neuropathy, dizziness, and fatigue are CNS effects that can occur when taking interferon alfa-2b. These should be reported to the provider, and teach the client to prevent injury from falls.
   D. Bone loss can occur from treatment with gonadotropin-releasing hormone agonists (leuprolide). Bone loss does not occur with interferon alfa-2b treatment.
   E. **CORRECT:** Depression and mental status changes can occur with interferon alfa-2b treatment. Assess the client for suicidal thoughts.

   Ⓝ *NCLEX® Connection: Pharmacological and Parenteral Therapies, Adverse Effects/Contraindications/Interactions*

Active Learning Scenario Key

Using the ATI Active Learning Template: Medication

THERAPEUTIC USES: Leuprolide is a gonadotropin-releasing hormone agonist that prevents testosterone production by stopping the release of luteinizing and follicle-stimulating hormones. It is used instead of surgical castration for clients who have advanced prostate cancer.

COMPLICATIONS
- Hot flashes (or flashes), decreased libido, gynecomastia
- Cardiac manifestations (dysrhythmias) and increased edema, which can lead to heart failure
- Decreased bone density, which can lead to fractures
- Disease flare, which means manifestations of the client's prostate cancer can worsen after a dose of the medication

NURSING INTERVENTIONS
- Monitor prostate-specific antigen and testosterone levels, which should both decrease with treatment.
- Bone density testing can be needed for some clients, as well as ECG if cardiac manifestations are present.

CLIENT EDUCATION
- Increase calcium and vitamin D in diet.
- Increase weight-bearing exercise to minimize bone loss.
- Report a flare in prostate manifestations to the provider.
- Report adverse effects (palpitations, edema, and hot flashes) to the provider.

Ⓝ *NCLEX® Connection: Pharmacological and Parenteral Therapies, Medication Administration*

ⓝ NCLEX® Connections

When reviewing the following chapters, keep in mind the relevant topics and tasks of the NCLEX outline, in particular:

Pharmacological and Parenteral Therapies

ADVERSE EFFECTS/CONTRAINDICATIONS/SIDE EFFECTS/INTERACTIONS

Identify actual and potential incompatibilities of prescribed client medications.

Notify the primary health care provider of side effects, adverse effects, and contraindications of medications and parenteral therapy.

Monitor for anticipated interactions among the client's prescribed medications and fluids.

Assess the client for actual or potential side effects and adverse effects of medications.

EXPECTED ACTIONS/OUTCOMES

Use clinical decision-making/critical thinking when addressing expected effects/outcomes of medications.

Evaluate client's response to medication.

MEDICATION ADMINISTRATION

Evaluate appropriateness and accuracy of medication order for client.

Review pertinent data prior to medication administration.

Administer and document medications given by parenteral routes.

Educate client about medications.

PARENTERAL/INTRAVENOUS THERAPIES: Evaluate the client's response to intermittent parenteral fluid therapy.

UNIT 12   MEDICATIONS FOR INFECTION

CHAPTER 41 *Principles of Antimicrobial Therapy*

Antimicrobial therapy is the use of medications to treat infections due to bacteria, viruses, or fungi. Antimicrobials (natural or synthetic) use selective toxicity to kill or otherwise control microbes without destroying host cells.

Changes in the DNA of micro-organisms, called conjugation, which produces resistance to multiple existing medications, mandates the continual creation of new antimicrobials.

Superinfection is a type of resistance that results when an antibiotic kills normal flora, thus favoring the emergence of a new infection that is difficult to eliminate.

METHODS OF ANTIMICROBIAL ACTIONS

- Destroying the cell wall that is present in bacteria but not in mammals
- Inhibiting the conversion of an enzyme unique for a particular bacterium's survival
- Impairing protein synthesis in the bacteria's ribosomes, which are never identical to mammalian cells
- Disrupting bacterial synthesis or function of DNA and RNA
- Inhibiting viral replication

CLASSIFICATION OF ANTIMICROBIAL MEDICATIONS

- Requires defining which microbes are susceptible to each medication
  - **Narrow-spectrum antibiotics,** to which only a few types of bacteria are sensitive
  - **Broad-spectrum antibiotics,** to which a wide variety of bacteria are sensitive
- Requires identifying the mechanism of action of each antibacterial medication
  - **Bactericidal medications** are directly lethal to the micro-organism.
  - **Bacteriostatic medications** slow the growth of the micro-organism, but the immune-system response of phagocytic cells (macrophages, neutrophils) actually destroys the bacteria.
- Multiple factors determine which medication providers prescribe for clinical use (antibacterial, antifungal, or antiviral medication).

- When selecting an antibiotic, 3 principal factors must be considered:
  - Identity of the causative agent
  - Sensitivity of the infecting organism to an antimicrobial
  - Other factors (location of infection, age, allergies, and immune status of host)

SELECTION OF ANTIMICROBIALS

IDENTIFICATION OF CAUSATIVE AGENT

Laboratory testing of body fluids (blood, urine, sputum, and wound drainage), identifies the micro-organism causing the infection.

Gram stain

Technicians examine an aspirate of the body fluid under a microscope to identify the micro-organisms directly.

Culture

Technicians apply the aspirate to a culture medium, where colonies of the micro-organism grow over several days. A culture is preferable when a gram stain does not yield a positive identification.
- Nurses should obtain specimens for culture prior to treatment with antimicrobials. ○EBP
- Nurses must collect fluid for culture carefully to prevent contamination.

SENSITIVITY OF A MICRO-ORGANISM TO AN ANTIMICROBIAL

For organisms commonly resistant, technicians test the sensitivity of the organism to various antimicrobials.
- **The disk diffusion test** (Kirby-Bauer test): The infecting organism is placed on several disks then impregnated with different antimicrobiotics. The size of the bacteria-free zone on the disk determines the degree of medication sensitivity.
- **Serial dilution** is a quantitative method using several test tubes with varying concentrations of the antimicrobial to determine the amount necessary to treat a specific infection.
  - **Minimum inhibitory concentration (MIC):** The lowest concentration of antibiotic that inhibits bacterial growth completely but does not kill the bacteria.
  - **Minimum bactericidal concentration:** The lowest concentration of the antibiotic that kills 99.9% of the bacteria.
  - Providers should adjust the antibiotic dosage to produce the concentration equal to or greater than the MIC of the same antibiotic.
- **Gradient diffusion** uses a disk and strips with varying concentrations of the same antibiotic. No further growth of bacteria identifies the essential antibiotic concentration.

HOST FACTORS

Immune system

- In people who have an intact immune system, an antimicrobial works with host defense systems to suppress micro-organisms. Providers prescribe either bactericidal or bacteriostatic antibiotics.
- People with immune-system compromise need strong bactericidal antibiotics, not bacteriostatic medication.

Site of infection

Some sites are difficult for antimicrobials to reach.
- Infections in cerebrospinal fluid, where the antimicrobials have to cross the blood-brain barrier (meningitis)
- Bacterial infiltration within the heart (endocarditis)
  - Infectious micro-organisms vegetate on the thrombus that develops on the injured endocardium.
  - New thrombus formation covers and conceals the micro-organisms, making it difficult for defense mechanisms and antibiotics to kill them.
- Purulent abscesses anywhere within the body due to poor blood supply
- Surgical removal of purulent drainage increases the effect of antimicrobials

Phagocytes that attack foreign objects (pacemaker, joint prosthesis, vascular grafts, heart valves, surgical mesh) become less able to destroy micro-organisms that colonize around the foreign object

Age

- Infants are at increased risk for antimicrobial toxicity due to undeveloped kidney and liver function, causing slow excretion of the medication.
- Older adult clients easily develop toxicity because of the reduction in medication metabolism and excretion. ©

Pregnancy

- Antimicrobials can harm a developing fetus by crossing over to the placenta. Qs
  - **Sulfonamides** can produce kernicterus, a severe neurologic disorder, in newborns.
  - **Gentamicin** causes hearing loss in infants.
  - **Tetracyclines** cause discoloration of developing teeth. Toxicity to these antibiotics is more likely during pregnancy.
- Lactation is usually a contraindication for antimicrobials because of possible danger to breastfeeding infants.

Presence of a previous allergic reaction

- Especially with penicillin
- Clients should not receive penicillin after an allergic reaction, narrowing the antibiotic choices for those clients.

41.1 Case study

Scenario introduction
Joe is a nurse in caring for Joline, who is a recent admission from her provider's office.

Scene 1
Joe: Hello Joline. My name is Joe, and I will be your nurse on the medical unit. I understand you have an area on the heel of your foot that your doctor is concerned about.

Joline: Yes, the nurse in the office told me it might be infected.

Joe: Do you have diabetes?

Joline: Yes, I have had diabetes for over 20 years.

Scene 2
Joe: Would it be okay if I inspect the area?

Joline: Certainly.

Joe: There is a great deal of drainage, and the area does have indications of infection.

Joline: Will I have to have antibiotics?

Joe: I will contact the provider who will be caring for you and I will let you know what they recommend for you.

Scenario conclusion
Joe contacts the provider and reports his findings.

Case Study Exercises

1. Joe is developing the plan of care for Joline. Which of the following actions is the nurse's priority?

   A. Administer antibiotic medication.

   B. Obtain a wound specimen for culture.

   C. Monitor the client for a superinfection.

   D. Teach the client about wound care.

2. Joe is reviewing the principal factors necessary for selecting an antibiotic. Which of the following should Joe recognize as necessary for antibiotic selection for Joline? (Select all that apply.)

   A. Identity of the causative agent

   B. Level of mobility

   C. Sensitivity of the infecting organism to an antimicrobial

   D. Allergies

   E. Location of infection

Combination therapy

Combining more than one antimicrobial can cause additive, potentiating, or antagonistic effects.
- To treat severe infections
- To treat infections from more than one micro-organism
- Prevents bacterial resistance from causing an infection (tuberculosis)
- Decreases the risk of toxicity by reducing the dosage of each medication
- Produces more effective treatment than using only one antimicrobial medication

Combining antimicrobials can cause adverse effects.

- Increased resistance to antimicrobials
- Increased cost of therapy **SDoH**
- More adverse or toxic reactions
- Antagonistic effects between a combination of two or more antimicrobials that results in decreased effectiveness.
- Increased risk for a superinfection

PROPHYLAXIS

- Indications for prophylactic use include prevention of the following.
  - Infections for clients undergoing gastrointestinal, cardiac, peripheral vascular, orthopedic, or gynecologic surgery
  - Sexually transmitted infections following sexual exposure
- Use antimicrobials for individuals who have the following.
  - Prosthetic heart valves prior to dental or other procedures because of the danger of bacterial endocarditis
  - Recurring urinary tract infections

PREVENTIVE MEASURES

- Perform hand hygiene before and after each client contact to prevent the spread of infection.
- Recognize invasive procedures that increase the risk of infection (indwelling urinary catheter, IV catheter, cardiac catheterization).
- Encourage prevention by having clients maintain an up-to-date immunization status. **SDoH**
- Instruct clients to take the full course of antimicrobials the provider prescribes to prevent medication resistance and recurrence of infection.
- Use infection-control procedures to prevent transmission of resistant micro-organisms. Practice infection-control principles (aseptic technique, standard and transmission-based precautions, and careful assignment of rooms within facilities).
- Evaluate the effectiveness of treatment.
  - Check post-treatment cultures to confirm that they are negative for micro-organisms.
  - Monitor clients for clinical improvement (clear breath sounds and resolution of fever).

Active Learning Scenario

A staff educator is providing information to a group of nurses about ways to prevent the spread of micro-organisms. What information should the educator include? Use the ATI Active Learning Template: Basic Concept to complete this item.

RELATED CONTENT: Determine one related concept.

UNDERLYING PRINCIPLES: Describe one related to the concept.

NURSING INTERVENTIONS: Identify five related to the concept.

Application Exercises

1. A nurse Is reviewing the medical record of a client who has manifestations of a urinary tract infection. The nurse should expect the provider to prescribe which of the following diagnostic tests to determine which microorganism is causing the infection?

   A. Blood WBC

   B. Blood creatinine

   C. Urine culture

   D. Urine specific gravity

2. A nurse is caring for a group of clients who are receiving antimicrobial therapy. The nurse should identify that which of the following clients is at risk for medication toxicity?

   A. A client who has a sinus infection

   B. An older adult client who has prostatitis

   C. A client who is postpartum and has mastitis

   D. A middle adult client who has a urinary tract infection

3. A nurse is teaching a group of nurses about antimicrobial therapy. The nurse should instruct that effective penetration of antibiotics can be impeded by which of the following conditions? (Select all that apply.)

   A. Meningitis

   B. An infected abscess

   C. Endocarditis

   D. Pneumonia

   E. Pyelonephritis

4. A nurse is caring for a group of clients. Which of the following clients should the nurse expect to receive prophylactic antimicrobial therapy? (Select all that apply.)

   A. Administer prophylactic antimicrobial therapy to clients who report exposure to a sexually transmitted infection.

   B. Administer prophylactic antimicrobial therapy to clients who are having orthopedic surgery.

   C. Instruct clients who have a prosthetic heart valve about the need for prophylactic antimicrobial therapy before dental work.

   D. Consult the provider for prophylactic antimicrobial therapy for clients who have recurrent urinary tract infections.

   E. Instruct clients to request prophylactic antimicrobial therapy immediately when they have an upper respiratory infection.

Application Exercises Key

1. C. **CORRECT:** When analyzing cues, the nurse should expect a provider prescription for a urine culture to identify the causative micro-organism and the sensitivity.

Ⓝ *NCLEX® Connection: Pharmacological and Parenteral Therapies, Medication Administration*

2. B. **CORRECT:** The nurse should analyze the findings and determine that an older adult client who has prostatitis and is receiving antibiotics is at risk for toxicity due to the age-related reduction in medication metabolism and excretion.

Ⓝ *NCLEX® Connection: Pharmacological and Parenteral Therapies, Adverse Effects/Contraindications/Interactions*

3. A. **CORRECT:** A nurse who is taking actions and teaching other nurses about antimicrobial therapy, should include that effective penetration of antibiotics, can be impeded in clients who have meningitis due to the need of the medication to cross the blood brain barrier which can block antibiotics from reaching the infective micro-organisms.
   B. **CORRECT:** The nurse should also note that purulent drainage and poor vascularity can impede penetration of an antibiotic to an infected abscess.
   C. **CORRECT:** Clients who have endocarditis might develop a bacterial vegetation which can impede penetration of an antibiotic.

Ⓝ *NCLEX® Connection: Pharmacological and Parenteral Therapies, Medication Administration*

4. A, B, C, D. **CORRECT:** The nurse should analyze the cues from the clients' history and expect to administer prophylactic antimicrobial therapy to clients who suspect exposure to a sexually transmitted infection, as well as clients who are having orthopedic surgery to prevent an infection.

Ⓝ *NCLEX® Connection: Pharmacological and Parenteral Therapies, Medication Administration*

Case Study Exercises Key

1. B. **CORRECT:** When analyzing cues and generating solutions, the nurse should plan to obtain a wound specimen for culture. When using the urgent vs. nonurgent approach to care, the nurse's priority action is to obtain a culture of the wound before initiating antibiotic therapy.

Ⓝ *NCLEX® Connection: Pharmacological and Parenteral Therapies, Expected Actions/Outcomes*

2. A, C, D, E. **CORRECT:** When analyzing cues regarding the principal factors for antibiotic therapy selection, the nurse should identify that identifying the causative agent, sensitivity of the infecting organism to an antimicrobial, location of the infections and allergies are all necessary factors to consider when determining correct antibiotic therapy.

Ⓝ *NCLEX® Connection: Pharmacological and Parenteral Therapies, Medication Administration*

Active Learning Scenario Key

Using the ATI Active Learning Template: Basic Concept

RELATED CONTENT: Preventive nursing measures

UNDERLYING PRINCIPLES: Controlling the spread of infection to staff and clients in a health care setting

NURSING INTERVENTIONS
- Perform hand hygiene before and after each client contact to prevent the spread of infection.
- Recognize invasive procedures that increase the risk of infection (indwelling urinary catheter, IV catheter, cardiac catheterization).
- Encourage prevention by having clients maintain an up-to-date immunization status.
- Instruct clients to take the full course of antimicrobials the provider prescribes to prevent medication resistance and recurrence of infection.
- Use infection-control procedures to prevent transmission of resistant micro-organisms.
- Evaluate the effectiveness of treatment.

Ⓝ *NCLEX® Connection: Pharmacological and Parenteral Therapies, Medication Administration*

CHAPTER 42

Antibiotics Affecting the Bacterial Cell Wall

Antibiotics that affect the cell wall are bactericidal. This group of antibiotics includes penicillins, cephalosporins, carbapenems, and monobactams.

Penicillins

SELECT PROTOTYPE MEDICATION: Penicillin G potassium, a narrow-spectrum medication for IM or IV use

OTHER MEDICATIONS
- **Narrow-spectrum**
  - Penicillin G benzathine for IM use
  - Penicillin V for PO use
- **Broad-spectrum**
  - Amoxicillin for PO use
  - Amoxicillin-clavulanate for PO use
  - Ampicillin for PO or IV use
- **Antistaphylococcal:** Nafcillin for IM or IV use (nafcillin, oxacillin)
- **Antipseudomonal (extended spectrum)**
  - Piperacillin tazobactam for IV use

PURPOSE

EXPECTED PHARMACOLOGICAL ACTION
Penicillins destroy bacteria by weakening the bacterial cell wall. Considered a beta-lactam antibiotic.

THERAPEUTIC USES
- Penicillins treat infections due to gram-positive cocci (*Streptococcus pneumoniae* [pneumonia and meningitis], *Streptococcus viridans* [infectious endocarditis], and *Streptococcus pyogenes* [pharyngitis]).
- Penicillins treat meningitis due to gram-negative cocci (*Neisseria meningitides).*
- Penicillins kill spirochetes (*Treponema pallidum)* which causes syphilis.
- Extended-spectrum penicillins (piperacillin, ticarcillin) are effective against organisms (*Pseudomonas aeruginosa*, *Enterobacter* species, *Proteus*, *Bacteroides fragilis*, and *Klebsiella).* Ticarcillin by itself is no longer available in the U.S., but ticarcillin in combination with clavulanic acid is available.
- Penicillins provide prophylaxis against bacterial endocarditis in at-risk clients prior to dental and other procedures.

COMPLICATIONS

Allergies, anaphylaxis

NURSING ACTIONS
- Interview clients for prior allergy.
- Observe for allergic reactions for 30 min following parenteral administration of penicillin. Immediate reactions occur between 2 to 30 min after administration; accelerated reactions occur within 1 to 72 hr; and delayed reactions occur within days to weeks.
- Ensure epinephrine and respiratory support equipment is easily accessible.

CLIENT EDUCATION: Wear an allergy identification bracelet. Because of cross sensitivity, being allergic to one penicillin should be considered allergic to all other penicillins.

Renal impairment

NURSING ACTIONS
- Monitor kidney function.
- Monitor I&O.

Hyperkalemia, dysrhythmias, hypernatremia

- **Hyperkalemia, dysrhythmias:** High doses of penicillin G potassium
- **Hypernatremia**: High doses of penicillin G sodium
- NURSING ACTIONS: Monitor cardiac status and electrolyte levels.

CONTRAINDICATIONS/PRECAUTIONS

Warnings
  - Pregnancy: Although safety not established, it has been used safely.
  - Lactation: Safety not established.
- A history of severe allergic reactions to penicillin, cephalosporins, or imipenem is a contraindication for penicillins. ⓠs
- Use cautiously for clients who have or are at risk for kidney dysfunction (clients who are acutely ill, older adults, or young children). ⓒ
- Clients who are allergic to one penicillin are cross-allergic to other penicillins and are at risk for cross-sensitivity to cephalosporins.

INTERACTIONS

Penicillin in the same IV solution as aminoglycosides inactivates the aminoglycoside.
NURSING ACTIONS: Do not mix penicillin and aminoglycosides in the same IV solution because penicillin inactivates the aminoglycoside.

Probenecid delays the excretion of penicillin.

NURSING ADMINISTRATION

- Instruct clients to report any findings of an allergic response (dyspnea, a skin rash, itching, and hives).
- Give IM injections cautiously to avoid injecting into a nerve or an artery. Can cause sensory and motor dysfunction, or neurotoxicity.

CLIENT EDUCATION

- Penicillin V, amoxicillin, and amoxicillin–clavulanate can be taken with meals. Take all others with 8 oz of water 1 hr before or 2 hr after meals. ⓆEBP
- Complete the entire course of therapy, even if manifestations resolve.
- Use an additional contraceptive method when taking penicillins, as penicillins can cause a decrease in effectiveness.

Cephalosporins

SELECT PROTOTYPE MEDICATION: Cephalexin, first generation

OTHER MEDICATIONS

- **First generation:** Cefazolin for IM or IV use
- **Second generation:** Cefaclor for PO use, cefotetan for IM or IV use
- **Third generation:** Ceftriaxone, cefotaxime for IM or IV use
- **Fourth generation:** Cefepime for IM or IV use
- **Fifth generation:** Ceftaroline for IV use- only cephalosporin that is effective against MRSA

PURPOSE

EXPECTED PHARMACOLOGICAL ACTION

- Cephalosporins are beta-lactam antibiotics, similar to penicillins, that destroy bacterial cell walls causing destruction of micro-organisms.
- Most cephalosporins are administered IV or IM because of decreased absorption from the GI tract.
- Cephalosporins comprise five generations. Each subsequent generation is
  ○ More likely to reach cerebrospinal fluid.
  ○ Less susceptible to destruction by beta-lactamase.
  ○ More effective against gram-negative organisms and anaerobes.

THERAPEUTIC USES
Cephalosporins are broad-spectrum bactericidal medications with a high therapeutic index that treat a wide variety of infections.

COMPLICATIONS

Allergy, hypersensitivity, anaphylaxis, possible cross-sensitivity to penicillin

NURSING ACTIONS

- If indications of allergy appear (urticaria, rash, hypotension, dyspnea), stop the cephalosporin immediately, and notify the provider.
- Question clients carefully about a history of allergy to a penicillin or another cephalosporin, and notify the provider if present.
- Acceptable for use with clients who have mild penicillin allergies.

Bleeding tendencies from cefotetan and ceftriaxone

NURSING ACTIONS

- Avoid use for clients who have bleeding disorders and for clients taking anticoagulants.
- Observe clients for bleeding.
- Monitor prothrombin and bleeding times. Delays in clotting can require discontinuation of the medication.
- Administer parenteral vitamin K.

Thrombophlebitis with IV infusion

NURSING ACTIONS

- Observe injection site for findings of phlebitis
- Rotate injection sites.
- Administer as a dilute intermittent infusion or slowly over 3 to 5 min and in a dilute solution for bolus dosing.

Renal insufficiency

NURSING ACTIONS: Give a lower dosage of most cephalosporins to prevent accumulation to toxic levels. Cephalosporins are mainly eliminated by the kidneys. One cephalosporin (ceftriaxone) is eliminated largely by the liver and dosage reduction is unnecessary for clients with renal impairment.

Pain with IM injection

NURSING ACTIONS: Administer IM injections deep into a large muscle mass (into the ventrogluteal site). Educate client about the possibility of pain at the injection site prior to administration.

Antibiotic-associated pseudomembranous colitis

NURSING ACTIONS

- Observe for diarrhea, and notify the provider if present.
- Stop the medication.
- Risk for developing clostridium difficile (C. difficile) by consuming broad-spectrum antibiotics.

CONTRAINDICATIONS/PRECAUTIONS

Warnings
- Pregnancy: Has been used safely.
- Lactation: Has been used safely.

NURSING ACTIONS
- Do not give cephalosporins to clients who have a history of severe allergic reactions to penicillins or cephalosporins. Qs
- Use cautiously with clients who have renal impairment or bleeding tendencies.

INTERACTIONS

Disulfiram reaction (intolerance to alcohol) occurs with simultaneous use of alcohol and either cefotetan or cefazolin.
CLIENT EDUCATION: Do not consume alcohol while taking these cephalosporins.

Probenecid delays renal excretion.
NURSING ACTIONS: Monitor I&O.

Calcium and ceftriaxone interaction: Do not administer together. Can cause the solutions to precipitate and lead to serious complications.

NURSING ADMINISTRATION

CLIENT EDUCATION
- Complete the entire course of therapy, even if manifestations resolve. QEBP
- Take oral cephalosporins with food.
- Store oral cephalosporin suspensions in a refrigerator.

Carbapenems

SELECT PROTOTYPE MEDICATION: Imipenem-cilastatin for IM or IV use

OTHER MEDICATIONS: Meropenem for IV use

PURPOSE

EXPECTED PHARMACOLOGICAL ACTION
Carbapenems are beta-lactam antibiotics that destroy bacterial cell walls, causing destruction of micro-organisms. They have very broad antimicrobial spectra.

THERAPEUTIC USES
- Their broad antimicrobial spectrum is effective for serious infections (pneumonia, peritonitis, and urinary tract infections) due to gram-positive cocci, gram-negative cocci, and anaerobic bacteria.
- Resistance develops from using imipenem alone to treat *Pseudomonas aeruginosa* infections. This pathogen requires a combination of antipseudomonal medications.
- To delay emergence of resistance, Carbapenems should be reserved for clients who cannot be treated with a more narrow-spectrum antibiotic.

COMPLICATIONS

Allergy, hypersensitivity, possible cross-sensitivity to penicillin or cephalosporins

NURSING ACTIONS
- Monitor for indications of allergic reactions (dyspnea, rashes, and pruritus).
- Question clients carefully about their history of allergy to a penicillin or other cephalosporin, and notify the provider if present.

Gastrointestinal upset (nausea, vomiting, diarrhea)

NURSING ACTIONS
- Observe for manifestations, and notify the provider if they occur.
- Monitor I&O.

Suprainfection

NURSING ACTIONS: Monitor for indications of colitis (diarrhea), oral thrush, black furry overgrowth on the tongue, and vaginal yeast infection.

CONTRAINDICATIONS/PRECAUTIONS

Warnings
- Pregnancy: Imipenem-cilastatin safety for use during pregnancy has not been established.
- Lactation: Imipenem-cilastatin safety for use during lactation has not been established.
- Use cautiously in clients who have renal impairment.

INTERACTIONS

Imipenem-cilastatin can reduce blood levels of valproic acid. Breakthrough seizures are possible.
NURSING ACTIONS: Avoid using together. If concurrent use is unavoidable, monitor for increased seizure activity and consider supplemental anti-seizure therapy.

NURSING ADMINISTRATION

CLIENT EDUCATION: Complete the entire course of therapy, even if manifestations resolve.

Other inhibitors of cell wall synthesis

SELECT PROTOTYPE MEDICATIONS
- Vancomycin for PO, IV, or rectal use. Commonly used in hospitals. Poor absorption through the gastrointestinal tract.
- Aztreonam, a monobactam, for IM or IV use
  - Used to treat C. difficile infections
  - Diarrhea common during use
- Fosfomycin for PO use
  - Given as a single dose for UTIs
  - Can cause diarrhea, headaches, vaginitis, drowsiness, and abdominal pain

- Televancin, for IV use
  - Used to treat gram positive bacteria
  - Can cause kidney toxicity and diarrhea (associated with clostridium difficile)
- Televancin, for IV use
  - Used to treat gram positive bacteria
  - Can cause kidney toxicity and diarrhea (associated with clostridium difficile)

PURPOSE

EXPECTED PHARMACOLOGICAL ACTION
This group of antibiotics destroys bacterial cell walls, causing destruction of micro-organisms.

THERAPEUTIC USES
- Treat serious infections due to methicillin-resistant *Staphylococcus aureus*, *Staphylococcus epidermidis*, and streptococcal infections.
- Treat antibiotic-associated pseudomembranous colitis due to *Clostridium difficile*.

COMPLICATIONS

Ototoxicity (rare and reversible)

NURSING ACTIONS
- Assess for indications of hearing loss.
- Monitor vancomycin trough levels so dosage adjustments can be made as needed.

CLIENT EDUCATION: Notify the provider if changes in hearing acuity develop.

Infusion reactions

Red man syndrome (related to rapid infusions): rashes, itching, flushing, tachycardia, and hypotension

NURSING ACTIONS: Administer vancomycin slowly over 60 min.

IM and IV injection-site pain, thrombophlebitis

NURSING ACTIONS
- Dilute medication according to pharmacy instructions.
- Rotate injection sites.
- Monitor the infusion site for redness, swelling, and inflammation.

Renal toxicity

NURSING ACTIONS
- Monitor I&O and kidney function tests.
- Monitor vancomycin trough levels.
- Major toxicity is renal failure.

CONTRAINDICATIONS/PRECAUTIONS

- An allergy to vancomycin is a contraindication. Qs
- Use cautiously for older adults and with clients who have renal impairment or hearing loss. C

42.1 Case study

Scenario introduction
Mary is a nurse caring for Ms. Young on the medical unit. Ms. Young has meningitis and Mary has received the prescriptions from Dr. Brown.

Scene 1
Mary: Good morning, Ms. Young, I have the prescriptions from Dr. Brown and one of them is to initiate antibiotic therapy with nafcillin.

Ms. Young: Will I have to have an IV for that?

Mary: No, I will administer this medication intramuscularly.

Scene 2
Mary: Before I administer the medication, I will need to review your medication history and then I will be back to talk with you.

Ms. Young: OK.

Scene 3
Ms. Young: I really hope this new medication will help me feel better.

Mary: The medication Dr. Brown has prescribed is a type of penicillin which is one that is specific for the treatment of meningitis.

Scenario conclusion
Mary talks with Ms. Young and goes to prepare for the medication administration.

Case study exercises

1. Mary is preparing to administer nafcillin IM to Ms. Young, a client who has meningitis. Which of the following actions should the nurse plan to take? (Select all that apply.)

   A. Select a 25-gauge, ½-inch needle for the injection.

   B. Administer the medication deeply into the ventrogluteal muscle.

   C. Ask the client about an allergy to penicillin before administering the medication.

   D. Monitor the client for 30 min following the injection.

   E. Tell the client to expect a temporary rash to develop following the injection.

2. Mary is monitoring Ms. Young for manifestations of a potential allergic reaction to the nafcillin. For which of the following manifestations should Mary observe as an indication of anaphylaxis? (Select all that apply.)

   A. Rash

   B. Fever

   C. Pruritus

   D. Wheezing

   E. Pain at injection site

INTERACTIONS

Increased risk for ototoxicity when taking vancomycin concurrently with another medication that causes ototoxicity (loop diuretics, ethacrynic acid, aminoglycoside antibiotics).

NURSING ACTIONS: Assess for hearing loss.

NURSING ADMINISTRATION

- Monitor vancomycin trough levels routinely after blood levels have reached a steady state.
- For clients who have renal insufficiency, creatinine clearance levels indicate IV dosage adjustments.

NURSING EVALUATION OF MEDICATION EFFECTIVENESS

Indications of effectiveness include the following.
- Reduction of manifestations (fever, pain, inflammation, and adventitious breath sounds).
- Resolution of infection

Case Study Exercises Key

1. B. **CORRECT:** Mary should administer nafcillin IM into a deep muscle mass (the ventrogluteal site) and plan to monitor Ms. Young for 30 min after the injection for an allergic reaction.
    C. **CORRECT:** Mary should plan to generate solutions for the administration of nafcillin to Ms. Young. Mary should begin by asking Ms. Young about an allergy to penicillin or other antibiotics before administering nafcillin. An allergy to another penicillin or to a cephalosporin is a contraindication for administering nafcillin.
    D. **CORRECT:** Mary should administer nafcillin IM into a deep muscle mass (the ventrogluteal site) and plan to monitor Ms. Young for 30 min after the injection for an allergic reaction.
    Ⓝ *NCLEX® Connection: Pharmacological and Parenteral Therapies, Medication Administration*

2. A, C, D. **CORRECT:** Mary should generate solutions and plan to monitor Ms. Young for manifestations of a potential anaphylactic reaction. Manifestations of anaphylaxis can include rash, pruritus, laryngeal edema, wheezing, and abdominal pain. If these manifestations occur, Mary should discontinue the nafcillin and contact Dr. Brown immediately.
    Ⓝ *NCLEX® Connection: Pharmacological and Parenteral Therapies, Medication Administration*

Application Exercises

1. A nurse is assessing a client who has a severe infection and has been receiving cefotaxime for the past week. Which of the following findings indicates a potentially serious adverse reaction to this medication that the nurse should report to the provider?

   A. Diaphoresis

   B. Epistaxis

   C. Diarrhea

   D. Alopecia

2. A nurse is obtaining a medication history from a client who is to receive imipenem-cilastatin IV to treat an infection. Which of the following medications the client also receives increases the risk for a medication interaction?

   A. Regular insulin

   B. Furosemide

   C. Valproic acid

   D. Ferrous sulfate

Active Learning Scenario

A nurse is administering vancomycin IV to a client who has a serious wound infection. What should the nurse teach the client about this medication? Use the ATI Active Learning Template: Medication to complete this item.

THERAPEUTIC USES: Identify for vancomycin for this client.

COMPLICATIONS: Identify two adverse effects the client should watch for.

NURSING INTERVENTIONS: Describe two nursing actions for clients receiving vancomycin.

Application Exercises Key

1. C. **CORRECT:** The nurse should analyze the cues from the assessment findings and determine that severe diarrhea can indicate the client has developed antibiotic-associated pseudomembranous colitis or *C. difficile*, which can be a life-threatening adverse reaction to cefotaxime. This finding requires reporting to the provider.

   Ⓝ *NCLEX® Connection: Pharmacological and Parenteral Therapies, Adverse Effects/Contraindications/Interactions*

2. C. **CORRECT:** The nurse should analyze the cues from the client's medical history and determine that Imipenem-cilastatin decreases the blood levels of valproic acid, an antiseizure medication, putting the client at risk for increased seizure activity. If the client must take these two medications concurrently, monitor for seizures.

   Ⓝ *NCLEX® Connection: Pharmacological and Parenteral Therapies, Adverse Effects/Contraindications/Interactions*

Active Learning Scenario Key

Using the ATI Active Learning Template: Medication

THERAPEUTIC USES: Vancomycin is an antibiotic that kills bacteria by disrupting their cell wall. The IV form treats serious infections due to methicillin-resistant *Staphylococcus aureus*, *Staphylococcus epidermidis*, and streptococci.

COMPLICATIONS
- Infusion reactions (red man syndrome: rashes, flushing, tachycardia, and hypotension)
- Ototoxicity (rare and reversible)
- Renal toxicity
- Thrombophlebitis at the IV site
- IM and IV injection-site pain

NURSING INTERVENTIONS
- Infuse vancomycin over at least 60 min/dose to prevent an infusion reaction.
- Monitor the IV site for redness, pain, or other manifestations of thrombophlebitis.
- Monitor I&O, and notify the provider for oliguria or other findings of acute renal injury.
- Monitor for hearing loss.
- Ask the client about allergy to antibiotics before administering the medication. Watch for allergic manifestations during and after the infusion.

Ⓝ *NCLEX® Connection: Pharmacological and Parenteral Therapies, Medication Administration*

CHAPTER 43

Antibiotics Affecting Protein Synthesis

Antibiotics affecting protein synthesis are bacteriostatic (tetracyclines and macrolides) or bactericidal (aminoglycosides) and are used to treat various respiratory, gastrointestinal (GI), urinary, and reproductive tract infections. These medications work by suppressing the replication and growth of the bacteria.

Tetracyclines

SELECT PROTOTYPE MEDICATION: Tetracycline

OTHER MEDICATIONS
- Doxycycline
- Minocycline
- Demeclocycline

PURPOSE

EXPECTED PHARMACOLOGICAL ACTION
Tetracyclines are broad-spectrum antibiotics that inhibit micro-organism growth by preventing protein synthesis (bacteriostatic).

THERAPEUTIC USES
Treats the following.
- Acne vulgaris (topically and orally)
- Periodontal disease (oral or topical)
- Rickettsia infections (typhus fever, Rocky Mountain spotted fever)
- STIs: *Chlamydia trachomatis*
- Brucellosis
- Pneumonia due to *Mycoplasma pneumonia*
- Lyme disease
- Anthrax
- GI infections due to *Helicobacter pylori* (peptic ulcer disease)
- UTIs

COMPLICATIONS

GI discomfort

Cramping, nausea, vomiting, diarrhea, and esophageal ulceration

NURSING ACTIONS
- Monitor for nausea, vomiting, and diarrhea.
- Monitor I&O.
- Suggest taking doxycycline and minocycline with meals, although food can reduce absorption.
- Avoid taking at bedtime to reduce the risk of esophageal ulceration.

Yellow or brown tooth discoloration, hypoplasia of tooth enamel

NURSING ACTIONS: Avoid administration to children younger than 8 years of age and to clients who are pregnant.

Hepatotoxicity (lethargy, jaundice)

NURSING ACTIONS: Avoid administration of high daily doses IV.

Photosensitivity

Increased skin sensitivity with UV light or sunlight can cause intense sunburn

CLIENT EDUCATION: Wear protective clothing and use sunscreen with an SPF of 30 or higher while outdoors in sunlight.

Suprainfection

Excessive growth of microbes that are potentially medication resistant can lead to pseudomembranous colitis (diarrhea), yeast infections of the mouth, pharynx, vagina, bowels

CLIENT EDUCATION: Notify the provider of diarrhea or manifestations of a yeast infection.

CONTRAINDICATIONS/PRECAUTIONS

Warnings
- Pregnancy:
  - If used during the last half of pregnancy, can cause permanent staining of teeth in the infant.
  - If client is pregnant or postpartum and has history of kidney disease, can cause increased risk for hepatoxicity
- Lactation: Contraindicated.
- Reproductive
  - Tetracyclines decrease the effectiveness of oral contraceptives. Clients should use an alternative or nonhormonal form of contraception.
  - Males (sex assigned at birth) clients who are prescribed minocycline should use a form of contraception while taking this medication.
- Use cautiously with liver and kidney disease. Doxycycline and minocycline are generally safe for clients who have kidney disease, because the liver, not the kidneys, eliminates these two tetracyclines.
- Not recommended for clients who are less than 8 years of age.

INTERACTIONS

Interaction with milk products, calcium and iron supplements, laxatives containing magnesium, and antacids causes formation of nonabsorbable chelates, thus reducing the absorption of tetracyclines.
NURSING ACTIONS: Ensure that any milk products and antacids are separated by at least 2 hours of tetracycline ingestion.
CLIENT EDUCATION: Take tetracyclines on an empty stomach with 8 oz water (1 hr before or 2 hr after meals). Clients may take tetracyclines with food if gastric distress occurs, but this will decrease absorption. Minocycline may be taken with food.

Doxycycline increase the risk of digoxin toxicity.
NURSING ACTIONS: Monitor digoxin level carefully if taking concurrently.

NURSING ADMINISTRATION

If this medication is given to treat an STD, clients should abstain from intercourse until they finish their medication, manifestations have resolved, and partners have been treated.

CLIENT EDUCATION
- Take tetracyclines (except for minocycline) on an empty stomach with 8 oz water. It may be taken with food if gastric distress occurs. Q_{EBP}
- Do not take tetracyclines just before lying down because it increases the risk of esophageal ulceration.
- Tetracyclines should be administered at least 1 hr before or 2 hr after ingestion of chelating agents.
- Complete the entire course of therapy, even though manifestations may resolve sooner.
- Utilize additional contraception.

NURSING EVALUATION OF MEDICATION EFFECTIVENESS

Indications of effectiveness include the following.
- A decrease in the manifestations of infection (fever, pain, inflammation, and adventitious breath sounds).
- Resolution of yeast infections of the mouth, vagina, and bowels
- Resolution of acne vulgaris

Macrolides

SELECT PROTOTYPE MEDICATION: Erythromycin

OTHER MEDICATION:
- Azithromycin
- Clarithromycin

PURPOSE

EXPECTED PHARMACOLOGICAL ACTION
Erythromycin slows the growth of micro-organisms by inhibiting protein synthesis (bacteriostatic), but it is bactericidal at high doses.

THERAPEUTIC USES
Treats the following.
- Infections in clients who have a penicillin allergy (for prophylaxis) against rheumatic fever and bacterial endocarditis
- Legionnaires' disease, *Bordetella pertussis* (whooping cough), and acute diphtheria (also eliminating the carrier state of diphtheria)
- Treats chlamydial infections (urethritis, cervicitis), pneumonia due to *Mycoplasma pneumoniae*, and streptococcal infections

COMPLICATIONS

GI discomfort (nausea, vomiting, epigastric pain)

NURSING ACTIONS
- Administer erythromycin with meals.
- Monitor for and report adverse GI effects.

Prolonged QT intervals

Causing dysrhythmias and possible sudden cardiac death

NURSING ACTIONS: Avoid use in clients who have prolonged QT intervals.

Ototoxicity with high-dose therapy

NURSING ACTIONS: Monitor for and report hearing loss, vertigo, and tinnitus.

CONTRAINDICATIONS/PRECAUTIONS

Warnings
- Pregnancy
  - Azithromycin: Contraindicated
  - Clarithromycin: Contraindicated.
- Lactation
  - Erythromycin: Use with caution
  - Azithromycin: Safety has not been established.
  - Clarithromycin: Contraindicated.
- Liver disease and QT prolongation are contraindications. Q_S

INTERACTIONS

Erythromycin inhibits the metabolism of antihistamines, theophylline, carbamazepine, warfarin, and digoxin, which can lead to toxicity.
NURSING ACTIONS: To minimize toxicity, avoid using erythromycin with medications that affect hepatic medication-metabolizing enzymes. If unavoidable, monitor liver function tests carefully for indications of toxicity.

Verapamil, diltiazem, HIV protease inhibitors, antifungal medications, and nefazodone inhibit the metabolism of erythromycin, which can lead to toxicity and cause tachydysrhythmias and possible cardiac arrest.
NURSING ACTIONS: Avoid concurrent use.

NURSING ADMINISTRATION

- If this medication is given to treat an STD, clients should abstain from intercourse until they finish their medication, manifestations have resolved, and partners have been treated.
- Hormonal contraceptive effectiveness decreases with various antibiotics and therefore it is recommended clients use a back-up method (a condom).
- Except for azithromycin, administer oral preparations on an empty stomach (1 hr before meals or 2 hr after) with 8 oz of water, unless GI upset occurs. Q EBP
- Administer erythromycin IV only for severe infections or for clients who cannot take oral doses.
- Carefully monitor the PT or INR of clients who take warfarin concurrently with erythromycin.
- Monitor liver function tests for therapy lasting longer than 2 weeks.

CLIENT EDUCATION: Complete the entire course of antimicrobial therapy, even if manifestations resolve sooner.

NURSING EVALUATION OF MEDICATION EFFECTIVENESS

Indications of effectiveness include the following.
- A decrease in the manifestations of infection (fever, sore throat, cough, inflammation, and adventitious breath sounds).
- Resolution of urinary tract manifestations
- Resolution of bacterial endocarditis (negative blood cultures, WBC counts within the expected reference range)

Aminoglycosides

SELECT PROTOTYPE MEDICATION: Gentamicin

OTHER MEDICATIONS
- Tobramycin
- Neomycin
- Streptomycin
- Paromomycin

PURPOSE

EXPECTED PHARMACOLOGICAL ACTION
Aminoglycosides are bactericidal antibiotics that destroy micro-organisms by disrupting protein synthesis.

THERAPEUTIC USES
- Treats aerobic gram-negative bacilli (*Escherichia coli*, *Klebsiella pneumoniae*, *Proteus mirabilis*, and *Pseudomonas aeruginosa*).
- Paromomycin (an oral aminoglycoside) treats intestinal amebiasis and tapeworm infections.
- Oral neomycin suppresses the normal flora of the GI tract preoperatively in preparation for colorectal surgery; topically, it treats infections of the eye, ear, and skin.
- Streptomycin can treat tuberculosis in combination with other medications, but newer and safer ones (ethambutol, rifampin, isoniazid) are preferable. Streptomycin also treats severe, uncommon infections (tularemia, plague, and brucellosis).

COMPLICATIONS

Ototoxicity

Cochlear damage (hearing loss), vestibular damage (loss of balance)

NURSING ACTIONS
- Monitor for tinnitus, headache, hearing loss, nausea, dizziness, and vertigo.
- Do baseline audiometric studies (hearing tests).
- Stop aminoglycoside if manifestations occur.

CLIENT EDUCATION: Notify the provider if tinnitus, hearing loss, or headaches occur.

Nephrotoxicity

Due to high total cumulative doses resulting in acute tubular necrosis (proteinuria, casts in the urine, dilute urine, elevated BUN, elevated creatinine)

NURSING ACTIONS
- Monitor I&O, BUN, and creatinine.
- Report hematuria and cloudy urine.

Intense neuromuscular blockade

Resulting in respiratory depression, muscle weakness

NURSING ACTIONS: Closely monitor use in clients who have myasthenia gravis, clients taking skeletal muscle relaxants, and clients receiving general anesthetics.

Hypersensitivity

Rash, pruritus, paresthesia of hands and feet, urticaria

NURSING ACTIONS: Monitor for allergic effects.

STREPTOMYCIN

Neurologic disorder

Peripheral neuritis, optic nerve dysfunction, tingling/numbness of the hands and feet

CLIENT EDUCATION: Report any manifestations to the provider promptly.

CONTRAINDICATIONS/PRECAUTIONS

Warnings
- Pregnancy
  - Tobramycin and streptomycin: Can cause congenital hearing loss.
  - Aminoglycosides: Safety has not been established. May cause fetal harm.
- Lactation: Aminoglycosides safety has not been established.
- Use cautiously with clients who have kidney impairment, hearing loss, and myasthenia gravis. Qs
- Use cautiously for clients taking ethacrynic acid (increases the risk for ototoxicity), amphotericin B, cephalosporins, vancomycin (increases the risk for nephrotoxicity), and neuromuscular blocking agents (tubocurarine).
- Clients who have kidney impairment should receive lower doses of aminoglycosides.
- Antibacterial and antifungal medications can kill the bacteria and yeasts in probiotic products; therefore, to help preserve probiotic activity, these preparations should be administered at least 2 hours after dosing with antibacterial or antifungal drugs.

INTERACTIONS

Penicillin inactivates aminoglycosides when in the same IV solution.
NURSING ACTIONS: Do not mix aminoglycosides and penicillins in the same IV solution.

Concurrent administration with other ototoxic medications (ethacrynic acid/loop diuretics) increases the risk for ototoxicity.
NURSING ACTIONS: Assess frequently for hearing loss with concurrent medication use.

Concurrent administration with skeletal muscle relaxants increases risk for developing neuromuscular blockade.

NURSING ADMINISTRATION

- Most aminoglycosides (gentamicin and streptomycin (IM only) are parenteral. Neomycin also has oral and topical formulations; tobramycin also has an inhalation formulation.
- Base acquisition of aminoglycoside levels on dosing schedules. QEBP
  - ONCE-A-DAY DOSING: It is only necessary to obtain a blood sample for measuring trough levels.
  - DIVIDED DOSES
    - **Peak:** 30 min after administration of aminoglycoside IM or 30 min after completion of an IV infusion
    - **Trough:** Right before the next dose

CLIENT EDUCATION: Complete the entire course of antimicrobial therapy, even if manifestations resolve sooner

NURSING EVALUATION OF MEDICATION EFFECTIVENESS

Indications of effectiveness include the following.
- A decrease in the manifestations of infection (fever, inflammation, and adventitious breath sounds)
- Resolution of urinary tract manifestations

Application Exercises

1. A nurse is providing teaching with a client who has a new prescription for tetracycline to treat a GI infection due to *Helicobacter pylori*. Which of the following client statements indicate understanding?

   A. "I will take this medication with 8 ounces of milk."

   B. "I will report if I start having diarrhea while taking this medication."

   C. "I can stop taking this medication when I feel completely well."

   D. "I can take this medication just before bedtime."

2. A nurse is caring for a client who is undergoing preparation for extensive colorectal surgery. Which of the following oral antibiotics should the nurse expect a prescription to administer specifically to suppress normal flora in the GI tract?

   A. Kanamycin

   B. Gentamicin

   C. Neomycin

   D. Tobramycin

3. A nurse is providing care for a client who has subacute bacterial endocarditis and is receiving several antibiotics, including streptomycin IM. For which of the following manifestations should the nurse monitor as an adverse effect of this medication?

   A. Tinnitus

   B. Urinary retention

   C. Constipation

   D. Complex partial seizures

4. A nurse caring for a client who is starting a course of gentamicin IV for a serious respiratory infection. For which of the following manifestations should the nurse monitor as an adverse effect of this medication? (Select all that apply.)

   A. Pruritus

   B. Hematuria

   C. Cardiac arrhythmia

   D. Difficulty swallowing

   E. Vertigo

5. A nurse is monitoring the administration of gentamicin by IV infusion at 0900. The medication will take 1 hr to infuse. When should the nurse recommend obtaining a blood sample for a peak blood level of gentamicin?

   A. 1000

   B. 1030

   C. 1100

   D. 1130

Active Learning Scenario

A nurse is teaching a client who has pneumonia and received a new prescription for oral erythromycin. What should the nurse teach the client about this medication? Use the ATI Active Learning Template: Medication to complete this item.

THERAPEUTIC USES: Describe the therapeutic use for erythromycin in this client.

COMPLICATIONS: Identify two adverse effects the client should monitor for.

NURSING INTERVENTIONS: Describe two diagnostic tests to monitor for clients taking erythromycin.

CLIENT EDUCATION: Include two teaching points for clients taking erythromycin.

Active Learning Scenario Key

Using the ATI Active Learning Template: Medication

THERAPEUTIC USES: Erythromycin inhibits protein synthesis in the cells of susceptible micro-organisms, usually gram-positive bacteria. Erythromycin can be either bacteriostatic or bactericidal, depending on the organism and on the medication's dosage. It also treats infections for clients who are allergic to penicillin.

COMPLICATIONS

- The most common adverse effects of erythromycin are GI manifestations, including abdominal pain, nausea, vomiting, and diarrhea.
- Hepatotoxicity with abdominal pain, anorexia, fatigue, and possibly jaundice can occur after 1 to 2 weeks of erythromycin therapy.
- Erythromycin can cause a prolonged QT interval on ECG, which can lead to potentially fatal tachydysrhythmias.
- Ototoxicity can occur with high doses, especially after prolonged periods.

NURSING INTERVENTIONS

- Monitor liver function tests for clients who take erythromycin over a period of several weeks.
- If the client is concurrently taking warfarin or digoxin with erythromycin, carefully monitor PT and INR or digoxin levels.
- Monitor WBC counts for effectiveness of erythromycin treatment.

CLIENT EDUCATION

- Take erythromycin on an empty stomach, 1 hr before or 2 hr after meals with 8 oz of water.
- Observe for adverse effects, and call the provider for severe GI distress, manifestations of liver toxicity, and ototoxicity.
- Take the entire course of the medication and not to stop when feeling better.

Ⓝ *NCLEX® Connection: Pharmacological and Parenteral Therapies, Medication Administration*

Application Exercises Key

1. A. The client should avoid taking this medication with milk because this can form a nonabsorbable chelate.
    B. **CORRECT:** The client should report and notify their provider of findings of diarrhea while taking tetracycline because this could indicate that client is developing a superinfection which is very serious. The client should take tetracycline on an empty stomach or with food.
    C. The client should take the full prescription of tetracycline and not stop the medication if they begin to feel well.
    D. Taking tetracycline in the morning helps prevent esophageal ulceration, which can occur if the client takes it just before lying down.

    Ⓝ *NCLEX® Connection: Pharmacological and Parenteral Therapies, Medication Administration*

2. C. **CORRECT:** To rid the large intestine of normal flora, the nurse should expect a prescription to administer neomycin which is an aminoglycoside that can be administered orally.
    A, B, D. Kanamycin, gentamicin, and tobramycin are aminoglycosides that does not pass through the GI tract, therefore, is not recommended for administration prophylactically for a client who is undergoing GI surgery.

    Ⓝ *NCLEX® Connection: Pharmacological Therapies, expected actions/outcomes*

3. A. **CORRECT:** Tinnitus/ringing of ears is an adverse effect of streptomycin which could indicate ototoxicity. Other adverse effects include headache, angioedema, muscle weakness, and stomatitis.
    B, C, D. Urinary retention, constipation, and complex partial seizures are not adverse effects of streptomycin.

    Ⓝ *NCLEX® Connection: Pharmacological and Parenteral Therapies, Adverse Effects/Contraindications/Side Effects/Interactions*

4. A. **CORRECT:** The adverse effects of gentamicin include paresthesia, hematuria, and vertigo. Paresthesia of the hands and feet, urticaria, rash, and pruritus are indications of a hypersensitivity reaction.
    B. **CORRECT:** Hematuria could indicate acute kidney toxicity.
    C, D. QT prolongation and difficulty swallowing are not adverse effects of gentamicin. QT prolongation can occur in clients who are taking macrolide antibiotics.
    E. **CORRECT:** Vertigo, ataxia, and hearing loss could indicate ototoxicity.

    Ⓝ *NCLEX® Connection: Pharmacological and Parenteral Therapies, Adverse Effects/Contraindications/Side Effects/Interactions*

5. A. The IV infusion should end at 1000, but that is not the time to collect a blood specimen for the peak blood level.
    B. **CORRECT:** The nurse should plan to obtain a peak blood level within 30 minutes after infusion. The infusion should end at 1000, therefore, 1030 is time recommended to obtain a peak blood level. The trough level should be obtained prior to next scheduled dose of the medication.
    C, D. Collecting the specimen for the peak blood level at 1100 or 1130 would yield an inaccurate peak level.

    Ⓝ *NCLEX® Connection: Pharmacological and Parenteral Therapies, Medication Administration*

UNIT 12   MEDICATIONS FOR INFECTION

CHAPTER 44 *Urinary Tract Infections*

Sulfonamides, trimethoprim, and urinary tract antiseptics are medications that treat urinary tract infections (UTIs). Others include penicillins, aminoglycosides, cephalosporins, fluoroquinolones, and a phosphoric acid derivative. These medications treat active infections and prevent recurrent infections for susceptible individuals. Typical regimens are a single-dose; a short course of 3 days; the traditional course of 7 days; or up to 14 days for severe infections.

Trimethoprim-sulfamethoxazole and nitrofurantoin treat uncomplicated cystitis. Fluoroquinolones treat UTIs resistant to trimethoprim-sulfamethoxazole and nitrofurantoin. Fosfomycin, which requires one dose, is a good alternative for clients who have difficulty with adherence. Qᴘᴄᴄ

Sulfonamides and trimethoprim

SELECT PROTOTYPE MEDICATIONS
- Trimethoprim-sulfamethoxazole
- Sulfadiazine
- Trimethoprim

PURPOSE

EXPECTED PHARMACOLOGICAL ACTION
Sulfonamides and trimethoprim inhibit bacterial growth by preventing the synthesis of a folic acid derivative, tetrahydrofolate. Folic acid is essential for the production of DNA, RNA, and proteins.

THERAPEUTIC USES
Trimethoprim-sulfamethoxazole treats the following.
- UTIs, which are most often due to infection with *Escherichia coli*
- Otitis media, chancroid (unlabeled use), pertussis, shigellosis, and Pneumocystis jirovecii pneumonia

COMPLICATIONS

Hypersensitivity

Including Stevens-Johnson syndrome

NURSING ACTIONS
- Do not administer trimethoprim-sulfamethoxazole to clients who have allergies to the following.
  - Sulfonamides (sulfa)
  - Thiazide diuretics (hydrochlorothiazide)
  - Sulfonylurea-type oral hypoglycemics (glipizide, glyburide)
  - Loop diuretics (furosemide)
- Stop trimethoprim-sulfamethoxazole at the first indication of hypersensitivity (rash).

Blood dyscrasias

Hemolytic anemia, agranulocytosis, leukopenia, thrombocytopenia, aplastic anemia

NURSING ACTIONS
- Obtain blood samples for baseline and periodic CBC counts to detect hematologic disorders.
- Observe for and instruct clients to report bleeding, sore throat, and pallor.

Crystalluria

Crystalline aggregates in the kidneys, ureters, and bladder, causing irritation and obstruction that causes acute kidney injury

NURSING ACTIONS
- Encourage adequate oral fluid intake (at least eight 8 oz glasses per day).
- Monitor urine output (should be at least 1,200 mL/day).

Kernicterus

Jaundice, increased bilirubin levels, neurotoxic for newborns

NURSING ACTIONS: Do not give trimethoprim-sulfamethoxazole to clients who are pregnant (during the first trimester or near term) or breastfeeding, or to infants younger than 2 months (due to the risk of kernicterus).

Hyperkalemia

NURSING ACTIONS: Monitor potassium levels.

CONTRAINDICATIONS/PRECAUTIONS

- **Warnings**
  - Pregnancy: Sulfonamides/trimethoprim is contraindicated due to the risk of kernicterus in infancy.
  - Lactation: Sulfonamides and trimethoprim are contraindicated due to the risk of kernicterus in infancy.
- Use cautiously in clients who have impaired kidney function (give lower dosages).
- Administer with caution to adults older than 65 years who take ACE inhibitors or angiotensin II receptor blockers because of the risk for hyperkalemia. Ⓒ

INTERACTIONS

Increased effects of warfarin, phenytoin, sulfonylurea oral hypoglycemics

NURSING ACTIONS
- Give lower dosages during trimethoprim-sulfamethoxazole therapy.
- Monitor laboratory levels (PT, INR, blood glucose, phenytoin levels).

NURSING ADMINISTRATION

- Hormonal contraceptive effectiveness decreases with various antibiotics and therefore it is recommended clients use a back-up method (a condom).

CLIENT EDUCATION
- Take trimethoprim-sulfamethoxazole on an empty stomach with 8 oz water.
- Complete the entire course of therapy, even if manifestations resolve sooner.

NURSING EVALUATION OF MEDICATION EFFECTIVENESS

Indications of effectiveness include the following.
- A decrease in the manifestations of UTI (frequency, burning, and dysuria)
- Negative urine cultures and lower WBC counts

Urinary tract antiseptics

SELECT PROTOTYPE MEDICATION: Nitrofurantoin

OTHER MEDICATIONS: Methenamine

PURPOSE

EXPECTED PHARMACOLOGICAL ACTION
Nitrofurantoin is a broad-spectrum urinary antiseptic with bacteriostatic and bactericidal action. It injures bacteria by damaging DNA.

THERAPEUTIC USES
- Acute UTIs
- Prophylaxis for recurrent lower UTIs

COMPLICATIONS

Gastrointestinal (GI) discomfort

Anorexia, nausea, vomiting, diarrhea

NURSING ACTIONS
- Administer nitrofurantoin with milk or meals.
- Reduce dosages, and use macrocrystal capsules.

Hypersensitivity reactions

With fever, chills, severe pulmonary manifestations (dyspnea, cough, chest pain, alveolar infiltrations)

CLIENT EDUCATION
- Stop taking the medication and to report these reactions.
- Pulmonary manifestations should subside within several days after stopping nitrofurantoin.
- Do not take nitrofurantoin again.

Blood dyscrasias

Agranulocytosis, leukopenia, thrombocytopenia, megaloblastic anemia, hepatotoxicity

NURSING ACTIONS
- Obtain blood samples for a baseline CBC and periodic blood tests including liver function tests.
- Monitor for and report easy bruising and epistaxis (nose bleeding).

Peripheral neuropathy

Numbness, tingling of the hands and feet, muscle weakness

NURSING ACTIONS: Do not administer to clients who have chronic kidney disease (increased risk for peripheral neuropathy).

CLIENT EDUCATION
- Report neuropathy.
- Avoid chronic use of nitrofurantoin.

Headache, drowsiness, dizziness

NURSING ACTIONS: Report these adverse effects.

CONTRAINDICATIONS/PRECAUTIONS

- **Warnings**
  - Pregnancy: Nitrofurantoin safety has not been established; avoid use during the third trimester.
  - Lactation: Nitrofurantoin can be used short-term; however, avoid breastfeeding for at least 4 to 6 hr after taking medication.
- Impaired kidney function and alteration in creatinine or creatinine clearance levels can decrease nitrofurantoin effects. Impaired kidney function increases the risk of toxicity because of the inability to excrete nitrofurantoin.
- Nitrofurantoin should not be administered to an infant under 1 month of age.
- Older adults with renal impairment should not receive nitrofurantoin. Ⓖ

NURSING ADMINISTRATION

CLIENT EDUCATION
- Nitrofurantoin turns urine rust-yellow to brown and can stain teeth.
- Take medication with food if adverse GI effects occur.
- Complete the entire course of therapy, even if manifestations resolve sooner.
- Avoid crushing, chewing, or opening capsules because of the possibility of tooth staining.

NURSING EVALUATION OF MEDICATION EFFECTIVENESS

Indications of effectiveness include the following.
- A decrease in the manifestations of UTI (frequency, burning, and dysuria)
- Negative urine cultures and lower WBC counts
- Resolution of GI disturbances (anorexia, diarrhea, nausea, and vomiting)

Fluoroquinolones

SELECT PROTOTYPE MEDICATION: Ciprofloxacin

OTHER MEDICATIONS
- Ofloxacin
- Moxifloxacin
- Levofloxacin
- Gemifloxacin

PURPOSE

EXPECTED PHARMACOLOGICAL ACTION
Fluoroquinolones are bactericidal due to inhibition of an enzyme necessary for DNA replication.

THERAPEUTIC USES
- Broad-spectrum antimicrobials treat a wide variety of micro-organisms (some gram-positive bacteria and gram-negative bacteria [Klebsiella and Escherichia coli]).
- Alternative to parenteral antibiotics for clients who have severe infections
- Urinary, respiratory, and GI tract infections; infections of bones, joints, skin, and soft tissues
- Prevention of anthrax for clients who have inhaled anthrax spores

COMPLICATIONS

GI discomfort (nausea, vomiting, diarrhea)

CLIENT EDUCATION: Tell clients to take the medication with food (with the exception of dairy products) if GI discomfort occurs.

Achilles tendon rupture

CLIENT EDUCATION
- Observe for and report pain, swelling, and redness at the Achilles tendon site.
- Stop taking ciprofloxacin and avoid exercise until the inflammation subsides.

Suprainfection (thrush, vaginal yeast infection)

CLIENT EDUCATION: Observe for and report manifestations of yeast infection (cottage-cheese or curd-like lesions on the mouth and genital area).

Phototoxicity (severe sunburn)

From direct and indirect sunlight and sun lamps, even with sunscreen use

CLIENT EDUCATION
- Avoid sun exposure and wear protective clothing outdoors in sunlight.
- Stop taking the medication if phototoxicity occurs.

CONTRAINDICATIONS/PRECAUTIONS

- **Warnings**
  - Pregnancy: Use fluoroquinolones only if the benefit to the client outweighs the risks to the fetus.
  - Lactation: Safety not established.
- Do not administer ciprofloxacin to children younger than 18 years of age (due to the risk of Achilles tendon rupture), unless the treatment is for Escherichia coli infections of the urinary tract or inhalational anthrax.
- Ciprofloxacin increases the risk for a Clostridium difficile infection because it destroys normal intestinal flora.
- Ciprofloxacin and several other fluoroquinolones can affect the CNS (dizziness, headache, restlessness, confusion). Use cautiously with older adults and with clients who have cardiovascular disorders. Ⓖ
- Older adults tolerate fluoroquinolone medication well, providing kidney function is within the expected reference range.

CLIENT EDUCATION: If taking this medication to treat an STD, abstain from intercourse until the medication is finished, manifestations resolve, and partners are treated.

INTERACTIONS

Cationic compounds (aluminum- or magnesium-containing antacids, iron salts, sucralfate, dairy products) decrease the absorption of ciprofloxacin.
NURSING ACTIONS: Administer cationic compounds 6 hr before or 2 hr after ciprofloxacin.

Plasma levels of theophylline can increase with concurrent use of ciprofloxacin.
NURSING ACTIONS: Monitor levels, and adjust dosages.

Plasma levels of warfarin can increase with concurrent use of ciprofloxacin.
NURSING ACTIONS: Monitor prothrombin time and INR, and adjust dosages.

NURSING ADMINISTRATION

- Ciprofloxacin is available in oral and IV formulations. Discontinue other IV infusions or use another IV site when administering ciprofloxacin IV.
- Give lower dosages to clients who have impaired kidney function.
- Administer ciprofloxacin IV in a dilute solution slowly over 60 min in a large vein. Ⓠ EBP
- For inhalation anthrax infection, give ciprofloxacin every 12 hr for 60 days.

CLIENT EDUCATION: Complete the entire course of therapy, even if manifestations resolve sooner.

NURSING EVALUATION OF MEDICATION EFFECTIVENESS

Indications of effectiveness include the following.
- A decrease in the manifestations of UTI (frequency, burning, and dysuria)
- Negative urine cultures and lower WBC counts
- No evidence of suprainfection

Urinary tract analgesic

SELECT PROTOTYPE MEDICATION: Phenazopyridine

PURPOSE

EXPECTED PHARMACOLOGICAL ACTION: The medication is an azo dye that functions as a local anesthetic on the mucosa of the urinary tract.

THERAPEUTIC USES: Relieves manifestations of burning with urination, pain, frequency, and urgency

NURSING ADMINISTRATION

- Acute kidney injury and chronic kidney disease are contraindications.
- It changes urine to an orange–red color.

CLIENT EDUCATION
- Urine can stain clothes.
- Take it with or after meals to minimize GI discomfort.

CONTRAINDICATIONS/PRECAUTIONS

- **Warnings**
  - Pregnancy: Safety not established.
  - Lactation: Safety not established.

COMPLEMENTARY THERAPIES

- Cranberry juice is used to prevent urinary tract infections (UTIs) and is not effective if the client has a UTI.
- Probiotics can help reestablish the intestinal flora for a client who has taken antibacterial and antifungal medications. However, antibacterial and antifungal medication can kill the bacteria and yeasts in probiotic products. Therefore, to help preserve probiotic activity, these preparations should be administered at least 2 hours after dosing with antibacterial or antifungal medications.

Application Exercises

1. A nurse reviewing a client's medication history notes an allergy to sulfonamides. The nurse should identify this allergy as a contraindication for taking which of the following medications?
   - A. Levothyroxine
   - B. Metoprolol
   - C. Acetaminophen
   - D. Glipizide

2. A nurse is teaching a client who has a new prescription for nitrofurantoin. Which of the following information should the nurse include? (Select all that apply.)
   - A. Observe for bruising on the skin.
   - B. Take the medication with milk or meals.
   - C. Expect brown discoloration of urine.
   - D. Crush the medication if it is difficult to swallow.
   - E. Expect insomnia when taking it.

3. A nurse is teaching a client who has a severe UTI about ciprofloxacin. Which of the following information about adverse reactions should the nurse include? (Select all that apply.)
   - A. Observe for pain and swelling of the Achilles tendon.
   - B. Watch for a vaginal yeast infection.
   - C. Expect excessive nighttime perspiration.
   - D. Inspect the mouth for cottage cheese-like lesions.
   - E. Take the medication with a dairy product.

Active Learning Scenario

A client who has a UTI has a prescription for phenazopyridine. What information should the nurse review? Use the ATI Active Learning Template: Medication to complete this item.

EXPECTED PHARMACOLOGICAL ACTION

THERAPEUTIC USES: Describe four.

CLIENT EDUCATION: Include three teaching points.

Application Exercises Key

1. D. **CORRECT:** The nurse should analyze cues from the client's medication history and determine that a sulfonamide allergy is a contraindication for taking some oral antidiabetic medications, including glipizide and glyburide. Hypersensitivity, including Stevens-Johnson syndrome, can result from taking glipizide and a sulfonamide concurrently.

   Ⓝ *NCLEX® Connection: Pharmacological and Parenteral Therapies, Adverse Effects/Contraindications/Interactions*

2. A. **CORRECT:** When taking action and teaching a client about a new prescription for nitrofurantoin, the nurse should include that bruising can indicate a blood dyscrasia, and the client should notify the provider if this occurs.
   B. **CORRECT:** The nurse should instruct the client that taking the medication with milk or meals can minimize GI discomfort from nausea, vomiting, anorexia, and diarrhea.
   C. **CORRECT:** The nurse should also inform the client that a brown discoloration of urine is a common adverse effect of nitrofurantoin.

   Ⓝ *NCLEX® Connection: Pharmacological and Parenteral Therapies, Medication Administration*

3. A. **CORRECT:** When taking actions and teaching a client about ciprofloxacin, the nurse should explain to the client that pain and swelling of the Achilles tendon can indicate an adverse effect of ciprofloxacin and should be reported to the provider immediately.
   B. **CORRECT:** The nurse should inform the client that a vaginal yeast infection as well cottage cheese-like lesions in the mouth can be an overgrowth of Candida albicans, which commonly occurs when taking ciprofloxacin and should be reported to the provider.
   D. **CORRECT:** The nurse should inform the client that a vaginal yeast infection as well cottage cheese-like lesions in the mouth can be an overgrowth of Candida albicans, which commonly occurs when taking ciprofloxacin and should be reported to the provider.

   Ⓝ *NCLEX® Connection: Pharmacological and Parenteral Therapies, Adverse Effects/Contraindications/Interactions*

Active Learning Scenario Key

Using the ATI Active Learning Template: Medication

EXPECTED PHARMACOLOGICAL ACTION: Phenazopyridine is an azo dye, which acts as a local anesthetic on the mucosa of the urinary tract. It is not an antibiotic.

THERAPEUTIC USES: Relieves urinary burning, urgency, pain, and frequency

CLIENT EDUCATION
- Acute kidney injury and chronic kidney disease are contraindications.
- It changes urine to an orange-red color.
- Tell clients that the urine can stain clothes.
- Instruct clients to take it with or after meals to minimize GI discomfort.

Ⓝ *NCLEX® Connection: Pharmacological and Parenteral Therapies, Expected Actions/Outcomes*

CHAPTER 45

Mycobacterial, Fungal, and Parasitic Infections

Mycobacterium tuberculosis is a slow-growing pathogen that necessitates long-term treatment. Long-term treatment increases the risk for toxicity, poor client adherence, and development of medication-resistant strains. Treatment for tuberculosis requires the use of at least two medications to which the pathogen is susceptible. Isoniazid and rifampin are two effective antituberculosis medications.

Metronidazole is the medication of choice for parasitic infections.

Antifungal medications belong to a variety of chemical families and are used to treat systemic and superficial mycoses.

Antimycobacterial (selective antituberculosis)

SELECT PROTOTYPE MEDICATION: Isoniazid

OTHER MEDICATIONS
- Pyrazinamide
- Ethambutol (bacteriostatic only to M. tuberculosis)
- Rifapentine

PURPOSE

EXPECTED PHARMACOLOGICAL ACTION
This medication is highly specific for mycobacteria. Isoniazid inhibits growth of mycobacteria by preventing synthesis of mycolic acid in the cell wall.

THERAPEUTIC USES
Indicated for active and latent tuberculosis

Latent: Isoniazid only daily for 9 months, or isoniazid with rifapentine once weekly for 3 months. (Contraindicated in children under age 2, clients who have HIV, pregnant clients, and clients resistant to either medication)

Active: Several antimycobacterial medications are used to treat a client who has active tuberculosis in order to decrease medication resistance. Treatment usually consists of a four-medication regimen often including isoniazid and rifampin.

The initial phase (induction phase) focuses on eliminating the active tubercle bacilli, which will result in noninfectious sputum. The second phase (continuation phase) works toward eliminating any other pathogens in the body. Length of treatment varies and can be as short as 6 months for medication-sensitive tuberculosis (2 months for the initial phase and 4 to 7 months for the continuation phase) or as long as 24 months for medication-resistant infections.

COMPLICATIONS

Peripheral neuropathy

Tingling, numbness, burning, and pain resulting from deficiency of pyridoxine, vitamin B6

NURSING ACTIONS: Administer 50 to 200 mg vitamin B6 daily. Prophylactic use of pyridoxine (vitamin B6) at 25 to 50 mg/day can decrease the risk of acquiring peripheral neuropathy. If peripheral neuropathy develops, it can be reversed by administering pyridoxine; however, higher doses are required.

CLIENT EDUCATION: Observe for manifestations and notify the provider if they occur.

Hepatotoxicity

Anorexia, malaise, fatigue, nausea, and yellowish discoloration of skin and eyes

NURSING ACTIONS
- Monitor liver function tests.
- Elevated liver function test results can result in the need to discontinue the medication.

CLIENT EDUCATION
- Observe for manifestations and notify the provider if they occur.
- Avoid consumption of alcohol.

CONTRAINDICATIONS/PRECAUTIONS

Warnings
- Pregnancy
  - Isoniazid, pyrazinamide, rifapentine: Safety has not been established
  - Ethambutol: Contraindicated; only take if the benefit to the client outweighs the risk to the fetus.
- Lactation
  - Ethambutol: Safe
  - Isoniazid: Safety has not been established

Isoniazid is contraindicated for clients who have liver disease.
NURSING ACTIONS
- Use cautiously in older clients and those who have diabetes mellitus or alcohol use disorder. Qs
- Isoniazid, pyrazinamide, ethambutol, and rifapentine are Pregnancy Risk Category C.

INTERACTIONS

Isoniazid inhibits metabolism of phenytoin, leading to buildup of medication and toxicity. Ataxia and incoordination can indicate toxicity.
NURSING ACTIONS: Monitor levels of phenytoin. Adjust dosage of phenytoin based on phenytoin levels.

Concurrent use of tyramine foods (aged cheeses, cured meats), alcohol, rifampin, and pyrazinamide increases the risk for hepatotoxicity.
NURSING ACTIONS: Monitor liver function.

CLIENT EDUCATION
- Avoid foods with high levels of tyramine.
- Avoid alcohol consumption.

NURSING ADMINISTRATION

- Usually administered orally. When given IM, warm to room temperature to ensure that the solution is free of crystals, and inject deeply into a large muscle.
- For active tuberculosis, direct observation therapy is done to ensure adherence. Qᴘᴄᴄ

CLIENT EDUCATION
- Consider using a second form of birth control (such as condom) if taking a hormonal contraceptive as various antibiotics can decrease their effectiveness.
- Take isoniazid 1 hr before or 2 hr after meals, with a full glass of water. If gastric discomfort occurs, take isoniazid with meals.
- Complete the prescribed course of antimicrobial therapy, even though manifestations can resolve before the full course is completed.

Broad-spectrum antimycobacterial (antituberculosis)

SELECT PROTOTYPE MEDICATION: Rifampin

PURPOSE

EXPECTED PHARMACOLOGICAL ACTION: Rifampin is bactericidal as a result of inhibition of protein synthesis.

THERAPEUTIC USES
- Rifampin is a broad-spectrum antibiotic effective for gram-positive and gram-negative bacteria.
- Rifampin is given in combination with at least one other antituberculosis medication to help prevent antibiotic resistance. Qᴇʙᴘ

COMPLICATIONS

Discoloration of body fluids

CLIENT EDUCATION: There is an expected orange color of urine, saliva, sweat, and tears.

Hepatotoxicity (jaundice, anorexia, and fatigue)

NURSING ACTIONS: Monitor liver function.

CLIENT EDUCATION
- Monitor for manifestations of anorexia, fatigue, and malaise, and notify the provider if they occur.
- Avoid alcohol.

Mild GI discomfort

Anorexia, nausea, and abdominal discomfort

NURSING ACTIONS: Abdominal discomfort is mild and usually does not require intervention.

Pseudomembranous colitis

CLIENT EDUCATION: Monitor and report fever, diarrhea, abdominal pain, or bloody stool. Discontinue medication if manifestations occur.

CONTRAINDICATIONS/PRECAUTIONS

- **Warnings**
  - Pregnancy: Use rifampin with caution.
  - Lactation: Use rifampin with caution.
  - Reproductive: When taking oral contraceptives, a nonhormonal form of birth control should be used while taking this medication.
- Use cautiously in clients who have liver dysfunction. Qˢ

INTERACTIONS

Rifampin accelerates metabolism of warfarin, oral contraceptives, protease inhibitors, and non-nucleoside reverse transcriptase inhibitors (NNRTIs) for HIV, resulting in diminished effectiveness.
NURSING ACTIONS
- Increased dosages of HIV medications are often necessary.
- Monitor PT and INR.
- Advise clients to use a non-hormonal form of contraception.

Concurrent use with isoniazid and pyrazinamide increases risk of hepatotoxicity.
NURSING ACTIONS
- Instruct clients to avoid alcohol consumption.
- Monitor liver function.

NURSING ADMINISTRATION

- Administer orally or by IV route.
- Administer oral rifampin 1 hr before or 2 hr after meals with a full glass of water. Absorption is decreased if given with food.
- Monitor kidney and liver function prior to and during treatment.

CLIENT EDUCATION

- Use a non-hormonal form of contraception.
- Complete the prescribed course of antimicrobial therapy, even though manifestations can resolve before the full course is completed.
- Body fluids may have a red-orange color which is an expected and non-harmful effect of the medication.
- Avoid the use of alcohol while taking this medication as it can increase the risk of liver damage.

NURSING EVALUATION OF MEDICATION EFFECTIVENESS

Depending on therapeutic intent, effectiveness is evidenced by the following.

- Improvement of tuberculosis manifestations (clear breath sounds, no night sweats, increased appetite, and no afternoon rises of temperature)
- Three negative sputum cultures for tuberculosis, usually taking 3 to 6 months to achieve

Antiprotozoals

SELECT PROTOTYPE MEDICATION: Metronidazole

PURPOSE

EXPECTED PHARMACOLOGICAL ACTION: Metronidazole is a broad-spectrum antimicrobial with bactericidal activity against anaerobic micro-organisms.

THERAPEUTIC USES

- Treatment of protozoal infections (intestinal amebiasis, giardiasis, trichomoniasis) and obligate anaerobic bacteria (*Bacteroides fragilis*, antibiotic-induced *Clostridium difficile*, *Gardnerella vaginalis*)
- Prophylaxis for clients who will have surgical procedures (vaginal, abdominal, colorectal surgery) and are high-risk for anaerobic infection
- Treatment of H. pylori in combination with tetracycline and bismuth subsalicylate in clients who have peptic ulcer disease

COMPLICATIONS

GI discomfort

Nausea, vomiting, dry mouth, and metallic taste

CLIENT EDUCATION: Observe for effects and to notify the provider. Take the medication with meals to reduce adverse effects.

Darkening of urine

CLIENT EDUCATION: This is a harmless effect of metronidazole.

CNS effects

Dizziness, headache, seizures, peripheral neuropathy, aseptic meningitis, encephalopathy

CLIENT EDUCATION

- Notify the provider if manifestations occur.
- Stop metronidazole.

CONTRAINDICATIONS/PRECAUTIONS

Warnings

- Pregnancy: Metronidazole contraindicated in the first trimester; safety not established during the second and third trimesters
- Lactation: Do not breastfeed for 24 hr after taking metronidazole; single dosing recommended.
- Use cautiously in clients who have blood dyscrasias, renal or hepatic impairment, seizures, or other neurological problems.

INTERACTIONS

Alcohol causes a disulfiram-like reaction (facial flushing, vomiting, dyspnea, tachycardia).
CLIENT EDUCATION: Avoid alcohol consumption.

Metronidazole inhibits inactivation of warfarin, phenytoin, and lithium.
NURSING ACTIONS: Monitor prothrombin time and INR, and phenytoin and lithium levels. Adjust dosages accordingly.

NURSING ADMINISTRATION

Administer by oral or IV route.

CLIENT EDUCATION

- Complete the prescribed course of antimicrobial therapy, even though manifestations can resolve before the full course is completed. Qᴘᴄᴄ
- Use condoms if using this medication for treatment of trichomoniasis.
- Hormonal contraceptive effectiveness decreases with various antibiotics, and therefore it is recommended to use a back-up method (a condom).
- If this medication is given to treat an STD, abstain from intercourse until the medication is finished, manifestations have resolved, and partners have been treated.

NURSING EVALUATION OF MEDICATION EFFECTIVENESS

Depending on therapeutic intent, effectiveness is evidenced by improvement of manifestations.

- Resolution of bloody mucoid diarrhea
- Formed stools
- Negative stool results for amoeba and giardia
- Decrease or absence of watery vaginal/urethral discharge
- Negative blood cultures for anaerobic organisms in the CNS, blood, bones and joints, and soft tissues

Antifungals

SELECT PROTOTYPE MEDICATIONS

- Amphotericin B (a polyene antibiotic for systemic mycoses)
- Ketoconazole (an azole for treating both superficial and systemic mycoses)

OTHER MEDICATIONS

- Flucytosine
- Nystatin
- Miconazole
- Clotrimazole
- Terbinafine
- Fluconazole
- Griseofulvin

PURPOSE

EXPECTED PHARMACOLOGICAL ACTION: Amphotericin B is an antifungal agent that acts on fungal cell membranes to cause cell death. Depending on concentration, these agents can be fungistatic (slows growth on the fungus) or fungicidal (destroys the fungus).

THERAPEUTIC USES

- Antifungals are the treatment of choice for systemic fungal infection (candidiasis, aspergillosis, cryptococcosis, mucormycosis) and nonopportunistic mycoses, (blastomycosis, histoplasmosis, coccidioidomycosis)
- Some antifungals treat superficial fungal infections: dermatophytic infections (tinea pedis [ringworm of the foot] and tinea cruris [ringworm of the groin]); candida infections of the skin and mucous membranes; and fungal infections of the nails (onychomycosis).

COMPLICATIONS

Infusion reactions

Fever, chills, rigors, and headache 1 to 3 hr after initiation

NURSING ACTIONS

- A test dose of 1 mg amphotericin B, infused slowly IV, can assess client reaction.
- Pretreat with diphenhydramine and acetaminophen. Qs
- Administer meperidine, and dantrolene.

Thrombophlebitis

NURSING ACTIONS

- Observe infusion sites for of erythema, swelling, and pain.
- Rotate injection sites.
- Administer in a large vein.

Nephrotoxicity

NURSING ACTIONS

- Obtain baseline kidney function (BUN and creatinine) and do weekly kidney function tests.
- Monitor I&O.
- Infuse 1 L of 0.9% sodium chloride IV on the day of amphotericin B infusion.

Electrolyte imbalance

NURSING ACTIONS

- Monitor electrolyte levels, especially potassium.
- Administer supplements for deficiencies.

Bone marrow suppression

NURSING ACTIONS: Obtain baseline CBC and hematocrit, and monitor weekly.

CONTRAINDICATIONS/PRECAUTIONS

Warnings
- Pregnancy
  - Amphotericin B: Safe
  - Fluconazole, miconazole, clotrimazole: Safety not established
- Lactation
  - Amphotericin B and ketoconazole: Contraindicated
  - Miconazole, clotrimazole: Safety not established
  - Fluconazole: Safe
- Antifungals are contraindicated in clients who have impaired kidney function due to the risk for nephrotoxicity. Qs
- Use antifungals with caution in clients who have anemia, electrolyte imbalance, and bone marrow suppression.

INTERACTIONS

Aminoglycosides (gentamicin, streptomycin, cyclosporine) have additive nephrotoxic risk when used concurrently with antifungal medications.
NURSING ACTIONS: Avoid use of these antimicrobials when clients are taking amphotericin B due to additive nephrotoxicity risk.

Antifungal effects of flucytosine are potentiated with concurrent use of amphotericin B.
NURSING ACTIONS: Potentiated flucytosine effects allow for a reduction in amphotericin B dosages.

Azole antibiotics increase levels of multiple medications, including digoxin, warfarin, and sulfonylurea antidiabetic medications.
NURSING ACTIONS: If concurrent administration is necessary, carefully monitor for toxicity.

NURSING ADMINISTRATION

- Amphotericin B is highly toxic and should be reserved for severe life-threatening fungal infections.
- Infuse amphotericin B slowly over 4 to 6 hr IV.
- Observe solutions for precipitation and discard if precipitates are present. Use a filter to prevent infusion of undissolved crystals. Kidney injury is lessened with administration of 1 L of 0.9% sodium chloride IV on the day of amphotericin B infusion. ⓆEBP
- Apply antifungals for topical use to treat superficial vulvovaginal candidiasis as vaginal suppository or cream.

CLIENT EDUCATION

- Consider using a second form of birth control (such as condom) if taking a hormonal contraceptive as various antibiotics can decrease their effectiveness.
- Complete the prescribed course of antimicrobial therapy, even though manifestations might resolve before the full course is completed.

NURSING EVALUATION OF MEDICATION EFFECTIVENESS

Depending on therapeutic intent, effectiveness is evidenced by the following.

- Improvement of findings of systemic fungal infections
- Improvement of findings of superficial infections (clear mucus membranes, clear nails, and intact skin)

45.1 Potential adverse effects

	AMPHOTERICIN B	METRONIDAZOLE	RIFAMPIN
Hyperglycemia	✓		
Hepatotoxicity			✓
Fever	✓		
Hypokalemia	✓		
Altered taste		✓	
Nausea	✓	✓	✓
Ataxia		✓	✓
Dark-colored urine			✓
Seizures		✓	

COMPLEMENTARY AND ALTERNATIVE THERAPIES

- By suppressing immune function (in response to long-term use), echinacea can compromise drug therapy of tuberculosis.
- Antibacterial and antifungal medications can kill the bacteria and yeasts in probiotic products. Therefore, to help preserve probiotic activity, these preparations should be administered at least 2 hours after dosing with antibacterial or antifungal medications.
- By eliminating intestinal flora, antibiotics may reduce conversion of isoflavones to their active form, thus reducing potentially positive effects of soy.
- Rifampin and St. John's Wort both induce CYP3A4 and P-glycoprotein which can cause interactions.

Application Exercises

1. A nurse is teaching a client who has active tuberculosis about the treatment regimen. The client asks why multiple medications are necessary. Which of the following responses should the nurse make?

   A. "Multiple medications decrease the risk for a severe allergic reaction."

   B. "Multiple medications reduce the chance that the bacteria will become resistant."

   C. "Multiple medications reduce the risk for adverse reactions."

   D. "Multiple medications decrease the chance of having a positive tuberculin skin test."

2. A nurse is caring for a client who has diabetes mellitus, pulmonary tuberculosis, and a new prescription for isoniazid. Which of the following supplements should the nurse expect to administer to prevent an adverse effect of INH?

   A. Ascorbic acid

   B. Pyridoxine

   C. Folic acid

   D. Cyanocobalamin

3. A nurse is administering IV amphotericin B to a client who has a systemic fungal infection. The nurse should monitor which of the following laboratory values? (Select all that apply.)

   A. Blood albumin

   B. Blood amylase

   C. Blood potassium

   D. Hematocrit

   E. Blood creatinine

Application Exercises Key

1. B. **CORRECT:** When taking actions and teaching a client about the treatment regimen for tuberculosis, the nurse should explain to the client that taking only a single medication to treat active tuberculosis can cause resistance to the medication. Taking multiple medications decreases this possibility from occurring.

   Ⓝ *NCLEX® Connections: Pharmacological and Parenteral Therapies, Medication Administration*

2. B. **CORRECT:** The nurse should plan to generate solutions to address the client who has diabetes and a prescription for isoniazid by expecting to administer pyridoxine. Pyridoxine is frequently prescribed along with INH to prevent peripheral neuropathy for clients who have increased risk factors (diabetes mellitus or alcohol use disorder).

   Ⓝ *NCLEX® Connections: Pharmacological and Parenteral Therapies, Expected Actions/Outcomes*

3. C, D, E. **CORRECT:** When taking actions while administering IV amphotericin B to a client, the nurse should evaluate the client for hypokalemia, which is a serious adverse effect of amphotericin B, by monitoring the client's potassium level.

   Amphotericin B can cause bone marrow suppression; therefore, the nurse should monitor the client's CBC and hematocrit count periodically.

   The nurse should also monitor the client's kidney function (with blood creatinine, BUN, and creatinine clearance) to evaluate the client for nephrotoxicity.

   Ⓝ *NCLEX® Connections: Pharmacological and Parenteral Therapies, Expected Actions/Outcomes*

Active Learning Scenario

A nurse in a public health department is teaching a client who has latent tuberculosis (TB) and a new prescription for isoniazid twice weekly for 6 months. What should the nurse teach the client about this medication? Use the ATI Active Learning Template: Medication to complete this item.

THERAPEUTIC USES: Describe the therapeutic use for isoniazid in this client.

COMPLICATIONS: List two adverse effects the client should watch for.

NURSING INTERVENTIONS: Describe one test to monitor for clients taking isoniazid.

CLIENT EDUCATION: Describe two teaching points for clients taking isoniazid.

Active Learning Scenario Key

Using the ATI Active Learning Template: Medication

THERAPEUTIC USES: A client who has latent tuberculosis has been infected by Mycobacterium tuberculosis and is at risk for (but has not yet developed) active tuberculosis. Some clients who have latent tuberculosis (those who are immunocompromised or who have recently immigrated to the U.S. from a country where active TB is common) can require treatment with isoniazid, with or without rifapentine, in order to prevent the onset of active TB. The client who has latent TB has a positive tuberculin test but a negative sputum culture and negative chest x-ray for TB. The client cannot infect others with tuberculosis unless the infection becomes active.

COMPLICATIONS
• Paresthesias in the extremities caused by vitamin B6 deficiency
• Hepatotoxicity

NURSING INTERVENTIONS: The client who starts isoniazid should have baseline liver function testing and be tested periodically throughout treatment.

CLIENT EDUCATION
• Teach the client to watch for paresthesias and to take pyridoxine daily to reverse the effect if they occur.
• Teach the client about indications of hepatitis (anorexia, fatigue, nausea, jaundice) and to notify the provider if these occur.
• Teach the client to take isoniazid as prescribed and not to stop until the entire course of treatment is completed.
• The client who has latent tuberculosis does not feel ill. The nurse should be sure that the client understands why it is important to continue with treatment.

Ⓝ *NCLEX® Connections: Pharmacological and Parenteral Therapies, Medication Administration*

UNIT 12   MEDICATIONS FOR INFECTION

CHAPTER 46 # Viral Infections, HIV, and AIDS

Most antiviral medications act by altering viral reproduction. Antiviral medications are only effective during viral replication. Therefore, they are ineffective when the virus is dormant.

The human immunodeficiency virus (HIV) is a retrovirus. A retrovirus must attach to a host cell to replicate. RNA is changed into DNA using the enzyme reverse transcriptase.

Antiretroviral agents are used to treat HIV infections. These medications do not cure HIV infection, but when taken as prescribed can reduce the viral load, thereby assisting with the reduction of the transmission of the virus. As HIV is not completely eradicated, clients should still be educated on strategies to reduce transmission. Antiretroviral agents act by preventing the virus from entering the cells (fusion/entry inhibitors and CCR5 antagonists). Others act by inhibiting enzymes needed for HIV replication (nucleoside reverse transcriptase inhibitors [NRTIs], non-nucleoside reverse transcriptase inhibitors [NNRTIs], protease inhibitors [PIs], and an integrase inhibitor [INSTI]). Skipping doses or taking decreased dosages of antiretroviral medications causes medication resistance and possible treatment failure.

Highly active antiretroviral therapy

- Highly active antiretroviral therapy (HAART) involves using three to four HIV medications in combination with other antiretroviral medications to reduce medication resistance, adverse effects, and dosages.
- HAART is an aggressive treatment method using three or more different medications to reduce the amount of virus and increase CD4 counts.
- Adherence to medication regimens are an important part of the program because missed doses of antiretroviral medication can promote medication resistance, which can cause treatment failure. SDoH
- In addition to HAART, clients who have HIV infection take additional medications to treat adverse effects of antiretrovirals and to treat or prevent secondary infections (pneumocystis pneumonia).

Antivirals

SELECT PROTOTYPE MEDICATIONS
- Acyclovir (oral, topical, IV)
- Ganciclovir (oral, IV)

OTHER MEDICATIONS
- Interferon alfa–2b
- Lamivudine
- Oseltamivir
- Ribavirin
- Amantadine
- Boceprevir
- Telaprevir

PURPOSE

EXPECTED PHARMACOLOGICAL ACTION: Acyclovir and ganciclovir prevent the reproduction of viral DNA and thus interrupt cell replication.

THERAPEUTIC USES
- Acyclovir is used to treat herpes simplex and varicella–zoster viruses.
- Ganciclovir is used for treatment and prevention of cytomegalovirus (CMV). Prevention therapy using ganciclovir is given for clients who have HIV/AIDS, organ transplants, and other immunocompromised states.
- Interferon alfa–2b and lamivudine are used to treat hepatitis B and C.
- Oseltamivir is used to treat influenza A and B.
- Ribavirin is used to treat respiratory syncytial virus, hepatitis C, and influenza (unlabeled use).
- Boceprevir and telaprevir are protease inhibitors used to treat hepatitis C virus.

COMPLICATIONS

Acyclovir

Phlebitis and inflammation at the site of infusion
NURSING ACTIONS
- Rotate IV injection sites.
- Monitor IV sites for swelling and redness.

Nephrotoxicity

NURSING ACTIONS
- Administer acyclovir infusion slowly over 1 hr.
- Ensure adequate hydration during infusion and 2 hr after to minimize nephrotoxicity by administering IV fluids and increasing oral fluid intake as prescribed.
- Use with caution in clients who have renal impairment or are dehydrated.

Mild discomfort associated with oral therapy: Nausea, headache, diarrhea
NURSING ACTIONS: Observe for manifestations and notify the provider.

Ganciclovir

Suppressed bone marrow: Including leukocytes and thrombocytes

NURSING ACTIONS
- Obtain baseline CBC and platelet count.
- Administer granulocyte colony-stimulating factors.
- Monitor WBC, absolute neutrophil, and platelet counts frequently during treatment.

CLIENT EDUCATION: Report manifestations of infection and bleeding, and avoid crowds or individuals who have respiratory infections.

Fever, headache, nausea, diarrhea
NURSING ACTIONS: Administer with food.

CLIENT EDUCATION: Report these findings.

CONTRAINDICATIONS/PRECAUTIONS

- **Warnings**
  - Pregnancy
    - Acyclovir: Safety not established
    - Ganciclovir: Contraindicated
  - Lactation
    - Acyclovir: Safety not established
    - Ganciclovir: Contraindicated
  - Reproductive
    - Acyclovir: No sexual activity should occur when lesions are present. Use a condom during sexual contact.
    - Ganciclovir: Clients should have pregnancy testing prior to starting the medication and use contraception during treatment and for 30 days following completion of the medication regimen. May cause infertility. Use a barrier contraceptive during treatment and for 90 days following completion of treatment.
- Acyclovir should be used cautiously in clients who have renal impairment or dehydration and clients taking nephrotoxic medications. Qs
- Use cautiously in older adults; infants younger than 6 months; and clients who have dehydration, renal insufficiency, or malignant disorders. Ⓖ

INTERACTIONS

Acyclovir

Probenecid can decrease elimination of acyclovir.
NURSING ACTIONS: Monitor for medication toxicity.

Concurrent use of zidovudine can cause drowsiness.
NURSING ACTIONS: Use with caution.

Ganciclovir

Cytotoxic medications can cause increased toxicity.
NURSING ACTIONS: Use together with caution.

NURSING ADMINISTRATION

CLIENT EDUCATION
- Complete the prescribed course of antimicrobial therapy, even though manifestations can resolve before the full course is completed.
- Use barrier contraception if using this medication.

Acyclovir

- Administer IV infusion slowly over 1 hr or longer.
- Clients who have healed herpetic lesions should continue to use condoms to prevent transmission of the virus.

CLIENT EDUCATION
- Expect relief of manifestations, but not a cure.
- For topical administration put on rubber gloves to avoid transfer of virus to other areas of the body. Qᴇʙᴘ
- Wash affected area with soap and water three to four times per day and keep the lesions dry after washing.
- Refrain from sexual contact while lesions are present.

Ganciclovir

- Administer IV infusion slowly, with an infusion pump, over at least 1 hr.
- Administer oral medication with food.
- Encourage extra fluid intake during therapy.
- Administer intraocular for CMV retinitis. Do not use contact lenses with medication.
- Avoid getting ganciclovir solution or powder on skin. Wash well if contact occurs.

NURSING EVALUATION OF MEDICATION EFFECTIVENESS

Depending on therapeutic intent, effectiveness can be evidenced by improvement of findings (genital lesions, decreased inflammation and pain, and improvement in vision).

Antiretrovirals: fusion/entry inhibitors

SELECT PROTOTYPE MEDICATION:
Enfuvirtide (subcutaneous)

PURPOSE

EXPECTED PHARMACOLOGICAL ACTION: Decreases and limits the spread of HIV by blocking HIV from attaching to and entering CD4 T cell

THERAPEUTIC USES: Treatment of HIV that is unresponsive to other antiretrovirals

COMPLICATIONS

Localized reaction at injection site
NURSING ACTIONS: Rotate injection sites. Monitor for swelling and redness.

Bacterial pneumonia
NURSING ACTIONS: Assess breath sounds prior to start of therapy. Monitor for manifestations of pneumonia (fever, cough, or shortness of breath).

Fever, chills, rash, hypotension
NURSING ACTIONS: Monitor for medication reaction. Discontinue and notify the provider.

CONTRAINDICATIONS/PRECAUTIONS

- **Warnings**
  - Pregnancy: Enfuvirtide is recommended for use for clients who have HIV. Clients who are pregnant and taking this medication should register in the Antiretroviral Pregnancy Registry.
  - Lactation: Breastfeeding is contraindicated for clients who have HIV.
- Enfuvirtide is contraindicated in clients who have medication hypersensitivity and for clients who are breastfeeding. Qs

INTERACTIONS

None significant

NURSING ADMINISTRATION

- Enfuvirtide is only administered subcutaneously. Rotate injection sites and avoid previous skin reaction areas. QEBP
- Bring the solution to room temperature before injection.
- Monitor for bacterial pneumonia.
- Monitor for systemic hypersensitivity reaction.

CLIENT EDUCATION:
- Take exactly as prescribed to minimize development of resistance.
- Notify the provider if pregnancy is suspected.

NURSING EVALUATION OF MEDICATION EFFECTIVENESS

Depending on therapeutic intent, effectiveness is evidenced by a reduction of manifestations and the client being free of opportunistic infection.

Antiretrovirals: CCR5 antagonists

SELECT PROTOTYPE MEDICATION: Maraviroc (oral)

PURPOSE

EXPECTED PHARMACOLOGICAL ACTION: Prevents HIV from entering lymphocytes by binding to CCR5 on cell membranes

THERAPEUTIC USES: Treats HIV infection in conjunction with other antiretroviral medications

COMPLICATIONS

Cough and upper respiratory tract infections
NURSING ACTIONS: Teach client to report respiratory findings.

CNS effects: Dizziness, paresthesias, orthostatic hypotension
CLIENT EDUCATION: Move carefully from lying or sitting to standing, and prevent injury caused by dizziness.

Hepatotoxicity: Jaundice, right upper quadrant pain, and nausea, often preceded by allergic reaction (hives, rash)
CLIENT EDUCATION: Stop maraviroc and notify provider for these findings.

Pseudomembranous colitis
NURSING ACTIONS: Monitor for and report diarrhea and bloody stools.

CONTRAINDICATIONS/PRECAUTIONS

- **Warnings**
  - Pregnancy: Maraviroc is recommended for use for clients who have HIV. Clients who are pregnant and taking this medication should register in the Antiretroviral Pregnancy Registry.
  - Lactation: Contraindicated for clients who have HIV
- Contraindicated in clients who have renal impairment Qs
- Use caution in clients who have existing cardiovascular disorders, renal or liver disease, dehydration, and orthostatic hypotension.
- Use caution in clients who are breastfeeding and in older adults. ©
- Maraviroc is recommended for use for clients who have HIV.

INTERACTIONS

Most protease inhibitors raise maraviroc levels.
NURSING ACTIONS: Adjust maraviroc dosage.

Rifampin, efavirenz, phenytoin, some other anticonvulsants, nafcillin, verapamil, azole antifungals, other antibiotics, and St. John's wort decrease maraviroc levels.
NURSING ACTIONS: Adjust maraviroc dosage.

NURSING ADMINISTRATION

- Administer orally in conjunction with other antiretroviral medications.
- Monitor liver function tests, blood pressure, and CBC at baseline and periodically during treatment.
- Notify provider if pregnancy is suspected.
- Take at regular intervals to maintain therapeutic blood levels.

NURSING EVALUATION OF MEDICATION EFFECTIVENESS

Decrease in manifestations of HIV infection and absence of opportunistic infections

Antiretrovirals: NRTIs

SELECT PROTOTYPE MEDICATION: Zidovudine

OTHER MEDICATIONS

- Didanosine
- Stavudine
- Lamivudine
- Abacavir

COMBINATION MEDICATIONS: Fixed medication dosages in one tablet or capsule

- Abacavir, lamivudine, dolutegravir
- Abacavir, lamivudine
- Lamivudine, zidovudine
- Tenofovir/emtricitabine

ROUTE OF ADMINISTRATION: Oral, IV

PURPOSE

EXPECTED PHARMACOLOGICAL ACTION: Reduces HIV manifestations by inhibiting DNA synthesis and thus viral replication

THERAPEUTIC USES: First-line antiretrovirals to treat HIV infection for short-term care.

COMPLICATIONS

Suppressed bone marrow: Zidovudine can cause suppressed bone marrow, resulting in anemia, agranulocytosis (neutropenia), and thrombocytopenia.

NURSING ACTIONS

- Monitor CBC and platelets.
- Teach the client to monitor for bleeding, easy bruising, sore throat, and fatigue.

Lactic acidosis
NURSING ACTIONS

- Monitor for indications of lactic acidosis (hyperventilation, nausea, and abdominal pain).
- Pregnancy increases the risk of lactic acidosis.

Nausea, vomiting, diarrhea
NURSING ACTIONS

- Take medication with food to reduce gastric irritation.
- Monitor fluids and electrolytes.
- Pancreatitis

Hepatomegaly/fatty liver
NURSING ACTIONS: Monitor liver enzymes.

CONTRAINDICATIONS/PRECAUTIONS

- **Warnings**
  - Pregnancy

- Zidovudine: Recommended for use for clients who have HIV
- Increased risk for lactic acidosis
- Clients who are pregnant and taking this medication should register in the Antiretroviral Pregnancy Registry.
  - Lactation: Contraindicated for clients who have HIV
- These medications are contraindicated in clients who have medication hypersensitivity.
- Use with caution in clients who have liver disease and bone marrow suppression.

INTERACTIONS

Probenecid, valproic acid, and methadone can increase zidovudine.
NURSING ACTIONS: Reduce dosage. Monitor for medication toxicity.

Ganciclovir or medications that decrease bone marrow production can further suppress bone marrow.
NURSING ACTIONS: Use together with caution. Monitor blood counts, and report sore throat or fever.

Clarithromycin can reduce zidovudine levels.
NURSING ACTIONS: Adjust dosage if needed.

Phenytoin can alter both medication levels.
NURSING ACTIONS: Monitor medication levels.

NURSING ADMINISTRATION

- Monitor for bone marrow suppression. Obtain baseline CBC and platelets at the start of therapy, and monitor periodically as needed. ⓠEBP
- Treat anemia with epoetin alfa or transfusions.
- Treat neutropenia with colony-stimulating factors.
- Teach client to take exactly as prescribed to minimize development of medication resistance.
- Notify provider if pregnancy is suspected.

NURSING EVALUATION OF MEDICATION EFFECTIVENESS

Depending on therapeutic intent, effectiveness is evidenced by a reduction of manifestations and absence of opportunistic infection.

Antiretrovirals: NNRTIs

SELECT PROTOTYPE MEDICATIONS

- Delavirdine
- Efavirenz

OTHER MEDICATIONS

- Nevirapine
- Etravirine
- Rilpivirine

ROUTE OF ADMINISTRATION: Oral

PURPOSE

EXPECTED PHARMACOLOGICAL ACTION: NNRTIs act directly on reverse transcriptase to stop HIV replication.

THERAPEUTIC USES
- Primary HIV-1 infection
- Often used in combination with other antiretroviral agents to prevent medication resistance

COMPLICATIONS

Rash: Can become serious and lead to Stevens-Johnson syndrome

NURSING ACTIONS
- Monitor for rash. Treat with diphenhydramine if prescribed.
- Notify the provider for fever or blistering.

Flu-like manifestations, headache, fatigue
NURSING ACTIONS
- Monitor for adverse reactions.
- Encourage rest and adequate oral fluid intake.

CNS manifestations: Dizziness, drowsiness, insomnia, nightmares (especially with efavirenz)

CLIENT EDUCATION
- These findings should decrease after first few weeks of therapy.
- Do not perform activities that require alertness until effects are known.

Nausea, diarrhea
NURSING ACTIONS: Take at night on an empty stomach.

CONTRAINDICATIONS/PRECAUTIONS

- **Warnings**
  - Pregnancy: Efavirenz can be used during pregnancy only if other options are considered. Clients who are pregnant and taking this medication should register in the Antiretroviral Pregnancy Registry.
  - Lactation: Contraindicated for clients who have HIV
  - Reproductive: Use a nonhormonal form of contraceptive during and at least 12 weeks after therapy.
- These medications are contraindicated in clients who have medication hypersensitivity or severe liver disease.
- Use with caution in clients who have liver or renal disease.

INTERACTIONS

Antacids can decrease absorption of delavirdine.
NURSING ACTIONS: Allow 1 hr between medications.

NNRTIs can increase effects of benzodiazepines, antihistamines, calcium channel blockers, ergot alkaloids, quinidine, warfarin, and others.
NURSING ACTIONS: Monitor for medication toxicity.

Rifampin and phenytoin can cause decreased levels of delavirdine.

NURSING ACTIONS: Do not use together.

Didanosine can reduce absorption of both medications.
NURSING ACTIONS: Allow 1 hr between medications.

NNRTIs can cause increase in sildenafil level.
NURSING ACTIONS: Monitor for hypotension and changes in vision. Use together with caution.

Efavirenz and delavirdine can decrease the effects of hormonal contraceptives.
CLIENT EDUCATION: Use a barrier form of contraception, (condoms) in addition to a hormonal contraceptive.

NURSING ADMINISTRATION

- Monitor for rash.
- Efavirenz may be given with a high-fat meal to increase absorption.

CLIENT EDUCATION
- Take exactly as prescribed and do not skip doses to minimize development of resistance. ⓠEBP
- Take NNRTIs exactly as prescribed to minimize medication resistance.
- Use a barrier form of contraception (condoms) in addition to a hormonal contraceptive.

NURSING EVALUATION OF MEDICATION EFFECTIVENESS

Depending on therapeutic intent, effectiveness is evidenced by a reduction of manifestations and absence of opportunistic infection.

Antiretrovirals: protease inhibitors

SELECT PROTOTYPE MEDICATION: Ritonavir

OTHER MEDICATIONS
- Saquinavir
- Indinavir
- Fosamprenavir
- Nelfinavir
- Lopinavir/ritonavir combination

ROUTE OF ADMINISTRATION: Oral

PURPOSE

EXPECTED PHARMACOLOGICAL ACTION: Protease inhibitors act against HIV-1 and HIV-2 to alter and inactivate the virus by inhibiting enzymes needed for HIV replication.

THERAPEUTIC USES
- Used to treat HIV infections
- Usually combined with one or two reverse transcriptase inhibitors.
- Ritonavir is usually given with other PIs to increase their effect.

COMPLICATIONS

Bone loss/osteoporosis
NURSING ACTIONS: Severe bone loss is treated with medications (raloxifene and alendronate).

CLIENT EDUCATION: Eat a diet high in calcium and vitamin D.

Diabetes mellitus/hyperglycemia
NURSING ACTIONS: Monitor blood glucose. Adjust diet and administer antidiabetic medications as prescribed.

CLIENT EDUCATION: Monitor for increased thirst and urine output.

Hypersensitivity reaction
NURSING ACTIONS: Monitor for rash. Notify the provider if rash develops.

Nausea and vomiting
CLIENT EDUCATION: Tell the client to take medication with food to reduce GI effects and increase absorption.

Elevated blood lipids
NURSING ACTIONS: Monitor for hyperlipidemia. Adjust diet.

Altered fat distribution
CLIENT EDUCATION: Warn clients of these effects.

CONTRAINDICATIONS/PRECAUTIONS

- **Warnings**
  - Pregnancy: Protease inhibitors safety has not been established. Clients who are pregnant and taking this medication should register in the Antiretroviral Pregnancy Registry.
  - Lactation: Contraindicated for clients who have HIV
  - Reproductive: Use of protease inhibitors can decrease the effectiveness of oral contraceptives. Clients should be encouraged to use an additional nonhormonal form of contraception during therapy.
- Use with caution in clients who have liver disease, pancreatitis, diabetes mellitus, AV block, and hypercholesterolemia.
- Contraindicated with many other medications. Advise the client to notify the provider before taking any new medications.

INTERACTIONS

All protease inhibitors (especially ritonavir) cause multiple medications (such as quinidine) to raise to toxic levels.
NURSING ACTIONS: Check any new medication with the list of medications that must be avoided in clients taking protease inhibitors.

Ritonavir can increase medication levels of sildenafil, tadalafil, and vardenafil.
NURSING ACTIONS: Use with caution. Reduce dosages as needed.

Ritonavir decreases levels of ethynyl estradiol in oral contraceptives.
NURSING ACTIONS: Instruct clients to use an alternative form of birth control.

Phenobarbital, phenytoin, carbamazepine, and St. John's wort all significantly reduce level of protease inhibitors.
NURSING ACTIONS: Avoid concurrent use, or adjust dosages.

Grapefruit juice can decrease metabolism of PIs.
CLIENT EDUCATION: Avoid grapefruit juice.

NURSING ADMINISTRATION

- Except for indinavir, take protease inhibitors with food to increase absorption.
- Administer with another antiretroviral to reduce the risk of medication resistance.

CLIENT EDUCATION
- Report all other medications, including over-the-counter and herbal medications, to the provider.
- Use a barrier form of contraception (condoms) in addition to a hormonal contraceptive.

NURSING EVALUATION OF MEDICATION EFFECTIVENESS

Depending on therapeutic intent, effectiveness can be evidenced by reduction of HIV manifestations and freedom from opportunistic infections.

Antiretrovirals: integrase inhibitors (INSTIs)

SELECT PROTOTYPE MEDICATION: Raltegravir (oral)

PURPOSE

EXPECTED PHARMACOLOGICAL ACTION: Interferes with the enzyme integrase to prevent HIV replication within the cell

THERAPEUTIC USES: A first-line treatment for HIV when combined with two or three other antiretroviral medications

COMPLICATIONS

Headache and difficulty sleeping
CLIENT EDUCATION: Notify the provider if these findings occur.

Skin rash: Can indicate Stevens-Johnson syndrome or other serious disorder (allergy)

NURSING ACTIONS: Notify the provider if a rash or other skin manifestations occur.

Liver injury: Anorexia, nausea, right upper quadrant pain, jaundice

NURSING ACTIONS
- Monitor liver function tests.
- Notify the provider for manifestations of liver injury.

Renal failure, hematuria
NURSING ACTIONS: Monitor for hematuria.

Suicidal ideation
NURSING ACTIONS: Notify the provider of suicidal thoughts.

CONTRAINDICATIONS/PRECAUTIONS

- **Warnings**
  - Pregnancy: Use only if the benefits to the client outweigh the risks to the fetus. Clients who are pregnant and taking this medication should register in the Antiretroviral Pregnancy Registry.
  - Lactation: Contraindicated for clients who have HIV
- Use cautiously in clients younger than 16 years, older adult clients, or clients who have existing liver disorders.

INTERACTIONS

Raltegravir can be decreased with concurrent use of rifampin or tipranavir/ritonavir.
NURSING ACTIONS: Increase raltegravir dosage if needed.

NURSING ADMINISTRATION

- Take raltegravir with or without food.
- Monitor baseline and periodic liver function tests and CBC.
- Teach the client to take the medication exactly as prescribed without skipping doses to prevent medication resistance.
- Notify the provider if pregnancy is suspected.

NURSING EVALUATION OF MEDICATION EFFECTIVENESS

Depending on therapeutic intent, effectiveness is evidenced by reduction of HIV manifestations and absence of opportunistic infections.

ALTERNATIVE AND COMPLEMENTARY THERAPIES

- By suppressing immune function (in response to long-term use), echinacea can compromise drug therapy of HIV infection.
- Garlic can reduce levels of saquinavir (a protease inhibitor used to treat HIV infection).
- St. John's Wort can reduce antiretroviral effects in clients taking protease inhibitors or non-nucleoside reverse transcriptase inhibitors.

Application Exercises

1. A nurse is teaching a client who is beginning highly active antiretroviral therapy (HAART) for HIV infection. Which of the following information should the nurse provide the client about how the client can minimize resistance?

    A. Take low dosages of antiretroviral medication.

    B. Take one antiretroviral medication at a time.

    C. Take medications at the same times daily without missing doses.

    D. Change the medication regimen when adverse effects occur.

2. A nurse is caring for a client who is receiving acyclovir. Which of the following actions should the nurse take?

    A. Administer a stool softener.

    B. Decrease fluid intake following infusion.

    C. Obtain BUN and creatinine prior to administration.

    D. Monitor client for hypotension.

3. A nurse is caring for a client who is taking ritonavir, a protease inhibitor, to treat HIV infection. The nurse should monitor for which of the following adverse effects of this medication?

    A. Increased TSH level

    B. Decreased ALT level

    C. Hypoglycemia

    D. Hyperlipidemia

4. A nurse is monitoring a group of clients who are taking antiviral medications. Sort the adverse effects by the medication that can potentially be the causative agent: zidovudine or ritonavir.

    A. Anemia

    B. Hyperglycemia

    C. Hyperlipidemia

    D. Lactic acidosis

    E. Pancreatitis

    F. Bronchospasm

Application Exercises Key

1. C. **CORRECT:** When taking actions and teaching a client beginning HAART for HIV infection, the nurse should emphasize the importance of taking each dose of medication exactly as prescribed. Missing even a few doses of antiretroviral medication can promote medication resistance, which can cause treatment failure.

   Ⓝ *NCLEX® Connection: Pharmacological and Parenteral Therapies, Medication Administration*

2. C. **CORRECT:** When taking actions for a client who is receiving acyclovir, the nurse should obtain the client's BUN and creatinine prior to administration. Acyclovir dosage may need to be altered for a client who has renal insufficiency.

   Ⓝ *NCLEX® Connection: Pharmacological and Parenteral Therapies, Medication Administration*

3. D. **CORRECT:** When taking actions, the nurse should monitor the client's cholesterol and triglyceride levels to observe for hyperlipidemia, a potential adverse effect of this medication.

   Ⓝ *NCLEX® Connection: Pharmacological and Parenteral Therapies, Expected Actions/Outcomes*

4. **ZIDOVUDINE:** A, D, E; **RITONAVIR:** B, C, F

   When taking actions and monitoring clients for adverse effects of antiviral medications, the nurse should identify that anemia, lactic acidosis, and pancreatitis are potential adverse effects of zidovudine. The nurse should identify that hyperglycemia, hyperlipidemia, and bronchospasm can be potential adverse effects of ritonavir.

   Ⓝ *NCLEX® Connection: Pharmacological and Parenteral Therapies, Medication Administration*

Active Learning Scenario

A nurse is caring for a client who is immunocompromised and has a new prescription for ganciclovir IV twice per day to prevent cytomegalovirus. What should the nurse teach the client about this medication? Use the ATI Active Learning Template: Medication to complete this item.

THERAPEUTIC USES: Identify for ganciclovir in this client.

COMPLICATIONS: Identify two adverse effects.

NURSING INTERVENTIONS: Describe two for clients taking ganciclovir and two tests the nurse should monitor.

Active Learning Scenario Key

Using the ATI Active Learning Template: Medication

THERAPEUTIC USES: Ganciclovir prevents reproduction of viral DNA and thus prevents viral cell replication. It is used to prevent or treat cytomegalovirus in clients who are immunocompromised.

COMPLICATIONS

- Minor discomforts (fever, headache, and nausea)
- Suppresses the bone marrow, causing a decrease in WBCs, especially granulocytes
- Causes thrombocytopenia frequently
- The client should report any discomforts and be sure to report new onset of fatigue, easy bruising, or sore throat.
- Advise the client to report manifestations of infection or bleeding and to avoid crowds or individuals who have respiratory infections.

NURSING INTERVENTIONS

- Monitor client blood counts, especially WBC, absolute neutrophil count, and thrombocyte count. Expect ganciclovir therapy to be interrupted for an absolute neutrophil count less than 500/mm³ or a thrombocyte count less than 25,000/mm³.
- Prepare to administer granulocyte colony-stimulating factors for a low absolute neutrophil count.
- Monitor I&O, and encourage the client to increase fluid intake.
- Avoid direct contact with the powder from oral ganciclovir or the IV solution, and wash well if contact occurs.
- Advise clients to use a barrier contraception (condoms) during treatment and for 3 months following treatment.

Ⓝ *NCLEX® Connection: Pharmacological and Parenteral Therapies, Medication Administration*

When reviewing the following chapters, keep in mind the relevant topics and tasks of the NCLEX outline, in particular:

Pharmacological and Parenteral Therapies

ADVERSE EFFECTS/CONTRAINDICATIONS/SIDE EFFECTS/INTERACTIONS

Notify the primary health care provider of side effects, adverse effects, and contraindications of medications and parenteral therapy.

Identify a contraindication to the administration of a medication to the client.

Provide information to the client on common side effects/adverse effects/potential interactions of medications, and inform the client of when to notify the primary health care provider.

MEDICATION ADMINISTRATION: Educate client about medications.

CHAPTER 47 *Complementary, Alternative, and Integrative Therapies*

There are numerous health care practices that are not a typical part of the conventional medical care, as well as those that have origins outside of usual Western practice. Often these approaches are referred to as alternative and complementary.

Alternative medicine refers to using a non-mainstreamed practice in place of conventional medicine.

Complementary medicine refers to using a non-mainstreamed practice together with conventional medicine.

When complementary approaches are coordinated with conventional treatments, the focus becomes emphasizing a holistic and client-focused approach to health care referred to as integrative health. It works to coordinate care between a variety of treatment options, providers, and institutions.

The current focus of research involving integrative health and medicine includes pain management for military personnel and veterans as well as the relief of manifestations in cancer clients and survivors.

Natural products and herbal therapies

Natural products and dietary herbal supplements are widely used but less tested and regulated than conventional medications. Dosages are less precise than for more regulated medications. Because different formulations are not standardized, it can be difficult to know which preparations can provide therapeutic effects.
- Exempt from FDA regulation and approval prior to marketing
- The Dietary Supplement Health and Education Act (DSHEA) of 1994 imposes restrictions on labeling. Supplement labels must state: "This product is not intended to diagnose, treat, cure, or prevent any disease."

Aloe, aloe vera

- Topically, aloe has anti-inflammatory and analgesic properties.
  - Soothes pain
  - Heals burns
  - Softens skin
- Orally, aloe has laxative effects.

ADVERSE EFFECTS AND PRECAUTIONS
- Skin preparations: Possible hypersensitivity
- Oral preparations: Possible fluid and electrolyte imbalances, abdominal cramping
- Avoid in clients who have kidney disorders and history of cardiac disorders.

INTERACTIONS: Interacts with digoxin, diuretics, corticosteroids, and antidysrhythmics

NURSING ADMINISTRATION: Teach clients to recognize manifestations of fluid and electrolyte imbalance if using as a laxative.

Black cohosh

- Acts as an estrogen substitute
- Treats manifestations of menopause
- Mechanism of action is unknown

ADVERSE EFFECTS AND PRECAUTIONS
- GI distress, lightheadedness, headache, rash, weight gain
- Avoid taking during pregnancy, especially the first two trimesters of pregnancy. Qs
- Limit use to no longer than 6 months due to lack of information regarding long-term effects.

INTERACTIONS
- Increases effects of antihypertensive medications
- Can increase effect of estrogen medications
- Increases hypoglycemia in clients taking insulin or other medications for diabetes

NURSING ADMINISTRATION: Question clients who take antihypertensives, insulin, hypoglycemic agents, or hormone therapy or clients who might be pregnant about possible use of black cohosh.

Echinacea

- Stimulates the immune system
- Decreases inflammation
- Topically heals skin disorders, wounds, and burns
- Possibly treats viruses (common cold, herpes simplex)
- Used to increase T lymphocyte, tumor necrosis factor, and interferon production

ADVERSE EFFECTS
- Bitter taste
- Mild GI manifestations or fever
- Allergic reactions, especially in clients who are allergic to plants (ragweed or others in the daisy family)

INTERACTIONS: With chronic use (more than 6 months), echinacea can decrease positive effects of medications for tuberculosis, HIV, or cancer.

NURSING ADMINISTRATION

- Echinacea is available in many forms, including dried roots, plants, extracts, and teas.
- Question clients who have tuberculosis, cancer, HIV, lupus erythematosus, and rheumatoid arthritis about concurrent use. Advise these clients to talk to the provider.

Feverfew

- Can block platelet aggregation
- Can block a factor that causes migraines
- Can decrease the number and severity of migraine headaches (does not treat an existing migraine)

ADVERSE EFFECTS AND PRECAUTIONS

- Mild GI manifestations
- Post feverfew syndrome can occur when abruptly discontinued, causing agitation, tiredness, inability to sleep, headache, and joint discomfort.
- Allergic reactions in clients allergic to ragweed or echinacea

INTERACTIONS: Can cause increased risk of bleeding in clients taking NSAIDs, heparin, and warfarin Qs

NURSING ADMINISTRATION

- Question clients about concurrent use of NSAIDs, heparin, and warfarin.
- Discontinue 2 weeks before elective surgery.

Garlic

- When crushed, forms the enzyme allicin
- Blocks LDL cholesterol and raises HDL cholesterol; lowers triglycerides
- Suppresses platelet aggregation and disrupts coagulation
- Acts as a vasodilator (can lower blood pressure)

ADVERSE EFFECTS: GI manifestations, bad breath, and body odor

INTERACTIONS

- Due to antiplatelet qualities, can increase risk of bleeding in clients taking NSAIDs, warfarin, and heparin
- Decreases levels of saquinavir (a medication for HIV treatment) and cyclosporine

NURSING ADMINISTRATION

- Question clients about concurrent use of NSAIDs, heparin, and warfarin.
- Have clients who are taking antiplatelet or anticoagulant medication, cyclosporine, or saquinavir contact their provider.

Ginger root

- Relieves vertigo and nausea
- Increases intestinal motility
- Increases gastric mucous production
- Decreases GI spasms
- Produces an anti-inflammatory and analgesic effect (arthritis and inflammatory conditions)
- Suppresses platelet aggregation
- Used to treat morning sickness, motion sickness, nausea from surgery
- Can decrease pain and stiffness of rheumatoid arthritis

ADVERSE EFFECTS AND PRECAUTIONS

- Use cautiously in clients who are pregnant because high doses can cause uterine contractions.
- Potential CNS depression and cardiac dysrhythmias with excessive ingestion

INTERACTIONS

- Interacts with medications that interfere with coagulation (NSAIDS, warfarin, and heparin)
- Can increase hypoglycemic effects of antidiabetic medications

NURSING ADMINISTRATION

- Question clients about concurrent use with NSAIDs, heparin, and warfarin.
- Monitor for hypoglycemia if the client takes insulin or other medication for diabetes.

Ginkgo biloba

- Promotes vasodilation: Decreases leg pain caused from occlusive arterial disorders
- Decreases platelet aggregation: Can decrease risk of thrombosis
- Decreases bronchospasm
- Increases blood flow to the brain: Claims to improve memory (dementia, Alzheimer's disease) have not been proven. Qᴇʙᴘ

ADVERSE EFFECTS AND PRECAUTIONS

- Mild GI upset, headache, lightheadedness, which can be decreased by reducing dose
- Should be avoided in clients at risk for seizures

INTERACTIONS

- Can interact with medications that lower the seizure threshold (antihistamines, antidepressants, and antipsychotics)
- Can interfere with coagulation

NURSING ADMINISTRATION

- Question clients regarding history of antidepressant use (imipramine), which causes a decrease in seizure threshold.
- Question clients about concurrent use with NSAIDs, heparin, and warfarin.

Glucosamine

- Stimulates cells to make cartilage and synovial fluid
- Suppresses production of cytokines that influence inflammation and cartilage destruction. This supplement is often taken with chondroitin.

ADVERSE EFFECTS AND PRECAUTIONS

- Mild GI upset (nausea, heartburn)
- Products that contain iodine may not always be a contraindication in clients who have a shellfish allergy. Further assessment may be needed.

INTERACTIONS: Avoid use if taking antiplatelet or anticoagulant medication due to increased risk of bleeding.

NURSING ADMINISTRATION: Question clients about concurrent use with NSAIDs, heparin, and warfarin.

St. John's wort

- Affects serotonin, producing antidepressant effects
- Used for mild to moderate depression
- Used orally as an analgesic to relieve pain and inflammation
- Applied topically to treat infection

ADVERSE EFFECTS

- Mild adverse effects, including dry mouth, lightheadedness, constipation, GI upset
- Skin rash with client exposure to sunlight
- Allergic skin reactions, especially in people allergic to ragweed and the daisy family of plants

INTERACTIONS

- Can cause serotonin syndrome when combined with other antidepressants, amphetamine, and cocaine
- Decreases effectiveness of oral contraceptives, cyclosporine, warfarin, digoxin, calcium channel blockers, steroids, HIV protease inhibitors, and some anticancer medications ⓆEBP
- Can accelerate the metabolism of many drugs, thus decreasing their effects

NURSING ADMINISTRATION

- Question clients taking any of the medications with which this substance interacts about concurrent use.
- Encourage clients using St. John's wort to prevent prolonged sun exposure and use sunscreen.

Saw palmetto

ADVERSE EFFECTS AND PRECAUTIONS

- Few adverse effects; can cause mild GI effects
- Contraindicated during pregnancy

INTERACTIONS

- Possible additive effects with finasteride
- Can interact with antiplatelet and anticoagulant medications

NURSING ADMINISTRATION

- Question clients about use before prostate-specific antigen tests.
- Question clients about concurrent use with aspirin, heparin, and warfarin.

Valerian

- Increases GABA to prevent insomnia (similar to benzodiazepines)
- Reduces anxiety related restlessness
- Drowsiness effect increases over time.

ADVERSE EFFECTS AND PRECAUTIONS

- Can cause drowsiness, lightheadedness, depression
- Risk of physical dependence

47.1 Case study

Scenario introduction

Susan is a nurse in a provider's office caring for Mr. Smith who is asking for a prescription for medical marijuana.

Scene 1

Mr. Smith: "My friend smokes marijuana and says it helps him control pain. Is there a way the doctor can prescribe it for me?"

Susan: "Can you tell me about the pain you are having that you feel the marijuana can help relieve?"

Mr. Smith: "I get a lot of headaches, and sometimes my joints ache too."

Scene 2

Susan: "I will make a note about your pain in your medical record, and we can discuss treatment options with your doctor."

Mr. Smith: "Since it is legal here now, it should be just like any other pain medicine, right?"

Susan: "There are still some legal issues surrounding the use of marijuana even in states that have legalized its use."

Scene 3

Mr. Smith: "I hear it is safe to use. Are there side effects from using it?"

Susan: "Yes, I will review these with you if you choose to use it for pain relief."

Mr. Smith: "Hi, Dr. Lawnton. The nurse and I were just talking about me getting some marijuana."

Scenario conclusion

Dr. Lawnton discusses the use of marijuana, and with the nurse, they discuss legal issues, potential adverse effects, and other treatment options that might work for Mr. Smith.

Case study exercises

1. Susan is discussing legal issues regarding the use of medical marijuana with Mr. Smith. Which of the following statements indicates an understanding of the information?

   A. A health care provider cannot write a prescription for medical marijuana.

   B. Medical marijuana is a Schedule V controlled substance in the United States.

   C. Pharmacies must obtain certification prior to dispensing medical marijuana.

   D. The FDA recognizes only the marijuana plant as a form of medicine.

2. Susan is teaching Mr. Smith about the potential adverse effects of smoking marijuana. Which of the following manifestations should the nurse include in the teaching? (Select all that apply.)

   A. Elevated heart rate

   B. Increased fertility

   C. Structural changes in the brain

   D. Development of asthma

   E. Increased urination

3. Susan is talking with Mr. Smith about the use of marijuana for pain control. What response should Susan give to Mr. Smith?

PRECAUTION

- Clients who have mental health disorders should use with caution.
- Should be avoided by clients who are pregnant or breastfeeding

INTERACTIONS: It is not known if valerian potentiates effects of CNS depressants.

NURSING ADMINISTRATION: Clients taking valerian should be warned about the possibility of drowsiness when operating motor vehicles and other equipment.

Integrative substances

Cannabis (medical marijuana)

- Cannabis is legal for medical use in 34 states, while 11 states have approved the use of recreational marijuana.
- Manufacturing, distributing and using cannabis for medical purposes is set forth in statutes and rules developed by each applicable jurisdiction.
- The term medical marijuana is used when referring to the treatment of manifestations of illness or other conditions using the whole, unprocessed marijuana plant or the basic extracts.
- Medical marijuana can be taken through several routes, including inhalation (smoking, vaporization) topical application, and ingestion (edible substances and beverages).
- As a Schedule I controlled substance in the United States, having a high potential for misuse, cannabis cannot be legally prescribed by health care providers, nor can it be dispensed from pharmacies.
- The FDA does not recognize nor approve the marijuana plant as a form of medicine. There are two–FDA approved medications (dronabinol, nabilone) which are derived from chemical components of marijuana that are prescribed to treat nausea and anorexia.
- Medical Marijuana Programs (MMPs) are typically regulated by the jurisdiction's department of health. The MMP defines the qualifying conditions and the type of provider who can certify clients.
  - Certified clients can only obtain cannabinoids from an authorized cannabis dispensary after registering with the MMP.

QUALIFYING CONDITIONS: Scientific evidence demonstrates benefits of cannabis use

- Cachexia
- Anorexia
- Chemotherapy-induced nausea and vomiting
- Pain (resulting from cancer or rheumatoid arthritis)
- Chronic pain (resulting from fibromyalgia)
- Neuropathies (resulting from HIV/AIDS, multiple sclerosis [MS], or diabetes)
- Spasticity (from MS or spinal cord injury)

ADVERSE EFFECTS AND PRECAUTIONS: There are no regulations regarding the quality and purity of medical cannabis. Adverse effects include:

- Increased heart rate, appetite
- Sleepiness, dizziness
- Decreased blood pressure, urination
- Dry mouth and dry eyes
- Hallucinations, paranoia, anxiety, impaired attention and memory
- Exacerbation of asthma, cardiac disease
- Possible dependency, leading to cannabis use disorder
- Exacerbation of alcohol or other substance dependencies

NURSING ADMINISTRATION

- Do not administer medical marijuana to a client unless jurisdiction laws specifically authorize nurses to do so.
- Determine if the client has a MMP designated caregiver who can assist the client with the medical use of cannabis.
- Promote client autonomy in the choice of medical cannabis as a treatment and avoid actions or statements that might be perceived as judgmental. Qᴘᴄᴄ

CLIENT EDUCATION: Effectiveness of the treatment can vary depending on the purity of the substance, and the route affects the time of onset of therapeutic effects. Effects can be seen 10 min following inhalation, compared to 30 to 60 min following ingestion.

Application Exercises

1. A nurse is caring for a client who requests information on the use of feverfew. Which of the following responses should the nurse make?
   - A. "It is used to treat skin infections."
   - B. "It can decrease the frequency of migraine headaches."
   - C. "It can lessen the nasal congestion in the common cold."
   - D. "It can relieve nausea of morning sickness during pregnancy."

2. A nurse is reviewing a client's current medications. The client states, "I also take ginkgo biloba." Which of the following medications has the potential to interact with ginkgo biloba?
   - A. Acetaminophen
   - B. Warfarin
   - C. Digoxin
   - D. Lisinopril

3. A nurse is caring for a client who has diabetes mellitus, has a fasting blood glucose of 50 mg/dL, and is taking herbal supplements. Which of the following herbal supplements should the nurse identify as the potential cause for the low blood glucose level?
   - A. Glucosamine
   - B. Saw palmetto
   - C. Ginger root
   - D. St. John's Wort

Active Learning Scenario

A nurse is educating a client about the use of the dietary herbal supplement St. John's Wort. What should the nurse include in the teaching? Use the ATI Active Learning Template: Medication to complete this item.

THERAPEUTIC USE: Describe the potential uses of this supplement.

COMPLICATIONS: Identify four potential adverse effects of this supplement.

MEDICATION INTERACTIONS: Identify four medication interactions that can occur with this supplement.

Application Exercises Key

1. B. **CORRECT:** When taking actions and responding to a client's questions, the nurse should respond that feverfew can be taken to decrease the frequency of migraine headaches, but it has not been proven to relieve an existing migraine headache.

   Ⓝ *NCLEX® Connection: Pharmacological and Parenteral Therapies, Medication Administration*

2. B. **CORRECT:** When taking actions and reviewing the client's medications, the nurse should identify that ginkgo biloba can suppress coagulation and increase the risk of bleeding or hemorrhage which is further increased if the client is taking an anticoagulant, such as warfarin.

   Ⓝ *NCLEX® Connection: Pharmacological and Parenteral Therapies, Adverse Effects/Contraindications/Side Effects/Interactions*

3. C. **CORRECT:** When taking actions and identifying the adverse effects of herbal supplements, the nurse should note that ginger root has the capability of lowering blood sugar and potentiating the hypoglycemic effects of diabetic medications.

   Ⓝ *NCLEX® Connection: Pharmacological and Parenteral Therapies, Adverse Effects/Contraindications/Side Effects/Interactions*

Active Learning Scenario Key

Using the ATI Active Learning Template: Medication

THERAPEUTIC USE
- Affects serotonin, producing antidepressant effects
- Mild depression
- Oral analgesic to relieve pain and inflammation
- Applied topically to treat infection

COMPLICATIONS
- Mild adverse effects, including dry mouth, lightheadedness, constipation, GI discomfort
- Skin rash with client exposure to sunlight

INTERACTIONS
- Can cause serotonin syndrome when combined with other antidepressants, amphetamine, and cocaine
- Decreases effectiveness of oral contraceptives, cyclosporine, warfarin, digoxin, calcium channel blockers, steroids, HIV protease inhibitors, and some anticancer medications

   Ⓝ *NCLEX® Connection: Pharmacological and Parenteral Therapies, Medication Administration*

Case Study Exercises Key

1. A. **CORRECT:** When evaluating Mr. Smith's understanding of the information provided regarding legal issues and marijuana use, Susan should identify that Mr. Smith understands the information when he tells her that his doctor is not able to legally write him a prescription for medical marijuana.

   Ⓝ *NCLEX® Connection: Pharmacological and Parenteral Therapies, Medication Administration*

2. A, C, D. **CORRECT:** When taking actions and teaching Mr. Smith about the potential adverse effects of marijuana, Susan should include that tachycardia, asthma development, and structural changes of the brain are potential adverse effects of marijuana.

   Ⓝ *NCLEX® Connection: Pharmacological and Parenteral Therapies, Adverse Effects/Contraindications/Side Effects/Interactions*

3. The use of cannabinoids for pain is not an approved use. There are some strains of marijuana that have been found useful for some types of pain relief; however, there is limited research on the use of marijuana for pain. It is also important to remind Mr. Smith that because marijuana is considered by the DEA to be a Schedule I substance, providers cannot prescribe the drug; they can only state that it "may be of benefit."

   Ⓝ *NCLEX® Connection: Pharmacological and Parenteral Therapies, Medication Administration*

References

ATI Nursing. (2022). *Engage fundamentals.*

Burchum, J.R. & Rosenthal, L.D. (2022). *Lehne's pharmacology for nursing care* (11th ed.). Elsevier.

Centers for Disease Control and Prevention. (2021, March 10). About Social Determinants of Health (SDOH). https://www.cdc.gov/socialdeterminants/about.html

Dudek, S.G. (2022). *Nutrition essentials for nursing practice* (9th ed.). Lippincott, Williams & Wolter.

Ford, S.M. (2018). *Roach's introductory clinical pharmacology* (11th ed.). Lippincott, Williams & Wolter.

Foster, A.A., Daly, C. J., Logan, T., Logan, R., Jarvis, H., Croce J., Jalal, Z., Trygstad, T., Bowers, D., Clark,B. , Moore, S. and Jacobs, D.M. (2021.) Addressing social determinants of health in community pharmacy: Innovative opportunities and practice models. *Journal of the American Pharmacists Association, 61*(5); doi.org/10.1016/j.japh.2021.04.022.

Frier, A., Devine, S., Barnett, F., Dunning, T. (2020). Utilizing clinical settings to identify and respond to the social determinants of health of individuals with type 2 diabetes—A review of the literature. *Health & Social Care in the Community, 28*(4):1119-1133. doi:10.1111/hsc.12932

Hinkle, J.L., Cheever, K.H., & Overbaugh, K.J. (2022). *Brunner & Suddarth's textbook of medical-surgical nursing* (15th ed.). Wolters Kluwer.

Hockenberry, M.J., Wilson, D. & Rodgers, C. (2019). *Wong's nursing care of infants and children* (11th ed.). Elsevier.

Ignatavicius, D.D., Workman, M.L., Rebar, C.R. & Heimgartner, N.M. (2021). *Medical-surgical nursing: Concepts for interprofessional collaborative care* (10th ed.). Elsevier.

Kiles, T., Jasmin, H., y Nichols, Haddad, R., Renfro, C.P. (2020, November). A scoping review of active-learning strategies for teaching social determinants of health in pharmacy. *American Journal of Pharmaceutical Education, 84*(11) 8241; DOI: 10.5688/ajpe8241

Lilley, L.L., Rainsforth Collins, S., & Snyder, J.S. (2020). *Pharmacology and the nursing process* (9th ed.). Elsevier.

Pagana, KD., Pagana, TJ., & Pagana, TN. (2022). *Mosby's manual of diagnostic and laboratory tests* (7th ed.). Elsevier.

Patel MR, Piette JD, Resnicow K, Kowalski-Dobson T, Heisler M. (2016). Social determinants of health, cost-related nonadherence, and cost-reducing behaviors among adults with diabetes: Findings from the national health interview survey. *Medical Care, 54*(8):796-803. doi:10.1097/MLR.0000000000000565

Potter, P.A., Perry, A. G., Stockert, P. A. & Hall, A.M. (2021). *Fundamentals of nursing* (10th ed.). Elsevier.

Vallerand, A.H. & Sanoski, C.A. (2021). *Davis's drug guide for nurses* (17th ed). F.A. Davis.

Basic Concept

STUDENT NAME _____

CONCEPT_____ REVIEW MODULE CHAPTER_____

Related Content
(E.G., DELEGATION, LEVELS OF PREVENTION, ADVANCE DIRECTIVES)

Underlying Principles

Nursing Interventions
WHO? WHEN? WHY? HOW?

ACTIVE LEARNING TEMPLATE: *Diagnostic Procedure*

STUDENT NAME _____

PROCEDURE NAME _____ REVIEW MODULE CHAPTER_____

Description of Procedure

Indications

Interpretation of Findings

CONSIDERATIONS

Nursing Interventions (pre, intra, post)

Client Education

Potential Complications

Nursing Interventions

Growth and Development

STUDENT NAME _____

DEVELOPMENTAL STAGE _____ REVIEW MODULE CHAPTER_____

EXPECTED GROWTH AND DEVELOPMENT

Physical Development	Cognitive Development	Psychosocial Development	Age-Appropriate Activities

Health Promotion

Immunizations	Health Screening	Nutrition	Injury Prevention

Medication

STUDENT NAME _____

MEDICATION _____   REVIEW MODULE CHAPTER_____

CATEGORY CLASS_____

PURPOSE OF MEDICATION

Expected Pharmacological Action

Therapeutic Use

Complications

Medication Administration

Contraindications/Precautions

Nursing Interventions

Interactions

Client Education

Evaluation of Medication Effectiveness

ACTIVE LEARNING TEMPLATE: *Nursing Skill*

STUDENT NAME _____

SKILL NAME _____ REVIEW MODULE CHAPTER _____

Description of Skill

Indications

CONSIDERATIONS

Nursing Interventions (pre, intra, post)

Outcomes/Evaluation

Client Education

Potential Complications

Nursing Interventions

System Disorder

ACTIVE LEARNING TEMPLATE:

STUDENT NAME _____

DISORDER/DISEASE PROCESS _____ REVIEW MODULE CHAPTER_____

Alterations in Health (Diagnosis)	Pathophysiology Related to Client Problem	Health Promotion and Disease Prevention

ASSESSMENT

Risk Factors	Expected Findings

Laboratory Tests	Diagnostic Procedures

SAFETY CONSIDERATIONS

PATIENT-CENTERED CARE

Nursing Care	Medications	Client Education

Therapeutic Procedures		Interprofessional Care

Complications

ACTIVE LEARNING TEMPLATE: *Therapeutic Procedure*

STUDENT NAME _____

PROCEDURE NAME _____ REVIEW MODULE CHAPTER_____

Description of Procedure

Indications

CONSIDERATIONS

Nursing Interventions (pre, intra, post)

Outcomes/Evaluation

Client Education

Potential Complications

Nursing Interventions

Concept Analysis

STUDENT NAME _____

CONCEPT ANALYSIS_____

Defining Characteristics

Antecedents

(WHAT MUST OCCUR/BE IN PLACE FOR CONCEPT TO EXIST/FUNCTION PROPERLY)

Negative Consequences

(RESULTS FROM IMPAIRED ANTECEDENT — COMPLETE WITH FACULTY ASSISTANCE)

Related Concepts

(REVIEW LIST OF CONCEPTS AND IDENTIFY, WHICH CAN BE AFFECTED BY THE STATUS OF THIS CONCEPT — COMPLETE WITH FACULTY ASSISTANCE)

Exemplars